THE CAUSATION OF RHEUMATOID DISEASE AND MANY HUMAN CANCERS
-A New Concept in Medicine-

In Memoriam
Roger Wyburn-Mason, M.D., Ph.D.
October 2, 1911-June 16, 1983

By Anthony di Fabio, June 18, 1983

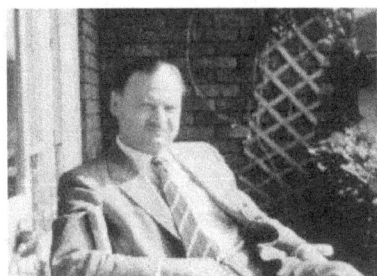

Roger Wyburn-Mason

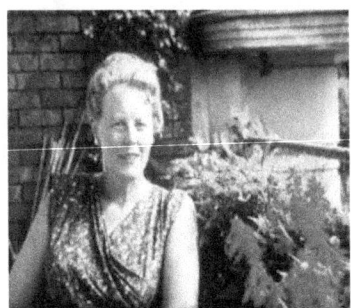

Joan Wyburn-Mason

Professor Roger Wyburn-Mason was curing folks of so-called incurable rheumatoid disease (including rheumatoid arthritis) way back in the 1960s. Folks in England, Australia, Canada, United States and on other continents would hear of his success from those cured. They'd contact him and he'd tell them how do achieve this wonderful result!

As you will see from the following mini-biography Roger was a brilliant scholar, researcher and world-famed nerve specialist until he publicly touted his successes when treating this crippling disease. Then he was suddenly ostracized by the know-it-all medical profession, according to his wife, Joan, in her *Dedication, Love and Humor: My Life With Professor Roger Wyburn-Mason*. [http://www.arthritistrust.org]

Although he resisted the idea that the *Amoeba chromatosa* was the sole cause of Rheumatoid Disease by a friend and world-renowned protozoologist, Vice Admiral Stamm, Professor Wyburn-Mason did finally accept the idea. While no one has yet been able to reproduce their laboratory findings, at least the treatment based upon their hypothesis works, curing folks worldwide when nothing else is [or was] available.

In fact, nothing else is available worldwide to this day, except the treatment that this foundation derived from Roger Wyburn-Mason's perhaps faulty hypothesis plus the treatment based on the work of Thomas McPherson Brown, M.D., claiming that a mycoplasm is the primary culprit.

To Dr. Wyburn-Mason's credit, he rescinded his belief that the Amoeba chromatosa was the essential cause of rheumatoid diseases. His assertions and objections to their review were reported in in the April 24, 1979 *Lancet*, as follows:

"Sir,

"Referring to your nine line review in your issue of April 7th. 1979 of my 479 page monograph *The Causation of Rheumatoid Disease and Many Human Cancers. A New Concept in Medicine*, 1978, I would like to draw your attention to the fact that the term "Amoeba chromatosa" to which you refer was used in a previous book by me published in 1964, but that in the monograph that you were supposed to be reviewing further work over 14 years described in this has shown that the organism is probably one or more species of Naegleria, and the term *Amoeba chromatosa* abandoned, but you fail to mention this. Your statement that my ideas should be refuted or confirmed is welcome, but if the monograph had been carefully read full details of the properties of the organism had also the names of the workers and establishments where the isolation of this organism has been confirmed would have been found. In a leading article in your own journal (1) on "Pathogenic free-living amoebae" you state "the discovery that free-living protozoa (including amoebae) are able to infect man and animals has revolutionized the very concept of parasitism". Why then should you be surprised at my discovery of an amoeba in the tissues? You also refer to the findings of Cursons et al. (2) using a direct fluorescent amoebic antibody test on the sera of 200 people in New Zealand, including new-born children, who found fluorescence in all, either with neat serum or with serum diluted up to 1/20 of Naegleria and 1/80 of Acanthamoebae, suggesting that all humans are or have been infected with one or more of these organisms, the new-born through the placenta. Furthermore using immunofluorescent amoebic antibody techniques the presence of these organisms in the tissues of both normal and diseased subjects has been confirmed by eminent workers in this field in this country and is described in my monograph. The markedly beneficial effects of various anti-amoebic drugs on cases of active rheumatoid disease described by me in this and confirmed in several countries throughout the world itself proves the causation of the disease is an amoeba

1

in the tissues.

"May I ask two questions - 1) why, if the monograph was going to be reviewed at all, was it not read carefully in order to follow the closely argued deductions and the effects of anti-amoebic drugs in rheumatoid disease ignored and the statement made that my ideas have not been taken seriously by most of the medical profession, this last is made because they have obviously not read it or attempted to confirm my findings? and 2) why do you find it impossible to believe the confirmed evidence of the presence of an amoeba in the body tissues from various sources which are before you in the monograph? Fortunately elsewhere in the world minds have been more receptive to new discoveries and the tremendous relief of suffering in cases of active rheumatoid disease by my discovery of the use of anti-amoebic drugs realised, appreciated and practiced.

"References.
"1. Wyburn-Mason, The Causation of Rheumatoid Disease and Many Human Cancers: A New Concept in Medicine, Iji Publishing Co, Tokyo, Japan
2. Pathogenic free-living amoebae. Leading Article, Lancet 1977, ii, 1165
3. Immunity to Pathogenic Free-Living Amoebae, Cursons R.T.M. Brown, T.J., Kays, E.A. Ibid, 1977, ii, 875"

When I was at last cured of this dreaded, crippling rheumatoid arthritis, I never dreamed of embarking on a worldwide challenge to professional rheumatologists, and the gigantic and ineffective Arthritis Foundation, and the American pharmaceutical industry that siphons S15,000,000,000 a year in the United States of America from the sick and the lonely, chiefly for aspirin substitutes and failed cancer chemicals that simply treat arthritic symptoms and not causes.

Somehow the Good Lord has seen fit to successfully guide my path -- along with other determined, sincere people -- to bring the good message to all --
There's a cure!
It's simple!
It's cheap!
It's available everywhere!
And here's how you do it!
My book *Rheumatoid Diseases Cured at Last* was monitored by Professor Roger Wyburn-Mason, and based on his original work, *The Causation o/ Rheumatoid Disease and Many Human Cancers - A new Concept in Medicine* (1978) [Also on the *Pre'cis* of the *Causation o/ Rheumatoid Disease and Many Human Cancers.*] My first arthritis book, published in

a hurry, was designed for the ailing to find hope, to convince them, to be carried to their family physician for further use where they would be treated. More often than not, the book was heaved into a nearby waste-basket by an angry, know-it-all authoritarian physician!

My small book, also launched *The Roger Wt burn-Mason & Jack M. Blount Foundation for Eradication of Rheumatoid Disease* (AKAs: *The Arthritis Trust of America* and *The Rheumatoid Disease Foundation*), which is now successfully off and running, millions of messages having already spread the word. Many fine humanity-conscious physicians and non-physicians are now members, or independent practitioners of life-saving, pain-relieving treatments, and working toward common goals set by Professor Roger Wyburn-Mason.

Since that beginning we've also published *The Art of Getting Well, Arthritis: Little Known Treatments,* and *Arthritis: Osteoarthritis and Rheumatoid Disease Including Rheumatoid Arthritis* -- all stemming from Dr. Wyburn-Mason's work.

Professor Roger Wyburn-Mason solved the riddle of one of man's oldest curses, so called "uncurable" rheumatoid diseases. He strived with every ounce of his great intellect to bring to all humanity his discoveries. We prayed to be there when he walked across the stage to receive his Nobel Prize, and other prizes that were his due -- but God, in his great wisdom, decided otherwise, and so we must accept.

To the famous names of Semmelweis, Jenner, Koch, Harvey, Ross, Lister, Pasteur, Ehrlich, Sister Kenny, and Roentgen we now add Wyburn-Mason -- a most brilliant, brave, humanity-loving man who pursued evil forces causing them to acknowledge that humanity need not always feel pain, suffering, depression and disillusionment.

What you will read in Wyburn-Mason's 468 page *The Causation of Rheumatoid Disease and Many Human Cancers* is a wonderful example of the detailed nature of medical/scientific analysis performed years earlier than the present "gold-standard," today's "double-blind" study.

Medical analysis in Wyburn-Mason's day required a great deal of knowledge, clinical experience, and wisdom. He often made fun of double-blind studies, claiming that one of his medical students invented it as a joke -- but that the world-wide medical audience took it seriously -- and, he said, it was OK for determining whether one aspirin substitute was better than another aspirin substitute, but could never replace true medical evaluation based upon human clinical experiences and their critical evaluation.

This book is a tribute to not just the man who wrote it, but also to those who roll up their sleeves and dig into human suffering with a passion to end it!

Some six weeks before his death I wrote, asking that he please include a summary of his professional life and writings.

Reluctantly, Professor Roger Wyburn-Mason sent this, his last letter, before the Good Lord called him on June 16, 1983.

"I was born in Monmouthsire, England. On my mother's side I am a descendent of Bishop Stephen Gardiner, who was Lord Chancellor of England, that is the most powerful person in the country after the Monarch in the reign of King Henry VIII, King Edward VI, Queen Mary the first and Queen Elizabeth the first. He conducted the marriage of King Philip II of Spain to Queen Mary the first of England in Winchester Cathederal, where he is buried in a magnificent tomb. My mother's cousin was the former Prime Minister of New Zealand, Mr. Nash. My godfathers were the greatest English Composer, Dr. Ralph Vaughan Williams of Cambridge University and now buried in Westminster Abbey, and the historian H.A.L. Fisher, the head of New College Oxford, both of whom held the decoration of Order of Merit (O.M.), the highest honour that can be bestowed by the Monarch.

"I attended a public school (a public school in England is the opposite of one in the United States, being privately as opposed to state owned and includes such distinguished Institutions as Eton, Harrow and Winchester Colleges). At the end of school years I took the necessary final examinations and gained the top marks in the whole of Great Britain and was awarded a State Scholarship and an Open Scholarship to Christ's College, Cambridge (founded in 1405 A.D.), where the poet John Milton and the great scientist Charles Darwin were also students. Here I occupied the same rooms as those of Darwin himself.

"At Cambridge I obtained double first class honours in the final examinations for the B.A. (Bachelor of Arts) degree. I also represented my University at Rugby football and Athletics. At the end of my period as an Undergraduate I remained in Cambridge as a Bachelor Fellow of the College and did research in pathology and particularly protozoology. I afterwards was awarded the degree of M.A. (Master of Arts) a higher degree and the only University scholarship awarded to graduates completing their clinical studies at a London Hospital where 1 finally obtained my M.B. (Bachelor of Medicine) and B. Chir. (Bachelor of Chirurgerie). I afterwards held the posts of Registrar (the equivalent of Instructor in America) in the foremost hospitals in London, namely the Middlesex Hospital, the Brompton Hospital for Chest Diseases, the National Heart Hospital, the National Hospital for Nervous Diseases and the Royal Marsden Hospital for Cancer. While at the Middlesex Hospital I took part in the first Clinical Trials of the first sulphonamide antibiotics. While working at the National Hospital for Nervous Diseases I wrote my thesis for the M.D. (Cambridge Degree -- This is a higher degree unlike it is in the United States and other countries). I also sat for M. R. C. P. (Member of the Royal College of Physicians) examination in which 1 obtained the top marks of all the candidates. My M.D. thesis was entitled "The vascular tumours and abnormalities of the spinal cord and its membranes" and received with acclaim as it was the first description of these matters. It was published as a monograph and has remained the standard work on this subject. While working at the National Hospital for Nervous Diseases I published a number of papers in medical journals and two of these described new diseases which have since been named after me and I am the only living doctor who has such a distinction. One of these conditions describes the presentation of cancer as a peripheral neuropathy, that is a disturbance of the nerves of the limbs before any other evidence of cancer is present. The other describes a congenital blood vessel disease of the skin of the forehead, the fundus of the eye, the optic nerve and the brain.

"I later was elected Research Fellow at the Royal Marsden Hospital for research into cancer and later Research Fellow at the Royal College of Surgeons of England, where I continued my research into the nature of cancer and first isolated from all human malignant tumours and from cases of rheumatoid arthritis an hitherto unknown, very small free-living amoeba. For this I received the Ph.D. degree.

"While working at the Royal Marsden Hospital I discovered that human tissues affected by herpes zoster (shingles) and by herpes simplex (cold sores) which are both due to virus infections, were liable to develop cancer of the skin at a later date. This was the first description of human cancer caused by a virus and it resulted in my invitation by the late Professor Duran-Reynals, who was working at Yale University on the viral cause of human cancer, to Yale to work with him as his assistant where I continued after his death. I later travelled to the Mayo Clinic and worked with [my friend] the late Dr. J.W. Kernohan, the neuropathologist.

"I became convinced that while viruses cause cancer in animals, they rarely do so in man. During these years I published many papers and monographs (books) on my researches, and as a result of these I was awarded the degree of Doctor of Science of Cambridge University (a rare honour) and elected a Fellow of my old College.

"After twenty years work on the new organism which I had discovered I was able to show that this was the cause of rheumatoid arthritis. Furthermore, infection with species of this organism in susceptible subjects seemed to be the cause of a large proportion of cases of human cancer, which can be prevented by taking appropriate substances which kill the organism. This work has all been described in a book entitled *The causation of rheumatoid disease and many human cancers - A new concept in Medicine,* and it has caused worldwide interest.

"After a time it became necessary for me to return to England where I continued my work in the laboratories and wards of the National Health Service.

"Among my publications are the following -

Books

The vascular tumours and abnormalities

Summary:
Roger Wyburn-Mason
M.A., M.D. Cambridge, England; Sometime Open Scholar, Christ's College, Cambridge, England,\; Formerly Gordon Jacob Research Fellow, Royal College of Surgeons, London, England; Fellow, Royal Marsden Hospital, London, Prophit Research, London, England; Formerly Associate Professor Microbiology and Lecturer, Yale University Medical School, U.S.A.; Member of High Table, Christ's College, Cambridge, England; Former Consultant Physician, Ealing, Hammersmith and Hounslow Health Authority (Teaching) London.

"It is in the very nature of things that the study of disease, to be effective, must begin as it must end with the disease itself, and that all knowledge applicable to human disease must owe its inspiration, directly or indirectly, to intimate contact with disease as this exists in living man."

Sir Thomas Lewis

4

THE CAUSATION OF RHEUMATOID DISEASE
AND MANY HUMAN CANCERS
A New Concept in Medicine

1978

Roger Wyburn-Mason

IJI Publishing LTD
Tokyo, Japan

Preface

Over the years there have been defined a number of agents which cause cancer in man. These are considered in the text. There has of late been enthusiasm for the virus theory, but all recent reviews have stressed the fact that there is no definite evidence that any cancer in man is due to a virus infection. In fact, Professor Boyland in 1969 expressed the view that in only about ten per cent of human cancer cases can causes, including viruses (if these are factors), be identified. The other 90 per cent are of unknown origin. Furthermore, many writers on the aetiology of cancer have stressed the fact that what is required in the search for the causes of human cancer are not increasing expenditure of money, but new ideas. The same applies to rheumatoid disease. This book puts forward such a new idea and shows how clinically and pathologically it fits the known facts about both rheumatoid disease and many cases of human cancer and related diseases. The text requires careful reading to follow the argument and the author asks the reader not to dismiss the idea without repeating the experimental observations described as occurred with the new ideas of Pasteur, Lister and Fleming.

Acknowledgements.

The observations recorded in the following pages were made by the author over the course of some twenty or more years working as a consultant physician and begun originally while holding appointments at the National Hospital for Nervous Diseases, Queen Square, London, and the Royal Marsden Hospital, London. The author was greatly helped on the clinical side by his various assistants, especially Dr. N.C. Dauda and Dr. M.A. Shaikh. I am also especially grateful to my surgical colleagues, including Mr. R. Burkitt, F.R.C.S. and Mr. O.D. Morris, F.R.C.S., who kindly allowed me free access for investigations to their cases of malignant disease, to Air Vice-Marshall W.P. Stamm, Director of the Amoebiasis Research Unit, Royal Free Hospital, London, for kindly carrying out the immunofluorescent staining of sections for free-living amoebae, to Dr. R.J. Goldacre of the Chester Beatty Research Institute, Royal Marsden Hospital, London, for helpful advice, to Mr. P.W. Payne, director of the South West Metropolitan Cancer Registry, for access to records of cancer cases, to Mr. S.A. Taylor, F.P.S., for much help and advice on pharmaceuticals and to Dr. G.I.M. Ross of the Pathological Laboratory, Ashford Hospital, Middlesex, who carried out many of the laboratory investigations on cases cited.

I should like to express my sincere thanks to Messrs. Champion Plugs and their Mr. Herbert Starley, who supplied a microscope, to British Insulated Callender Cables Ltd. (BICC) and their Mr. Reynolds, who kindly constructed and supplied an apparatus to aid in the isolation of limax amoebae from living tissue and to Bayer Pharmaceuticals of Germany, who kindly supplied the drug Clotrimazole.

Lastly, and very specially I should like to thank my wife "Poppi", without whose endless hours of typing and retyping, tirelessness and encouragement over the years these observations would never have seen the light of day and to Dr. T. Koba of Tokyo through whose generosity this book was published.

Richmond,
Surrey,
England.

Printed by Ishi Publishing Company
Miyasaka Building 37 Nihonbashihoncho
Chao-ku Tokyo 103 Japan

Your Notes

Contents

Part I
"Collagen" and "Auto-immune" Disease

Chapter I

INTRODUCTION

The continuous spectrum of 'collagen" and "auto-immune" disease

I, i) The overlap of "collagen" diseases with one another

The term rheumatoid arthritis is given to a condition in which arthritis is the presenting symptom, but in fact any tissue in the body may be involved in this generalized disease (Sinclair and Cruikshank, 1956; Hart, 1969, 1970; Haslock et al., 1970; Boyle and Buchanan, 1970; Gardner, 1972) and indeed arthropathy may be minimal or absent. The term rheumatoid arthritis is a misnomer and rheumatoid disease is a preferable description. Rheumatoid disease may be present at birth, appear in childhood as Still's disease, which is uncommon before six months of age and common at the age of 1-3 years, or occur at any time in life, but especially about the time of the menopause in women.

Rheumatoid arthritis, systemic lupus erythematosus, dermatomyositis (polymyositis), scleroderma or primary systemic sclerosis and polyarteritis nodosa have been grouped as the so-called "collagen" diseases. Every combination and gradation of these diseases one into another may occur (Jager, 1950; Tuffanelli and Winkelmann, 1962; Harvey, 1967; Kantor et al., 1969; Austen, 1971; Thompson 1974) and all may be associated with Raynaud's phenomenon (Lessof and Coffman, 1971). Transitional forms of systemic lupus erythematosus, dermatomyositis and scleroderma were reported by Tuffanelli and Winkelmann (1962), Kierland (1964) and Sharp et al. (1972). Dermatomyositis (polymyositis) or scleroderma, into which the former may develop, may be associated with other collagen diseases, such as rheumatoid arthritis and systemic lupus erythematosus (Keil, 1940; Heathfield and Williams, 1960; Kierland, 1964; Becker et al., 1965; Rose and Walton, 1966; Pitkeathly and Coomes, 1966; Chorzelski and Jablonska, 1970).

Various forms of *vasculitis* may accompany rheumatoid arthritis, systemic lupus erythematosus and dermatomyositis or polymyositis (see Ball, 1954; Talbott and Ferrandis, 1956; Miller et al., 1962; Sokoloff, 1964; Alarcon-Segovia and Brown, 1964; Harvey, 1967; Gardner, 1972). The arterial system is susceptible to four forms of the disease.

1) A necrotizing arteritis distributed in the viscera and involving both medium sized or microscopic arteries. These changes are those of polyarteritis nodosa.

2) A subacute arteritis.

3) An intimal cell hyperplasia (endarteritis obliterans), which may lead to gangrene.

4) Thrombotic micro-angiopathy (see Gardner, 1972).

The venules may be similarly affected. Such lesions are common in kidneys, heart, gastro-intestinal tract, liver, lungs, adrenals, testes, brain and peripheral nerves. The endarteritis may lead to pulmonary arteriolar involvement, pulmonary hypertension and cor-pulmonale. The vascular changes may occur in the absence of other obvious signs of rheumatoid arthritis or collagen disease. They are a specific manifestation of rheumatoid and collagen diseases and may be fulminant. In one of the author's cases diffuse arteritis developed 20 years after the onset of rheumatoid arthritis. The obliterative endarteritis may

Addendum: Kirby J., and Munro D.D. Proc. R. Soc. Med., 1977, 70, 748. report a case with overlap of several collagen diseases. Ramos-Niembro F., Alancon-Segovia D. and Hernandez-Ortiz J. Arth. Rheum. 1979, 22, 43. discussed 28 cases of mixed connective tissue disease with arthropathy, SLE, Scleroderma or polymyositis with positive rheumatoid factor in the serum. MCTD is also discussed in Mixed Connective tissue disease-- a decade of growing pains, Alarcon-Segovia D. J. Rheumatol. 1981, 8 535-540.

occur in digital vessels and result in Raynaud's manifestations or lead to gangrene or cutaneous lesions of the nailfold, nail edge and pulps of the fingers and toes. *Raynaud's phenomenon* may be a feature of any type of collagen disease and rheumatoid arthritis (Lessof and Coffman, 1971) or of any disease with which these may be associated (see below), such as hypothyroidism and diabetes mellitus (Raynaud's disease, Leading Article, Brit. med. J., 1972, 3, 782).

Yet again *Sjogren's syndrome* or *Mikulicz's disease*, which is the same condition except for enlargement of the salivary and lacrimal glands in the latter case (see below), may complicate any of the collagen diseases (Hoffbrand and Beck, 1965; Halberg et al., 1965; Bloch et al., 1966; Macsween et al., 1967; Robinson, 1967).

Diffuse lymphocytic thyroiditis, that is Hashimoto's thyroiditis without goitre, is the basic lesion of primary myxoedema (Williams and Doniach, 1962). Spontaneous myxoedema and Hashimoto's thyroiditis are variants of the same pathological process (Smart and Owens, 1961; Euchanan and Harden, 1965). It is now considered that lymphocytic goitre and thyrotoxicosis are two facets of the same disease. Spontaneous transitions from thyrotoxicosis to Hashimoto's thyroiditis and to myxoedema are seen in a small percentage of patients with thyrotoxicosis observed over several years (Doniach and Roitt, 1969). Again any form of "collagen" disease may be associated with lymphocytic thyroiditis, myxoedema or thyrotoxicosis. Rheumatoid arthritis with Hashimoto's thyroiditis or focal thyroiditis was described by Buchanan et al. (1961) and Becker et al. (1963, 1965), while systemic lupus erythematosus associated with Hashimot':::; thyroiditis was reported by White et al. (1961), Mahaux: et al. (1961) and Becker et al. (1965). Leonardt (1964) and Winkelmann et al. (1968) described systemic lupus erythematosus associated

with rheumatoid arthritis, lupoid hepatitis, Sjogren's syndrome, scleroderma, dermatomyositis, polyarteritis or Hashimoto's thyroiditis. Systemic scleroderma associated with Hashimoto's thyroiditis, Sjogren's syndrome or cirrhosis of the liver was reported by Tuffanelli and Winkelmann (1962). Furthermore, Hashimoto's thyroiditis and dermatomyositis (polymyositis) may be found together (Sharvil, 1958; Becker et al., 1965). Lastly Hashimoto's thyroiditis and Sjogren's syndrome may co-exist (Heaton, 1959; Vazquez (quoted by Bloch et al., 1960), Bunim, 1961; Doniach and Roitt, 1968; Bloch, 1969; Shearn, 1971). Thus, there exist transitional, overlap or combined syndromes involving systemic lupus erythematosus, rheumatoid arthritis, primary systemic sclerosis, dermatomyositis (polymyositis), polyarteritis nodosa, Hashimoto's thyroiditis, myxoedema and thyrotoxicosis and Sjogren's syndrome or any of these conditions may occur alone.

I, ii) Organ specific "auto-immune" diseases and their association with "collagen" diseases

Any combination of focal or diffuse thyroiditis (Hashimoto's thyroiditis) with or without hypothyroidism or thyrotoxicosis, "idiopathic" atrophy of the adrenal cortex leading to Addison's disease and atrophic gastritis with or without pernicious anaemia may occur together (Williams and Doniach, 1962; Anderson et al., 1967; Irvine, 1968, Goudie, 1968). Atrophic gastritis in association with Hashimoto's thyroiditis, myxoedema or thyrotoxicosis was described Wilkinson (1940), Tudhope and Wilson (1960, 1962), McNicol (1961), Markson and Moore (1962), Doniach et al. (1963) and Raitt and Doniach (1969). Not only Hashimoto's thyroiditis, but also thyrotoxicosis may exhibit significant association with pernicious anaemia with its associated atrophic gastritis (Furszyfer et al., 1971). In these diseases there may be found auto-antibodies to thyroid constituents, gastric parietal cells and intrinsic factor and to adrenal cortical cells, but a low incidence of non-specific complement-fixing antibodies, such as antinuclear factor (ANF) and rheumatoid factor (RF). Such diseases of the thyroid and adrenal glands and gastric mucosa may also be associated with the changes of chronic active hepatitis with similar cellular infiltration progressing to cirrhosis of the liver of postnecrotic type (Williams and Doniac'h, 1962; and see below). The affected tissues in Hashimoto's thyroiditis, "idiopathic" atrophy of the adrenal cortex and atrophic gastritis all show infiltration with lymphocytes and often plasma cells with the formation of germinal centres identical with those found in the joint capsules in cases of rheumatoid disease.

The tendency of Hashimoto's or focal thyroiditis to be combined with various collagen diseases has been stressed. The author has seen a number of cases of Hashimoto's thyroiditis with widespread vasculitis. Short et al. (1957) found hyper- or hypo-thyroidism in 33 per cent of cases of rheumatoid arthritis. Becker et al. (1963) found a ten-fold incidence of rheumatoid arthritis in patients with Hashimoto's thyroiditis as compared with controls. Buchanan (1965) also noted the association of the two. Gardner (1969) in a pathological study of 142 cases of rheumatoid arthritis found 17 (12 per cent) with evidence of thyroiditis. He found thyroiditis and thyroid fibrosis are frequent in elderly rheumatoids.

Longcope (1928) reports the association of thyrotoxicosis and Addison's disease with scleroderma. Idiopathic Addison's disease co-existing with rheumatoid disease was described by Irvine (1968).

Partridge and Duthie (1963) report a five-fold higher frequency of pernicious anaemia with its associated atrophic gastritis in cases of rheumatoid arthritis when compared with controls. Wintrobe (1967) records that pernicious anaemia is associated with rheumatoid arthritis in 5 per cent of cases. Siurala et al. (1965) also report the frequent association of atrophic gastritis with collagen disease. Edstrom (1939) found 18.5 per cent of 432 patients with rheumatoid arthritis had histamine fast achlorhydria indicative of atrophic gastritis. Bieder and Wigley (1964) report that 10 per cent of 20 cases of rheumatoid arthritis had pernicious anaemia and Ghazi (1972) found 5 per cent of cases of pernicious anaemia had rheumatoid arthritis and one of these cases also had diabetes and myxoedema and one case of pernicious anaemia had myxoedema. There was a high incidence of RF in the serum in cases of pernicious anaemia. Fenyohazi et al. (1970) report that in 18 cases of rheumatoid arthritis 11 showed gastric mucosal atrophy, severe in 5 and with inflammatory changes in 7 as compared with 2 in controls, neither of which showed inflammatory changes. In the last 20 cases of pernicious anaemia seen by the author, apart from the presence of gastric parietal cell and intrinsic factor auto-antibodies, ANF was also present in the serum in 11 cases.

The author is grateful to Dr. N.C. Dauda for the following data. He examined 100 successive cases of moderate or severe rheumatoid arthritis admitted to a geriatric unit for the presence of associated diseases. They included 90 females and 10 males of ages ranging from 66-86 years. Symptoms of rheumatoid arthritis had been present for up to 20 years. The associated diseases found were as follows:—

1) Dermatomyositis-scleroderma . . 1
2) Systemic lupus erythematosus . . 2
3) Sjogren's syndrome 12
4) Psoriasis and Sjogren's syndrome 1
5) Diabetes mellitus 12
6) yxoederna 15
7) Rheumatoid heart disease 18
8) Coeliac disease 1
9) Atrophic gastritis with iron deficiency anaemia 14
10) Atrophic gastritis with pernicious anaemia 8

11) Polycythaemia with achlorhydria 2
12) Paget's disease of bone 16
13) Post-necrotic cirrhosis of the
    liver 2
14) Parkinsonism 10
15) Motoneurone disease 1
16) Hepa'tosplenomegaly 4
17) Asthma developing into chronic
    bronchitis 11
18) Carcinoma 16

The carcinomata were distributed as follows:-

Bronchus .... 4 cases all in
Stomach .... 5 non-smokers.
Senile breast 1
Pancreas 1
Body of uterus 1
Kidney 1
Colon and rectum 3

Thus, in this series atrophic gastritis, with or without pernicious anaemia or polycythaemia, was present in 24 cases (24 per cent) , while myxoedema, the end result of lymphocytic thyroiditis, was present in 15 cases (15 per cent).

Three cases illustrating the essentially common aetiology of the manifestations of collagen and auto-immune disease observed by the writer are the following:-

Case 1 Female, aged 64 years. Developed menarche only at the age of 17 years, but her periods were always scanty, lasting only 1-3 days. The menopause occurred at the age of 37 years. She failed to conceive. At the age of 28 years S'he developed *diabetes mellitus,* which was controlled by diet and insulin, the requirements of which gradually increased over the years. About the age of 36-38 years *vitiligo* appeared over the neck, wrists and trunk. At the age of 48 years she developed classical *rheumatoid arthritis* accompanied by *S jogren's syndrome* with a markedly raised E.S.R., hypergammaglobulinaemia and a strongly positive RF, but no ANF in the serum. The axillary hair was absent, but . pubic hair was of normal distribution. X-rays showed marked rheumatoid changes in the joints. At the age of 51 years she

found a mass in the left breast which was removed and proved to be an area of *cystic mastitis.* At the age of 59 years she developed both *myxoedema* and *pernicious anaemia.* Investigations showed a P.B.I. of less than 1 J·l·G per cent, complete achlorhydria, a low vitamin Bl2 content of the serum, a normal urinary oestrogen output and the following auto-antibody tests:- immunofluorescent tests thyroid cytoplasm + +; gastric parietal cells +; mitochondria rat kidney tubule, negative; intrinsic factor +, thyroglobulin tanned R.B.C. agglutination test positive, 1 in 25,000; thyroid C.F.T. positive>! in 1024, immunofluorescent test against steroid-producing cells of rabbit ovary, negative. Immunofluorescent antibodies against adrenal cortical cells, negative. A tentative diagnosis of Hashimoto's thyroiditis was made. There was no evidence of hypo-adrenalism and all tests of adrenal function were within normal limits. She was treated with L-thyroxin and vitamin B12 injections. At the age of 61 years she developed paralysis agitans. A diagnosis of rheumatoid arthritis, Sjogren's syndrome, cystic mastitis, Hashimoto's thyroiditis and myxoedema, pernicious anaemia and atrophic gastritis, diabetes mellitus, vitiligo and primary gonadal failure was made.

Case Z Female, aged 69 years. Menarche aged 12 years. Periods became scanty and irregular at the age of 35 years and ceased at 42 years. Aged 42 years onset of *intrinsic asthma,* which remained and developed into *bronchitis* with *asthma.* Aged 52 years onset of severe *rheumatoid arthritis* for which she received treatment during the next 5 years. Aged 55-61 years she developed *recurrent papillomata* of the bladder, for which she was treated repeatedly by fulguration. At the age of 67 years she developed *diabetes* and *myxoedema* and at the age of 69 years a gradually spreading *neuropathy.* At this time she was found to have *Sjogren's syndrome* as well as signs of burnt-out rheumatoid arthritis and radiographs showed extensive

Paget's disease of bone and calcified *fibroids*. *Achlorhydria* was present and a moderate degree of iron deficiency anaemia. The E.S.R. was raised and the serum contained ANF, thyroid and gastric parietal cell antibodies. A diagnosis of rheumatoid arthritis, Sjagren's syndrome, myxoedema, atrophic gastritis, diabetes mellitus, intrinsic asthma and chronic bronchitis, primary gonadal failure, Paget's disease of bone, fibroids and recurrent papillomata of the bladder was made.

The essential close relationship of rheumatoid arthritis and systemic lupus erythematosus is shown in the following , case:-

Case 3 Male, aged 34 years. He presented with morning stiffness and painful swelling of the hands, later flitting from joint to joint and pains in the neck of 6 months duration. Examination showed hot, swollen joints of the fingers, wrists, feet, ankles and knees. Enlarged nodes were present in the posterior triangles in both sides of the neck with psoriasis over the trunk, elbows, knees and shins. Investigations showed a raised E.S.R., a strongly positive Rose-Waaler test, but no lupus erythematosus cells or ANF in the blood. The W.B.C. was 7,500 per cu. mm.

He was treated with butazolidine 100 mgms. t.d.s. with considerable improvement in the joint symptoms over the course of the next six months, at the end of which time the E.S.R. had fallen to normal, but morning stiffness of the joints persisted. One year later he developed a butterfly erythema of the face and hands. The blood, however, showed no lupus erythematosus cells. He was then given camoquin 200 mgms. daily. Within 24 hours he felt extremely ill with severe anorexia, nausea, faintness on standing, a flushed feeling and extreme thirst. The camoquin was stopped after 7 days, but his condition became worse and he developed diarrhoea, severe frontal headache, pain and redness of the eyes, sweating and rigors. Examination showed a temperature of 101-104°F, a very

ill-looking, flushed individual, a dry mouth, cracked lips, severe conjunctivitis, swollen eyelids, erythema multiforme on the face, abdomen and fronts of the thighs. The liver was enlarged two fingers breadth. Investigations now showed W.B.C. 1,300 per cu. mm., polymorphs 78 per cent, lymphocytes 22 per cent. The bone marrow showed increase in the plasma cells, the urine contained protein, red blood cells and casts and the blood now showed large numbers of lupus erythematosus cells and the RF was still strongly positive. ANF was now present in the serum. He was treated with prednisolone and his condition slowly improved, the erythema waxing and waning and the W.B.C. count gradually returned to normal. The lupus erythematosus cells disappeared from the blood.

In this case the patient evidently exhibited a hypersensitivity to camoquin which, however, changed the picture from that of rheumatoid arthritis to one of acute systemic lupus erythematosus.

Thus, the same pathological changes as found in the joints in cases of rheumatoid disease may be found in those organs affected by so-called "auto-immune" diseases and there is evidence of an *overlapping incidence and association between so-called organ-specific (auto-immune) and the collagen (non-organ specific auto-immune) diseases,* though it has been suggested that this is less common than that between the diseases in each of the two groups (Anderson et al., 1967). The two groups of diseases form a continuous spectrum of which they represent the two extremes. Thus *"auto-immune diseases" affecting single tissues can be regarded as the specific manifestations of rheumatoid disease as it affects certain internal organs and that all collagen and auto-immune diseases represent manifestations of a single disorder.* These conclusions will be amplified in the following pages.

I, iii)   Serological changes in collagen and auto-imtnune disease

Addendum: Crisp, A.J., Hoffbrand, B.I., J. Roy.Soc. Med. 1980, 73, 60-61, report a case of Sjogren's syndrome which developed ulcerative colitis with negative RA, ANF and autoantibodies in the blood. The patient was treated with prednisolone and sulphasalazine and afterwards developed rheumatoid arthritis, tender subcutaneous patches and nodules on the face, scalp and limbs with surrounding hair loss. The serum ANF was now positive. Skin biopsy showed vasculitis. She then developed pyrexia, chest pain and an enlarged cardiac shadow and bilateral basal pleural effusions. The serum ANF and RF were now positive. The sulphasalazine was stopped and antibiotics and steroids given with speedy recovery and the patient remained well for 4 years.

Addendum: Brooks, A.P. and Paulley, J.W. Brit. Med. J., 1980, 280, 480, describe the case of a male patient with antibody positive hypothyroidism and hypertension who was given hydrallazine and afterwards developed polyarthralgia, fever, malaise, chest pains, haemoptosis, vasculitis, anaemia, raised ESR and ANF in the serum. Symptoms regressed with withdrawal of hydrallazine.

In the various collagen diseases with or without Hashimoto's thyroiditis and SjBgren's syndrome a hypergammaglobulinaemia of polyclonal type may occur and there are commonly found various abnormal factors in the serum in a proportion of cases. These include the so-called rheumatoid factor (RF), a macroglobulin or M-antiglobulin, the significance of which is not clear, and the antinuclear factor (ANF) (non-organ-specific auto-antibodies) and a host of serum antibodies capable of reacting with the patients own tissues (organ-specific auto-antibodies). These include thyroglobulin antibodies and complement fixing-antibodies to various human organs and tissues, such as gastric mucosa, thyroid and adrenal cortical cells, intrinsic factor (Hift et al., 1973), auto-haemolysins, bodies giving false positive tests for infectious mononucleosis (Horwitz et al., 1973), syphilis and cryoglobulins (Halberg et al., 1965; Harvey, 1967). Lupus erythematosus cells may be present in the blood in any of these conditions, but especially in lupus erythematosus. Sometimes, however, in otherwise completely classical rheumatoid disease no abnormal factors are found in the serum throughout the illness.

In cases of idiopathic Addison's disease, atrophic gastritis or Hashimoto's thyroiditis occurring alone or in combination one with another, auto-antibodies against thyroglobulin or thyroid or gastric parietal or adrenal cortical cells or intrinsic factor (Hift et al., 1973) (organ-specific auto-antibodies) may or may not be present in the serum whichever organ is primarily affected (Carpenter et al., 1964; Irvine, 1968). ANF and RF show a low incidence in these diseases when they occur in the absence of obvious collagen disease (Halberg et al., 1965; Brown, 1966). Serological overlap between systemic lupus erythematosus, rheumatoid arthritis and thyroid auto-immune diseases exists in many cases (Hijmans et al., 1961), while Carpenter et al. (1964) in 15 cases of idiopathic Addison's disease found two who

had a positive Rose-Waaler test and one with ANF in the blood. *In general it may be said that all of the abnormal serum antibodies, both non-organ and organ-specific, found in association* with *collagen* diseases *are manifestations of the rheumatoid* process. The same may be true of the same organ-specific and non-organ-specific auto-antibodies found in cases of Hashimoto's thyroiditis, atrophic gastritis or idiopathic Addison's disease whether occurring associated with clinical manifestations of collagen disease or not. It must be stressed that RF may be absent but ANF or organ-specific auto-antibodies may be present in some cases of both active rheumatoid arthritis and other collagen diseases, while in some cases of burnt-out rheumatoid arthritis all auto-antibodies both organ and non-organ-specific may be absent from the serum. Furthermore, the proof of the existence of a so-called "auto-immune" disease affecting an organ can really only be made histologically and not by means of the presence or not of specific auto-antibodies against the cells of the organism in the serum as has been the tendency of some workers.

Not only do these abnormal antibodies occur in subjects of the collagen or auto-immune diseases, but they tend to appear in normal subjects, their incidence increasing with age, for example RF and thyroid auto-antibodies (Anderson et al., 1967). They also occur in families of such patients and in these they may be unassociated with any physical disturbance or organic lesions. Thyroid antibodies may be detected in about 10 per cent of the population (Fowler et al., 1970).

I, iv) Familial incidence of collagen and auto-immune diseases

Any one of the diseases considered above may occur in several members of a family. A familial aggregation of collagen diseases has been reported in systemic lupus erythematosus (Leonardt, 1964; An-

Addendum: Montiero, E., Ceboleiro. C. and Galvas-Teles, D. Lancet, 1979, 2. 797 report that in 90 cases of adult rheumatoid arthritis, 13 of juvenile rheumatoid arthritis and 27 of ankylosing spondylitis 18%. 27% and 17% respectively of anti microsomalthyroid antibodies were demonstrated by immunofluorescence.

sell and Lawrence, 1964; Holborow and Johnson, 1964; Siegel et al., 1965), rheumatoid arthritis (Stieber et al., 1953; Short et al., 1957), thyroiditis (Hall et al., 1963) and pernicious anaemia (Wallace, 1969). Familial studies also support the possibility that a genetically determined causal factor is concerned in atrophic gastritis and pernicious anaemia. The genetic factor in pernicious anaemia was considered by Wallace (1969). He posed the question as to whether such clusters of cases could also be environmentally determined. Holman (1963) points out that in any family there may occur a range of connective tissue disorders and abnormal blood auto-antibodies, but no lesions in some members of a family although the antibodies are present. A case of dermatomyositis with positive ANF in the serum, whose father had systemic lupus erythematosus and sister rheumatoid arthritis, was reported by Williams (1965). It would appear that several collagen and related diseases have a genetic basis (Rowley and Jenkins, 1962; Birch and Rowell, 1965). The subject of genetics and auto-immune disease is considered fully in the volume, Auto-immunity and Genetics, 1968, Blackwell Scientific Publications, Oxford.

I, v) Dermatomyositis (polymyositis)

Polymyositis may occur 1) alone, 2) with skin lesions (dermatomyositis) and minor evidence of collagen disease, 3) with severe collagen disease, for example rheumatoid arthritis, systemic lupus erythematosus, ankylosing spondylitis and systemic sclerosis and 4) with malignant disease (Haethfield and Williams, 1960; Rose and Walton, 1966). The case of a youth of 18 years with dermatomyositis and with ANF in the serum and whose father suffered from systemic lupus erythematosus and the father's sister from rheumatoid arthritis was reported by Williams (1965). Dermatomyositis may merge into scleroderma and not only affects the skin and muscles, but

many other tissues. Apart from the muscles and skin, every other tissue may be involved in cases of dermatomyositis. Rheumatoid nodules may be found around the joints and in viscera. There may be involvement of the eyes (exophthalmos, oedema of the lids and iritis), fingers and toes (Raynaud's phenomena), mucosa of the upper respiratory passages and of the bronchi, the lungs and pleura leading to effusions, the blood vessels (arteritis), the heart leading to cardiac dysfunction and pericardiaJ effusions, the mucous membrane of the gastrointestinal tract leading to stomatitis and gastro-enteritis, and the salivary and lacrimal glands leading to Sjogren's syndrome. Splenomegaly, lymphadenopathy and peripheral neuropathy may be found and involvement of the central nervous system producing mental confusion, psychoses and dementia (Talbott and Ferrandis, 1956). Cases of dermatomyositis with severe rheumatoid granulomatous myocarditis and thymoma were reported by Mendelow and Jenkins (1954), Waller et al. (1957), Langston et al. (1959) and Rundle and Sparks (1963). The blood often shows an eosinophilia (Talbott and Ferrandis, 1956). In a personally observed case (Case 4) with onset at 36 years atrophic vaginitis developed at the age of 42 years, while another patient, aged 24 years, developed Sjogren's syndrome and Hashimoto's thyroiditis three years after the onset of dermatomyositis.

Winkelman et al. (1968) in an important paper from the Mayo Clinic reported on 289 cases of dermatomyositis of which 28 had the disease for 4 years or more. They showed that the condition may be precipitated by various factors, such as operations, intercurrent infections, etc. In one of the author's patients (Case 5) the operation of hysterectomy for fibroids precipitated the appearance of the condition and later the operation of gastrectomy for peptic ulcer resulted in its dramatic disappearance. When a malignant lymphoma developed 8 years later the dermatomyositis did not

-17

Addendum: Reid. J.M. and Murdoch, R., Brit. Heart. Journ. 1979. 41. 628-629 report a case of complete heart block occurring 4 years after the onset of polymyositis.
Addendum: Dermatomyositis associated with fibrosing alveolitis was described by Plowman, P.N. and Stableforth, D.E. (Proc. R. Soc. Med., 1977. 70. 738). Another case of dermatomyositis without apparent myositis, but complicated by fibrosing alveolitis was reported by Fernandes, L. and Goodwill, C.T., J. Roy. Soc. Med., 1979, 72, 777.

reappear. Winkelmann et al. found that dermatomyositis may come and go on several occasions and, if the patient develops malignant disease, dermatomyositis may or may not reappear or, if already present, it may disappear. Malignant disease may develop *many years after* the onset of dermatomyositis. On the other hand dermatomyositis and malignant disease may develop *at the same time* or dermatomyositis may occur *after* the onset of malignancy. In some cases this may be an appreciable period. Simpson (1953) reported a case of successful treatment of carcinoma of the breast who developed dermatomyositis six years after-wards without recurrence of the cancer. When co-incident in time, successful removal or treatment of the cancer may, it is said, occasionally cause regression or disappearance of the symptoms of dermatomyositis (Talbott and Ferrandis, 1956), which may return with the recurrence of the tumour, but this appears to be rare. The development of a tumour appears to be only one of a number of factors which may precipitate the appearance of latent dermatomyositis or if it is present, may cause its disappearance.

Cases of polymyositis may become chronic and "burnt out". Christensen and Rosse! (1964) found that in such cases some of the muscles showed the changes of muscular dystrophy and elsewhere chronic myositis. The distinction between the two conditions may then become difficult or impossible. This finding explains the occurrence of some cases of muscular dystrophy occurring sporadically.

I, vi)   Sjogren's syndrome (sicca syndrome) and Mikulicz's disease

SjtJgren's syndrome is almost always a manifestation of rheumatoid disease. The following considerations apply only to such cases and not to those rare cases due to other causes, such as sarcoidosis.

Sjtigren's syndrome and Mikulicz's disease are clinically and histologically the same condition (Goodwin, 1952; Morgan and Castleman, 1953; Morgan, 1954; Bunim, 1961, Bunim et al., 1964; Seifert and Geiler, 1967; Von Schultess, 1968). For references to this condition see Sjogren (1951), Bunim (1961), Futcher (1959), Heaton (1962) and Shearn (1971). Bertram (1967) collected 32 cases of this condition. A recent extensive monograph by Shearn (1971) reviews the present knowledge of the syndrome and reports on 80 cases, while Whaley et al. (1973 a, b) analysed a series of 171 cases. The otolaryngeal aspects are considered by Doig et al. (1971). In this condition the lacrimal and salivary glands are heavily infiltrated with lymphocytes and sometimes with plasma cells, often with the formation of germinal follicles. This results in compression of the gland cells with later fibrosis and sometimes obstruction and cystic dilatation of the ducts. The only difference between Sjogren's syndrome and Mikulicz's disease is the enlargement of the affected glands found in the latter. Sometimes only one of the salivary glands is enlarged. The condition may present with recurrent painless swelling of the salivary glands (autoimmune parotitis), which later becomes permanent. Familial cases occur (Shearn, 1971). Secondary bacterial infection may ensue. The glandular lesions are identical with those found in the thyroid gland in Hashimoto's or focal thyroiditis. In some cases the cellular infiltration of the salivary glands may not involve the whole of the gland, but have a focal distribution. Waterhouse and Doniach (1966) found such focal lymphocytic infiltration of the salivary glands in 16 of 17 cases of rheumatoid arthritis and considered this to be Sjogren's syndrome in minature. *Sjogren's syndrome is to be regarded as part of the rheumatoid disease complex* (Ericson and Sundmark, 1970). Bloch et al. (1965) found that in patients with Sjogren's syndrome with or without associated rheumatoid arthritis hypergammaglobulinaemia was common and RF, ANF and thyroid auto-antibodies were frequently present in the serum and the direct Coombs test positive in a quarter of the cases. Lupus erythematosus cells were present in 10 per cent of cases. Thyroid auto-antibodies occurred in the absence of thyroid disease. MacSween et al. (1967) in a series of cases of Sjogren's syndrome found auto-antibodies to salivary duct epithelium in 13 of 20 cases without rheumatoid arthritis and in **I I** of 17 associated with rheumatoid arthritis and in 34 of 129 patients with rheumatoid arthritis alone. J'he authors concluded that the antibodies in these cases are a manifestation of the rheumatoid process. In Sjogren's syndrome the blood may show an eosinophilia (Futcher, 1959; Pearson, 1961; Shearn, 1971) and the salivary mucus may be infiltrated with eosinophils (Pearson, 1961).

Every gradation between Sjogren's syndrome, Mikulicz's disease and enlargement of the salivary glands due to the presence of benign lympho-epithelial lesions (adenalymphoma, lymphocytic tumours or papillary cystadenolymphomatosum) are found (Lloyd, 1946; Godwin, 1952; Morgan, 1954; Orloff, 1956; Von Schultess, 1968; Sprinkle and Yarington, 1968). According to Cruikshank (1965), however, a benign epithelial lesion is to be distinguished from adenolymphoma in that it is not associated with collagen disease. These tumours tend to be symmetrical, solid or cystic and a broad spectrum from the solid to the alveolar and cystic may be seen. They consist of areas of lymphocytic infiltration with epithelial metaplasia of the alveolar element. The tumour is usually benign, but may recur after removal.

In cases of Sjogren's syndrome there tends to occur a generalised dessication due to atrophy and hypofunction of the exocrine glands in all parts of the body. In addition the endocrine glands may also be involved. **It** is commonly associated with rheumatoid arthritis, Felty's syndrome, systemic lupus erythematosus (Mackay

and Burnet, 1963; Steinberg and Tala!, 1971), psoriatic arthropathy (Whaley et al., 1973), Raynaud's phenomena (Heaton, 1962), scleroderma, polymyositis (myopathy), polyarteritis or vasculitis, lymphadenopathy and splenomegaly, hepatomegaly,Hashimoto's thyroiditis with or without thyrotoxicosis or myxoedema, active chronic hepatitis, postnecrotic or biliary cirrhosis, skin disturbances (ichthyosis acquisita, vitiligo), pneumonitis, chronic pulmonary fibrosis, heart lesions of various kinds, hypoglycaemia (Pearson, 1961), diabetes mellitus, atrophic gastritis, achlorhydria (60 per cent of cases), pernicious anaemia, chronic pancreatitis often with calicification in the gland, coeliac disease (Pittman and Holub, 1965; Shearn, 1971), ulcerative colitis (Recant and Lacey, 1964; Shearn, 1971), nephropathy, auto-immune haemolytic anaemia, purpura, paraproteinaemia or Waldenstrom's macroglobulinaemia and polyneuropathy and certain other neurological disturbances.

In cases of Sjogren's syndrome the diminished secretion of the lacrimal and salivary glands involves not only the main, but also the accessory lacrimal and salivary glands (Whaley et al., 1968). This results in a dryness of the mouth and eyes and may be followed by or associated with atrophy of the oral, palatal and pharyngeal mucosa (atrophic glossitis, stomatitis and pharyngitis), which is thin and the tongue loses its papillae. Fissures appear at the angle of the mouth (angular stomatitis). These changes are associated with lymphocytic infiltration of the affected submucosa. This condition may be complicatd by rampant dental caries or by periodontitis (Shearn, 1971; Boyle and Buchanan, 1971). The same loss of secretion may extend to involve other tissues with atrophy of surfaces lubricated by local mucus secretion and accompanied by lymphocytic infiltration of the submucosa. This may affect the nasal mucosa resulting in dryness of the nose and crusting, epistaxis and anosmia (atrophic rhinitis) and nasal septal perforation and sinusitis (Hughes and Whaley, 1972). This change may extend to the lining of the Eustachian tube and middle ear leading to chronic adhesive salpingitis and otitis, adhesions between the tympanic membrane and bony wall of the middle ear and obstruction of the Eustachian tube (Doig et al., 1971) with conduction deafness.

The atrophic changes may affect the mucosa of the oropharynx and larynx which is covered by thick tenacious mucus secretion infiltrated with eosinophils (Pearson, 1961). This is associated with soreness, and dryness of the throat and hoarseness (pharyngo-laryngitis sicca). The mucosal atrophy may extend from the pharynx to affect the oesophagus, leading to atrophic oesophagitis, the submucous glands being diffusely infiltrated with lymphocytes and plasma cells, to postcricoid narrowing and the presence of mucoidal webs identical with those in the Paterson-Kelly syndrome and to dysphagia (Doig et al., 1971).

Sjogren's syndrome may be associated with Hashimoto's or focal thyroiditis, in which the changes in the thyroid gland are identical with those in the lacrimal and salivary glands. This may result in atrophy and fibrosis of the thyroid. Both hyperthyroidism and hypothyroidism may occur and clinical thyroid disease has been reported in 6-13 per cent of cases of Sjogren's syndrome (Bloch et al., 1965). Diabetes associated with Sjogren's syndrome was reported by Pearson (1961), Bertram (1967) and Shearn (1971).

The skin may be dry and flake and sweating is diminished. The sweat glands are infiltrated by lymphocytes. This condition is known as *ichthyosis acquisita*. It occurs in the absence of myxoedema or diabetes. The hair may be dry and sparse or localized alopecia may be seen. There may be atrophic changes in the nails.

Atrophy and drying up of the secretions of the vulva leading to atrophic vulvitis and vaginitis (vulvo-vaginitis sicca) may cause dyspareunia. The submucosa is in-filtrated with lymphocytes involving the secretory glands.

In the breast (an exocrine gland) there may be found areas in which the acini are surrounded with lymphocytes and this is followed by fibrosis, producing localized tumour-like formations (Sokoloff, 1966) and often dilatation of the ducts and cyst formation. These changes are identical with the early stages of cystic mastitis and closely resemble those occurring in the salivary glands.

The mucosal atrophy of the oesophagus may extend to the stomach leading to atrophic gastritis with achlorhydria and sometimes pernicious anaemia (Bertram, 1967; Wegelius et al., 1970). The gastric mucosa shows severe lymphoid infiltration. In 4 patients with Sjogren's syndrome Wegelius et al. (1970) found all had achlorhydria, 3 pernicious anaemia and 1 atrophic gastritis alone. Two had longstanding rheumatoid arthritis and all 4 a high titre of RF in the serum. Sjogren's syndrome may also be associated with coeliac disease (Pittman and Holub, 1965; Shearn, 1971) in which atrophy of the small intestinal mucosa (villus atrophy) occurs and the submucosa shows a lymphocytic infiltration. Sjogren's syndrome may also be accompanied by ulcerative colitis (Recant and Lacey, 1964; Shearn, 1971). Fenster et al. (1964) found that clinical or morphological involvement of the pancreas may complicate Sjogren's syndrome and found mild functional involvement in 4 of 11 patients with the syndrome. Shearn (1971) confirmed these findings and in one case found at autopsy a heavy lymphocytic infiltration of the stroma of the pancreas, identical with that in the salivary and lacrimal glands. Whaley et al. (1970) stressed the association of liver disease with Sjogren's syndrome. Golding (1970) examined an unselected group of patients with "auto-immune" liver disease and found Sjogren's syndrome was present in nearly 40 per cent of patients with active chronic hepatitis, 65 per cent of those with primary biliary cirrhosis and 26 per cent of those with cryptogenic cirrhosis. Read (1970) in the same article reports a spectrum of auto-immune liver disease in cases of rheumatoid arthritis and Sjogren's syndrome. Sjogren's syndrome accompanied by active chronic hepatitis or post-necrotic cirrhosis is reported by Urban and Carrott (1959), Shearn (1971) and Whaley et al. (1973 b). There may be intense lymphocytic infiltration of the liver in such cases. Such liver disease occurring with Sjogren's syndrome may also be associated with scleroderma (Morgan, 1973) or with rheumatoid arthritis, haemolytic anaemia, renal tubular acidosis and interstitial nephritis (see below).

Sjogren's syndrome may be associated with renal tubular acidosis and with interstitial lymphocytic inflammatory infiltrates of the kidney leading to fibrosis, the changes resembling those found in the salivary and lacrimal glands. Such an association occurs in 20-25 per cent of Sjogren's syndrome (Talalet al., 1968). The glomeruli are spared (McCurdy et al., 1967; Tu et al., 1968; Mason and Golding, 1970 a, 1970 b; Zalin et al., 1970; Shioji et al., 1970; Shearn, 1971; Farid and Evered, 1971). Renal tubular acidosis may be combined with Sjogren's syndrome with or without rheumatoid arthritis (Farid and Evered, 1971), hepatosphmomegaly (McCurdy et al., 1967), lymphocytic thyroiditis, biliary cirrhosis (Tu et al., 1968) or chronic active hepatitis. Glomerular disease may occur in some cases of Sjogren's syndrome (Whaley et al., 1973 b).

The mucosal atrophy of the pharynx and larynx may extend to the trachea and bronchi and the lungs may be similarly involved giving rise to the same lesions as those associated with rheumatoid arthritis, including pneumonitis, fibrosing alveolitis, pleuritis, asthma and bronchospasm (Heaton, 1959) and chronic bronchitis and leading to a tendency to respiratory infections. Nodular parenchymal disease may be seen in the lung, the nodules being composed of lymphocytes, plasma and reticulum cells and often giant cells with germinal centres. All these changes are identical with those found in rheumatoid arthritis. The heart may be affected and rheumatoid nodules may be seen in the myocardium, pericardium and endocardium as in rheumatoid arthritis. Various conduction disturbances may be observed.

Finally Sjogren's syndrome may be associated with neurological disturbances. These include peripheral neuropathy, trigeminal sensory neuropathy, epilepsy, cerebrovascular accidents, psychoneurosis and mental disturbances. These changes have been variously ascribed to vasculitis affecting the peripheral nerves or the brain may exhibit perivascular lymphocytosis in the cerebral vessels or vasculitis (Sheldon, 1939; Ramage and Kinnear, 1956; Heaton, 1959; Pearson; 1961; Shearn, 1971).

Sjogren's syndrome is not uncommonly associated with Waldenstrom's macroglobulinaemia (Shearn, 1971). Allergic reactions are common, drug reactions occurring in up to 63 per cent of cases (Shearn, 1971; Whaley et al., 1973 b).

The author had under his care an Anglo-Indian patient (Case 6) a man of 64 years, who nine years previously developed severe rheumatoid arthritis followed by Sjogren's syndrome, myxoedema, atrophic rhinitis and tracheo-bronchitis, atrophic oesophagitis leading to dysphagia, fibrosing alveolitis and heart failure due to rheumatoid granulomatous myocarditis. The serum contained RF and ANF in high concentration. He died suddenly of deep vein thrombosis in the leg and pulmonary embolism.

Shearn (1971) observes that Sjögren's syndrome is a manifestation of a generalized disease, which appears to be infective in nature. . He likens it to syphilis in its protean manifestations and compares it to the latter before the discovery of Treponema pallidum. The statement that the epithelial lesions in the mouth are due to lack of saliva is untenable, since xerostomia can occur without their development.

Addendum: Rheumatoid nodules formation within the choroid plexus. Report of a second case. Kim RC, Collins, GH, Paris, JE. Arch PatholLab Med 1982, 106, 83 - 84

Again the statement often made that atrophy of other mucosal surfaces is due to lack of mucus is also untenable. The atrophy of mucous surfaces like that of exocrine glands is associated with submucous lymphocytic infiltration. As has been said Sjogren's syndrome is nearly always a manifestation of rheumatoid disease as must be the conditions with which it is associated.

I, vii) Periarteritis nodosa, polyarteritis or necrotizing angeitis, vasculitis and collagen disease

This condition is often referred to as a disease to be distinguished from hypersensitivity angeitis, allergic granulomatous angeitis, cranial arteritis and rheumatic arteritis. It is not a disease, however, but a pathological change which is found in association with collagen, including rheumatoid, diseases. Every tissue in the body may be involved by the changes which have already been considered above. Small vessels and venules as well as arteries are also affected, that is, it is a vasculitis rather than a purely arterial change and this vasculitis also includes an endarteritis. The changes tend to be associated with certain acute manifestations of the collagen diseases, such as asthma, urticaria, fever, sweating and a blood eosinophilia occurring in recurrent bouts. When these are present, the cases merge into the condition of disseminated eosinophilic collagen disease (see below). Such cases are generally thought to be due to an infection (Harvey, 1967). It must again be emphasized, however, that periarteritis is not in itself a disease, but a manifestation of a disease and, if periarteritis is the result of an infection, then so must the collagen diseases be.

I, viii) Venous thromboses and rheumatoid disease

It has been stressed above that the venous system may be involved in the vasculitis of collagen disease. Bowie et al. (1963) draws attention to the occurrence of venous thromboses in cases of systemic lupus erythematosus. Gardner (1969) in 142 autopsies on rheumatoid arthritic cases found 13 cases (9 per cent) with venous thromboses. A patient of the author's, a woman aged 73 years, had suffered from a rodent ulcer of the nose for 6 years, for which no treatment was given. She then developed a venous thrombosis of the left leg, for which she was treated with phenylbutazone. This precipitated the appearance of systemic lupus erythematosus with polyarthropathy. The blood contained numerous lupus erythematosus cells, RF and ANF. Achlorhydria was present. Another patient, a woman aged 86 years, suffered from a deep vein thrombosis of one leg and was found to have a serum R.A. latex fixation test of one in 4096.

I, ix) Rheumatoid nodules or granulomata

Visible rheumatoid nodules or granulomata may occur in 20-30 per cent of rheumatoid arthritic patients at some time in the course of the disease and are most characteristic. They may be single or multiple. Similar nodules may occur in systemic lupus erythematosus and dermatomyositis (Short et al., 1957; Dubois et al., 1972). They range in size from microscopic to up to seven centimetres in diameter. They consist of granulomata with focal collections of lymphocytes, often in relation to an area of arteritis with a central necrotic area. Giant cells are rare. They occur especially at sites exposed to pressure or stress, such as over bony prominences like the olecranon; over the ischial and femoral tuberosities; in relation to the bases of the phalangeal and metacarpal bones; at the site of pressure when holding a pen; attached to joint capsules; over tendons in tendon sheaths; in the scalp and occiput, abdominal wall, tongue,

-:- 22-

Addendum: Benign rheumatoid nodules may occur in children. Roggins DL, Moore, TL, Naguwa SM Clin. Rheumatol. 1982, 1/2104-111 In the absence of obvious rheumatoid disease.
Addendum: Rheumatoid nodules also occur in systemic sclerosis (Bywaters, E.G.L., Journ. Rheumatol., 1979, 6, 243-246)

pharynx, larynx, lungs and pleura, peritoneum, splenic capsule, sclera, over the bridge of the nose (at the site of pressure of spectacles) and at the antihelix of the ear (Gardner, 1967, 1972; Boyle and Buchanan, 1971), on periostea, in the breast, loose subcutaneous tissue, synovial membranes, the upper layers of the integument, the dura mater, the subdural and extradural spaces and the base of the heart valves. Similar lesions occur in the myocardium and in the lung substance and other viscera, in the connective tissue between bundles of skeletal muscle and in the sheaths of peripheral nerves. The author has observed these lesions occurring in the pulp of the finger tips and also in the substance of the lips, where they may come and go. Occasionally these nodules may occur both in children and adults as the only sign of rheumatoid disease (Boyle and Buchanan, 1971). The granulomatous structure of the nodules resembles that of tuberculosis, mycoses or other infective granulomata and suggests the infective and generalized nature of rheumatoid disease. Gardner (1972) states that their structure appears directed against a repelled chemical or extrinsic microbiological agent.

Rheumatoid nodules may be found in the absence of signs or symptoms of rheumatoidtoid arthritis. Berardelli et al. (1972) describe ten cases of children with isolated rheumatoid nodules, but without other evidence of juvenile rheumatoid arthritis. When examined 2-16 years after their appearance, RF was present in the serum.

I, x) Disseminated eosinophilic collagen disease

The condition of disseminated eosinophilic collagen disease has been defined by Engfeldt and Zetterström (1956), Bousser (1957), Odeberg (1965), Pierce et al. (1967) and Benvenisti and Ultmann (1969) who review previously reported cases. This condition had been described under various names before. It is related to rheumatoid arthritis, systemic lupus erythematosus, dermatomyositis, vasculitis or periarteritis and has some of the features of each condition. The disease process may be acute, subacute or chronic. In children it is not usually fatal, whereas in adults it is. In acute cases the onset is sudden with severe generalized malaise, high pyrexia, sweating and often drenching night sweats. These symptoms accompanied by other manifestations of the disease may recur with varying severity throughout the illness. In addition there may be evidence of involvement of any organ of the body, varying from case to case. These include skin lesions, such as pruritus, rashes of various types, urticaria, scaly erythema, vesicular exanthemata, lesions like those of dermatomyositis or systemic lupus erythematosus and alopecia. The joints, especially peripheral, may be painful and swollen like those in rheumatoid arthritis. The muscles may be painful and weak as in dermatomyositis. There may be signs and symptoms of peripheral neuropathy, oedema of face, hands and feet, asthmatic attacks with pulmonary infiltration constituting Löffler's syndrome and pneumonia, lymphadenopathy, splenomegaly, hepatomegaly, cardiac involvement with pancarditis, renal involvement, orchitis, intestinal involvement with abdominal pains and vomiting and injection of the conjunctivae, thrombophlebitis and cerebral disturbances of various types, such as confusion, delusions, epilepsy and coma. The blood exhibits a raised E.S.R. and hyperglobulinaemia. Heterophil antigen may be found in the serum. There is usually an increasing anaemia, sometimes preceded by erythrocytosis. The anaemia may be of acute haemolytic "auto-immune" type. There is a marked leucocytosis largely due to a very high *eosinophilia*, usually without the presence of immature eosinophils. Occasionally in some long-standing cases immature eosinophil precursors may be present in the blood and in some cases neutrophil precursor cells, constituting a mye- loid leukaemic change. There may be thrombocytopenia. Death usually occurs from heart failure.

At autopsy the changes vary with the duration of the disease. They consist essentially of vasculitis, endarteritis, thrombotic changes with infarction and areas of focal necrosis or focal eosinophilic granulomata. The larger vessels may show intimal necrosis and fibrous obliteration. All the tissues exhibit heavy infiltration with mature eosinophils, and also with lymphocytes, plasma cells and sometimes histiocytes in various admixtures. These changes are particularly seen in the heart. The liver may show centro-lobular necrosis and healed peri-arteriolar vasculitis in the periportal spaces. The skeletal muscles show myositic changes and focal infiltration with lymphocytes and eosinophils, especially round the vessels, closely resembling the changes in other collagen diseases, especially systemic lupus erythematosus and polyarteritis. Similar changes are present in all other organs of the body, including lymph nodes, spleen, pancreas, salivary glands and endocrines. The lymph nodes frequently exhibit the changes of chronic inflammation or reactive hyperplasia, though they are also heavily infiltrated with eosinophils. The marrow is hypercellular, exhibits marked eosinophilia and often granulocytic hyperplasia, the predominant granulocyte being the myelocyte. Moderate plasmacytosis may be seen. Charcot-Leyden crystals may occur in the tissues. The changes are consistent with a chronic inflammation or an early myelo-proliferative disorder (Pierce et al., 1957).

Examples of this condition are the following cases:-

Case 7 Female, aged 23 years. Family and past history irrelevant. She developed a sudden influenzal-like illness with rhinitis, sore throat, pyrexia of 101°F and profuse sweating and two days after the onset went into severe status asthmaticus, became de-

lirious and confused and remembered nothing for a week. The temperature reached 103°F. The lungs exhibited severe bronchospasm and a blood count at this time showed W.B.C. 29,000 per cu. mm. of which 70 per cent were mature eosinophils and the E.S.R. was 35 mms. per hour. Her mental state gradually improved and she then complained of severe pain, stiffness and swelling of the peripheral joints, severe muscular tenderness and weakness, intense paraesthesiae in the extremities, swelling of the salivary glands and tenderness over the thyroid gland. Examination showed a markedly injected pharynx, oedema of the eyelids, generalized rhonchi and signs of bronchospasm in the chest, tender, swollen parotid salivary and thyroid glands, severe swelling and tenderness of the peripheral joints, marked muscular weakness and tenderness, loss of all tendon reflexes and sensory impairment in the peripheries of the limbs. The W.B.C. showed a total of 44,000 per cu. mm., 65 per cent being eosinophils. Repeat chest X-rays revealed wandering pulmonary infiltrations. An E.C.G. showed well-marked ST segment deviation in all leads. RF was absent from the serum. She continued to run an irregular temperature and had attacks of asthma and urticaria of varying length and periods of confusion and occasinally epileptic attacks. The pain and swelling of the joints, muscle tenderness and salivary gland swelling persisted during the next six months and the W.B.C. count ranged between 40,000 and 98,000 per cu. mm. of which up to 85 per cent were eosinophils. The E.S.R. reached 65 mm. per hour. The sputum also contained large numbers of eosinophils. After six months the arthropathy, muscular weakness and peripheral neuropathy had advanced to the state of the typical appearance of advanced rheumatoid deformity with severe muscular wasting and contractures. She now developed a sterile abscess of the left parotid gland and incision of the abscess yielded a large amount of bacteriologically sterile pus composed almost entirely of eosinophil leucocytes. She then began to complain of dryness of the eyes and mouth and Schirmer's test showed almost complete absence of tear formation. The serum now showed strongly positive tests for RF and ANF and thyroid auto-antibodies. During the next 18 months her asthma continued irregularly. Skeletal muscle biopsy showed heavy infiltration of the interfibrillary spaces with eosinophils and evidence of vasculitis. Repeat E.C.G.'s continued to show ST segment deviation in all leads and after 9 months the blood urea reached 107 rpgms. per cent. She eventually died of cardiac failure 25 months after the onset.

Autopsy revealed oedema and generalized eosinophilic and lymphocytic infiltration and focal necrosis of all organs, including myocardium, lungs, endocrines, liver, pancreas, kidneys, salivary glands and muscles and atrophy of the constituent cells. There was generalized evidence of arteritis of the larger vessels and endarteritis of the smaller ones. A diagnosis of disseminated eosinophilic collagen disease or of rheumatoid arthritis with peripheral neuropathy, myositis, Sjogren's syndrome with heart, lung, liver and kidney involvement, asthma and urticaria accompanied by eosinophilia was made.

Case 8 Female, aged 62 years. Three years previously she developed a "frozen" right shoulder. She gave a 6 months history of bouts of dyspnoea even at rest without cough, of easy exhaustion, a constant feeling of heat and also nocturnal sweating. Examination showed a healthy looking, but dyspnoeic woman with slight tachycardia, a pyrexia of 99.4oF and scattered adventitiae in both lung bases. Severe bilateral hallux valgus and overriding of the toes was present. A chest X-ray showed areas of consolidation in both lung fields, especially on the right side. E.S.R.=60 mm. per hour. W.B.C. 6,500 per cu. mm. Neutrophils 84 per cent. Lymphocytes 12 per cent. Eosinophils 4 per cent. Sputum contained commensals only. Dur-

ing the next two months she ran an irregular pyrexia reaching 100.8°F with general muscle aching, bouts of dyspnoea, night sweats and wandering shadows in both lung fields. She gradually developed an anaemia with Hb 60 per cent and the W.B.C. rose to 25,000 per cu. mm. and the eosinophils reached 28 per cent. The E.S.R. rose to 86 mm. per hour. No parasites, cysts or ova were found in the stools. Tests for trichinosis were negative. Complement fixation tests for mycoplasma pneumoniae, psittacosis, K.G.V. and Q fever were negative. No cold agglutins were detected in the blood. The RF was weakly positive in the serum. Muscle biopsy showed interfibrillary collections of monocytes and eosinophils and evidence of arteritis. There was no response to antibiotics or hetrazan. The symptoms, radiological changes and other disturbances gradually disappeared over the next 3 months. Except for pains in the neck and across the shoulders she remained well for the next 18 months and then developed attacks of urticaria in various parts of the body and painful swelling of the joints of the hands and feet accompanied by morning stiffness. The eosinophilia in the blood returned and reached 20 per cent of a total W.B.C. of 10,500 per cu. mm. The RF was now strongly positive in the serum.

Various cases have been reported which show merging of disseminated eosinophilic collagen disease into "eosinophilic leukaemia" or subacute granulocytic leukaemia with eosinophilia even in some cases lymphomatous changes in the lymphoid tissue and chloroma or myeloblastoma in the marrow (Benvenisti and Ultmann, 1969) or carcinoma elsewhere in the body (Boone, 1969). Most authors do not consider that such a condition as true eosinophilic leukaemia exists. They regard the eosinophilia and granulocytic changes seen in disseminated eosinophilic collagen disease as leukaemoid reactions. In a great number of cases features suggesting "eosinophilic leukaemia", granulocytic leukaemia, collagen disease and lymphoma have been present together in the same case raising the question as to whether a common aetiologic factor causes all these phenomena (Odeberg, 1967). Moreover, there is no clear cut *pathological difference between benign bronchial asthma with eosinophilia, U)ffler's syndrome and disseminated eosinophilic collagen* disease.

Aetiologically disseminated eosinophilic collagen disease has been thought to be either allergic or auto-immune in nature, that is an allergic-immunity reaction, or a combination of these. It is, however, highly significant that as pointed out in several papers an almost identical condition may be seen in cases of parasitic infestations, such as trichiniasis, ascariasis or toxacara (visceral larva migrans) infection or in cases of animal filariasis affecting man in Eastern countries. However, no such parasite has been found in disseminated eosinophilic collagen disease. Such phenomena as the pyrexia, profuse sweating, urticaria, pruritus, eosinophilia and the occurrence of granulomata, lymphadenopathy and splenomegaly accompanying the eosinophilia are highly suggestive that the condition is related to infestation by an unknown parasite. This applies not only to the collagen disease itself, but also to the granulocytic leukaemic changes and the development of lymphoma, chloroma and myeloblastomata in the marrow found in some cases.

I, xi) Generalized symptoms 1DC1.uding oedema, as manifestations of collagen disease

Fatigue, anorexia, fever and weight loss are common in all collagen diseases suggesting an infective a ology. Oedema of feet, hands or orbits is often found in cases of rheumatoid arthritis, systemic lupus erythematosus, dermatomyositis and disseminated eosinophilic collagen disease. Its aetiology has not been explained. Amyloidosis is also a common feature of long-standing rheumatoid disease (see Duthie, 1969). The occurrence of all these phenomena favour the view that the disease is a chronic infection.

I, xii) Psoriasis and arthropathy

Psoriasis may accompany arthropathy, so-called psoriatic arthropathy, which appears to be a distinct form of rheumatoid disease. The RF is usually absent from the serum and the course of the disease is different from that of rheumatoid arthritis. Psoriasis, however, may also be associated with classical rheumatoid arthritis (Short et al., 1957; Robinson, 1971) and psoriasis occurs in 5-10 per cent of casec of rheumatoid arthritis. Hellgren (1969) found a mathematical association between the two. Whether the skin disease is a manifestation of rheumatoid disease is not yet clear. Psoriasis and Sjogren's syndrome occurred in a classical case of rheumatoid arthritis in the geriatric series already quoted (see also Whaley et al., 1973). Another of the author's patients (Case 9) with long-standing psoriasis developed pernicious anaemia and lupoid hepatitis and later cerebral tumour. Psoriasis combined with post-necrotic cirrhosis has been seen by the author on two occasions, and psoriatic arthropathy in association with polycythaemia vera in another (Case 10). Thus, psoriasis may in some way be a manifestation of collagen auto-immune disease.

I, xiii) Ankylosing spondylitis and collagen disease

Ankylosing spondylitis differs from rheumatoid disease affecting the spine both clinically and radiologically, though in both the heart may be affected. However, rheumatoid arthritis may occasionally be combined with ankylosing spondylitis (Huskisson, 1970; Hart, 1970). In a man of 53 years observed by the author psoriasis began at 18 years of uge and ankylosing spon-

Addendum : Rheumatoid lymphoedema. Kyle VM, de Silva M, Hurst G. ClinicalRheumatology 1982, 1/2 126·7. This occurs in upper limbs due to abnormalities of the lymphatics resulting from lymphangitis secondary to the inflammatory process of the disease. The demonstration of lymphatic channel on wrist arthrography in rheumatoid disease with particular reference to associated lymphoedema. Wu g, Whitehouse GH, Littler TR, Lwasowe Hosp. LiverpoolUK. Rheumatol. Rehabil1982, 21, 65-71.

dylitis at 27 years. At the age of 48 years he developed peripheral joint disease in the hands and knees and at 51 years Raynaud's phenomenon. RF was present in the blood and typical X-ray changes of ankylosing spondylitis were present. This appears to be a transitional case between rheumatoid arthritis, psoriatic arthropathy and ankylosing spondylitis.

Summary of Chapter I

To summarize the above observations it appears that-

1) there exists a continuous spectrum of diseases in which every transition from and combination of one collagen disease, including rheumatoid arthritis, with another and with the most acute form of this type of disease, namely disseminated eosinophilic collagen disease,

2) every tissue in the body may be affected in these conditions to a varying degree, and may exhibit evidence of vasculitis,

3) Sj5gren's-Mikulicz's syndrome is a special manifestation of collagen disease,

4) there exists every combination of any form of collagen disease with any type of "auto-immune" disease affecting specific tissues and any combination of "auto-immune" diseases in different tissues may be found (see later),

5) in cases of "auto-immune" disease of a tissue occurring apparently in isolation involvement of other tissues may often be found, if sought carefully.

6) various organ and non-organ-specific auto-antibodies may or may not exist in the serum regardless of the type of "collagen" or "auto-immune" disease present.

Aetiologically rheumatoid arthritis has long been thought to be the result of an infection (see later). The consensus of opinion on the aetiology of that manifestation of "collagen" diseases known as Sj5gren's syndrome is that it is an infection highly reminiscent of syphilis, while the evidence from consideration of the nature of that form of collagen disease known as disseminated eosinophilic collagen disease is that it represents the effects of an unknown parasitic infestation. The features of rheumatoid nodules are highly suggestive of infection by a microbiological agent.

Chapter II

The manifestations of "collagen" and "auto-immune" diseases as they affect specific organs and tissues

In this chapter the manifestations of "collagen" and "auto-immune" diseases as they affect different organs and tissues will be considered. Stress has already been laid on the fact that rheumatoid disease, systemic lupus erythematosus, dermatomyositis and scleroderma and the associated vasculitis and in particular disseminated eosinophilic collagen disease may affect every tissue in the body, though sometimes the brunt of the disease falls especially on certain organs. In the pages that follow various conditions are considered as regards their possible relationship to "collagen" and "auto-immune" diseases. Burkitt (1970) suggests that common or related causes may be suspected for diseases that have similar geographical distributions and tend to occur together in the same patient. Morris (1964) states that "one of the paths of progress in medicine is to define and refine syndromes among the undifferentiated mass of clinical data by discovering that apparently unrelated phenomena have the same cause". In other wordcertain conditions associated with .<;;ollagen or auto-immune diseases "may be considered as due to a single cause" or they are guilty of being auto-immune diseases by association. Statisticians may criticize the conclusions reached on the ground that controls were not used in assessing such relationships in the following pages, for example whether the incidence of malignant disease in cases of rheumatoid arthritis is higher than in controls. Reasons will be given in the course of the argument why any "controls" used in these circumstances are quite unacceptable. Recourse must be made to different principles.

Siurala et al. (1965) studied 71 cases of collagen disease, including rheumatoid arthritis, ankylosing spondylitis, systemic lupus erythematosus, dermatomyositis, scleroderma, polyarteritis nodosa and some undetermined cases with respect to the presence of disease of the gastro-intestinal tract. They found superficial gastritis in 11, atrophic gastritis in 13, subtotal or total villous atrophy of the small intestine in 6 and inflammatory changes only in 9 cases. There was intestinal malabsorption giving rise to coeliac disease in 7 patients, three of whom had systemic lupus erythematosus. They found no difference in the changes in the mucosa of the small intestine from those of adult coeliac disease. In two cases the malabsorption responded to a gluten-free diet. Five patients had typical clinical signs and other evidence of chronic pancreatitis. One case developed cancer of the colon. Two cases suffered from hyperthyroidism, one from hypothyroidism, two from diabetes mellitus and five from chronic hepatitis. Liver function tests were abnormal in 33 patients and liver biopsy showed fatty changes in 3, acute hepatitis in 3 and chronic hepatitis in 2 cases. Fenyohazi et al. (1970) in 18 patients with rheumatoid arthritis found 11 with gastric mucosal atrophy, severe in 5 cases and with inflammatory changes in 7. Only 2 of a control series showed atrophy and none inflammatory changes. Pettersson et al. (1970) in 24 patients with rheumatoid arthritis found 16 showed malabsorption, due to intestinal amyloidosis in 4 cases while the rest showed villous atrophy of the small intestine.

II, i) Involvement of the spinal and other joints

Rheumatoid arthritis can affect any or all of the synovial joints of the body. It may be followed by osteo-arthritis in the affected joints, such as the knees. Rheumatoid disease of the spine is well described by Boyle and Buchanan (1971), Ball (1971) and Ball and Sharp (1971). The changes are to be distinguished from those of osteo-arthritis and ankylosing spondylitis. Rheumatoid spondylitis occurs especially in juvenile rneumatoid arthritis. The cervical spine is frequently involved in 'cases of rheumatoid disease. The changes can be divided into two categories.

a) Subluxation of the atlanto-axial joint.

b) Changes below C2 vertebra. These occur frequently and lead to pain in the neck, which is increased by movement and coughing, and to restricted movements. Radiologically there are found multiple narrowed intervertebral spaces with little or no osteophyte formation. These changes are characteristic and narrowing of the higher spaces between C2 and 3 and C3 and 4 vertebrae is almost pathognomonic. Subluxation of vertebrae at any level is not uncommon as are erosions of the apophyseal joints and rheumatoid spondylitis at other levels is shown by multiple disc narrowing or by subluxation or spondylolisthesis.

Other parts of the spine may be involved in cases of rheumatoid arthritis in association with peripheral joint disturbances in 14 per cent of cases (Short et al., 1957; Gardner, 1972). As with the cervical spine the disease affects the apophyseal joints and the intervertebral discs. Rheumatoid sacro-iliac disease may also occur.

Rheumatoid disease of the *cryo-arytenoid joints* is not uncommon and may lead to laryngeal ankylosis. In some cases this may be associated with involvement of the neighbouring pharyngeal and laryngeal mucosa (Gardner, 1972) or atrophic laryngitis and this again occurs in association with Sjogren's syndrome (personal observation). Similarly the changes associated with rheumatoid *temporo-mandibular arthritis* may extend outwards and involve the neighbouring parotid gland leading to auto-immune parotitis or Sjogren's syndrome as observed by the author in several cases.

In the feet rheumatoid disease is manifested by the development of *hallux valgus* (Boyle and Buchanan, 1971). This may be of minor degree or severe and accompanied by overriding of the other toes.

The *manubria-sternal joints* may also be involved in cases of rheumatoid disease (Gardner, 1972).

II, ii) Rheumatoid disease and fibrositis

Primary fibrositis affects chiefly the neck, shoulders, lower back and chest areas. The condition may be associated with early rheumatoid arthritis, especially when this involves the cervical spine. As in rheumatoid arthritis the symptoms are worse after rest and on waking. Definite "trigger" spots may be found and biopsy of these areas has been reported as showing a lymphocytic infiltration. This condition, whether occurring with or in the absence of rheumatoid arthritis, appears to be a manifestation of rheumatoid disease affecting the soft tissues.

II, iii) Rheumatoid disease and tendons

Tendon disease and tendon sheath disease is common in rheumatoid disease (see Gardner, 1972). Microscopically the lesions are irregular in distribution. They may show granulomatous changes and a structure like that of a rheumatoid nodule. Spontaneous tendon rupture may occur.

II, iv) Rheumatoid disease and bursitis

Rheumatoid synovitis may affect bursae and form swellings or "cysts" often near or communicating with joints. This is probably the explanation of ganglia and Baker's cysts. Such cysts show an inflamed synovium which exhibits cellular infiltration with lymphocytes and plasma cells and sometimes lymphoid follicles. Olecranon and tendo Achilles bursitis is common in cases of rheumatoid arthritis and secondary infection may occur. Other bursae may be involved also, for example the supra-spinatus and the infrapatellar in patients who kneel. This suggests pressure may play a part in their localization.

II, v) The diseases associated with Hashimoto's (auto-immune) thyroiditis

In Hashimoto's (auto-immune or lymphocytic) thyroiditis the gland is heavily infiltrated with lymphocytes and sometimes with plasma cells and histiocytes with the formation of germinal follicles. Hashimoto's thyroiditis may be associated clinically with hyperthyroidism, hypothyroidism or euthyroidism and may end in myxoedema or in nodular goitre due to irregular fibrosis in the gland. Diffuse thyroiditis, that is Hashimoto's thyroiditis without goitre, is the fundamental lesion of myxoedema (Williams and Doniach, 1962). Hashimoto's thyroiditis is sometimes accompanied by a regional lymphadenopathy (Blackburn and O'Gorman, 1961; Reinlein and Navarro, 1967). Thyroid auto-antibodies of various types may be present in high concentration in the blood and there is frequently a hypergammaglobulinaemia, while ANF, RF and gastric parietal cell antibodies may also be found.

Reference has been made above to the fact that Hashimoto's thyroiditis or diffuse or focal changes in the gland of the same nature without enlargement may be associated with rheumatoid arthritis, systemic lupus erythematosus, dermatomyositis and polymyositis and with atrophic gastritis with or without pernicious anaemia and idiopathic Addison's disease. The author has had under his care two cases of Hashimoto's thyroiditis developing myxoedema and associated with widespread vasculitis and the presence of ANF and a high titre of thyroid auto-antibodies in the serum. A similar case was reported in the Clinico-Pathological Conference, 1962, and nt a Medical Staff Round at the Royal Postgraduate Medical School in 1965 a case of thyroiditis with Addison's disease and arteritis was shown. Hashimoto's thyroiditis may also be associated with Sjogren's syndrome (Heaton, 1959; Vazquez, quoted by Bloch et al., 1960; Mackay and Burnet, 1963; Doniach and Roitt, 1968; Bloch, 1969; Shearn, 1971; Whaley et al., 1973, b). In Sjogren's syndrome the pathological changes in the salivary and lacrimal glands are identical with those in the thyroid gland. Hashimoto's thyroiditis may also be associated with thymic hypertrophy in which pathological changes similar to those in the thyroid and with germinal centres form in the thymus with or without tumour formation (see below). Becker et al. (1965) in a review of 155 patients with Hashimoto's thyroiditis at the Mayo Clinic found 36 (23 per cent) had other diseases associated with it. Mackey and Burnet (1963) also describe associated diseases in adults and Kuitunen et al. (1971) record them in c'hildren. These diseases comprise rheumatoid arthritis, systemic lupus erythematosus, polymyositis, scleroderma, atrophic gastritis with or without pernicious anaemia, coeUac disease, idiopathic Addison's disease, diabetes, glomerulo-nephritis, nephrosis, idiopathic cirrhosis of the liver, Paget's disease of bone, myasthenia gravis, ulcerative colitis, acute acquired haemolytic anaemia and thrombocytopenic purpura and atopic disease (Kuitunen et al., 1971).

II, vi) Thyrotoxicosis as an auto-immune disease

Addendum: Hamilton, D.V. (J.R. Soc. Med., 1978, 71, 147) describes a woman of 68 with SL.E. with rheumatic symptoms, myxoedema due to Hashimoto's thyroiditis and atrophic gastritis and pernicious anaemia. Her mother was crippled with rheumatoid arthritis and the patient's twin brothers have Hashimoto's thyroiditis and one diabetes

It is now considered that lymphocytic (Hashimoto's) thyroiditis and thyrotoxicosis are interrelated and are two facets of the same disorder (Doniach and Roitt, 1969; Furszyfer et al., 1970). The thyroid gland in cases of thyrotoxicosis may show varying degrees of lymphocytic infiltration and lymph follicle formation and the changes of Hashimoto's thyroiditis may even be present. As with Hashimoto's thyroiditis and hypothyroidism, so thyrotoxicosis is not infrequently associated with rheumatoid arthritis, systemic lupus erythematosus (Short et al., 1957; Siurala et al., 1965; Furszyfer et al., 1970), with pernicious anaemia (Furszyfer et al., 1971, Lit.) or Sjogren's syndrome (Shearn, 1971) and may be accompanied by lymphadenopathy, hepatomegaly or splenomegaly. Patients with thyrotoxicosis frequently show thyroid auto-antibodies in the blood and the same incidence of gastric parietal cell antibodies as do patients with Hashimoto's thyroiditis and myxoedema. Furthermore, there is an association with chronic gastritis and pernicious anaemia and probably with idiopathic Addison's disease (Frederickson, 1957; Gasteau et al., 1964; Anderson et al., 1967; Furszyfer et al., 1970) as in cases of Hashimoto's thyroiditis. In addition diabetes mellitus also tends to occur with a greater frequency than would be expected in cases of thyrotoxicosis. Fatourechi et al. (1971) in considering hyperthyroidism associated with the histologic features of Hashimoto's thyroiditis found that in patients with hyperthyroidism due to Graves' disease the histologic features in the thyroid gland may vary from the classic pathological changes of Graves' disease to those typical of Hashimoto's thyroiditis and these two conditions may represent a single disease entity. In 5 of 24 patients with Hashimoto's and thyrotoxicosis diabetes was present and in 5 others there was a family history of diabetes. Thyrotoxicosis has thus been stated to be a member of the auto-immune "club". It seems highly probable that thyrotoxicosis is a manifestation of an "auto-immune" disease similar to Hashimoto's thyroiditis and myxoedema (Anderson et al., 1967). It may be associated with the presence in the blood of long acting thyroid stimulator (L.A.T.S.) in a proportion of cases. L.A.T.S. may, in fact, be a thyroid auto-antibody and is an IgG globulin.

II, vii) Collagen and auto-immune disease and other endocrine glands

Consideration has already been given to the involvement of the thyroid gland (Hashimoto's thyroiditis) and the cortex of the adrenal glands (idiopathic Addison's disease) in the lymphocytic and often plasma cell infiltration with germinal centre formation in the histological changes of cases of collagen disease, such as rheumatoid arthritis. In other cases the same histological changes occur simultaneously in the two endocrine glands and in the gastric mucosa when atrophic gastritis with or without pernicious anaemia is also present. However, other endocrine glands and tissues may also be involved in such cases.

a) "Collagen and auto-immune" disease and the parathyroid glands

Idiopathic hypoparathyroidism is probably an "auto-immune" disease (see Blizzard, 1969). In certain cases the parathyroid glands show changes like those found in the adrenal cortex in cases of idiopathic Addison's disease and in the thyroid in cases of lymphocytic thyroiditis and are replaced by fibrous tissue, fat and collections of lymphocytes. These are commonly associated with similar changes in other tissues, including a number of endocrine glands constituting so-called multiple or polyendocrinopathy (see below). In other cases *hyperparathyroidism* has been recorded as a result of a parathyroid adenoma associated with rheumatoid arthritis (Howell, 1972). Richards (1971) described a patient who suffered from Raynaud's phe-

-31

Addendum: Blizzard, R.M., Clee, D., ft Davis, W., Clin. Exp. Immunol. 1966, 1, 119, reported idiopathic hypoparathyroidism, Addison's disease, diabetes mellitus and ovarian failure together. E monds, O.E·Sau.ers,, A., Sturrock, R.D., J. Roy. Soc. Med., 1979, 72, 856·8, described a case of rheumatOid arthntls wlth SJogren s syndrome and hypoparathyroidism.

nomenon (a symptom of collagen disease) for years and later developed a parathyroid adenoma and carcinoma of the thyroid.

b) "Auto-immune disease" and the pituitary gland

It appears that the pituitary gland, like the thyroid, parathyroids and adrenals, may be involved in "auto-immune" disease. Thus, Hume and Roberts (1967) described a case of pernicious anaemia with atrophic gastritis, lymphocytic thyroiditis and hypopituitarism associated with Addison's disease. The anterior pituitary and thyroid showed acinous atrophy, fibrosis and lymphocytic infiltration like the gastric mucosa. A similar case of progressive hypopituitarism and Hashimoto's thyroiditis in which the adrenals could not be found was described by Goudie and Pinkerton (1962). Sheehan and Summers (1949) record many cases of chronic fibroid lesions of the anterior pituitary exhibiting lymphocytic infiltration and often associated with atrophy and lymphocytic infiltration of the thyroid. Such changes constitute the chronic hypophysitis responsible for certain cases of hypopituitarism (see Selye, 1947; Sheehan and Summers, 1949; Christy, 1967) and are identical in nature with the "idiopathic" atrophy of the thyroid and adrenals seen in cases of spontaneous myxoedema and idiopathic Addison's disease. Such observations point to the pituitary gland as being involved in the lymphocytic infiltration and later fibrosis which may affect the thyroid and adrenal glands in "auto-immune" and "collagen" diseases.

c) Collagen and auto-immune diseases and multiple (poly-)endocrinopatbies

In so-called multiple or poly-endocrinopathy idiopathic hypoparathyroidism may be found associated with idiopathic Addison's disease, diabetes, atrophic gastritis and pernicious anaemia, Hashimoto's thyroiditis, thyrotoxicosis or hypothyroidism, post-necrotic cirrhosis, alopecia universalis, vitiligo, premature menopause and steator-

rhoea. Polyarthropathy may also be found (Stickler et al., 1965 (literature); Doniach and Roitt, 1969; Doniach et al., 1972; Ellwood et al., 1972). Stickler et al. review the literature. Cases tend to be familial (Hall and Stanbury, 1967). In addition to the above changes there may be found kerato-conjunctivitis, enamel hypoplasia of the teeth in the young affected patient, and gonadal failure and moniliasis due to a defect in cell mediated immunity are common. RF and other antibodies, including those against thyroid, are commonly present in the serum (Levy et al., 1971). A case in which idiopathic hypoparathyroidism was associated with diabetes mellitus, cirrhosis and steatorrhoea was reported by Stickler et al. (1965). Doniach et al. (1972) describe a mother and son with such a condition. The mother aged 40 years developed psoriasis at the age of 7 years, premature greying of the hair and alopecia aged 11 years, diabetes mellitus, vitiligo and melanoderma at 14 years and later iron deficiency anaemia and achlorhydria indicative of atrophic gastritis, transient polyarthritis, myxoedema, latent pernicious anaemia and possibly partial atrophy of the adrenal glands and the blood contained antibodies to thyroid, gastric oarietal cells, intrinsic factor and adrenal ortical cells. No account of the occurrence of RF is found in the report, but the patient suffered from polyarthritis for a while. The son, aged 15 years was a diabetic from the age of 4 years and developed myxoedema, atrophic gastritis and o:::ular myasthenia and his blood contairted antibodies to thyroid, gastric parietal cells and intrinsic factor. Ellwood et al. (1972) described a young brother and sister. The P-irl developed chronic keratitis, early ortal cirrhosis, hypoparathyroidism, Addison's disease, moniliasis, alopecia areata and failed to develop pubertal changes. The boy exhibited chronic keratitis, hypoparathyroidism, portal cirrhosis and the blood from both contained antibodies against adrenal, rabbit ovarian, testicular

Addendum: Botazzo, G.F. and Doniach, D., J. Roy. Soc. M d., 1978, 7, 43. and Gle son et l., Arch._ a h. Lab. Med., 1978, 102, 46, also describe cases of lymphocytic hypophysltls either associated With thyroiditis, gastritis or adrenalitis or with unexplained arthralgias.

and placental tissues.

It appears that svch cases are manifestations of collagen and auto-immune diseases.

d) Collagen and "auto-immune" disease and primary diabetes mellitus

Primary diabetes mellitus occurs in about 12-14 per cent of the population of this country (see Sonksen, 1972). Its incidence increases with age. Over the age of 70 years as many as 50 per cent of the population may be affected. Similar figures have been found in U.S.A (Sonksen, 1972). The incidence differs in different parts of the world and different groups in the United States, probably related to environmental rather than racial differences. As with other diseases heredity and obesity play a part in its causation, but environmental factors are as important as genetic in its aetiology (Sonksen, 1972). Doubts have been expressed as to whether the severe insulin-dependent juvenile acute onset and the mature onset milder type of the disease are the same (Leading Article, Lancet, 1971, 1, 583). Many cases of diabetes mellitus are now often regarded as belonging to the group of auto-immune diseases (Asherson, 1965; Anderson et al., 1967; Leading Article, Lancet, 1970, ii, 193; Irvine et al., 1970; Nerup et al., 1970). Whittingham et al. (1971) conclude that all cases of primary diabetes are examples of auto-immune disease. However, as will be seen later this may not be true of cases in young patients.

Pathologically there is occasionally evidence of "auto-immune" disease of islet tissues in some patients with diabetes mellitus (Anderson et al., 1967) and lymphocytic infiltration of the pancreatic islets (typical of auto-immune disease) has been described in children dying of diabetes (LeCompte, 1958) and in other cases (D'Agostino and Balin, 1963; Gepts, 1965; Bondy, 1971). In most cases, however, the pancreas shows few, if any, changes in the early stages of disease.

In uncomplicated cases of diabetes mel-

litus there is convincing evidence of an increased incidence of thyroid microsomal antibodies. Diabetes mellitus is also fairly common in cases of idiopathic Addison's disease, thyrotoxicosis, Hashimoto's thyroiditis (Pettit et al., 1961; Landing et al., 1963; Gharib and Gastineau, 1969), hypothyroidism, hypoparathyroidism, vitiligo, atrophic gastritis with or without pernicious anaemia (Gunther, 1965; de Mowbray, 1965; Unger et al., 1969; Irvine, 1970), Sjogren's syndrome (Pearson, 1961; Bruce et al., 1970; Shearn, 1971) or in association with hypoparathyroidism, Addison's disease and thyroid disease with RF and auto-antibodies in the serum in the so-called multiple or polyendocrinopathy (Levy et al., 1971). Davies (1971) described a girl of 10 years with myxoedema, atrophic gastritis and diabetes mellitus. Munichoodappa and Kozac (1970) report that the association of diabetes and pernicious anaemia is well recognized. Pernicious anaemia was found in 36 of 11,144 cases of diabetes, all of which showed achlorhydria, 9 had subacute combined degeneration, 1 had thyrotoxicosis, 2 hypothyroidism and 3 had polycythaemia. It occurs with marked frequency in Schmidt's syndrome (thyroid and adrenal insufficiency) (Carpenter et al., 1966). Diabetes mellitus with idiopathic Addison's disease and cirrhosis was described by Saba (1964). MacGregor (1972) mentions a patient suffering from Addison's disease, Hashimoto's thyroiditis, pernicious anaemia and diabetes mellitus. Diabetes may be associated with coeliac disease (Green et al., 1962; Sleisenger, 1967) or with cirrhosis (Besanc;on t al., 1966; Conn, 1971). It may also be associated with acanthosis nigricans (see below).

Thus, diabetes is commonly found in association with one or more auto-immune disorders, but, as is natural with such common diseases, it also occurs in association with rheumatoid arthritis and other collagen diseases. There have been anumber of conflicting reports as to the exist-

Addendum: Dr. M.C.J. Rudolf at the Annual American Diabetes Association, 1980, reported from the Yale Regional Center of the Connecticut Program for Children with Diabetes (International Medical News Service, 1980) a group of diabetic children developing the adult form of rheumatoid arthritis with positive RF or significant titers of antinuclear antibodies or mitochondrial antibodies in 6 or 7 children. These clinical and serological features were often associated with auto-immune disorders related to SLE, Type I diabetes pellitus is often associated with auto-immune thyrogastric disorders as they were in the above cases, six of the 7 patients had organ-specific antibodies to either thyroid microsomes, tyroglobulin, parietal or adrenal cells. Six children had the HLA alleles DRw3 or DRw4 which have been associated with HSKS for type I diabetes mellitus and RA.

ence of a special relationship between diabetes and rheumatoid arthritis. In Cases 1 and 2 described above diabetes was one of a number of "auto-immune" manifestations which accompanied rheumatoid disease. Weigl (1970, Literature) reports a positive association of rheumatoid arthritis with diabetes mellitus. In the 100 cases of rheumatoid arthritis in the geriatric unit reported above diabetes was found in 12 cases (12 per cent), a higher incidence than in the general population of this age group. In cases of rheumatoid arthritis treated with corticosteroids diabetes may develop and often persists after withdrawal of the hormone. It is generally thought that corticosteroids unmask a latent tendency to the disease. (A similar unmasking of latent diabetes may be seen in some patients who develop thyrotoxicosis or hypercortico-adrenalism). Williams (1968) and Good (1971) describe an increased incidence of diabetes in cases of systemic lupus erythematosus and Bruce et al. (1970, Literature) comment on its association with collagen disease, including rheumatoid arthritis and dermatomyositis. Sjogren's syndrome, a manifestation of rheumatoid arthritis, has also been reported as associated with diabetes (Pearson, 1961).

Thus, in the majority of cases of diabetes evidence of collagen or "auto-immune" disease is present, but no pancreatic changes are found, at any rate in early cases. Valiance-Owen (1966) has, therefore, suggested that diabetes is due to the presence of a circulating antagonist to insulin, which eventually leads to islet cell failure by exhausting the .S-cells. An infective aetiology for diabetes has been suggested in relation to Coxsackie B4 virus infection, but this has not been substantiated (Sonksen, 1972). The question will be considered in a later section.

II, viii) Collagen or auto-immune diseases and thymic lesions

This subject is considered by Marshall and White (1962), Marshall (1964) and Maldonado et al. (1964) and the association of thymic lesions with myasthenia gravis by Downes et al. (1966). Thymic lesions are of two types.

a) Hypertrophy with the appearance of germinal centres in the medulla. The thymic enlargement and histology may be compared with that found in the thyroid in Hashimoto's thyroiditis, with which it may be associated.

b) Hypertrophy with tumour formation, which in structure may be that of a lymphoma, lympho-epithelioma or a spindle-cell tumour and which is associated with the presence of germinal centres. Often a spindle-cell tumour may be associated with a granulomatous stroma with plasma cells, lymphocytes, giant cells and eosinophils (Lattes, 1962).

Thymic hypertrophy with or without tumour formation may occur in association with the following conditions (Hall, 1968).

1) Rheumatoid arthritis (see Marshall and White, 1962, Webster, 1975).

2) Systemic lupus erythematosus or discoid lupus erythematosus (Good, 1962; Alar on-Segovia et al., 1963; Larsson, 1963; Mackay et al., 1964; Singh, 1969; Delmas Marsalet et al., 1969).

3) Dermatomyositis or polymyositis (Rundle et al., 1963; Klein et al., 1964; Bouduelle et al., 1965). Dermatomyositis with severe rheumatoid granulomatous myocarditis was associated with thymoma in the cases cited by Mendelow and Jenkins (1954), Waller et al. (1957), Langston et al. (1959) and Rundle and Sparks (1963). The case of Langston et al. (1959) also had lymphocytic thyroiditis, splenic hyperplasia and bilateral ovarian cysts.

4) Sjogren's syndrome with or without hepato-splenomegaly, hyperglobulinaemia and purpura, that is Waldenstrom's disease (Lattes, 1962; Birch et al., 1964; Whaley et al., 1973. b).

5) Thyroid lesions exhibiting small round cell infiltration with or without thy-

rotoxicosis. This includes Hashimoto's thyroiditis (Daly and Jackson, 1964; Simpson, 1964).

6) Idiopathic Addison's disease (McEachern and Parnell, 1948).

7) Acromegaly (McEachern and Parnell, 1948).

8) Lupoid hepatitis (Linke, 1965).

9) Auto-immune haemolytic anaemia.

10) Thrombocytopenic purpura.

11) Hypergammaglobulinaemic purpura (Waldenstrom's disease) or hypogamma-globulinaemia (Mallinson, 1971, Paice, 1975).

12) Pure red cell aplasia or hypoplasia or pancytopenia. Dawson (1972) reported a case of Hashimoto's thyroiditis associated with pancytopenia and thymoma.

13) Acquired hypogammaglobulinaemia persisting after thymectomy (Peterson et al., 1965; Tan, 1974, b).

Following direct injection of antigen into the thymus, but not elsewhere into the body, germinal centres and other cellular reactions are induced in the gland resembling those found in the above diseases (Marshall and White, 1962). Thus, this suggests that the thymic changes are a response to the presence of an antigenic stimulus. It seems, therefore, that the above changes in the thymus form a manifestation of rheumatoid disease and its accompanying disturbances in various bodily tissues.

II, ix) Myasthenia gravis and collagen and auto-immune disease

Both types of thymic lesion described above may be accompanied by the symptoms of myasthenia gravis. This has been described when the thymic lesion is accompanied by signs of rheumatoid arthritis (Marshall and White, 1962; Simpson, 1964), systemic lupus erythematosus (Rowland, 1971), dermatomyositis (Talbott and Ferrandis, 1956), Raynaud's disease (Simpson, 1964), Sjogren's syndrome

(Whaley et al., 1973, b), Hashimoto's thyroiditis (Simpson, 1964; Becker et al., 1965), hyperthyroidism or myxoedema (Simpson, 1964), Addison's disease (Osserman, 1969), atrophic gastritis±pernicious anaemia (Simpson, 1964; Howard et al., 1965; Downes et al., 1966; Coreino et al., 1971), allergy and carcinoma (Simpson, 1964). A case of myasthenia gravis with Hashimoto's thyroiditis and pernicious anaemia was reported by Singer and Sahay (1966) and other cases of myasthenia with nephritis, hepatitis, ulcerative colitis or pemphigus were reported by Simpson (1964). A case in which vitiligo, myasthenia gravis, rheumatoid arthritis and auto-immune haemolytic anaemia occurred sucessively was described by Durance (1971). Lenormand et al. (1972) reported the case of a woman of 56 years who developed myasthenia, which regressed after a year. Eleven years later she was found to have an erythroblastopenia and a thymoma, which was removed. After drug treatment the erythroblastopenia disappeared. Later manifestations of systemic lupus erythematosus and chronic active hepatitis appeared. The patient died of cirrhosis three years after the first signs of blood disease appeared. Beutner et al. (1968) describe two cases of myasthenia gravis, one with malignant thymoma, pemphigus erythematosus and a butterfly rash and one with pemphigus vulgaris and they noted three other such cases in the literature. Non-organ or organ-specific antibodies may be found in the blood, including antibodies against striated muscle (see Leading Article, Brit. med. J., 1965, i, 879). While antibodies to striated muscle may be present with thymomas in association with myasthenia, the majority of patients with myasthenia do not show them.

It would appear that thymic changes of the nature described and myasthenia are part and parcel of collagen and "auto-immune" disease. Strauss (1965) points out "that though auto-immune processes appear to be intimately associated with pathogenic mechanisms in myasthenia gravis . . . . . . no sound evidence can currently justify the assumption that these (muscle) "antibodies" directly produce the well-known symptoms, signs and pharmacological responses of myasthenia gravis, either at the myoneural junction or elsewhere".

Cases may occur at all ages and even at birth (congenital myasthenia) and transitorily in infants born of myasthenics (neonatal myasthenia). The latter indicates that some substance is present in the maternal circulation which passes the placenta to produce the condition in the offspring and interferes in some way with the liberation or production of acetylcholine at nerve endings in muscle.

The Eaton-Lambert syndrome and auto-immune disorders.

Not only myasthenia, but the *Eaton-Lambert syndrome* may be associated with *auto-immune disorders,* such as hypothyroidism and pernicious anaemia (Gutmann et al., 1972).

II, x) Collagen and auto-immune diseases and cryptogenic fibrosing alveolitis

In cases of rheumatoid disease various lung lesions are described, among which are pleuritis with or without effusions, pleural rheumatoid nodule formation, nodule formation in the lungs, fibrosing alveolitis and cystic change (honeycombing), bronchiectiasis and bronchiolitis. In addition pulmonary necrotizing arteritis and vascular intimal proliferation are found (see Gardner, 1972). The nodular formations in the lungs are identical with rheumatoid nodules. They may by progression tend to fuse and result in massive pulmonary fibrosis. Caplan described pneumoconiosis in coal miners suffering from rheumatoid arthritis. The mildly irritant effects of dust are apparently sufficient to make the lungs a major focus of rheumatoid involvement (Caplan's syndrome). Sjogren's syndrome has been seen to be associated with similar lung lesions to those of rheumatoid disease as well as with atrophic tracheo-bronchitis (see Shearn, 1971).

Apart from rheumatoid arthritis and Sjogren's syndrome cryptogenic fibrosing alveolitis is frequently associated with other collagen diseases, including systemic lupus erythematosus, dermatomyositis or polymyositis (Scadding, 1969), scleroderma and systemic sclerosis and arteritis (Aronoff et al., 1955; Lee and Brain, 1962; Tomasi et al., 1962; Leading Article, Lancet, 1964, i, 1202; Livingstone et al., 1964; Turner Warwick, 1965; Sandbank et al., 1966; Leading Article, Brit. med. J., 1968, i, 199; Karlish, 1969; Scadding, 1969; Sperryn, 1971; Turner Warwick, 1973). Lee and Brain (1962) describe 3 cases of fibrosing alveolitis with rheumatoid arthritis. Karlish (1969) describes a case of Sjogren's syndrome, which 3 years later developed fibrosing alveolitis with a positive RF in the blood. Non-specific and specific auto-antibodies may be present in the blood in a high proportion of cases of fibrosing alveolitis (Turner Warwick and Doniach, 1965; Mackay and Ritchie, 1965). The former authors studied 48 cases, of whom 14 had rheumatoid arthritis. Auto-antibodies as shown by one or more tests were present in 32 cases, most of them being of non organ-specific nature. These occurred even though rheumatoid arthritis was not present. No auto-antibodies to the lung were demonstrated. Apart from collagen disease fibrosing alveolitis has been reported associated with Hashimoto's thyroiditis (Turner Warwick and Doniach, 1965), with pernicious anaemia (Turner Warwick, 1973) and with auto-immune haemolytic anaemia (Mackay and Ritchie, 1965). Fibrosing alveolitis with coeliac disease was present in 3 of 24 patients with coeliac disease studied by Smith et al. (1971). Turner Warwick (1968) has reported active chronic hepatitis, sometimes progressing to post-necrotic cirrhosis, in association with fibrosing alveolitis. Another patient developed ulcerative colitis 5 years after respiratory symptoms began. Fibrosing alveolitis associated with ulcerative colitis was also reported by Scadding (1969). A patient of the author's, aged 72 years, had fibrosing alveolitis, diabetes, Hashimoto's thyroiditis myxoedema and atrophic gastritis and developed Hodgkin's disease. In a case shown at a Medical Staff Round at Hammersmith Hospital, a patient with rheumatoid arthritis developed Raynaud's phenomenon, then scleroderma and fibrosing alveolitis and finally hepatitis and anaemia with ANF and lupus erythematosus cells in the blood. In cases of fibrosing alveolitis Haddad and Massaro (1969) describe atypical epithelial cell proliferation in the terminal air spaces, which become either cuboidal or columnar or show squamous metaplastic or stratification changes and later malignancy supervenes.

II, xi) The heart in rheumatoid and other collagen diseases

Descriptions of the cardiac pathology in collagen diseases are given by Talbott and Ferrandis (1956) and Duthie (1969). The heart in cases of rheumatoid disease and systemic lupus erythematosus may exhibit granulomatous endocarditis, the lesions resembling the subcutaneous nodules; diffuse chronic endocarditis; active or subacute granulomatous myocarditis, arteritis; and active or healed pericarditis. Rheumatoid granulomata are common in the heart and cardiac enlargement frequent. Specific focal granulomatous myocarditis may occur in 1-3 per cent of cases of rheumatoid arthritis (Sokoloff, 1963). Identical changes may be associated with Sjögren's syndrome (Shearn, 1971). Luckey (1967) states that myocarditis frequently occurs in cases of vasculitis and collagen and connective tissue disorders. In cases of dermatomyositis an identical granulomatous myocarditis may occur (Langston et al., 1959;

Rundle and Sparks, 1963). Fairfax (1977) reviews the immunological aspects of chronic heart block and points out its frequent association with known auto-immune disease, such as diabetes, vitiligo and hypothyroidism and rheumatoid arthritis and systemic lupus erythematosus. In cases of scleroderma fibrosis of the myocardium and pericardium may also be found (Busdorff, 1939; Talbott and Ferrandis, 1956). The author had under his care a patient already mentioned (Case 6), aged 64 years, who developed in combination rheumatoid arthritis, Sjögren's syndrome, atrophic rhinitis, atrophic tracheobronchitis and oesophagitis, fibrosing alveolitis and rheumatoid granulomatous myocarditis. Thus all parts of the heart may be involved in collagen diseases.

II, xii) Rheumatoid disease and coronary occlusion

Mention has just been made of the vasculitis, including arteritis, occurring in the heart in collagen diseases. This would be expected to predispose to coronary occlusion. The question as to whether rheumatoid arthritis predisposes to coronary occlusion has been raised, but no definite answer has been forthcoming (Leading Article, Brit. med. J., 1970, 1, 707). However, a number of cases of coronary arteritis resulting in cardiac infarcts occurring in cases of rheumatoid disease are on record (Gardner, 1972). There would, therefore, appear to be little doubt of such an association.

Fowler et al. (1970) and Bastenie at al. (1970) both describe cases of auto-immune thyroiditis developing coronary artery disease. The latter ascribe both the thyroiditis and coronary artery disease to a common unknown factor. The former consider that associated hypothyroidism leads to an abnormal lipid state and this again to arterial disease.

Recently it has been suggested (Mathews et al., 1974; Lancet, 1975, 1, 208) that membrane reactive auto-antibodies cause endothelial proliferation and thus predispose to hypertension and that circulating immune complexes comprising auto-antibodies of the IgG class and auto-antigens initiate platelet aggregation and increased vascular permeability, thus predisposing to thrombosis and atherosclerosis. The antiglobulin action of RF may increase the effect of membrane-reactive auto-antibodies and organ-specific auto-antibodies may play a part.

II, xiii) Collagen and auto-immune disease and liver disease

Short et al. (1957) and Boyle and Buchanan (1971) report that "liver failure" may occur in cases of rheumatoid disease. Short et al. (1957) in their monograph report various changes occurring in the liver in cases of rheumatoid arthritis, including the presence of periportal inflammation with infiltration of lymphocytes, plasma cells and histiocytes, central necrosis, hepatitis, acute yellow atrophy and cirrhosis. Siurala et al. (1965) reporting on the digestive tract in 71 cases of various collagen diseases studied the liver in 64 of their patients using various clinical tests and in some cases by liver biopsy. They found the clinical tests abnormal in 33 of the 64 cases. Liver biopsy was normal in 3 cases, showed fatty changes in 3, acute hepatitis in 3 and chronic hepatitis in 2 c es. Sherlock (1968) described *rheumatoid disease* associated with active chronic hepatitis and focal necrosis. Leftovits and Farrow (1955) found histological changes in the liver in 2 of 15 patients with rheumatoid arthritis. Whelton (1970) described rheumatoid arthritis or arthralgias in association with chronic active hepatitis in 23 of 83 patients with the latter and refers to other reports in the literature. Of 19 patients with arthralgias the R.A. latex test was positive in 15 of 16 cases, the Rose-Waaler test was positive in 7 of 17 and ANF was present in the serum of 16 of

19 patients. Lupus erythematosus cells were present in the blood in 6 patients. In cases without arthralgias the R.A. and ANF tests were positive in %-% of the cases. He also referred to similar findings in the literature. Blendis et al. (1969) in 12 patients with Felty's syndrome found 8 with disturbance of liver function and in 5 the liver showed lymphocytic infiltration of sinusoids and portal tracts with portal tract fibrosis. One patient was later found to have a macronodular cirrhosis and in others true cirrhosis was found. *Felty's syndrome* accompanied by cirrhosis has also been reported (Leading Article, Brit. med. J., 1971, 4, 379). In cases of *juvenile rheumatoid arthritis* Sury and Vesterdal (1969) found chronic hepatitis in I of 21 autopsies and hepatomegaly in 8 of 151 cases. Schaller et al. (1970) in 5 children with juvenile rheumatoid arthritis and massive hepatomegaly found 4 showed periportal collections of lymphocytes and hyperplasia of Kupffer cells.

The same liver changes are found in other collagen diseases. Chronic active hepatitis developing into postnecrotic cirrhosis has been reported as occurring in association with *systemic lupus erythematosus* by Mackay et al. (1956), Talbott and Ferrandis (1956), Mackay and Wood (1963), Leonardt (1964), Alar on-Segovia et al. (1965) and Winkelmann et al. (1968). *Scleroderma* in association with post-necrotic cirrhosis of the liver following acute hepatitis was described by Flack and Bruschke (1958) and also by Bartholomew et al. (1964). Two cases of scleroderma developing biliary cirrhosis were reported by Murray-Lyon et al. (1970) one by Morgan (1973) and another by August (1974). Reynolds et al. (1971) describe cases of biliary cirrhosis with scleroderma and Raynaud's phenomenon. A case of rheumatoid arthritis developing scleroder-matous changes, chronic fibrosing alveolitis and chronic active hepatitis with lupus erythematosus cells and ANF in the blood was shown at a Clinical Meeting at Hammersmith Hospital in 1966. A case of polymyositis developing hepatitis was reported by Greenberger et al. (1965). Systemic lupus erythematosus with liver cirrhosis and ulcerative colitis occurring together was described by Galbraith et al. (1964). Read (1970) recorded a spectrum of "auto-immune" liver disease, including active chronic hepatitis and primary biliary cirrhosis and other liver disease associated with systemic disorders, such as rheumatoid arthritis and Sjögren's syndrome. Golding (1970) in the same meeting reported on an unselected group of patients with "auto-immune" liver disease. Sjögren's syndrome was present in nearly 40 per cent of patients with active chronic hepatitis, in 65 per cent of those with primary biliary cirrhosis and 25 per cent of those with cryptogenic cirrhosis. Whalley et al. (1970) found clinical and/or biochemical evidence of liver disease in 6 per cent of patients with Sjögren's syndrome without rheumatoid arthritis, 1.5 per cent of patients with Sjögren's syndrome and rheumatoid arthritis and 0.66 per cent with rheumatoid arthritis alone. Sjögren's syndrome may be associated with chronic active hepatitis, post-necrotic cirrhosis or biliary cirrhosis (Shearn, 1971). Post-necrotic cirrhosis associated with lupus erythematosus cells and ANF in the blood and hypergammaglobulinaemia may occur in cases of chronic active hepatitis leading to post-necrotic cirrhosis in the absence of signs of disease of other organs, so-called lupoid hepatitis (Mackay et al., 1956; Talbott and Ferrandis, 1956; Doniach et al., 1966). Thus, there is abundant evidence of a spectrum of liver disease occurring in association with the collagen diseases.

Liver disease may also occur in association with "auto-immune" diseases. Williams and Doniach (1962) described active chronic hepatitis progressing to cirrhosis accompanying any of the triad of lymphocytic thyroiditis, atrophic gastritis and idiopathic Addison's disease. Hashimoto's thyroiditis or focal thyroiditis associated with active chronic hepatitis or post-necrotic cirrhosis was described by Luxton and Cooke (1956), Buchanan et al. (1962) and Becker et al. (1965), while Hashimoto's thyroiditis combined with lupoid hepatitis (active chronic) was reported by Hijmans et al. (1964). Addison's disease with hepatic cirrhosis was reported by Saha (1964). Mackay and Burnet (1963) describe active chronic hepatitis, lupoid hepatitis and primary biliary cirrhosis as occurring in association with lymphocytic thyroiditis and with other auto-immune diseases. The author had under his care (Case 11) a man aged 46 years, who presented with symptoms of thyrotoxicosis and mild jaundice, in whom the blood showed abnormal liver function tests indicative of hepatitis and ANF and large numbers of lupus erythematosus cells, but no other auto-antibodies. Liver biopsy showed the changes of chronic active hepatitis. Cases of multiple endocrinopathy with widespread evidence of "auto-immune" disease may also exhibit portal cirrhosis as described above. Simpson (1964) described hepatitis with myasthenia and Turner Warwick (1968) reported fibrosing alveolitis with chronic liver disease (chronic active hepatitis or interlobar hepatitis). In some cases the changes progress to cirrhosis. Sherlock (1968) records active chronic hepatitis as occurring before or after the onset of ulcerative colitis. In cases of ulcerative colitis Perrett et al. (1971) found that post-necrotic cirrhosis, biliary cirrhosis or chronic active hepatitis may occur. Conn et al. (1971) also found true diabetes in association with liver cirrhosis. This is to be distinguished from an abnormal glucose tolerance test associated with liver damage which disappears after caval anastomoses and Besançon et al. (1966) found diabetes was present in 50 of 633 cirrhotics. In 30 of these the cirrhosis was not the cause of the hyperglycaemia and true diabetes existed. Finally nodular regenerative hyperplasia of the liver may occur in Felty's syndrome

(Blendis et al., 1974).

Thus, there appears ample evidence to associate certain liver lesions with rheumatoid arthritis, Felty's syndrome, juvenile rheumatoid arthritis, Sjogren's syndrome and other collagen diseases and with various auto-immune diseases. These liver lesions consist of chronic active hepatitis, biliary cirrhosis and many cases of post-necrotic cirrhosis. The histological changes in the liver consist of lymphocytic and sometimes plasma cell infiltration and pro-liferation of histiocytes like the changes in other tissues in rheumatoid disease. These tend to occur especially in the periportal areas.

II, xiv) Collagen disease and chronic cholecystitis

The cause of chronic cholecystitis not preceded by acute disease is unknown. The onset of symptoms may be insidious or they may be absent. In cases of uncom-plicated chronic cholecystitis the micro-scopical changes involve the entire gall bladder and often the bile ducts. The wall of the gall bladder shows groups of lym-phocytes and occasionally large numbers of plasma cells and eosinophils as well as a more diffuse infiltration (Boyd, 1961). The folds of mucosa are thickened owing to oedema. In the later stages there is an abundant formation of granulation tissue causing great thickening of the walls of the organ. These changes are typical of those found in the mucosae of other hollow organs affected by rheumatoid disease. Marked proliferation of the mucosa leads to the formation of deep clefts which pene-trate down to or even through the muscu-laris like carcinoma (Rokitansky-Aschoff sinuses) and polypoid and adenomatoid change and epithelial metaplasia of the mucosa may be found. These have been suggested as premaligna nt changes. Fre-quently gall stones develop secondarily.

According to Short et al. (1957) gall bladder disease of this type occurs in as many as 15 per cent of cases of rheumatoid arthritis. In some cases there is found a close clinical and temporal relationship between the various manifestations of col-lagen or auto-imm une disease and chronic cholecystitis. These are exemplified by the following cases in the author's experience:-

Table I

Case I, 1   Male, aged 50 years. He developed within two yea rs *systemic lu pus erythematosus, pernicious anaemia, polyarteritis* and chronic cholecystitis with gall-stones.

Case I, 2   Female, aged 46 years. She developed within a few years *rheu mat oid arthritis, severe eczema, H ashimoto's thyroiditis, thyroto xicosis, unilat eral exophthalmos, dia-betes* and ch ronic cholecystitis with gall-stones. The serum contained thyroid auto-antibodies and RF was strongly positive.

Case I, 3   Male, aged 55 years. Operation for chronic cholecystitis *6* years previously. Now developed *S jogren's syndrome,* well-marked *rheumatoid* changes in the f eet and *exo phthalmic o pht halmo plegia.* ANF was present in the serum, but no other au to-antibodies. P.B.I. was normal.

Case I, 4   Female, aged 58 years. Moderate smoker over many years. Aged 31 years hyste ·ec-tomy for *fibroids.* Aged 33 years oophorectomy for *benign cyst o f le ft ovary.* Aged 42 years cholecystectom y for ch ronic cholecystitis. Aged 56 years operation for *right c ystic mastitis.* Examination showed severe *rheumatoid art hritis* of feet and carcinoma of the bronchus. *Achlorh yd ria* and RF found in the seru m. One brother died of cerebral glioma aged 47 years and another broth er died of carcinoma of the bronchus aged 65 years.

Case I, 5   Male, aged 80 years. Aged 40 years cholecystectomy for chronic cholecystitis and gall stones. Now severe *rheumatoid arthritis, at rophic gastritis* and carcinoma of the stomach. *Achlorhydria,* all serum auto-antibody tests negative.

Table I (continued)

Case I, 6   Female, aged 65 years. Aged 52 years cholecystectomy for chronic cholecystitis. Now crippled with severe *rheumatoid arthritis*. Has extensive squamous carcinoma pf the scalp.

Case I, '''   Female, aged 67 years. Aged 57 years onset of severe *rheumatoid arthritis*, for which under continuous treatment since. Aged 61 years operation for chronic cholecystitis. Aged 65 years onset of *myxoedema* and *diabetes*. Now multiple squamous carcinoma of face and trunk.

Case I, 8   Male, aged 84 years. Aged 65 years cholecystectomy for chronic cholecystitis and gall stones. Aged 80 years rodent ulcer of nose. Now *ichthyosis acquisita*, well-marked *rheumatoid arthritis* of feet and carcinoma of the stomach.

Case I, 9   Female, aged 75 years. Aged 40 years hysterectomy for *fibroids* and left benign *ovarian cyst* removed. Aged 46 years operation for chronic cholecystitis and gall stones. Aged 65 years carcinoma of the right breast, mastectomy. Six months ago acute onset of *rheumatoid arthritis* followed by malignant melanomatosis. Primary unknown. *Achlorhydria*. All serum auto-antibodies negative.

Case I, 10   Female, aged 67 years. Severe *Raynaud's* phenomena since her twenties. Aged 41 years cholecystectomy for chronic cholecystitis. Aged 59 years *rheumatoid arthritis* of hands, wrists, elbows and shoulders. Cervical spondylitis and now carcinoma of the bronchus. Serum contained ANF+ and RF+.

Case I, 11   Female, aged 57 years. Aged 45 years onset of moderately severe *rheumatoid arthritis* affecting hands, shoulders and feet. Aged 48 years cholecystectomy for chronic cholecystitis. Aged 50 years removal of benign uterine polyp. Aged 55 years onset of *ulcerative colitis*. Now *pseudomucinous cystadenoma of the left ovary* and metastatic spread of carcinoid of the ileum. *Achlorhydria*, gastric parietal cell antibodies in the serum.

See also Case VI, 34. (later) A significant case was that of a woman of 56 years in which severe seropositive arthritis began 3 years previously. Shortly afterwards she began to complain of symptoms of chronic cholecystitis, confirmed at operation. After a further two years fibroids were diagnosed.

Thus, it appears that in many cases chronic cholecystitis occurs in subjects who exhibit or later develop manifestations of collagen or auto-immune disease. Thus, chronic cholecystitis occurring in the absence of pre-existing acute disease may well be part of the spectrum of collagen and auto-immune disease clinically and histologically.

The same pathological process as occurs in the gall bladder and cystic ducts may be found in the bile ducts producing the condition known as obliterative or stenosing or sclerosing cholangitis and biliary cirrhosis, which has been shown to be part of the same collagen and auto-immune disease spectrum. Thus, Waldram et al. (1975) describe two siblings both with Sjogren's syndrome, chronic pancreatitis

(see below, often an "auto-immune" disease) and sclerosing cholangitis. In one case the liver was enlarged and there was a blood eosinophilia.

II, xv) Collagen disease and chronic pancreatitis

Chronic relapsing pancreatitis and many other cases of chronic pancreatitis are distinct from 1) the chronic pancreatitis found associated with diseases of the biliary tract which often show acute exacerbations, 2) those associated with chronic alcoholism and 3) the changes following acute pancreatitis. In cases of chronic "relapsing" pancreatitis and cases of chronic pancreatitis arising without other cause the pancreas becomes infil-

Addendum: Descamps, Ch., Gillain, P., Van Heuverzwyn, P. et al. Acta gastro-ent. belg., 1977, 40. 55. describe a case of ulcerative colitis with cholecystitis and progressive sclerosing cholangitis. They point out that ulcerative colitis is often associated with coeliac disease, chronic active hepatitis, biliary cirrhosis (all auto-immune dieseases), sclerosing cholangitis and cholangiocarcinoma.

trated with lymphocytes and plasma cells. Germinal centres may form (Willis, 1967) and later fibrosis occurs often with dilatation of the ducts and cyst formation giving rise to the condition of "cirrhosis" of the pancreas. Eventually they may result in the development of diabetes and steatorrhoea and calcification may occur in the organ. It will be noted that the cellular infiltration, fibrosis and cyst formation present in many cases of chronic pancreatitis is identical with that found in salivary, lacrimal and thyroid glands in the collagen diseases, while the occurrence of chronic relapsing disease resembles the recurrent swelling of the salivary glands in "auto-immune" parotitis.

Mackay and Burnet (1963) suggest that chronic pancreatitis is an auto-immune disease. Siurala et al. (1965) found 5 cases of chronic pancreatitis in 71 cases (7 per cent) of collagen diseases. Hollander et al. (1960) also mention chronic pancreatitis as occurring in cases of rheumatoid arthritis, while Harvey (1967) refers to chronic pancreatitis as occurring in cases of systemic lupus erythematosus and systemic sclerosis. Whaley et al. (1973, b) described two cases of rheumatoid arthritis with Sjagren's syndrome, chronic pancreatitis and steatorrhoea with calcification of the pancreas. One case was associated with pernicious anaemia. Fenster et al. (1964) and Shearn (1971) found that clinical or morphological evidence of involvement of the pancreas may be found in cases of Sjogren's syndrome. The former found mild functional involvement in 4 of 11 patients with Sjagren's syndrome. At autopsy in a case of Sjogren's syndrome Shearn (1971) discovered a heavy lymphocytic infiltration of the pancreatic stroma. A lymphocytic pancreatitis may be <:ssociated with Hashimoto's thyroiditis, thyrotoxicosis, Sjagren's syndrome and portal cirrhosis in cases of lipodystrophy with insulin-resistant diabetes (Taylor and Honeycutt, 1961). Chronic pancreatitis (cirrhosis) may also be associated with cirrhosis of the liver (Besan on et al., 1966).

It appears possible that the changes of chronic pancreatitis, including those of the relapsing type, arising in the absence of gall-stones, biliary tract disease, acute pancreatitis and alcoholism, may well constitute a manifestation of a collagen disease. The gland may become calcified.

II, xvi)   Collagen and auto-immune disease and the kidney

The kidney may be affected in cases of systemic lupus erythematosus, rheumatoid arthritis and systemic sclerosis (Hollander et al., 1960; Duthie, 1969). The vasculitis of collagen disease may also be seen in the kidneys and so-called "lupoid" nephritis is described in association with systemic lupus erythematosus. In cases of rheumatoid arthritis the kidney is frequently involved. In some cases this shows a papiilary necrosis, thought to be due to medication, but the organ may be involved in other ways. Chronic pyelonephritis is common (Boyle and Buchanan, 1971; Gardner, 1972). Rheumatoid lesions may also involve the kidney. Rheumatoid "glomerulitis" and rheumatoid kidney with interstitial changes have been described (Gardner, 1972; Whaley et al., 1973, b). Gulata and Vaishnova (1971) in 23 cases of rheumatoid arthritis found 5 cases of interstitial and/or vascular lesions on renal biopsy. Mackey and Burnet (1963) also describe glomerulo-tubular disease associated with rheumatoid arthritis. Such a case is exemplified by Case 12 below. The kidney may also be involved in cases of Sjogren's syndrome (see above), Hashimoto's thyroiditis (Luxton, 1957; Becker et al., 1965) or myasthenia gravis (Simpson, 1964). In these conditions the kidney shows lymphocytic infiltration of the interstitial tissues, the glomeruli usually being spared. The interstitial fibrosis leads to renal failure and hypertension.

42

A case in which renal involvement occurred in a case of rheumatoid disease with evidence of involvement of various internal organs is reported below.

Case 12 Male, aged 59 years. At the age of 27 years sudden onset of painful swelling of the fingers, wrists, elbows, knees, ankles and feet with marked morning stiffness. These symptoms persisted in spite of treatment and gradually increased in severity. Six months after the onset he developed the first of numerous attacks of oedema of hands, feet and eyelids, during which the joints became increasingly swollen and in which heavy proteinuria and hypertension were detected. After 3 years he was found to have typical rheumatoid nodules around the elbows and knees and particularly affecting the periostea. Some were also found on the heads of the metacarpals. He gradually developed established hypertension and the nodules became larger. In later years he also developed a very high colour, marked bowing of the tibiae and pains in the lumbar region. In the last 5 years there had appeared a recurrent lipoma of the under surface of the left heel, which had required removal on 3 occasions, and had also developed typical attacks of gout.

Examination. Advanced signs of rheumatoid arthritis affecting the hands, wrists, elbows, shoulders, knees, ankles and feet. Very large, soft, painless, rheumatoid nodules were present around the elbows, over the left fifth metacarpal head and around the knees. These felt like lipomata. The blood pressure was 240f140 mm. The blood count showed Hb of 134 per cent, PCV 62 per cent, W.B.C. 15,000 per cu. mm., platelets 900,000 per cu. mm., E.S.R. 60 mm. per hour., X-rays of the chest showed an enlarged heart, especially of the left ventricle, and of the spine, pelvis, femora and tibiae the typical changes of Paget's disease. The urine contained 500 mgms. per cent protein. The Rose-Waaler and latex fixation tests were strongly positive. ANF + +. Thyroid auto-antibodies strongly positive. Serum uric acid 12.4 mgms. per cent. Serum alkaline phosphatase 31 K.A. units per cent. Excision of several of the large rheumatoid nodules showed either the features of a lipoma with well-marked areas of lymphocytic infiltration or of a typical rheumatoid nodule. Renal biopsy showed abnormal glomeruli with increased cellularity, capsular adhesions and slight capsular proliferation. Advanced interstitial fibrosis was present with lymphocytic infiltration and some tubular atrophy. Multiple foci of collagenous degeneration and necrosis surrounded by histiocytes and small multinucleate cells were seen, a reaction typical of rheumatoid nodules. The picture was that of a focal and local glomerulo-tubular nephritis not typical of type I glomerular nephritis, arteritis or systemic lupus erythematosus. No amyloid was seen in a rectal muscle biopsy.

In this patient, therefore there existed rheumatoid arthritis, polycythaemia vera, Paget's disease of bone, focal glomerulo-nephritis with hypertension, gout secondary to polycythaemia and multiple lipoma formation. The renal changes are noteworthy.

Renal tubular acidosis has also been found associated with auto-immune thyroiditis. (Mason and Golding, 1970 a); with Sjogren's syndrome (Shearn, 1971) ; with Sjogren's syndrome, auto-immune liver disease, fibrosing alveolitis and hypergammaglobulinaemic purpura (Waldenstrom's macroglobulinaemia) ; with auto-immune thyroiditis and peripheral neuropathy (Mason and Golding, 1970 b); with non-organ specific auto-immune disease, such as hepatosplenomegaly (McCurdy et al., 1967; Tala! et al., 1968); with rheumatoid arthritis, Sjogren's syndrome, lymphadenopathy, hypochromic anaemia and an erythematous rash (Farid and Evered, 1971); with fibrosing alveolitis, Sjogren's syndrome and primary biliary cirrhosis (Mason et al., 1970 b; Zalin et al., 1970); and with Sj5gren's syndrome,. lymphocytic thyroiditis and biliary cirrhosis (Tu et al., 1968) . Renal tubular acidosis leads to generalized osteomalacia and nephrosclerosis.

To summarize, the kidney is frequently involved in cases of "collagen" and "auto-immune" disease. The organ usually exhibits interstitial lymphocytic infiltration with sparing of the glomeruli, though these may also be affected and later fibrosis occurs. Clinically there may be hypertension and renal failure or renal tubular acidosis leading to osteomalacia and nephrosclerosis.

II, xvii) Collagen and auto-immune disease and associated skin lesions

According to Wiener (1947) in cases of rheumatoid arthritis there may occur urticaria, eczema, ichthyosis acquisita, psoriasis, dermatitis herpetiformis, lupus erythematosus, pemphigus, papular and annular eruptions, figurate erythema and alopecia. In cases of systemic lupus erythematosus there may also occur light sensitivity of the skin, urticaria, bullous eruptions and alopecia. Again, in cases of dermatomyositis the skin exhibits a n erythema or dermatitis and often light sensitivity. In cases of ulcerative colitis pigmentation, dryness of the skin, ichthyosis acquisita, erythema, urticaria, pruritus, psoriasis, parapsoriasis and alopecia and in cases of cirrhosis or of thyrotoxicosis urticaria may be features.

These skin lesions, of course, may also occur not obviously associated with collagen or auto-immune diseases. Many types of such chronic skin diseases, such as eczema, psoriasis, lichen planus, seborrhoeic dermatitis, urticaria, ichthyosis acquisita, parapsoriasis, pemphigus, dermatitis herpetiformis and bullous eruptions show an infiltration of the dermis with lymphocytes and plasma cells and often with eosinophils and an eosinophilia may occur not only locally, but also in the blood and other tissues (see Wintrobe, 1966). Many

of these skin lesions show gradations from one to the other and different types may be present in the same patient. These les:ons occurring unassociated with other diseases differ in no way from the same skin lesions accompanying generalized collagen diseases. Such patients often show Kohner's phenomenon, that is typical skin lesions develop in an area of pressure or trauma in a subject of one of the above-named diseases, pointing to the *existence in all areas of the skin and body of a factor responsible for the lesion.* Further consideration will now be given to certain of these skin lesions.

a) Ichthyosis acquisita

In the section on Sjogren's syndrome the tendency for the skin to become dry and flake and for the drying up of the sweat due to a lymphocytic infiltration of the sweat glands was described. This condition is known as ichthyosis acquisita to distinguish from congenital ichthyosis. It is typical of rheumatoid infection and may occur in one-third of cases of rheumatoid arthritis (see Short et al., 1957). It may also be associated with thyrotoxicosis (Readett, 1964).

b) Alopecia universalis and areata

Alopecia universalis or areata may be associated with "auto-immune" diseases and are now considered "auto-immune" manifestations. They are discussed in "Textbook of Immunopathology" (1969), edited by Miescher, P.A. and Mtiller-Eberhard, H., Grune and Stratton, New York. Alopecia is not uncommon in systemic lupus erythematosus (Mackay and Burnet, 1963; Copeman and Taylor, 1970), rheumatoid dis ase (Fig. 1) dermatomyositis and scleroderma (Talbott and Ferrandis, 1956), Sjogren's syndrome (Shearn, 1971) and also in thyrotoxicosis (V. Basedow, 1840). Alopecia may also occur in multiple (poly-) endocrine disease (see above). Auto-antibodies to the thyroid or other tissues are regularly found in cases of alopecia universalis and areata. In two cases of the author's alopecia universalis

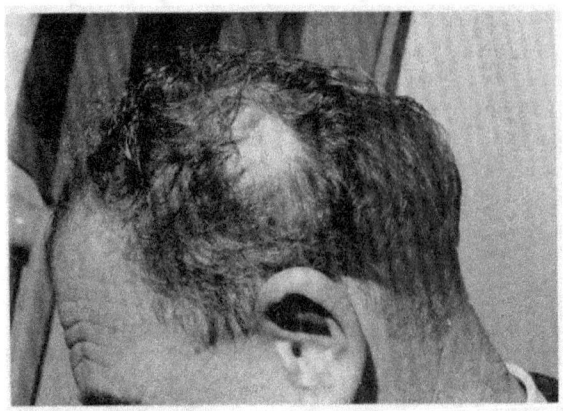

Fig. 1

Fig. 1 Alopecia areata occurring as a manifestation of seropositive rheumatoid disease. The alopecia disappeared after successful treatment of the joint condition.

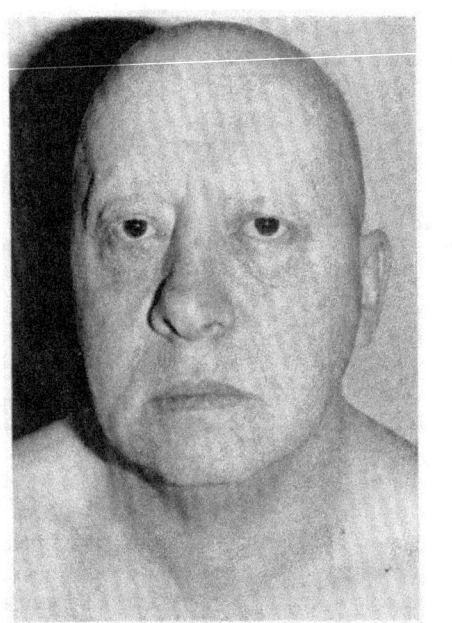

Fig. 2-A

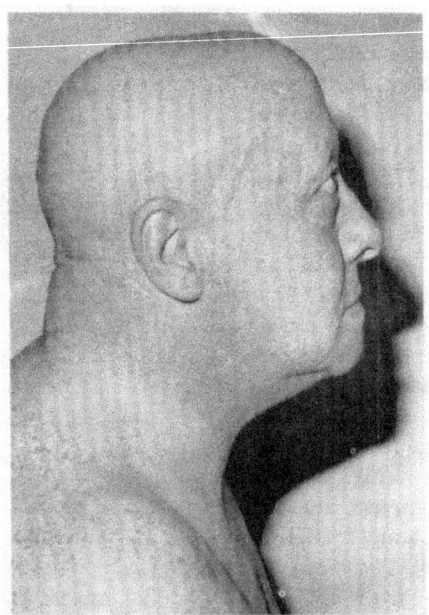

Fig. 2-B

Fig. 2 Alopecia universalis accompanied by a very high titre of thyroid auto-antibodies in the serum and followed by the development of malignant lymphoma (Case 13, or VII. 14.).

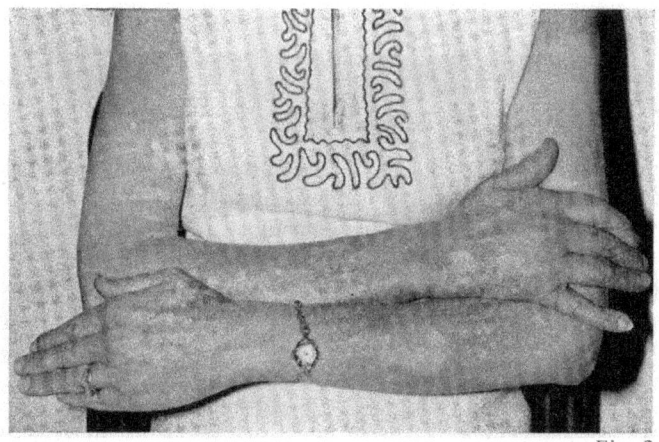
Fig. 3

Fig. 3 Vitiligo in a subject of seropositive rheumatoid disease.

was associated with an extremely high titre of thyroid auto-antibodies in the absence of evident thyroid disease. One of these presented as a case of schizophrenia, the other (Case 13 and VII, 14) developed malignant lymphoma.

c) Vitiligo (leucoderma) and melanoderma

Whenever it occurs, vitiligo tends to be associated with areas of increased pigmentation (mela noderma). There is considerable evidence that vitiligo occurs more frequently in patients with auto-immune disease as compared with controls. Thus, it is not uncommon in mature-onset diabetes mellitus (Dawber, 1968). It is also known to be associated with thyroid disease (hyper- and hypo-thyroidism), pernicious a naemia, diabetes, idiopathic Addison's disease, rheumatoid arthritis (Durance, 1961; Lerner, 1967; Cunliffe et al., 1968) (Fig. 3), idiopathic hypoparathyroidism a nd alopecia areata (Leading Article, Lancet, 1971, 2, 1298). De Mowbray (1965) described a case of Addison's disease with vitiligo, pernicious anaemia, hypothyroidism and diabetes mellitus. Brostoff et al. (1969) reported that patients with vitiligo showed a tendency to increased auto-antibody formation against adrenal, thyroid and gastri c parietal cells.

A case which successively developed vitiligo, myasthenia gravis, sero-positive rheumatoid arthritis and auto-immune haemolytic anaemia was described by Durance (1971). Howitz and Schwartz (1971) report on 102 patients with vitiligo. Twenty had achlorhydria of which 8 had pernicious anaemia. (Achlorhydria is almost always due to atrophic gastritis). Diabetes was present in 4 cases of which 2 also had pernicious anaemia and 6 patients had thyroid disease. Three of these had been operated on for thyrotoxicosis and 2 of these had pernicious anaemia. 3 had myxoedema. 2 of which were due to Hashimoto's thyroiditis. They refer to previous reports of the association of vitiligo with diabetes and thyroid disease. The au thor has observed it associated with sero-positive rheumatoid arthritis in 3 cases. In one case (Case 14). a woman of 81 years suffering from long-standing rheumatoid arthritis and myxoedema was found to be a diabetic and showed melano-dermatous areas on the face and neck and cardiomyopathy. In Case 1 rheumatoid atrhritis, Sjogren's syndrome, diabetes, pernicious anaemia, Hashimoto's thyroiditis and sca nty periods were associated with vitiligo. Whaley et al. (1973. b) also describe vitiligo accompanying Sjogren's syndrome.

Thus, vitiligo and melanoderma would appear to be a manifestation of rheumatoid-auto-immune disease.

d) Pemphigus erythematosus and vulgaris and pemphigoid

Pemphigus erythematosus has been thought to be a bullous type of lupus erythematosus. It has been grouped as an "auto-immune" condition (Beutner, 1969). It has been found in association with myasthenia gravis or with thymoma and then ANF may be found in the serum. Pemphigus erythematosus has also been described in association with systemic lupus erythematosus. Hausmanowa-Petmsewicz et al. (1969) reported the case of a myasthenic who developed systemic lupus erythematosus and pemphigus erythematosus after thymectomy. Holdstock and Oleesky (1970) described a case of coeliac disease with vasculitis in the skin producing lesions resembling systemic lupus erythematosus and pemphigus erythematosus.

Myasthenia gravis with pemphigus vulgaris was described by Simpson (1964) and Beutner et al. (1968) discussed the possibility that pemphigus erythematosus and vulgaris may be combined with systemic lupus erythematosus.

Thus, both pemphigus erythematosus and vulgaris may be associated with rheumatoid disease or its various manifestations.

Salo and Rasanen (1972) adduce evidence indicating that pemphigoid is a manifestation of rheumatoid disease or systemic lupus erythematosus. In 23 patients with pemphigoid 5 had severe mutilating rheumatoid arthritis. Ten of 19 patients had IgG type of ANF and 5 had RF in the serum.

e) Acanthosis nigricans

The condition of acanthosis mgncans was reviewed by Halpert et al. (1957), Curth et al. (1962) and Anscombe et al. (1967). It may affect several members of a family. It not only affects the skin, but also the oral, oesophageal, vaginal and rectal mucosae. The hair is usually destroyed in the affected regions. The underlying corium is infiltrated with lymphocytes and often plasma cells and eosinophils. Acanthosis nigricans occurring in the absence of associated malignant disease has been called "pseudo" or benign acanthosis nigricans, though histologically and clinically it is the same as when associated with malignancy. Pseudo-acanthosis nigricans may occur in association with hypothyroidism, idiopathic Addison's disease, mature onset diabetes mellitus, obesity, lipodystrophy (lipo-atrophy) with diabetes, lupoid hepatitis as well as with hypogonadism (Curth, 1936; Robinson and Tasker, 1947; Winkelmann et al., 1960; Brown et al., 1966; Brown and Winkelmann, 1968; Bruce et al., 1970; Wheeler, 1971). Brown et al. (1966) in 72 patients with benign acanthosis nigricans found 19 had endocrine diseases, 5 had diabetes mellitus, 2 had idiopathic Addison's disease, 2 Stein-Leventhal syndrome, 1 total lipodystrophy and 1 each with systemic lupus erythematosus, ulcerative colitis or hepatitis. Several showed hypertrichosis, amenorrhoea, moon-face, abdominal striae and hyperglycaemia. In addition to the association of the condition with such "auto-immune" diseases as the above it has been described in association with widespread systemic sclerosis with a positive RF in the blood (Clinico-Pathological Conference, Brit. med. J., 1966, ii, 1642). In two personally observed cases of acanthosis, one with cancer of the stomach and another of the ovary, RF and thyroid auto-antibodies were present in the serum, while another woman of 70 years with seropositive rheumatoid arthritis developed acanthosis nigricans and later cancer of the stomach. The author has also observed pseudo-acanthosis nigricans in a case of long-standing rheumatoid arthritis. In another case (Case 15, VI, 31, or X, 23) a woman developed acanthosis nigricans at 35 years of age and then Sjogren-Mikulicz's syndrome, atrophic stomatitis, falling of the teeth, uterine fibroids and then active chronic hepatitis and chronic lymphatic leukaemia and the serum contained a high titre of RF, paraprotein and cold agglutinins. It would appear, therefore, that in its associations acanthosis nigricans is probably a manifestation of coHagen or auto-immune disease.

A familial form of the condition has been described and may be present at birth or develop during childhood (Curth, 1936). Congenital forms may be associated with Von Recklinghausen's disease, arachnodactyly, achondroplasia and certain lesions of the central nervous system. As stated in many cases of the disease malignant disease may be present or develop after a period. In other cases no cancer develops, but cancer may be present in other members of the family.

f) Dennatitis herpetifonnis

This skin condition may also affect the gums and may be associated with pyrexia and a blood eosinophilia of up to 50 per cent. (Pemphigoid is possibly a senile type of dermatitis herpetiformis). Fraser (1970) and Kumar (1973) point out the definite association of dermatitis herpetiformis with thyrotoxicosis and pernicious anaemia and often the presence of thyroid and gastric parietal cell antibodies in the serum in this skin condition. Dermatitis herpetiformis is also frequently associated with malabsorption and partial villous atrophy in the small intestine. In one of the author's cases of this condition pernicious anaemia was also present and ANF, gastric parietal cell a uto-antibodies and intrinsic factor antibodies were found in the serum. Another personal case (Case 16) of dermatitis herpetiformis exhibited also atrophic glossitis, achlorhydria, pernicious anaemia and coeliac disease with gastric parietal cell auto-antibodies and ANF in the serum. Asherson (1973) reported the case of a man of 24 years who at the age of 8 years developed hypothyroidism due to thyroiditis and afterwards recurrent infections due to acquired hypogammaglobulinaemia. Gas-

tric parietal cell and thyroid auto-antibodies were present in the serum. (No reference to RF and ANF is made). He then developed arthropathy, achlorhydria, pernicious anaemia, malabsorption due to partial villous atrophy of the small intestine and dermatitis herpetiformis. Kumar et al. (1973) describe the case of a woman aged 48 years, who underwent thyroidectomy for thyrotoxicosis at the age of 23 years and developed thereafter dermatitis herpetiformis, achlorhydria, pernicious anaemia, arthropathy and malabsorption due to partial villous atrophy of the small intestine. The serum contained thyroid, gastric parietal cell and intrinsic factor auto-antibodies. No reference is made as to whether RF or ANF were present. Dermatitis herpetiformis has also been reported as developing in cases of controlled adult coeliac disease (Mayou-White, 1969). Many authors remark on the fading of the enteropathy associated with dermatitis herpetiformis into that of true adult coeliac disease and on the similarities of dematitis herpetiformis and coeliac disease (Fry, 1971; Engquist and Pock-Steen, 1971). An "auto-immune" basis for the skin lesions of dermatitis herpetiformis has been suggested. The pyrexia and high blood eosinophilia suggest the possibility of a parasitic infection as being the cause.

II, xviii) Collagen and auto-immune disease and allergic manifestations

The skin, nasal mucosa and the trachea, bronchi, lungs and pleurae have been seen to be involved in many cases of collagen disease, such as disseminated eosinophilic collagen disease and rheumatoid disease, and in Sjogren's syndrome. As seen above bouts of asthma and urticaria are frequent in cases of disseminated eosinophilic disease. Chronic bronchitis, intrinsic asthma and urticaria may be features of cases of rheumatoid disease (Wiener, 1947; Short et al., 1957; Spenser, 1968; Shearn, 1971)

Addendum: Acne link with arthritis. Davis DE et al. J. Rheumatol1981 8 2 317-320. Acne may be linked with rheumatoid arthritis.

and other collagen diseases (Talbott and Ferrandis, 1956). Again, attacks of asthma and urticaria with eosinophilia in the blood are common in collagen diseases in which polyarteritis is a feature. Statistical differences in the incidence of allergies -such as asthma, hay-fever and urticaria, in cases of rheumatoid arthritis and controls have been considered in the book by Short et al. (1957). In some cases an alternation between the manifestations of rheumatoid arthritis and asthma have been reported, especially by Jarvinen (1950). Other studies have shown an increased incidence of allergies in cases of rheumatoid arthritis, for example dermatitis. In the series of 100 cases of rheumatoid arthritis at a Geriatric Unit 11 (11 per cent) suffered from asthma and chronic bronchitis. Sjogren's syndrome may likewise be associated with chronic rhinitis or bronchospasm (Heaton, 1959) and tracheo-bronchitis. In cases of Sjogren's syndrome allergic reactions to various drugs are very common and occur in 63 per cent of cases of Sjogren's syndrome (see Boyle and Buchanan, 1971; Shearn, 1971). In any of these conditions the nasal and bronchial mucosa are infiltrated with lymphocytes, plasma cells and often eosinophils and exhibit oedema and swelling as in typical cases of intrinsic asthma. Eosinophilia may occur in the blood, sputum and bone marrow.

"Auto-immune" diseases may likewise be associated with asthma. In cases of juvenile Hashimoto's and lymphocytic thyroiditis Saxena and Crawford (1962) found a 50 per cent incidence of allergic manifestations, such as hay-fever, eczema and urticaria. Atopic disease and lymphocytic thyroiditis was described by Kuitunen et al. (1971). Readett (1964) found eczema and related skin diseases (pompholyx, pruritus, urticaria, seborrhoeic eczema and ichthyosis) are much more common (33 per cent) in cases of thyrotoxicosis than in controls (3.2 per cent). Many relatives have eczema or thyroid disease or both. Simpson (1964) describes myasthenia associated with allergy. Urticaria may occur in cases of ulcerative colitis (Wiener, 1947). Green and Lim (1971) review the literature and describe two cases of intrinsic asthma and idiopathic Addison's disease occurring together. Both showed a blood eosinophilia. In the first case ANF was present in the serum, but no RF or organ-specific auto-antibodies. In the second case the adrenals could not be found at autopsy. Harris and Collins (1971) report two further cases of this association and Del Rio et al. (1971) another case. Carryer et al. (1960) in 481 patients with Addison's disease found 27 with asthma, hay-fever, allergic rhinitis or drug reactions appearing with the first symptoms of Addison's disease. Polycythaemia vera ca5es are also predisposed to develop asthma and chronic bronchitis.

With such common conditions as asthma, rhinitis and urticaria and the various manifestations of collagen-auto-immune disease the two groups of conditions could well be associated purely by chance, but in some cases as in Case 2 the occurrence of intrinsic asthma among a spectrum of collagen and auto-immune diseases may be significant. The following cases have been observed:-

Table II

Case II, 1   Female, aged 26 years. Intrinsic asthma and hay-fever as a child and irregularly since. Four years ago simultaneous onset of *Hashimoto's disease* with acute *myxoedema* and *cystic mastitis* of left breast. Serum contained " very high titre of thyroid auto-antibodies. Mother and son had hay-fever.

Case II, 2   Female, aged 65 years. Eight years history of recurrent asthma. Six years later developed *myxoedema* and mental symptoms. Admitted in status asthmaticus, but euthyroid. Left-sided *exophthalmos.* Thyroid auto-antibodies absent.

-49-

Table II (continued)

Case II, 3   Male, aged 72 years. Aged 62 years operation for *chronic cholecystitis* and mixed gall stones. For 8 years subject to attacks of giant urticaria. *Sjogren's syndrome* present for 2 years. Well marked changes of *rheumatoid arthritis* in feet and fingers and bilateral exophthalmos. Euthyroid, achlorhydria. Serum contained ANF.

Case II, 4   Female, aged 62 years. Exhibited severe allergy to many drugs for years. Six years previously onset of *severe rheumatoid arthritis* and 2 years later onset of *dryness of mouth and eyes* and painless enlargement of *right parotid gland* with involvement of both tempera-mandibular joints. Recent onset of right carpal tunnel syndrome, enlargement of thyroid gland and spontaneous bruising. Now allergic to penicillin, tetracycline and phenobarbitone. Schirmer's test positive in both eyes. Found *to be myxoedematous.* P.B.I. less than 1 -tG per 100 mls. Serum contained RF, ANF, and thymid auto-antibodies in high concentration.

Case II, 5   Female, aged 64 years. Aged 60 years simultaneous onset of eczema, *thyrotoxicosis* and shoulder pains. X-rays showed rheumatoid changes in cervical spine. Thyroid auto-antibodies **++**.

Case II, 6   Male, aged 30 years. Onset of obesity. Severe asthma and rhinitis aged 26-7 years followed by *diabetes* at 30 years.

Case II, 7   Female aged 39 years. Two years ago simultaneous acute onset of *rheumatoid arthritis, polymyositis* and intrinsic asthma with marked eosinophilia in the blood.

Case II, 8   Male aged 30 years. Simultaneous onset of *rheumatoid arthritis* and severe asthma.

Case II, 9   Female aged 42 years, Eight years history of intrinsic asthma, the onset coinciding with the appearance of *thyrotoxicosis.* An area of *cystic mastitis* developed in the upper part of the right breast.

Case II, 10   Female aged 58 years. Recent simultaneous onset of *thyrotoxicosis* and severe intrinsic asthma with residual bronchitis.

Case II, 11   Female aged 38 years. Simultaneous onset of symptoms of intrinsic asthma and *ulcerative colitis.*

Case II, 12   Female aged *69* years. Fifteen years history of instrinsic asthma accompanied by *rheumatoid arthritis* followed by the development of *auto-immune haemolytic anaemia, Waldenstrom's macroglobulinaemia* and *systemic lupus erythematosus.* .. ...

Case II, 13   Male aged 48 years. Simultaneous onset of severe intrinsic asthma and *coeliac disease* with eosinophilia in blood and sputum. Serum rontained RF and thyroid auto-antibodies.

Case II, 14   Male aged 50 years. Simultaneous onset of severe chronic rhinitis and *diabetes* with blood eosinophilia.

Case II, 15   Female aged 45 years. Raynaud's phenomenon for 9 years. Six years previously sudden onset of severe chronic rhinitis. Recent development of *thyrotoxicosis* associated with eosinophilia in the blood and thyroid auto-antibodies in the serum. Treatment of the thyrotoxicosis had no effect on the rhinitis.

Case II, 16   Female aged 30 years. Eight years history of intrinsic 'lsthma and recent onset of *thyrotoxicosis* with a high titre of thyroid auto-antibodies in the blood.

Case II, 17   Female aged 48 years. Ten years history of intrinsic asthma. Recent development of *myxoedema* due to *Hashimoto's thyroiditis* with a very high titre of thyroid auto-antibodies in the serum. Treatment of the myxoedema had no effect on the asthma.

Case II, 18   Female aged 75 years. At the age of 65 years suddenly developed asthmatic attacks and three years later *thyrotoxicosis,* which was treated by radio-active iodine. This was followed by the development of a chromophobe pituitary adenoma and then by *ulcerative colitis* and finally by idiopathic *Addison's disease.* No signs of rheumatoid arthritis. Serum contained ANF and RF, but no gastric parietal cell, thyroid or adrenal auto-antibodies. *Achlorhydria.*

Table II (continued)

Case II, 19   Female aged 72 years. Intrinsic asthma since age of 20 years. Aged 60 years developed severe *rheumatoid arthritis*. Aged 70 years *myxoedema* appeared. Serum contained ANF, thyroid auto-antibodies. Developed carcinoma of right breast.

Case II, 20   Male aged 47 years. Chronic rhinitis and chestiness with attacks of asthma since childhood. Severe *rheumatoid arthritis* aged 27 years. Aged 42 years carcinoma of the thyroid.

Case II, 21   Female aged 46 years. Suffered from *psoriasis* and asthma for many years. Seven years previously she developed iron deficiency anaemia and found to have *achlorhydria (atrophic gastritis)*. Three years ago developed *myxoedema* and pain and swelling in various joints *(rheumatoid arthritis)*, and «t this time onset of first symptoms of multiple sclerosis. RF and thyroid auto-antibodies **+**.

Case II, 22   Female aged 55 years. Intrinsic asthma since teens. Aged 40 years hysterectomy for *fibroids*. Onset of gout. Aged 42 years removal of area of *cystic mastitis* in left breast. Taking steroids for asthma for last *15* years. On trying to stop steroids onset of fulminant *rheumatoid arthritis*. Serum ANF and RF **+**.

Case II, 23   Female aged 39 years. Indian from Tanzania. In England 11 years. Eight years history of chronic rhinitis, intrinsic asthma and migraine and now *atrophic gastritis* and iron deficiency anaemia. Calcified *fibroids* present. Achlorhydria. Gastric parietal cell auto-antibodies **+**.

Case II, 2{   Female aged 21 years. Chronic rhinitis and intrinsic asthma for 8 years. *Raynaud's phenomenon* for two years.

In all the above cases intrinsic asthma leading to chronic bronchitis, allergic and chronic rhinitis and urticaria often with eosinophilia and often with allergic reactions to drugs occurred in subjects exhibiting at some time evidence of collagen and auto-immune disease or auto-antibodies in the serum. These allergic manifestations seem to form part of this group of diseases. In cases of intrinsic asthma there is frequently an eosinophilia in the bronchial mucosa, sputum and blood and Hall et al. (1966) found a significantly higher incidence of thyroid and gastric parietal cell auto-antibodies, ANF and RF in the serum than in cases of extrinsic asthma or healthy subjects. The same symptoms and histological changes in the nasal and bronchial mucosae occur in association with collagen and auto-immune diseases, in infestations by certain parasites, such as filariasis and ascaris and in cases of tropical eosinophilia, thought to be due to animal filariasis. *This suggests that the possibility that in some cases both intrinsic asthma, urticaria and rhinitis and the col-lagen and auto-immune diseases could be due to infection by an unknown parasite.*

II, xix)   Collagen and auto-immune disease of the breast

Like all other tissues all exocrine and endocrine glands appear to be involved to a varying degree in cases of collagen disease. This is best known in cases of Sjogren's syndrome, in which the lacrimal and salivary glands, thyroid, parathyroids, adrenals, pituitary, pancreas, thymus, liver and the bronchial and gastro-intestinal secretory glands may be involved. The breast is an exocrine gland and like other exocrines would be expected to be involved in collagen and auto-immune disease. In Sjogren's syndrome localized tumour-like formations of infiltrative lymphoid tissue may involve the secretory tissue of the breast (Sokoloff, 1966). Subcutaneous or deeper rheumatoid nodules may also affect the breast and involve the glandular tissue. The glandular tissue of the breast may also be involved in cases of sclero-

–51

derma or be affected by arteritis. Shelly and Huxton (1960) described the case of a woman with progressive breast hypertrophy, migrating urticarial skin lesions and generalized pigmentation, dense collections of lymphoid cells in the diseased breast tissue, lupus erythematosus cells in the blood, hypergammablobulinaemia, false positive blood tests for syphilis and a favourable response to steroids.

The condition of cystic mastitis may occur in women at any time from about 30 years of age or even less to well past the menopause or later, but especially about the latter time. The condition often oc-'curs in *one breast only or in one small segment of a breast*. The cause is unknown. Hormonal factors have been thought to play a part. A powerful argument against hormonal factors playing any part in causing the changes is their occurrence in one breast only or in one small segment of a breast, whereas, if hormonal factors are responsible, the whole of both breasts would be expected to be involved. The earliest changes in the breast in this condition consist of an infiltration with lymphocytes and plasma cells and this is followed by the formation of cellular connective tissue surrounding the ducts and lobules and between the acini, which are often compressed and degenerate, eventually leading to progressive fibrosis and cystic dilatation of the ducts. These changes closely resemble those changes in the salivary glands in cases of Sjogren's syndrome and in the pancreas in many cases of chronic pancreatitis and, in fact, they are identical with those described in the breast in association with Sjogren's syndrome by Sokoloff (1966) and mentioned above. Numerous or solitary cysts may form and intraduct epitheliosis and papillomatosis may develop in the cysts and often malignant change. The condition is certainly premalignant, though to what degree is uncertain. It is very common at autopsy and is often undetectable clinically (see Evans, 1966).

The early changes in the breast are typical of those of collagen-auto-immune disease. Mackay and Burnet (1963), in fact, suggested cystic mastitis might be an auto-immune disease. In the author's experience cystic mastitis may develop in association with or during the course of cases of collagen-"auto-immune" disease. These are exemplified by the following cases of cystic mastitis seen by the author in a general *Medical* clinic during a period of three and a half years.

Table III

Case III, 1   Female, aged 27 years. Indian. Resident in England for 6 years. Simultaneous onset of *Hashimoto's thyroiditis* and cystic mastitis of upper inner quadrant of left breast. No RF, ANF or auto-antibodies in the serum.

Case III, 2   Female, aged 69 years. Aged 33 years onset of *rheumatoid arthritis,* for which
(Case VI, 2)   under continuous treatment for many years. Aged 37 years hysterectomy for *fibroids* and also removal of adenoma of the right side of the *thyroid.* Aged 42 years two separate operations on a) the upper outer and b) lower inner quadrant of the right breast for cystic mastitis. Aged 44 years dyspareunia due to *atrophic vaginitis* and now carcinoma of the stomach. *Achlorhydria,* ANF, RF and gastric parietal and thyroid auto-antibodies absent from the serum.

Case III, 3   Female, aged 51 years. Onset of *rheumatoid arthritis* at 45 years. Under continuous treatment since. Aged 50 years developed lumps in the upper parts of both breasts. The right was found to be due to cystic mastitis and the left to cystic mastitis becoming carcinomatous. At this time her periods were still present. At the age of 51 years she developed carcinoma of the cervix treated by radiation. The serum showed RF and gastric parietal cell auto-antibodies.

Table III (continued)

Case ill, 4   Female, aged 58 years.   Aged 34 years partial thyroidectomy for *thyrotoxicosis*. Menopause aged 48 years.   Aged 58 years she noticed lumps in both breasts.   Pre-operatively found to have lupus erythematosus cells + + in the blood and ANF, RF and thyroid antibodies + + in the serum.   Bilateral mastectomy carried out. Right breast showed only cystic mastitis, the left cystic mastitis, and an undifferentiated carcinoma.   Immediately post-operatively developed *acute arthropathy*.

Case III, 5   Female, aged 60 years.   Aged 50 years onset of *acute rheumatoid arthritis* and painful swelling of the right breast.   Under treatment ever since.   Aged 51 years removal of an area of cystic mastitis in right breast.   Aged 55 years cystic mastitis and intraduct carcinoma in right breast.   Aged 60 years developed carpal tunnel syndrome and *myxoedema*.   Free acid present in the stomach.   Serum contained ANF +.

Case 111, 6   Female, aged 39 years.   Simultaneous onset of *thyrotoxicosis* and cystic mastitis of right breast confirmed by mastectomy.   Serum contained thyroid auto-antibodies +.

Case III, 7   Female, aged 42 years.   *Acute rheumatoid arthritis* aged 18 years.   Aged 40 years bilateral cystic mastitis simultaneously.   Now has oligodendroglioma of right temporal lobe with well-marked *rheumatoid arthritic* changes in hands.   ANF, RF and auto-antibodies absent from serum.

Case III, 8   Female, aged 79 years.   Aged 49 years removal of area of cystic mastitis from left breast.   Aged 69 years onset of severe *rheumatoid arthritis* and under continuous treatment since.   Now lymphosarcoma of left orbit.   Investigations showed *achlorhydria* and serum contained RF, ANF + + and gastric parietal cell antibodies.

Case III, 9   Female, aged 46 years.   Simultaneous onset of *rheumatoid arthritis* and cystic mastitis of lower outer quadrant of left breast.   Periods still regular.   Serum RF negative.

Case III, 10   Female, aged 52 years.   Suffered from *thyrotoxicosis* for last two years and during this time she developed cystic mastitis of the upper outer quadrant of the left breast.   Serum contained ANF + and thyroid auto-antibodies + +.   Daughter suffered from thyrotoxicosis and diabetes.

Case III, 11   Female, aged 37 years.   Area of cystic mastitis upper outer quadrant right breast. Investigations showed serum contained thyroid auto-antibodies.

Case III, 12   Female, aged 68 years.   Aged 43 years cystic mastitis of upper part of left breast. Aged 45 years carcinoma of outer part of right breast.   Bilateral mastectomy.   Aged 45 years menopause and generalized *arthropathy* lasting 2·3 years, settling after prolonged treatment.   Aged 54 years E.S.R. found markedly raised and remaining so over the next !O years, when onset of myelomatosis.   Serum showed ANF + and thyroid antibodies + prior to the development of myelomatosis.

Case III, 13   Female, aged 42 years.   Onset of *thyrotoxicosis* three years previously.   This remained untreated and during this three years noticed recurrent hard slightly tender swellings affecting parts of both breasts and which tended to come and go.   Eventually one persisted in the lower outer quadrant of the left breast and became cystic.   Removal showed an area of cystic mastitis with well-marked lymphocytic infiltration.   She then developed menorrhagia and after a year urinary retention found to be due to the presence of huge *fibroids*.   Operation revealed also the presence of bilateral serous *ovarian cysts*.   Serum contamed thyroid antibodies and ANF.

Case III, 14 (same as Case II, 1)   Female, aged 26 years.   *Intrinsic asthma* as a child and irregularly since.   Four years previous to being seen simultaneous onset of *Hashimoto's thyroiditis, myxoedema* and cystic mastitis in the left breast.   Thyroglobulin R.B.C. agglutination test ▮ in 250,000.

Table III (continued)

Case III, 15   Female, aged 31 years. One years history of prominence and lid-lag of the right eye *(unilateral exophthalmos)*. Euthyroid. Eight months later cystic mastitis of area of left breast. Serum contained no auto-antibodies.

Case **III,** 16   Female, aged 69 years. Menarche aged 17 years. Periods *always scanty.* Menopause aged 43 years. Aged 55 years hysterectomy for *fibroids* and lumps in the peripheries of both breasts found due to *cystic mastitis.* This was accompanied by mild *peripheral arthropathy.* Aged 60 years *diabetes* found. Aged 69 years lymphadenopathy in right groin. Biopsy showed reticulosarcoma. Examination revealed mild *rheumatoid arthritis* changes in fingers, wrists, ankles and feet. *Achlorhydria,* ANF +, thyroid +, gastric parietal cell antibodies +. Incomplete CFT platelet antibodies present.

Case **III,** 17   Female, aged 63 years. Under treatment for 10 years for *rheumatoid arthritis.* Lumps in both breasts found recently. Right cystic mastitis, left carcinoma. Daughter had carcinoma of the breast and one brother carcinoma of the bladder.

Case III, **18**   Female, aged 58 years. Moderate smoker many years. Aged 31 years hysterectomy
(same as   for *fibroids.* Aged 33 years oophorectomy for benign cyst of *left ovary.* Aged 42
Case I, 4)   years cholecystectomy for *chronic cholecystitis.* Aged 56 years operation for right cystic mastitis. Examination showed severe *rheumatoid arthritis* of feet and presence of carcinoma of the bronchus. Achlorhydria and RF + were present. One brother died of cerebral glioma aged 47 years and one brother died of carcinoma of the bronchus aged 65 years.

Case **III,** 19   Female, aged 63 years. Bilateral cystic mastitis operation aged 24 years. Breast nodular since. Aged 40 years hysterectomy for *fibroids.* One *ovary* removed for benign cyst. Aged 61 years *diabetes* found. Now carcinoma of left breast and colon. One brother is a diabetic. Her husband died of carcinoma of the prostate and sarcoma of the right upper arm.

Case III, 20   Female, aged 55 years. Intrinsic *asthma* since her teens. Aged 40 years hysterec-
(same as   tomy for *fibroids.* Onset of gout. Aged 42 years operation for removal of area of
Case II, 22)   cystic mastitis in the left breast. On steroids for asthma for last 15 years. On trying to stop steroids onset of fulminant *rheumatoid disease.* Serum ANF and RF +.

Case III, 21   Female, aged 49 years. Hysterectomy for *fibroids* aged 38 years. Aged 42 years operation for *cystic mastitis.* Now has carcinoma of the pyloric end of the stomach, marked *rheumatoid arthritis* of the feet and *ichthyosis acquisita.* Achlorhydria and gastric parietal cells were found.

See also Cases VI, 12, VI, 42, and VI. 71.

In Case 1 described above the patient developed cystic mastitis in the course of a life in which very numerous manifestations of the spectrum of collagen-auto-immune disease appeared at intervals, including diabetes, vitiligo, rheumatoid arthritis, Sj<igren's syndrome, myxoedema, permctous anaemia, atrophic gastritis, Hashimoto's thyroiditis and primary gonadal failure.

In the above cases localized areas of cystic mastitis have occurred in subjects who are suffering, have suffered from or later develop collagen and/or auto-immune diseases. In subjects in which no clinical history or evidence of the existence of such disease is found at first examination, the blood may contain auto-antibodies. Most cases of diabetes mellitus are due to "auto-immune" disease. Lender et al. (1977) point out the increased incidence of cystic mastitis and breast cancer in a diabetic female population.

Cystic mastitis thus appears to be part of the spectrum of collagen-auto-immune disease as it affects the breast. The lym·

phocytic and plasma cell infiltration around the acini and ducts of the breast and the subsequent fibrosis and change in the acini and ducts appear to form part of the manifestations of collagen-auto-immune disease as found in all other glandular tissues in the body.

II, xx) Collagen and auto-immune disease and lymphadenopathy and splenomegaly

Enlargement of the lymph nodes and the malphighian corpuscles of the spleen is not uncommon in cases of rheumatoid disease (Gardner, 1966), systemic lupus erythematosus and dermatomyositis (Marshall, 1956). These usually show the changes described as chronic inflammation, reactive hyperplasia or lymphoid histiocytic follicular reticulosis. The changes may be confused with those of lymphoma. They resemble those of chronic infections. Motulsky et a!. (1952) found that in cases of rheumatoid arthritis 50-75 per cent had palpable lymph nodes up to 3 ems. in diameter and these formed part of a systemic disease. In 20 per cent of cases the spleen was palpable. In both Felty's disease and Still's disease (juvenile rheumatoid arthritis), variations of rheumatoid arthritis, the lymphadenopathy and splenomegaly are in the foreground. Generali:z;ed lymphadenopathy and splenomegaly may also occur in cases of thyrotoxicosis or Sjogren's syndrome (see above). A similar lymphadenopathy may be found in the lymph nodes adjacent to the thyroid gland in cases of Hashimoto's thyroiditis (Blackburn and O'Gorman, 1961; Reinlein and Navarro, 1967).

Such observations are strongly in favour of an infectious cause of the collagen-auto-immune diseases.

Collagen and auto-immune disease and enlarrement of the tonsils and adenoids

Enlargement of the tonsillar and adenoidal lymphoid tissue which exhibits the changes of reactive hyperplasia is a very common finding in cases of rheumatoid di-

sease and in cases of the latter these may be a long history of tonsillitis followed by exacerbation of the disease. Th is association is so well recognized that removal of the tonsils and adenoids as treatment in cases of rheumatoid disease has long been practiced. Enlargement of these lymphoid organs appears to form part of this generalized lymphoid hyperplasia found in many cases of collagen-auto-immune disease.

Follicular appendicitis

The normal appendix contains lymphomatous tissue in the submucosa. In chronic inflammation of the appendix without obstruction the organ often shows marked hyperplasia of the lymphoid tissue, large lymphoid follicles and lymphocytic infiltration in the wall of the organ, especially in the subserosa and submucosa and the mucosa is swollen and oedematous. This is known as follicular appendicitis. It may be followed by fibrosis.

In Case 17, a man, aged 55 years, developed diabetes and later upper abdominal pain. Laparotomy showed the presence of chronic pancreatitis. Histologically the gland exhibited infiltration with lymphocytes and fibrosis with dilatation of the ductules, which showed proliferation of the lining cells. The fibrosis involved the islets. At operation the appendix was also removed and this showed lymphoid hyperplasia. Later he developed balanitis and generalized joint pains and swelling and increasing stiffness. X-rays showed rheumatoid changes in the cervical spine. There was achlorhydria. At first all antibody tests were negative, but four years later RF and thyroid antibodies were present. Another patient (Case VI. 65) developed various manifestations of collagen and auto-immune disease and also follicular appendicitis. Such cases suggest the possibility that collagen and auto-immune disease which affect the lymphoid tissue throughout the body may involve the appendix in the form of follicular appendicitis.

II, xxi)   Collagen and auto-immune disease and the alimentary tract

Any part of the alimentary tract may be affected in association with collagen or auto-immune diseases.

a) The upper digestive tract

It has been seen that atrophic gastritis appears to be an auto-immune disease. The association of atrophic gastritis with or without pernicious anaemia with thyroiditis, adrenalitis or collagen disease (Siurala et al., 1965; Fenyohazi et al., 1970) has already been stressed. Siurala et al. in 71 cases of various types of collagen disease found superficial gastritis in 11 and atrophic gastritis in 13. In 18 patients suffering from rheumatoid arthritis Fenyohazi et al. (1970) found 11 with gastric mucosal atrophy, severe in 3 and with inflammatory changes in 7 cases. Hollander et al. (1960) described atrophic oesophagitis and chronic inflammation of the small intestine \Vith death from chronic diarrhoea in cases of rheumatoid arthritis. At a Medical Staff Round at Hammersmith Hospital there was shown a case of rheumatoid arthritis with Sjogren's syndrome and atrophic oesophagitis and gastritis. Systemic lupus erythematosus likewise may be associated with severe glossitis or Plummer-Vinson syndrome (Mackay and Burnet, 1963). In Case 6 mentioned above rheumatoid arthritis, Sjogren's syndrome, atrophic stomatitis, pharyngitis, oesophagitis and gastritis and tracheo-bronchitis, fibrosing alveolitis and rheumatoid granulomatous myocarditis occurred together in the same patient.

The "auto-immune" disease, atrophic gastritis, may likewise be associated with diabetes and hypothyroidism, superficial and atrophic glossitis, angular stomatitis, atrophic oesop'hagitis and pharyngitis and the formation of a postcricoid web (Paterson-Kelly or Plummer-Vinson syndrome) or with coeliac disease (Jacobs and Kilpatrick, 1964). This syndrome may be accompanied by hypochromic or pernicious anaemia and may also be associated with kraurosis vulvae (Phoads, 1940). The administration of iron in these cases may relieve some of the symptoms temporarily and correct the anaemia, but the atrophic lesions still come and go (Jacobs and Kilpatrick, 1964).

Post-cricoid webs in the oesophagus occur especially in association with iron-deficiency anaemia, angular stomatitis, glossitis, edentia, thyroid disease, especially myxoedema, gastric atrophy, pernicious anaemia, polycythaemia, ulcerative colitis, Sjogren's syndrome and rheumatoid arthritis. Thyroid auto-antibodies are commonly present in the blood (Chisholm et al., 1971). There is a high incidence of malignant disease (12 per cent) in the upper gastro-intestinal tract. When iron-deficiency anaemia is present, irrespective of the presence of a web, gastric parietal auto-antibodies occur in a high proportion of cases (Chisholm et al., 1971). One of the author's patients, a woman of 46 years. had undergone partial thyroidectomy for thyrotoxicosis 8 years previously and was now euthyroid, but had severe iron-deficiency anaemia, a post-cricoid web, free acid in the gastric secretions and RF and thyroid and gastric parietal cell auto-antibodies in the serum. These atrophic changes in the upper alimentary tract and the post-cricoid web are identical with those which may be found in these organs in cases of Sjogren's syndrome (see Shearn, 1971) when they form part of the general failure of mucosal secretions. The diseases associated with post-cricoid webs, including carcinoma of the upper gastro-intestinal tract, may occur in relatives of the patient (Chisholm et al., 1971). Thus, it appears that atrophy of the gastro-intestinal tract from the mouth to the stomach is to be grouped with the collagen-auto-immune diseases.

b) Collagen disease and the gums and teeth

In cases of Sjogren's syndrome with dryness of the mouth it has been mentioned that stomatitis and gingivitis are common. There may be acute pyorrhoea and rampant dental caries (see above). This may also occur in cases of rheumatoid arthritis with or without Sjogren's syndrome. So common are such changes in cases of rheumatoid arthritis that in the past poor teeth were removed in the mistaken idea that local infection was a causative factor in the disease. Gingival involvement may also lead to rapid and severe dental caries in cases of systemic lupus erythematosus (Mackay and Burnet, 1963). Attention was also drawn by Chisholm et al. (1971) to the association of edentia from premature falling of the teeth in association with post-cricoid webs in the oesophagus, angular stomatitis, glossitis, atrophic gastritis with or without iron deficiency or pernicious anaemia, thyroid disease, etc. It appears, therefore, that the ·health of the teeth suffers as a result of collagen-auto-immune diseases affecting the mucosa of the mouth, including the tongue and gums.

c) Coeliac disease

In cases of coeliac disease the mucosa of the jejunum and small intestine show a dense ipfiltration of the lamina propria with lymphocytes and plasma cells as in auto-immune diseases. All the lymphoid tissue in the body may be atrophic, including the Peyer's patches. The condition may or may not be gluten-sensitive (Booth, 1970) and in the latter case a thick layer of collagen may be found beneath the enterocytes in the gut (Booth, 1970). In gluten-sensitive cases successful treatment does not cause the cellular infiltration to disappear. In contrast to the normal mucosa there is an interference with the maturation of the enterocytes at the bottom of the crypts in the jejunum and small intestine in cases of coeliac disease. The normal process has been compared with haemopoiesis in the marrow (Doniach and Shiner, 1960). The changes in the mucosa in cases of coeliac disease may thus be compared with those in the bone marrow in myeloid leukaemia. There is no evi-

dence to support an enzyme deficiency as being responsible for this disease, nor of any genetic factor (Booth, 1970).

It has been seen above that in the series of cases of collagen disease described by Siurala et al. (1965) the typical atrophic changes of coeliac disease were present in the mucosa of the jejunum and small intestine in some cases and some of these had symptoms of coeliac disease and a proportion were gluten-sensitive. Petersson et al. (1970), Hall (1971) and Dyer et al. (1971) also describe similar cases. In some of the cases malabsorption is due to amyloidosis (Petersson et al., 1970). Another such case was described by Stephen and Shiner (1971). In this the serum ANF and latex fixation tests were negative and IgA was absent. Still's disease with massive hepatomegaly and coeliac disease was reported by Millen (1971). The occurrence of episodes of arthritis in cases of coeliac disease is also referred to by Bywaters and Ansell (1969) and ankylosing spondylitis associated with coeliac disease is described by Flavell Matts (1958). Evidence of malabsorption occurs in about a quarter of cases of active rheumatoid arthritis and the jejunal mucosa may show infiltration with lymphocytes and plasma cells but no other change according to Leading Article (Brit. med. J., 1972, 2, 187). In the series of 100 cases of rheumatoid arthritis collected at the geriatric unit and mentioned above there was also found one case of severe rheumatoid arthritis which developed coeliac disease. Sjogren's syndrome associated with coeliac disease has also been reported (Pittman and Holub, 1965; Shearn, 1971; Lancaster-Smith and Strickland, 1971) and the Plummer-Vinson syndrome associated with coeliac disease is mentioned by Jacobs and Kilpatrick (1964). A patient of the author's, a woman of 72 years, had suffered from rheumatoid arthritis for 15 years. She then developed myxoedema, atrophic gastritis. microcytic anaemia, coeliac disease and osteoporosis. Another patient, aged 60 years, developed coeliac disease at the same time as her only sibling and her mother developed rheumatoid disease. She herself had atrophic gastritis. Yet another patient, a female of 60 years, developed simultaneously the symptoms of Hashimoto's thyroiditis, proven histologically, and those of gluten-sensitive coeliac disease. She was hypothyroid, the blood contained thyroid auto-antibodies in high titre and her intestinal symptoms responded completely to a gluten-free diet. Below is described a case under the author's care in which long-standing rheumatoid arthritis was followed by the development of coeliac disease and later by Hodgkin's disease (Case 18).

Case 18 Male, aged 44 years on first attendance. Onset of severe rheumatoid arthritis affecting hands, wrists, elbows, knees, ankles and feet at the age of 34 years. Over the next 5 years had been in various hospitals and had various forms of treatment, including two course of gold injections. At the end of this time his condition had gradually deteriorated and it was then noticed that he had a mild generalized lymphadenopathy. Biopsy of a supraclavicular lymph node was reported as showing only reactive hyperplasia. He then developed marked dryness of the mouth and eyes. At the age of 40 years severe painless diarrhoea appeared, the stools being bulky and contained green vegetables and beans unchanged in passage through the gut. The stools floated in the pan. He also became markedly anaemic and this required repeated blood transfusions. The lymph nodes waxed and waned in size. Over the next year he had a series of boils. He then came under the author's care. Examination at that time showed severe rheumatoid arthritic deformities of the 'hands and feet, pale mucosae, marked dryness of the mouth, signs of conjunctivitis, marked wasting and slight generalized lymphadenopathy without enlargement of the liver or spleen. Investigations showed a strongly positive Rose-Waaler and latex

fixation test in the blood and achlorhydria. Schirmer's test showed almost complete lack of tears. The faecal fat secretion averaged 9.8 grams per day (steatorrhoea). The folic acid absorption test showed a marked failure of absorption, though the vitamin B12 absorption test was normal. The glucose tolerance test was normal, but the xylose absorption test showed a grossly diminished absorption. A barium swallow, meal and follow through showed pooling of the barium with multiple fluid levels in the small intestine. The serum iron was 40 mgms. per 100 mls. A blood count showed a megaloblastic anaemia with a haemoglobin of 9.4 mgms. per cent. The plasma proteins were albumin 2.9 G, globulin 3.5 G, E.S.R. was 85 mms. per hour. Serum electrolytes normal, alkaline phosphatase normal. Gastric parietal cell antibodies positive. A bone marrow smear showed severe megaloblastic change. Vitamin B12 administration gave no reticulocyte response. He was then started on folic acid 40 mgms. daily, which produced a rapid improvement in his anaemia, a reticulocyte response of up to 20 per cu. mm. and some improvement in his general condition. The lymphadenopathy subsided. He was then given gluten-free diet and there was a rapid disappearance of the diarrhoea and the haemoglobin rose to 91 per cent and the E.S.R. fell to 20 mm. per hour. A diagnosis of coeliac disease was made. He remained well on this regime for 4 years apart from the arthritic symptoms. He then began to run a fever and to lose weight. The enlarged lymph nodes in the neck reappeared and both liver and spleen became grossly enlarged. At this time the joints were much less painful. Moreover, he began to sweat and feel generally weak and the diarrhoea recurred in spite of continuing the gluten-free diet. At this time examination showed a pale, thin man with bilateral ankle oedema, severe rheumatoid deformity of the hands, wrists, feet and ankles, rheumatoid nodules on the elbows and small discrete lymph nodes 2 ems. in diameter on both sides of the neck, in both axillae, groins and femoral areas and there was a large palpable right external iliac mass. The spleen was enlarged 8 ems. downwards and 6 ems. from the midline and the liver 5 ems. downwards. Biopsy of a right axillary lymph node showed the typical changes of Hodgkin's disease. The pattern of the lymph nodes was completely destroyed and replaced by a picture composed of large reticulum cells with lymphocytes and a few plasma cells, eosinophils and polymorphs. There was an evenly distributed increase in reticulin.

He was repeatedly treated with prednisolone, chlorambucil, folic acid, radiotherapy and blood transfusions with variable decrease in the size of the liver, spleen and lymph nodes and intermittent fever and sweats. The diarrhoea, however, persisted for the rest of his life. The patient died 5 years after the diagnosis of Hodgkin's disease was made.

At autopsy the following positive findings were noted: – An emaciated middle-aged man, with mild clubbing of the fingers and toes and the signs of severe rheumatoid arthritis affecting the hands, wrists, elbows, ankles and feet. Rheumatoid nodules were present around the wrists and elbows. The lacrimal and salivary glands were very hard and fibrosed and sections showed infiltration with lymphocytes and fibrosis. The thyroid gland was fibrosed. There was massive lymph node enlargement on both sides of the neck, especially at the root, and in the anterior and posterior mediastinum, these being up to 3 ems. in diameter, firm and white, some showing areas of necrosis. Dense adhesions were present over both lungs to the chest wall and to the pericardium. The pericardial space was obliterated by adhesions. The lungs were gritty on palpation and sections showed small foci of fibrosis surrounded by focal emphysema. In addition there were larger areas of dense fibrosis up to 3 ems. in diameter (rheumatoid nod-

ules). Overlying some of the patches of fibrosis the pleura was thickened, glistening and white. The spleen was mildly enlarged, rubbery and brown and weighed 260 grams, the cut surface being smooth. The stomach showed gross atrophy of the mucosa and the duodenum, jejunum and small intestine showed gross flattening and complete atrophy of the villi typical of coeliac disease. The intestine down to the pelvic colon was infiltrated from without by firm white tumour nodules in several areas. The adrenal gland showed small areas of invasion by white tumour tissue as did the cortex of both kidneys and the hilum of the right kidney. There was massive enlargement of para-aortic lymph nodes forming one solid tumour mass invading the pancreas, spinal column, both psoas muscles and the mesentery. There were some minute tumour nodules on the cerebral arachnoid.

Histologically the lacrimal and salivary glands were completely infiltrated with lymphocytes with lymph follicle formation. The thyroid gland showed patchy infiltration of lymphocytes and plasma cells. The lamina propria of the stomach and small intestine showed similar infiltrations. The tumours showed typical changes of Hodgkin's disease with large reticulum cells and many lymphocytes. No amyloidosis was present.

A diagnosis of rheumatoid arthritis, Sjogren's syndrome, focal lymphocytic thyroiditis, atrophic gastritis, coeliac disease with complete villous atrophy of the small intestine and generalized Hodgkin's disease was made.

Another patient, a woman of 28 years at the onset of rheumatoid arthritis, later developed many lupus erythematosus cells in the blood, which also contained RF and ANF in high titre. Five years later she developed chronic pyelonephritis for which unilateral nephrectomy was carried out. After a further five years pernicious anaemia was diagnosed and she was found to have achlorhydria and gastric parietal cell antibodies in the blood. She then developed gluten-sensitive coeliac disease. Yet another patient, a man of 66 years, suffering from seropositive rheumatoid disease for 6 years also developed pernicious anaemia with gastric parietal cell auto-antibodies in the blood and was found to have symptomless coeliac disease as shown by jejunal biopsy and tests for malabsorption. The malabsorption disappeared when the patient was given a gluten-free diet. Henriksson et al. (1976) describe adult coeliac disease with polymyositis.

It has been concluded above that dermatitis herpetiformis appears to be a manifestation of rheumatoid disease and may be associated with other manifestations of this condition and with partial or complete villous atrophy of the small intestinal mucosa and that the enteropathy associated with dermatitis herpetiformis fades into that of true adult coeliac disease.

In a case of coeliac disease shown at a Medical Staff Round at Hammersmith Hospital in 1967 the patient developed pernicious anaemia and later Raynaud's phenomena and arthralgia and some years afterwards jejunal mucosal atrophy associated with malabsorption. A rash developed especially after exercise and then lymphadenopathy in the axillae and groins, vasculitis in the skin, cryoglobulinaemia and the serum showed a very strongly positive RF. Booth (1970) mentions 3 cases and Creamer and Pink (1967) 1 case of coeliac disease with extensive arteritis in various parts of the body. Doe et al. (1972) describe 4 cases of adult coeliac disease with vasculitis and cryoglobulinaemia.· Two cases showed Raynaud's phenomenon. In one, necrotizing vasculitis of skin and muscle was found. RF and direct antiglobulin tests were positive in the 3 patients in which the tests were carried out. Holdstock and Oleesky (1970) also describe a case of coeliac disease with vasculitis in the skin resembling systemic lupus erythematosus and also pemphigus erythematosus, thought by many to be an auto-immune disease. In a personally observed case of coeliac disease lupus erythematosus lesions occurred in the skin, RF and ANF were present in the serum and widespread arteritis was found at autopsy. Lancaster-Smith and Strickland (1971) studied 23 patients with adult coeliac disease. One showed the presence of Sjogren's syndrome, one had a past history of thyrotoxicosis and two suffered from fibrosing alveolitis. In three cases RF was present in the serum and in three others thyroglobulin antibodies were present. Seah et al. (1971) in 31 patients with adult coeliac disease found ANF in thE: serum in two, gastric parietal cell antibodies in four, thyroid microsomal antibodies in three, thyroglobulin antibodies in one and mitochondrial antibodies in two.

Apart from rheumatoid arthritis and other collagen diseases coeliac disease may also be found associated with or follow the development of "auto-immune" diseases, such as diabetes (Hamilton et al., 1961; Green et al., 1962; Wruble and Kaiser, 1964; Visakorpi, 1969) in the absence of diabetic neuropathy. Either disease may antedate the other. Visakorpi reported five cases of this association and states that 4 per cent of coeliacs exhibit diabetes. Scott and Losowsky (1975) described coeliac disease in association with 14 other different diseases. Kuitunen et al. (1971) reported auto-immune thyroiditis associated with coeliac disease in children. Dermatitis herpetiformis may accompany partial or complete villous atrophy of the small intestine (see above). Coeliac disease may also be associated with idiopathic hypoparathyroidism, hypothyroidism, idiopathic Addison's disease, atrophic gastritis with pernicious anaemia, post-necrotic cirrhosis and ulcerative colitis (Salem and Truelove, 1965) in every conceivable combination (Craig et al., 1955; Reisner and Ellsworth, 1955; Jackson, 1957; Williams and Wood, 1959; Morse et al., 1961; Taybi and Keale, 1962; Kunim et al., 1963; Stickler et al.,

1965; Goudie et al., 1969). Pernicious anaemia with gastric parietal cell and intrinsic factor auto-antibodies in the serum and atrophic gastritis were present in two personal cases of the disease, in one of which ANF was also present in the blood. Again coeliac disease may be associated with fibrosing alveolitis (Wood and Mason, 1970; Scadding, 1970; Lancaster-Smith and Strickland, 1971; Smith et al., 1971). The last named described three cases, in two of which thyroid auto-antibodies were present in high concentration in the serum. Scadding recorded one case and Wood and Mason two in which thyroid auto-antibodies and RF were present in the blood. In the Clinico-pathological Conference (1970, Brit. med. J., 3, 207) coeliac disease was associated with post-necrotic cirrhosis, the Rose-Waaler and latex fixation tests in the serum were strongly positive. In the discussion which followed another case of this association was mentioned. In the Clinico-pathological Conference (1970, Brit. med. J., 2, 711) adult coeliac disease associated with "auto-immune" Addison's disease was described. Vasculitis was present in the skin and RF in the blood. No antibodies to the adrenal gland, gonads, thyroid or stomach cells were present. The patient developed carcinoma of the breast. A patient of the author's, a girl aged 15 years, presented with a 6 years history of recurrent painless swelling of the parotid glands and a 5 years history of recurrent arthritis of various joints. The RF in the serum was strongly positive and ANF was present, but submandibular salivary gland antibodies were absent. Her brother, now aged 18 years, had suffered from gluten-sensitive coeliac disease since the age of 5 years. All auto-antibody tests on his serum were negative. At the age of 21 years the patient's sister also developed coeliac disease and the serum showed a strongly positive RF. There was a marked history of rheumatoid arthritis in the family. In another of the author's patients (Case 19) there was a

simultaneous onset of coeliac disease and intrinsic asthma in an adult and the serum contained RF and thyroid antibodies. In 4 other patients under the author's care peripheral neuropathy associated with symptomless coeliac disease confirmed by small intestinal biopsy was present. In one of these cases, a woman aged 55 years, her sister and mother both developed severe rheumatoid arthritis. Another case also suffered from thyrotoxicosis and later developed abdominal lymphoma. A third case suffered from Hashimoto's thyroiditis confirmed by biopsy and with a high serum titre of thyroid auto-antibodies. The fourth case showed thyroid and gastric parietal auto-antibodies in the serum and achlorhydria.

The clinical associations of coeliac disease described above suggests very strongly that the condition is at any rate in some patients a manifestation of collagen and "auto-immune" disease. The atrophic condition of the mucosa of the small intestine and the submucosal infiltration with lymphocytes and often plasma cells is similar to the atrophic condition of the mucosa of the mouth, tongue, oesophagus, pharynx and stomach with which coeliac disease may be associated and all of which may be complications of rheumatoid disease, including Sjögren's syndrome. Coeliac disease would thus form part of the spectrum of collagen-auto-immune disease and, like other manifestations of this spectrum, it may rapidly respond to steroids (Booth, 1970).

The question of the auto-immune nature of coeliac disease was raised by Truelove and Wright (1948) and Perlman and Broberger (1969). An IgA deficiency in the blood in some cases of the disease was reported by Mawhinney and Tomkin (1971) and Stephen and Shiner (1971). This is secondary, since it usually disappears with treatment with a gluten-free diet (Booth, 1970). In other cases an excess of IgA and IgM-containing lymphocytes in the jejunal mucosa has been reported (Asquith et al., 1969; Booth, 1970). Little (1972) estimated the serum levels of IgA, IgG and IgM in members of families with more than one member with coeliac disease. These were normal except for an isolated IgA deficiency in one healthy subject. This does not support the hypothesis that IgA deficiency is a major factor in the pathogenesis or inheritance of coeliac disease.

Malabsorption and small intestine mucosal atrophy due to "Mediterranean" lymphoma and associated with parasitic infection

Hoskins et al.. (1967) describe 6 cases infested with Giardia Iamblia complicated by the malabsorption syndrome, in two of which the jejunal mucosa showed moderate or severe atrophy during the infestation. The other four patients showed milder mucosal abnormalities. Immunoglobulin deficiency was present in the two severe cases. The affected mucosa showed a mononuclear infiltrate and trophozoites were found within the luminal space close to the brush border, but not invading the mucosa. Other observers, however, have reported the organism *within* the jejunal epithelial cells and the lamina propria. Treatment of the infestation with atebrine, an antiprotozoal drug, cured the malabsorption and the mucosal atrophy disappeared. It was thought that in the two cases showing immunoglobulin deficiency this had facilitated the infestation. Rambaud et al. (1968) described the malabsorption syndrome among non-Ashkenazy Jews and Israeli Arabs, in whom there was found involvement of the whole length of the small intestine and stomach by proliferation of lymphocytes and plasma cells in the lamina propria accompanied by mucosal atrophy. The epithelium had largely disappeared. No parasites were found in the stools or in the biopsy specimens. Neither the blood nor bone marrow showed eosinophilia. The serum and urine, however, contained an abnormal IgA and the condition has been referred to as alpha-chain disease. At first their patient, how-

ever, responded favourably to metronidazole (Flagyl, an antiprotozoal drug) . Doe et al. (1970) described a similar case in which the nasal mucosa and bone marrow also exhibited the diffuse plasma cell infiltration and the protein abnormalities were present in the blood, urine and saliva. In their case, however, there was a marked eosinophilia in the blood, though no parasites were found in the gut. The abnormal protein originated in the plasma cells in the gut wall. Scotto et al. (1970) report similar cases from Paris. Pena et al. (1970) reported another from Spain.

This condition of Mediterranean lymphoma was thought at first to be confined to Arabs, non-Ashkanazy Jews and Pakistanis, but cases have now been reported from other parts of the world. In other cases known as heavy-chain disease a similar condition has been associated with the presence in the serum and urine of a polypeptide similar to a fragment of IgG globulin and the clinical picture of a malignant lymphoma with lymphadenopathy, splenomegaly and sometimes hepatomegaly. Brandborg et al. (1970) describe 6 cases and refer to others in the literature in which steatorrhoea with a flat small intestinal mucosa appeared to be due to infiltration of the mucosa with the coccidial protozoon, Isopora, found widespread throughout the animal kingdom. In many such cases the blood shows an eosinophilia. Da Costa (1971) recalls that infestation by Strongyloides stercoralis or hookworms may also cause flattening of the small intestinal mucosa and malabsorption, sofrietimes with a dense inflammatory infiltrate in the lamina propria of the small intestine.

It, thus, appears that many of the features of coeliac disease can be produced by protozoal and other parasitic infections. A subtotal villous atrophy of the small intestinal mucosa may result from pulmonary and intestinal tuberculosis and disappears with appropriate chemotherapy (Fung et al., 1970).

d) Ulcerative colitis

In cases of ulcerative colitis the colonic mucosal lesions are continuous and snow at first a perivascular infiltration with lymphocytes and plasma cells and later foreign body giant cells and eosinophils. The lesions are the same as those found in "auto-immune" diseases. Emphasis has been laid on the granulomatous nature of the lesions (Almy, 1961). Ulcerative colitis may be characterized by fever and all the signs of an acute infection. Its possible "auto-immune" nature has frequently been suggested (see Truelove and Wright, 1968). Thus, it may be found associated with many of the collagen or "auto-immune" diseases. It may be accompanied by peripheral arthropathy in 10-15 per cent of cases (Hollander et al., 1960; Zetzel, 1967). Many workers do not distinguish this from rheumatoid arthritis. Others deny that this is true rheumatoid arthritis (Robinson, 1967). This arthropathy can be separated into three groups (Zetzel, see also Short et al., 1957; Wright and Watkinson, 1966). In the first group the changes are those of rheumatoid arthritis or spondylitis and RF is present in the serum. This has the typical X-ray changes of rheumatoid arthritis in the joints. The severity of the arthritis does not parallel that of the colitis and may persist after removal of the colon. In the second group there is arthralgia only, varying in severity with the colitis, affecting peripheral and sacro-iliac joints and relieved by subsidence of the colitis or colectomy. RF is absent from the serum. In the third group there is a "toxic" arthritis appearing simultaneously with episodes of colitis, affecting chiefly the larger joints and relieved by improvement in the colitis. RF is absent in the blood. In still other cases ankylosing spondylitis may be found (Kinsella et al., 1970). Galbraith et al. (1964), Alarcon-Segovia et al. (1965), Brown et al. (1966) and Wright and Truelove (1966) report the association of systemic lupus erythematosus with ulcerative colitis.

Alarcon-Segovia et al. (1965) report 8 cases and cite 11 more from the literature, five of these cases had hepatitis. Galbraith et al. (1964) report systemic lupus erythematosus with ulcerative colitis and cirrhosis. Ulcerative colitis with scleroderma ho.ve been described together (Bicks et al., 1958), ulcerative colitis with scleroderma and thymoma by Miller (1971), ulcerative colitis with scleroderma, alopecia areata and vitiligo by Thompson (1974) and Tan (1974 (b)) and alopecia and ulcerative colitis by MUller and Winkelmann (1963). Sjogren's syndrome associated with ulcerative colitis was reported by Recant and Lacey (1964) and Shearn (1971).

Apart from collagen diseases, ulcerative colitis may be associated with "auto-immune" diseases. Chisholm et al. (1971) report the association of auto-immune disease of the mouth and oesophagus or thyroid with ulcerative colitis. In a personally observed case a woman of 45 years (Case 20) thyrotoxicosis preceded by 15 years the development of ulcerative colitis and there were thyroid auto-antibodies in the serum. In another case, a man, ulcerative colitis began at the age of 19 years and he developed thyrotoxicosis with ocular myopathy at 50 years and rheumatoid arthritis at 55 years when thyroid auto-antibodies were found in the serum. The author observed two other cases in which ulcerative colitis was associated with thyrotoxicosis. Hashimoto's disease with a marked blood eosinophilia was accompanied by ulcerative colitis in cases reported by White et al. (1961) and Brierly and Spears (1962) and ulcerative colitis with Hashimoto's thyroiditis by Becker et al. (1965) and Wright and Truelove (1966). Ulcerative colitis may also be associated with myasthenia gravis (Simpson, 1964; Wright and Truelove, 1966; Miller, 1971). In another patient of the author's, a Kenyan Indian, a man aged 50 years (Case 21), living in this country for the last 12 years, very extensive vitiligo, which began in Kenya, preceded the development of ulcerative colitis by some 15 years and diabetes by 16 years. The serum contained thyroid auto-antibodies. Tan (1974 a) described a case of ulcerative colitis with myasthenia gravis, atypical lichen planus, alopecia areata and vitiligo with splenomegaly and LE cells in the blood. Turner Warwick (1968) describes a case of fibrosing alveolitis in which ulcerative colitis developed five years later. Scadding (1969) also records similar cases. Ulcerative colitis associated with pernicious anaemia was reported by Edwards and Truelove (1964) and Wright and Truelove (1966). Ulcerative colitis with coeliac disease was described by Salem et al. (1964). A personal case of ulcerative colitis (Case 22) was associated with pernicious anaemia and achlorhydria and the blood contained thyroid and gastric parietal cell auto-antibodies in high concentration. In Case II. xvii, 1 a woman of 63 years, developed intrinsic asthma followed by thyrotoxicosis and pituitary chromophobe adenoma then ulcerative colitis and finally primary Addison's disease. Ulcerative colitis may also be associated with lupoid hepatitis (Mackay and Wood, 1962; Read et al., 1963; Wright and Truelove, 1966). It may also be accompanied by cirrhosis of the liver (Edwards and Truelove, 1964; Holdsworth et al., 1965; Leading Article, Brit. med. J., 1965, ii, 495). Edwards and Truelove (1964) found 16 cases of cirrhosis, usually of post-necrotic type, in 624 patients with ulcerative colitis and Holdsworth et al. (1965) 20 of 519 cases. Holdsworth et al. (1965) report four types of liver damage in cases of ulcerative colitis. One type had inactive post-necrotic cirrhosis, which was preceded by long-standing colitis. A second type had "active" cirrhosis histologically like juvenile cirrhosis. There was a short interval between the two diseases. However, liver disease may precede the ulcerative colitis by months or years (Robinson, 1967; Sherlock, 1968). The commonest change in the liver is an infiltration of the portal tracts with lympho-

cytes. Some have attributed this to portal bacteraemia (Leading Article, Lancet, 1970, 2, 402), but this does not explain how the liver disease may antedate the bowel symptoms. Perrett et al. (1971) review the literature on the liver in ulcerative colitis and found pericholangitis, post-necrotic cirrhosis, biliary cirrhosis and chronic active hepatitis may occur. They found infection with bacteria played no part. These types of hepatitis and cirrhosis are of the auto-immune type already considered. In 300 cases of ulcerative colitis ANF was present in 8.9 per cent and thyroglobulin auto-antibodies in 10.8 per cent. Wright and Truelove (1966) report that there are commonly high eosinophil counts in the blood and colonic mucosa in this condition, especially in relapse. Cases of ulcerative colitis' may develop amyloidosis (Forshaw and Moorhouse, 1964) as do cases of rheumatoid arthritis. Thus, ulcerative colitis may be associated with either collagen or "auto-immune" diseases and would appear to belong to this spectrum of diseases.

II, xxii) Collagen diseases and peritonitis

In cases of disseminated eosinophilic collagen diseases all the serous membranes, including the peritoneum, may be affected. Systemic lupus erythematosus and rheumatoid arthritis may cause inflammatory changes in the pericardium and pleura and in synovia, such as those of joints, tendon sheaths and bursae. Moreover, as described above, rheumatoid nodules may affect the peritoneum. It seems logical to suppose that collagen diseases could also produce a chronic peritoneal inflammation and adhesions and which, when pericardium and pleura are also involved, would constitute a polyserositis. It is possible that some cases of sugar icing of the spleen and liver with a similar involvement of the heart and lungs may be so produced, though this is usually thought to be due to tuberculosis. Gardner (personal communication, 1972) states that at autopsy on 142 cases of rheumatoid arthritis he found peritoneal adhesions in 10 and 8 cases with acute peritonitis and he had records of 3 cases of retroperitoneal abscess in cases of rheumatoid arthritis. He raises t he question as to whether this may go on to produce retroperitoneal fibrosis.

II, xxiii) Collagen and auto-immune disease and clubbing of fingers and toes

Clubbing of the fingers and toes is best known to occur in cases of congenital heart disease, congenital cystic disease of the lung, chronic lung infections, bacterial endocarditis and intrathoracic tumours. However, it may also occur in :-

1) some cases of rheumatoid arthritis and systemic lupus erythematosus (Short et al., 1957; Boyle and Buchanan, 1971).

2) some cases of intrinsic asthma

3) some cases of thyroid disease

4) some cases of coeliac disease

5) some cases of cirrhosis of the liver

6) some cases of ulcerative colitis

7) some cases of endocrine disease (Abrahams, 1960) .

It would thus appear to result in some cases from collagen-auto-immune disease in its various forms.

II, xxiv) Collagen diseases and the eye

Involvement of the lacrimal gland in cases of Sjogren's syndrome has been described above. It predisposes to recurrent conjunctivitis and blepharitis. Apart from Sjogren's syndrome in cases of rheumatoid arthritis, including Still's disease and systemic lupus erythematosus, the eye may exhibit *iridocyclitis* (Smiley, 1973) involving the uveal tract and also the sclera may show the lesions of *episcleritis (scleromalacia perforanes)* (Talbott and Ferrandis, 1956) and histologically these

lesions are identical with rheumatoid subcutaneous nodules. The retina may be damaged secondarily. These eye lesions may precede those of rheumatoid arthritis by many years. In some cases no evidence of rheumatoid arthritis ever develops, but the serum contains RF (see below) . Hurd et al. (1970) point out that in cases of rheumatoid arthritis, in addition to the above changes, *kerato-conjunctivitis, choroidal nodules* and *exudative detachment of the retina* may occur. Kerato-conjunctivitis is also a feature of auto-immune multi- (poly) -endocrine lesions (see above). According to Dublin (1954) the vasculitis which occurs in the collagen diseases may involve the retinal, optic and choroid arterioles with or without focal necrosis and perivascular lymphocytic infiltrations and exudates. These changes resemble those of hypersensitive retinopathy and papilloedema may occur.

II, xxv) Collagen and auto-immune diseases and malignant exophthalmos (endocrine exophthalmos)

This condition has been considered an "auto-immune" phenomenon (see Mackay and Burnet, 1963; Werver, 1972). The orbital tissues, including fat, ocular muscles and lacrimal glands, are oedematous and infiltrated with lymphocytes and plasma cells and localized germ follicles may develop. (These changes are also a regular finding in Graves' disease without eye changes or exophthalmos). Later the ocular muscles may atrophy and fibrosis may occur. The eye itself may exhibit papilloedema or panophthalmitis. This condition can occur in subjects in which the thyroid gland has been completely removed and has also developed in patients who have had complete pituitary ablation for mammary cancer (Baron and Gurling, 1959). It cannot, therefore, result from either pituitary or thyroid gland secretions in excess. It may be strickly unilateral

Addendum : Boss JM Peachey RDG, Easty DL, Thomsitt J. Peripheral corneal melting syndrome with psoriasis. A report of two cases. Brit. med. J., 1981, 282, 609-10. The syndrome consists of marginal corneal thinning, sometimes to the extent of perforation. It is often seen in rheumatoid arthritis, Sjogren's syndrome, polyarteritis nodosa or psoriasis.

Addendum: Retinal vasculitis may occr in RD and SLE or in the absence of these diseases with RF in the serum. It is possibly due to raised concentration of circulating immune complexes. Retinal vasculitis in RA. Martin MFR, Scott DGI, Gilbert C, Dieppe PA, Easty DL. Brit med J 1981 282 1745-6.

or more marked on one side, a factor pointing to a local rather than a humoral causation. It may occur in the absence of obvious endocrine disease or in association *with* hyper- or hypo-thyroidism or Hashimoto's thyroiditis and in addition has been described in association with diabetes, Addison's disease, Cushing's syndrome and cirrhosis of the liver (Brain, 1959; Harvard, 1972). The author has observed its development after local unilateral orbital trauma and bilaterally in a patient suffering from pernicious anaemia, who was euthyroid, but had thyroid auto-antibodies in the serum. He has also observed a woman of 46 years (Case 23), who developed rheumatoid arthritis followed 12 years later by Hashimoto's thyroiditis with thyrotoxicosis and severe unilateral exophthalmos. The last-named increased following thyroidectomy and later she also developed diabetes, severe eczema and underwent an operation for chronic cholecystitis and gall stones. The ocular disturbance became so severe as to constitute malignant exophthalmos and require tarsorraphy. In the serum the thyroid auto-antibodies and RF were strongly positive. In Case 24, a male of 55 years, when aged 49 years had a cholecystectomy for chronic cholecystitis and gall stones. He now shows Sjt>gren's syndrome, well-marked rheumatoid changes in the feet and exophthalmic ophthalmoplegia. The serum P.B.I. was normal. ANF but no thyroid auto-antibodies were present in the serum. Such cases and the histological changes in the orbit are in favour of exophthalmic ophthalmoplegia being a manifestation of rheumatoid disease.

II, xxvi) Collagen disease and the ear

a) The pinna

The pinna may exhibit rheumatoid nodules (see below) and may, therefore, be involved in the rheumatoid process.

b) Nerve deafness is now recognized as resulting from rheumatoid disease, even in the absence of salicylate therapy (Gardner, 1972).

c) Aural arthritis The joints between the ossicles of the middle ear may perhaps be affected in some cases of rheumatoid arthritis (Gardner, 1972) leading to conduction deafness.

d) Chronic adhesive otitis and salpingitis

In cases of chronic adhesive otitis and salpingitis there occurs an atrophy of the mucosa of the middle ear and Eustachian tube with failure of mucus secretion. As a consequence the tympanic membrane adheres to the medial wall of the middle ear and the lumen of the Eustachian tube becomes blocked. These processes may result in a dysplasia of the mucosal lining of the tube and inner ear, which may become squamous in character and may result in the development of a cholesteatoma of the inner ear.

Clinically it manifests itself by conduction deafness of slow onset and the tympanic membrane can be seen *to* be indrawn and adherent to the medial wall of the middle ear. Eustachian catheterization may in early cases relieve the deafness, but afterwards is ineffective. These changes are not infrequently an extension of the changes of atrophic rhinitis from the nasal mucosa along the Eustachian tube to the middle ear. In some cases this atrophic rhinitis can be observed to be associated with Sjogren's syndrome or with other complications of this syndrome, such as atrophic pharyngitis, laryngitis, tracheo-bronchitis, oesophagitis a nd gastritis (see above). The author has also observed this condition as complicating rheumatoid arthritis in a number of cases and, in the absence of other causes, it would appear to be part of rheumatoid disease.

e) "Catarrhal" deafness

The pharyngeal and nasal mucosa and that of the Eustachian tube may exhibit chronic inflammatory changes and oedema, often accompanied by swelling and chronic inflammatory changes in the tonsils and adenoids as part of collagen and auto-immune disease affecting the upper respiratory tract. This often precedes the atrophic changes mentioned above. Not infrequently this leads to a chronic form of conduction deafness. In less severe cases slowly progressive conduction deafness develops with age in association with various manifestations of collagen diseases and constitutes so-called catarrhal deafness. This change is the fundamental disturbance in presbyacusis.

It appears, therefore, that deafness of different types is a frequent manifestation of collagen and auto-immune disease. This may well have been so in the case of the deafness of Beethoven, who suffered from ulcerative colitis with liver disease over many years.

II, xxvii) Collagen and "auto-immune" disease, the central nervous system and peripheral nerves

It has been mentioned above that the dura mater may exhibit rheumatoid nodules in rheumatoid disease and these may occur extradurally and subdurally too. Within the central nervous system itself widespread changes may be found in the collagen diseases. They are found in the cortex, corpus striatum, subthalamic nuclei and the substantia· nigra. Usually the brain-stem is only slightly involved. These are described at length by Dublin (1954). They consist of :–

1) Epithelioid and reticulum cell inflammatory reaction with varying admixture of lymphocytes with or without necrosis.

2) Vascular changes consisting of endarteritis of the smaller arterioles with obliterative proliferation of the vascular epithelium with perivascular lymphocytic infiltration leading to thrombosis and areas of infarction. The venules may be involved and these changes may extend to cause thrombosis of the dural sinuses.

3) Fibrinoid necrosis of the vessel walls and of collagen change seen especially in

systemic lupus erythematosus.

In all such cerebral disturbances accompanying collagen or auto-immune disease the cerebrospinal fluid may contain an increased amount of protein and a few lymphocytes and may show an irregular gold reaction (Dublin, 1954).

In cases of systemic lupus erythematosus, rheumatoid arthritis and Sjogren's syndrome, dermatomyositis, etc., these changes produce many different *neurological symptoms,* which include diplopia, nystagmus, hemiplegia, hemianaeathesia "f and hemianopia (Sheldon, 1939; Dublin, 1954; Ramage and Kinnear, 1956; Heaton, 1959, 1962; Shearn, 1971). An observation which may or may not be significant is that of the association of paralysis agitans with rheumatoid arthritis. In Case 1 described above, which exhibited menstrual disturbance, diabetes, rheumatoid arthritis, Sjogren's syndrome, myxoedema and pernicious anaemia, the patient eventually developed Parkinsonism, while of the 100 cases of rheumatoid arthritis in the geriatric unit series cited previously no less than 10 developed it.

Migraine frequently results from long-sustained contraction of skeletal muscles about the face, scalp and neck (Plum, 1971). Reference has been made above to the involvement of the cervical spine in cases of rheumatoid disease and with this there is associated spasm of the cervical muscles. In addition fibrositis of the cervical tissues is a common manifestation of rheumatoid disease. Migraine is thus a frequent accompaniment of rheumatoid disease and in the experience of the author, can often be dramatically relieved in such cases by the administration of anti-rheumatoid drugs, such as chloroquine.

In addition various *mental disturbances* may exist in association with these pathological changes in the brain in cases of rheumatoid arthritis (Duthie, 1969), dermatomyositis (Talbott and Ferrandis, 1956) and Sjogren's syndrome (Pearson, 1961; Shearn, 1971). These mental dis-

Addendum: Relapsing polychondritis. This condition appears to be "auto-immune" in nature (Clayton, R.N. and Hoffenberg, R., Brit. med. J., 1978, 2. 999). It may affect aural, nasal, trachael and articular cartilage producing deafness and arthropathy. It may be associated with Hashimoto's thyroiditis with myxoedema, goitre, expohthalmos and ophthalmoplegia. diabetes mellitus, vitiligo and arthropathy. Auto-antibodies to human cartilage, thryoglobulin, intrinsic factor and gastric parietal cells may be present in the serum.

turbances include anxieties, obsessional and paranoid reactions and psychotic states. Dublin (1954) described headache, photophobia, irritability, delirium, clouding of the sensorium, delusions, hallucinations, intellectual deterioration, convulsions and coma. Pearson (1961) and Shearn (1971) both described epilepsy, mental changes and psychoneurosis accompanying Sjogren's syndrome. Simpson (1964) reported epilepsy or psychoses accompanying myasthenia. Coeliac disease developing schizophrenia was described by Lancaster-Smith and Strickland (1970). Alopecia universalis may also be accompanied by mental changes and in the author's experience may be associated with schizophrenia as already mentioned.

A case under the author's care appears to show the importance of collagen-auto-immune disease in the production of mental disturbances. A man aged 55 years gave a history of being withdrawn during adolescence and given to fantasies and sexual perversions. Intellectually he was above average. He was called up into the army and discharged 3 years later with anxiety symptoms, periods of amnesia and wild sexual thoughts and perversions. He had periods of depression. At the age of 42 years *vitiligo* appeared and rapidly became generalized and at the age of 52 years he was found to have Arlie's syndrome with absence of the left ankle jerk. He showed profuse sweating. Examination at this time showed well-marked obsessional traits, depression and hyperidrosis, complete loss of pigment from the skin, an absent left ankle jerk, drooping of the left shoulder, tilting of the head to the right and atrophy of the posterior cervical muscles. The cerebrospinal fluid contained 100 mgms. of protein per cent, the W.R. was negative; F.B.I. 6.4 *JLg* per cent; the serum showed the presence of thyroid and gastric parietal cell auto-antibodies; achlorhydria was present, blood count and E.S.R. were normal. This patient appears to show the association of neurological

and mental disturbance with collagen-auto-immune disease.

A *mononeuropathy* may occur in cases of rheumatoid arthritis, systemic lupus erythematosus or Sjogren's syndrome (Hills, 1967; Kalkreider and Talal, 1969; Shearn, 1971). This is usually attributed to an arteritis of the vasa nervorum. Nerve deafness is now recognized as a complication of rheumatoid disease, even in the absence of salicylate therapy (Gardner, 1972).

A *symmetrical peripheral neuropathy* may also occur in any of the collagen diseases, including rheumatoid arthritis, systemic lupus erythematosus, scleroderma, polymyositis (see Dublin, 1954) and in association with Sjogren's syndrome (Hills, 1967; Kalkreider and Talal, 1969; Shearn, 1971) or in association with various mixed "auto-immune" diseases (Mason and Golding, 1970 a). This neuropathy may involve the autonomic nervous system as well as the peripheral nerves. Unlike the mononeuropathies the symmetrical peripheral neuropathy in this condition is not necessarily due to arteritis of the nutrient vessels of the peripheral nerves, but to other causes (Scott, 1969; Chamberlain and Bruckner, 1970). An arteritis of the nutrient vessels of the nerve does not explain the involvement of the autonomic system which may occur in these conditions. Furthermore, an identical peripheral neuropathy occurs in association with auto-immune diseases not accompanied by arteritis (Mason and Golding, 1970 a). Shearn (1971) mentions that infiltrations of the nerve sheaths with lymphocytes may be observed, corresponding with the changes found in other tissues in collagen and auto-immune diseases, while Gardner (1969) observes that rheumatoid nodules may involve the peripheral nerves, Duthie (1954) records that the peripheral nerves show obliterative proliferation of the endothelium of the small arteries supplying the nerves and also regular interstitial infiltration of the nerves with lymphocytes, especially about the vessels, and occurring diffusely in the nerves. Beckett and Dinn (1972) report that segmental demyelination of the peripheral nerves appears to be a fundamental nerve abnormality in rheumatoid arthritis. Only in more severe cases with superimposed arterial occlusion does Wallerian degeneration appear.

The *Guillain-Barre syndrome* is generally considered to be a form of auto-immune disease and may be found in association with other forms of auto-immune disease, such as thyrotoxicosis in one of the author's cases (Case 25).

In diabetes mellitus, which appears in many cases to be associated with collagen or auto-immune disease, a symmetrical peripheral polyneuropathy may also occur. This also affects the autonomic system. This again is to be distinguished from the mononeuropathy ascribed to vascular lesions in a nutrient vessel to the affected nerve. However, in this condition also the symmetrical peripheral polyneuropathy has been ascribed to vasculitis of the vessels supplying the peripheral nerves. If the disturbance is of long-standing, the nerves show segmental demyelination as in cases of rheumatoid arthritis. These changes are commonly said to be found in long-standing severe or poorly controlled diabetes (Hills, 1967), but this is by no means always the case. The condition may worsen despite adequate treatment of the diabetes. These diabetic peripheral neural lesions may be identical in nature with those occurring in other collagen-auto-immune diseases, such as rheumatoid arthritis. It is tempting to suppose that the symmetrical peripheral neuropathy is related to the causative agent of the collagen-auto-immune disease.

U, xxviii) Collagen and auto-immune disease and various disorders of the blood

In collagen and auto-immune diseases changes in the blood corpuscles are very varied.

A. Changes in the red corpuscles include:-

a) Hypochromic normocytic anaemia
This is due to depression of erythropoiesis in the bone marrow.

b) Hypochromic microcytic anaemia
This is due to iron deficiency and is usually associated with atrophic gastritis.

c) Pernicious anaemia
Pernicious anaemia is a complication of atrophic gastritis, which is itself one of the best known "auto-immune" diseases. As has been seen it can occur in association with any other form of "auto-immune" or collagen disease.

d) Auto-immune haemolytic anaemia
Auto-immune haemolytic anaemia may occur associated with the collagen-auto-immune diseases, including rheumatoid arthritis, systemic lupus erythematosus, arteritis, scleroderma, dermatomyositis, Sjogren's syndrome (Shearn, 1971), thymic hypertrophy and tumours, ulcerative colitis, cirrhosis, fibrosing alveolitis (Mackay and Ritchie, 1065), Hashimoto's thyroiditis (Becker et al., 1965) and hypert hyroidism (Dacie, 1962; see Young, 1967; Wintrobe, 1967) and with paraproteinaemia (see below). In other cases this type of anaemia may occur in the absence of evidence of collagen-auto-immune disease. The spleen may be enlarged and a direct Coombs test in the serum may be positive. The blood contains auto-antibodies to red blood corpuscles or to other organs or RF or ANF or cryoglobulins may be present (Tan and Chaplin, 1968). Eventually some form of collagen-auto-immune disease may appear. This type of anaemia may antedate the development of the collagen-auto-immune disease by months or years. In one of the author's cases, a woman of 65 years, (Case 26), a persistent auto-immune haemolytic anaemia had been present for 12 years. Achlorhydria was present. The blood contained cryoglobulins, thyroid auto-antibod-

ies in high concentration and RF. After 10 years she developFd polyarteritis and 2 years later she died of carcinoma of the stomach, which showed at rophic gastritis. Auto-immune haemolytic anaemia of a similar type may occur in many infections, including malaria, when they are also associated w ith splenomegaly, suggesting the possibility that collagen-auto-immune diseases with their associated auto-immune haemolytic anaemia may also be infective in origin.

e) Chronic "idiopathic" pure red cell aplasia

Pure red cell aplasia is discussed by Mitchell (1973). It may occur following exposure to certain chemicals or drugs or infections and in cases of uraemia and may complicate haemolytic anaemias.

Chronic "idiopathic" pure red cell aplasia has been thought to be of "auto-immune" origin (see Mitchell). In adults it has been described in association with benign thymomas (see above, and Wintrobe, 1967) and it may also occur in the absence of thymoma. In both cases there is a selective depression of erythropoiesis, but leucopenia and/or thrombocytopenia may develop later. a) In the former group myasthenia may also be present. Thymectomy usually has no effect on the anaemia. In one case thymectomy was followed three years later by pure red cell aplasia. Thus, the anaemia does not seem to be due to the tumour. In view of the relationship of thymic tumours to collagen-auto-immune disease described above and the usual persistence of the anaemia after thymectomy it would seem that the red cell aplasia like the thymic tumours may be evidence of an "auto-immune" disease. b) In the second group splenomegaly may be present and various "auto-immune" manifestations may be seen, such as an auto-immune haemolytic anaemia (Eisemann and Damashek, 1954) or the presence of ANF in the serum (Vilan et al., 1971), or immunosuppressive therapy may be beneficial or curative (Vilan et al., 1971;

(Literature)). l'his again suggests that the bone marrow disturbances are "auto-immune" in nature. In either type of red cell aplasia the basis would seem to be related to "auto-immune" disease.

B. Changes in the white blood cells

Changes in the number of white blood corpuscles in the blood are also of varying nature (see Wintrobe, 1967). Commonly in cases of rheumatoid arthritis t here occurs:-

a) A *neutrophil leucocytosis* typical of many infections.

b) In other cases, especially in cases of Felty's syndrome and systemic lupus erythematosus, there is found a *neutro phil leucopenia.*

c) In some cases of rheumatoid arthritis and also in association with lymphocytic thyroiditis and thyrotoxicosis a *lymphocy*tosis can be observed. Such a change again is one which may be observed in many different infections.

d) Conversely there may be a *lymphopenia,* seen especially in the pancytopenia of Felty's syndrome and systemic lupus erythematosus.

e) Again a monocytosis may sometimes be observed in cases of rheumatoid arthritis.

f) The blood may show an *eosinophilia* of up to 43 per cent in cases of rheumatoid arthritis (Short et al., 1957; Wintrobe, 1967). In cases of disseminated eosinophilic collagen disease (see above) an extreme eosinophilia may be found. A high eosinophilia is not uncommon in the collagen diseases when polyarthritis is present (Wintrobe, 1967). A similar eosinophilia is common in dermatomyositis and also in Sjogren's syndrome, where it occurs also in the oral mucus. In cases of pernicious anaemia an eosinophilia of up to 60 per cent may occur, even before the introduction of liver therapy (Levine and Ladd, 1921; Wintrobe, 1967). A high eosinophilia may occur in various "auto-immune" skin diseases, including pemphigus, dermatitis herpetiformis, psoriasis

Addendum: Pure red cell aplasia may be associated with SLE, thymoma, autoimmune hypothyroidism or multiple endocrine i nsufficiency.

and ichthyosis acquisita (Wintrobe, 1967). An eosinophilia may also occur in other manifestations of collagen-auto-immune disease, such as ulcerative colitis (Wright and Truelove, 1966) and Paget's disease (Whitby and Britton, 1950). Hashimoto's thyroiditis with ulcerative colitis and a high blood eosinophilia was described by Brearley and Spiers (1962). Eosinophilia may also be found in cases of Waldenstrom's macroglobulinaemia (Osserman, 1971) (see below). In cases of disseminated eosinophilic collagen disease the blood changes may develop into those of chronic myeloid leukaemia with or without chloroma, myeloblastoma or lymphoma.

C. Changes in the number of thrombocytes

a) *Thrombocytopenia:* with purpura and sometimes with splenomegaly or auto-immune haemolytic anaemia (Evans syndrome) may occur in various collagen diseases (see Wintrobe, 1967), including systemic lupus erythematosus (Taylor, 1970) and Sjogren's syndrome (Futcher, 1959; Pearson, 1961; Shearn, 1971). In cases of systemic lupus erythematosus and Felty's syndrome thrombocytopenia forms part of a pancytopenia. In some cases the thrombocytopenia may antedate by a considerable period signs of collagen disease. Levine and Shearn (1964) showed that 23 per cent of cases of thrombocytopenic purpura had evidence of systemic lupus erythematosus. Thrombocytopenia may also occur in cases of Hashimoto's thyroiditis (Becker et al., 1965), thyrotoxicosis, aplastic anaemia, pernicious anaemia, auto-immune haemolytic anaemia and myelofibrosis (Wintrobe, 1967). In some cases the associated purpura may come and go and such cyclic thrombocytopenia associated with multiple auto-antibodies in the serum was reported by Brey et al. (1969). Thus, thrombocytopenia is not uncommonly a manifestation of collagen and auto-immune disease.

b) *Thrombocytosis* (thrombocythaemia). This may occur in cases of rheumatoid arthritis and other collagen diseases and cases of polycythaemia (Wintrobe, 1967). The author has observed a case of Hashimoto's thyroiditis in which thrombocytosis occurred.

D. Changes in all the blood cells at the same time

a) Pancytopenia

In cases of Felty's syndrome or systemic lupus erythematosus there may occur an *anaemia, leucopenia* and *thrombocytopenia* due to depression of haematopoiesis as well as hypersplenism. Pancytopenia arising in the absence of exposure to chemicals, toxins or known infections is commonly a manifestation of a collagen disease. These changes may merge into those of leukaemia. Rosenthal et al. (1974) found specific IgG antibodies against white blood cells in 13 of 15 patients with Felty's syndrome. They suggested the antibodies were responsible for the neutropenia and a similar mechanism for the frequently associated thrombocytopenia.

b) Polycythaemia vera (erythraemia)

Polycythaemia vera is to be distinguished from polycythaemia secondary to anoxia and from that sometimes found secondary to certain tumours. In the last type polycythaemia appears to be due to liberation from the tumour of an erythropoietin-like substance and disappears with removal of the tumour. Polycythaemia vera is often associated with leucocytosis and thrombocytosis and the bone marrow shows hyperplasia of all the blood-forming elements. Occasionally, however, the polycythaemia is associated with leucopenia or thrombocytopenia. There is no evidence that excess of erythropoietin in the cirulation is responsible for this condition (Wintrobe, 1967). Polycythaemia vera may be accompanied by hypertension or splenomegaly and by non-alcoholic cirrhosis, presumably due to engorgement of the blood vessels of the liver.

Sometimes evidence of "auto-immune" disease may precede or accompany the

-71

Addendum: Waugh, D., Ibels, L. Malignant scleroderma associated with autoimmune neutropenia. Brit. med. J., 1980, 280, 1577-8 reported a case of scleroderma developing autoimmune neutropenia and mentioned that autoimmune haemolytic anaemia, thrombocytopenia and pancytopenia may occur in patients with scleroderma.

condition. Thus, Zadek (1927) reported its association with thyrotoxicosis. There is a significant association with atrophic gastritis and pernicious anaemia (Freund, 1919; Galt et al., 1952; Hinz, 1957; Engel and Stickney, 1962; Busse and Paulyn, 1965; Douglas and Rifkind, 1966; Wintrobe, 1967; England et al., 1968; Hume and Adams, 1968; Watkins, 1970). Up to 1968 more than 40 cases of this association had been reported. Polycythaemia may be preceded by, alternate with, be associated with or end in atrophic gastritis with pernicious anaemia. Hume and Adams (1968) studied 16 cases of polycythaemia, of which 2 had pernicious anaemia. They found a generally low acid secretion in the stomach in their cases and an achlorhydria in the two cases with pernicious anaemia. In three cases, including the two with pernicious anaemia, gastric parietal cell auto-antibodies were present in the blood. They point to a tendency to the development of atrophic gastritis in this condition. Up to 1968 more than 40 cases of polycythaemia associated with perntclous anaemia in the literature up to that time in 35 the polycythaemia became apparent after the treatment of pernicious anaemia. They found the incidence of gastric parietal cell auto-antibodies was not significantly increased as compared with controls, but they did not investigate the occurrence of other serum auto-antibodies. In the series of diabetics investigated by Munichoodatta and Kozac (1970) there occurred three cases of diabetes associated with pernicious anaemia developing polycythaemia. Polycythaemia may also be accompanied by Mikulicz's syndrome (Aird, 1958).

Richmond et al. (1956) report a significant increase in normal red cell precursors in the bone marrow in cases of rheumatoid arthritis. In the 100 cases of rheumatoid arthritis in the geriatric series reported previously, two were associated with polycythaemia and achlorhydria was present in both. In Case 12 of rheumatoid arthritis accompanied by nephritis, hypertension, Paget's disease of bone and multiple lipomata polycythaemia was also present. Chisholm et al. (1971) described the association of post-cricoid oesophageal webs and "auto-immune" diseases affecting the mouth and thyroid with polycythaemia vera.

The author investigated every case of polycythaemia vera observed over a number of years both as regards the clinical association of the condition and as regards the presence of achlorhydria (indicative of atrophic gastritis) and of various serum auto-antibodies, including RF, A NF, gas·tric parietal cells and thyroid auto-antibodies of various types and the level of the P.B.I. in the serum. They are briefly summarized below in Table IV.

Of the 40 cases all showed clinical evidence of some associated collagen or a uto·immune disease perhaps only in the presence of achlorhydria indicative of atrophic gastritis or in the presence of various organ specific or non-specific auto-antibodies in the serum. One case had had an operation for fibroids, one for bilateral benign ovarian cysts and one for an adenoma of the larynx. Two developed carcinoma of the bronch us and one of t he stomach. One case of seropositive rheumatoid arthritis, aged 50 years, was found to have polycythaemia, the blood haemoglobin level being 20.8 G per 100 mls and the PCV 61 per cent. He was treated with aspirin and prednisolone 5 mgms. twice daily for a year. The joint manifestations gradually disappeared and with this the blood haemoglobin level fell to 15.0 G per 100 mls. The evidence is in accord with the conclusion that polycythaemia vera is usually associated with evidence of collagen or auto-immune disease and is "guilty by association" of being part of the spectrum of these diseases.

E. Von Willebrand's disease

Poole-Wilson (1972) describes a case of systemic lupus erythematosus which developed Von Willebrand's disease and cites

Table IV

Case	Sex	Age	Presentation	Associated collagen and auto-immune	Presence of benign or malignant tumour	Presence of achlorhydria	Serum auto-antibodies
IV, 1	M	62	One years history of generalized pains and mild *arthropathy*.			+	ANF
IV, 2	F	77	Acute bronchitis. Mild *rheumatoid arthritis*.	Operation for *thyrotoxicosis*.		+	Thyroid
IV, 3	M	55	Dyspnoea. Known polycythaemia for 10 years. Recurrent attacks of bronchitis.				ANF
IV, 4	M	65	Hypertensive heart failure. Atrial fibrillation. *Rheumatoid nodules, mild rheumatoid arthritic deformity.*			+	ANF
IV, 5	M	69	Recurrent peptic ulcer symptoms	*Thyroidectomy for thyrotoxicosis aged 45 years. Aged 45–9 years acute rheumatoid arthropathy.*	Adenoma of the larynx		Thyroid
IV, 6	M	50	Oedema of feet. Polyarthropathy.	*Chronic active hepatitis. Mild rheumatoid arthritis.*		+	Thyroid Gastric parietal cell
IV, 7	F	62	Heart failure. Cerebral thrombosis. *Iron deficiency anaemia* found. Treatment resulted in polycythaemia.			+	RF Thyroid Gastric parietal cell
IV, 8	M	68	Moderate cigarette smoker. Ten years history of gout. Developed hypertension and recurrent thrombophlebitis.		Carcinoma of right lower lobe bronchus.		ANF Thyroid Gastric parietal cell
IV, 9	F	45	*Acute rheumatoid arthritis*. Irregular periods.		Aged 28 years operation for bilateral benign ovarian cysts.		RF
IV, 10	M	50	Under treatment for moderately severe *rheumatoid arthritis* for 10 years.	During disease developed *leucoderma* of wrists and neck and *alopecia areata*.			RF Thyroid

Table IV (continued)

IV. 11	F	59	Known polycythaemia for ten years. Recurrent epistaxes, haematemesis and thrombophlebitis. Mild *rheumatoid arthritis* present.	Operation for fibroids three years previously	+	Thyroid Gastric parietal cell
IV. 12	M	53	Recurrent peptic ulcer symptoms for 15 years. Later gout. Splenomegaly present.		+	Gastric parietal cell
IV. 13	M	53	*Psoriasis* for 20 years with mild *arthropathic symptoms*.			Thyroid ANF
IV. 14	M	54	Prostatism. Treated with Vitamin with development of polycythaemia.	Diagnosed as *pernicious anaemia* aged 57 years. Only intermittent treatment.	+	Thyroid B_{12} Gastric parietal cell
IV. 15	M	46	Recurrent thrombophlebitis during which found to have splenomegaly.	*Iron deficiency anaemia* treated with iron tablets and developed polycythaemia and postnecrotic cirrhosis	+	ANF Gastric parietal cell
IV. 16	M	70	Twenty years history of *pernicious anaemia*. Sporadic treatment. Presented with macrocytic anaemia and mild *hypothyroidism*. Treatment resulted in polycythaemia.		+	Thyroid Gastric parietal cell
IV. 17	M	70	Cerebral thrombosis. Found to be polycythaemic.	*Diabetes*	+	ANF Thyroid Gastric parietal cell
IV. 18	F	48	Known polycythaemic since age of 30 years. Presented with purpura and found to be hypertensive with polycythaemia.		+	ANF Thyroid Gastric parietal cell
IV. 19	M	71	Known polycythaemic for 20 years. Presented with dyspnoea and found to be suffering from *Pernicious anaemia*.	*Alopecia universalis* since aged 30 years. *Chronic active hepatitis* discovered.	+	ANF Gastric parietal cell
IV. 20	M	53	Jaundice		—	Very high titre of **thyroid**

Table IV (continued)

Case	Sex	Age	Clinical	Diagnosis	Notes		Antibody
IV. 21	M	50	Routine examination.				Thyroid
IV. 22	F	66	Eight years history of dyspnoea	*Pernicious anaemia* alternating with polycythaemia		+	Gastric parietal cell
IV. 23	M	53	Recurrent attacks of kerato-conjunctivitis	*Diabetes*			Thyroid
IV. 24	M	49	Left hemiplegia				ANF
IV. 25	F	55	Non-smoker. Known severe polycythaemia for 8 years.		Now had bronchial carcinoma	+	ANF / Thyroid
IV. 26	M	60	Under active treatment for moderately *severe rheumatoid arthritis* for 3 years.	*Psoriasis* for many years.		+	RF-it
IV. 27	M	81	Dysplasia found to be due to coco-phageal pouch. Long-standing moderately *severe rheumatoid arthritis* present.			+	ANF
IV. 28	F	55	Headache				RF / Thyroid
IV. ??	?	??	Hands and feet showed well-marked *rheumatoid arthritis.*			+	
IV. 30	M	62	History of two coronary thromboses			+	Gastric parietal cell
VI. 31	M	42	Headaches	*Psoriasis* since aged 14 years, *joint pains and swelling*			
IV. 32	F	55	Known polycythaemic for 10 years.	*Intrinsic asthma* for 5 years			RF / Thyroid
IV. 33	M	58	Dyspnoea on exertion				Thyroid
IV. 34	M	69	Tiredness and sleepiness	*Myxoedema* after treatment of which developed polycyth-aemia			Thyroid

<table>
<tr><td colspan="5">Table IV (continued)</td></tr>
<tr><td>IV, 35</td><td>Headache and dyspnoea</td><td></td><td>+</td><td>ANF</td></tr>
<tr><td>IV, 36</td><td>Headache</td><td></td><td>+</td><td>Thyroid</td></tr>
<tr><td>IV, 37</td><td>Recurrent polycythaemia since aged 34 years. Recurrent peptic ulcer symptoms.</td><td></td><td></td><td>RF
ANF</td></tr>
<tr><td></td><td>Long history of polycythaemia presenting with digestive disturbance</td><td>Carcinoma of stomach</td><td>+</td><td>Thyroid
Gastric parietal cell</td></tr>
<tr><td></td><td>Farm worker. Always high colour. Multiple keratoses on face and neck. Eight years ago rodent ulcer of left chest. Now polycythaemia. Rheumatoid arthritis of knuckles.</td><td></td><td>+</td><td>ANF</td></tr>
<tr><td></td><td>Indian Sikh. Myxoedema. Gout. Hypertension. Chronic dermatitis. Polycythaemia.</td><td></td><td></td><td>Thyroid</td></tr>
</table>

6 cases from the literature.

F. Myelofibrosis **and** myelosclerosis

Myelofibrosis and myelosclerosis are characterized by fibrotic or sclerotic bone marrow, in which the marrow spaces are replaced by a loose, fairly cellular connective tissue. The bones surrounding the marrow show increase in the number of bony trabeculae. *In* the connective tissue a few small islands of haemopoietic tissue often persist. The spleen is usually enlarged, sometimes enormously, and in some cases a generalized lymphadenopathy is present. Anaemia is usual or sometimes polycythaemia exists. The number of blood leucocytes may be normal or greatly elevated and immature forms may b present. Thrombocytopenia may be found. Immature myeloid cells are present in the spleen, liver and lymph nodes in the acute blastic phase of the disease. The enormous splenic enlargement may antedate other changes by many years (15 in one of the author's cases), even when the bone marrow is cellular and myelofibrosis may be a late development. Removal of the spleen is not followed by the disastrous consequences which would be expected if the organ was compensating for bone marrow destruction. Some cases of polycythaemia have terminated in myelofibrosis (Green et al., 1953; Wintrobe, 1967; Moore, 1967) or pernicious anaemia may later develop into myelofibrosis (Blackburn et al., 1968).

It has been postulated (see Wintrobe, 1967) that the marrow changes represent a mesenchymal reaction to injury or necrosis and an analogy with cirrhosis of the liver has been drawn. Only rarely is a cause for the myelofibrosis found, such as exposure to radiation, benzine, fluorine 0r phosphorus or tuberculosis or carcinomatous metastases in the marrow. In the "idiopathic" cases it would seem significant that cases may develop in subjects of preexisting polycythaemia or pernicious anaemia, suggesting a relationship to collagen and auto-immune disease and the splenomegaly which may be found early in the absence of myelofibrosis suggests the possibility of an infective agent as producing the splenic enlargement and the damage to the bone marrow.

G. Allergic (Henoch-Schonlein) purpura

Allergic or Henoch-Schonlein purpura is considered by Wintrobe (1967) and its features in adults by Cream et a!. (1970). Any tissue may be affected by the purpura and in addition there may be oedemas, angioneurotic oedema, urticarial wheals, rheumatoid pains, asthma and a blood eosinophilia, tenderness and joint swelling, headaches and pyrexia. Histologically the affected tissues exhibit perivascular collections of lymphocytes and a necrotizing arteriolitis, changes which are typical of those occurring in collagen diseases and, in fact, the condition has been related to polyarteritis and collagen diseases. In adult patients followed by Cream et a!. (1970) many of them later exhibited manifestations of collagen auto-immune disease. These manifestations included the presence of RF in the blood; Raynaud's phenomenon and hyperglobulinaemia; widespread visceral vasculitis; RF and ANF in the serum; elevated IgM in the serum; chronic hepatitis, cryoglobulinaemia and immune complex nephritis; late appearing polyarthritis with positive lupus erythematosus cells and ANF in the blood. No haemopoietic disturbances are present, but the oedemas and purpuras appear to result from an increased capillary permeability. It has been found that an abnormal factor is present in the serum and this gives rise to purpura experimentally.

The onset of symptoms may be precipitated by certain foods and infections and by hypersensitivity to various agents. A girl of 17 years with this disease under the author's care had a severe allergic reaction to penicillin, which was also shown by her two brothers and her mother. Both brothers suffered from intrinsic asthma and were allergic to aspirin and other substances.

It appears that allergic purpura may, in fact, be a feature of collagen and auto-immune disease in which damage to the capillary walls occurs.

II, xxix) Collagen and auto-immune disease and the bone marrow

In cases of polycythaemia there is increase in activity of all cell elements in the bone marrow in contrast to the decrease in such activity in cases of pancytopenia. In cases of collagen and auto-immune disease the marrow may also exhibit an infiltration with eosinophils, especially noteworthy in cases of disseminated eosinophilic collagen disease, but also in other manifestations of these conditions in whic.h a blood eosinophilia is found. *Lymphoid follicles* are also abnormally frequent in the marrow in cases of rheumatoid arthritis (Gardner, 1968). A *plasmacytosis* as well as immature plasma cells may be found in the bone marrow accompanied by diffuse hypergammaglobulinaemia or monoclonal gammopathy in the blood may be found in the following conditions (Evans, 1966; Gardner, 1968, 1972; Wegelius et al., 1970; Osserman, 1971):-

1) Chronic infections, such as tuberculosis, syphilis, osteomyelitis and in infections mononucleosis, where they are a response to chronic antigenic stimulation.

2) Cases of rheumatoid arthritis and systemic lupus erythematosus.

3) Cirrhosis of various types.

4) Hodgkin's disease and myelomatosis.

This raises the possibility that collagen diseases (and, in fact, Hodgkin's disease and myelomatosis) may be due to a chronic infection.

II, xxx) Collagen and "auto-immune" disease and paraproteinaemia

Polyclonal hypergammaglobulinaemia is commonly found in chronic infections and occasionally in such infections the poly-

Addendum: Acquired haemophilia. Leading Article, Lancet 1981, i, 255. This condition may occur especially in elderly females. There is a well recognized association with autoimmune or allergic diseases, including rheumatoid art hritis and other collagen-vascular diseases, cancer, pemphigus, ulcerative colitis and asthma or as a side effect of drug therapy. The blood contains a circulating anticoag ulant with special activity against Factor VIII in the blood. It is an antibody usually of the IgG class and evidently arises in response to the organism producing rheumatoid and autoimmune diseases. Acquired haemophilia. Duran-Suarez JR, Pigrau-Serrallach C, Bosch-Gil JA, Triginer-Boixeda J, Lancet 1981, i, 723. report that 46 of 6,000 patients had circulating anticoagulants. (against Factor VIII in 27) 8 of these 27 patients had acquired haemophilia and the rest had other diseases, including active chronic hepatitis, SLE and cancer.

clonal type may change into a monoclonal type with a significant M-band (Hallen, 1966; Hobbs, 1966). Wintrobe (1967) and Osserman (1971) report such a monoclonal hypergammaglobulinaemia (paraproteinaemia) or macroglobulinaemia as occurring in chronic infections, such as tuberculosis, syphilis, congenital syphilis, kala-azar, toxoplasmosis and malaria. A macroglobulinaemia of monoclonal type was found. in a case of juvenile syphilis reported by Fran ois et al. (1966). This disappeared after treatment of the disease. These blood changes are accompanied by plasmacytosis in the bone marrow. Polyclonal hypergammaglobulinaemia is also common in collagen diseases and Hashimoto's thyroiditis. Moreover, in some cases of rheumatoid arthritis, systemic lupus erythematosus and arteritis discrete (monoclonal) gammaglobulin M-components similar to those found in myelomatosis may be found in the serum by electrophoresis (Hallen, 1966). Dryll et al. (1969) found such an abnormal protein present in the serum in 6 cases of rheumatoid arthritis and 2 of scleroderma. In no case were there any signs of myeloma. In one case of rheumatoid arthritis lasting 30 years the results of electrophoresis changed from polyclonal hypergammaglobulinaemia to those of an abnormal monoclonal IgM. Zawadski and Benedek (1969) report 8 cases of rheumatoid arthritis with asymptomatic paraproteinaemia (monoclonal) and one case with heavy-chain disease and one with Waldenstrom's macroglobulinaemia. Zawadski et al. (1969) described the case of a male negro of 42 years who developed rheumatoid arthritis and at the age of 51 years heavy-chain disease. No malignant tumour was found. Druet et al. (1969) found 7 cases of sero-positive rheumatoid arthritis with a monoclonal gammopathy and Hallen (1966) records a similar condition in a case of rheumatoid arthritis with Sjogren's syndrome. Sirridge (1960), Gothani et a!. (1965) (2 cases), McFarlan and Nwokolo (1966), Miller (1967), Goldenburg et al.

(1969) (2 cases) and Wegelius et al. (1970) all describe similar cases of rheumatoid arthritis with paraproteinaemia or macroglobulinaemia developing at a later date. In Zawadski and Benedek's series of 8 cases the onset of symptoms of rheumatoid arthritis antedated the finding of paraproteinaemia by 1-14 years. Wintrobe (1967) also records Bence-Janes proteinuria as occurring in some cases of systemic lupus erythematosus. Meltzer and Franklin (1966) describe cases of systemic lupus erythematosus, rheumatoid arthritis and other collagen diseases with paraproteinaemia and with RF and ANF in the blood. Bonomo et al. (1970) report 5 cases of Waldenstrom's macroglobulinaemia with cryoglobulinaemia and very high levels of RF in the serum associated with IgM paraproteinaemia. In almost all the above cases the RF present in the blood in high concentration was associated with the IgM fraction. Shearn (1971) mentions that Waldenstrom's macroglobulinaemia may be associated with rheumatoid arthritis, Raynaud's phenomena, myositis, arteritis, nephropathy or the presence of lupus erythematosus cells in the blood. Linquette et al. (1967), Oka (1969) and Warin (1973) report patients with scleroderma who exhibited paraproteinaemia.

Sjogren's syndrome, which is a manifestation of rheumatoid disease, may also be associated with the presence in the serum of monoclonal immunoglobulin spikes of the 7S variety or with macroglobulinaemia with or without Bence-Janes proteinuria (Shearn, 1971; Grundy, 1971). Talal and Bunim (1964) followed 58 patients with Sj5gren's syndrome over 4 years and one developed Waldenstrom's macroglobulinaemia. Nover and Glees (1966) recorded a similar case. Talal et al. (1967) report on 8 patients with Sjogren's syndrome of which 2 developed macroglobulinaemia and Wegelius et al. (1970) one with heavy-chain disease. Bousser et al. (1961) report 2 cases of Sjogren's syndrome associated with Waldenstrom's macroglobulinaemia. In one of these Sjogren's syndrome was found when the patient was examined for purpura. The Rose-Waaler test was negative and no lupus erythematosus cells were found in the blood. In the second case the Sjogren's syndrome dominated the picture. These authors state that 15 other cases have been reported in which Sjogren's syndrome was associated with Waldenstrom's macroglobulinaemia and refer also to 2 cases of Milmlicz's disease associated with the same condition. They note the frequency of Sjogren's syndrome in cases of Waldenstrom's macroglobulinaemia as occurring in 17 of 76 cases. Sjogren's syndrome combined with Hashimoto's thyroiditis and Waldenstrom's macroglobulinaemiawas also reported by Vazquez (1960). Mention has been made above of the occurrence of Waldenstrom's macroglobulinaemia in association with thymic hypertrophy or thymic tumours, which appear to be manifestations of rheumatoid disease; or with Sjogren's syndrome; renal tubular acidosis, fibrosing alveolitis and auto-immune disease combined together (Mason et al., 1970 b; Zalin et al., 1970). Gumpel (1971) described a case of Sjogren's syndrome, pulmonary fibrosis (fibrosing alveolitis) and Waldenstrom's macroglobulinaemia with immune paresis. Hallen (1966) and Hobbs (1966) report paraproteinaemia as occurring in cases of arteritis and cirrhosis of the liver, while Zawadski and Edwards (1970) describe hypergammaglobulinaemia of polyclonal type developing into monoclonal type in some cases of cirrhosis, chronic hepatitis and biliary tract disease. Both Hallen and Hobbs report the occurrence of paraproteinaemia in cases of atrophic gastritis with pernicious anaemia. Pauders and Leeksma (1963) described cases of atrophic gastritis with pernicious anaemia in which Waldenstrom's macroglobulinaemia appeared. Kjeldson et al. (1969) reported paraproteinaemia with two M components occurring in a case of pernicious anaemia. Paget's disease devel-

oping macroglobulinaemia was reported by Jacottet and Ramel (1965) and Osserman (1958). Paraproteinaemia also was reported by the above as occurring in cases of coeliac disease and polycythaemia vera (Dittmar et al., (1968). The blood changes may be accompanied by Bence-Janes proteinuria. Blajchman et al. (1969) described paraproteinaemia in cases of auto-immune haemolytic anaemia. Three cases of rheumatoid disease with paraproteinaemia are now described.

Case 27 Female, aged 69 years. One brother died of carcinoma, organ unknown. For the last 15 years she had suffered from intrinsic asthma and painful swelling of the fingers, wrists, toes and ankles. Two years previously she developed herpes zoster of the left chest. For 18 months she had complained of rapid tiring and ex·haustion, shortness of breath, bouts of ankle swelling and more recently of slight haemoptyses and jaundice.

Examination Mucosal pallor, severe rheumatoid arthritic deformaties of the hands, wrists, feet and ankles. Palmar erythema and thickening of the left clavi·cle. Spleen enlarged three fingers breadth and liver two fingers breadth. No lymphadenopathy.

Investigations Blood count Hb 9.0 grams per cent., W.B.C. 10,500 per cu. mm., 50 per cent polymorphs. Normocytic anaemia present. Marked rouleaux formation. Serum bilirubin 3.0 mgms. per cent. Direct Coombs test strongly positive. No increase in cold agglutinins in the serum. Lupus erythematous cells + ++. ANF + + . RF + + +. E.S.R. 138 mms. per hour. No Bence-Janes protein in urine. W.R. and Kahn reactions negative. Total serum protein 9.8 G. per 100 mls. Albumin 4.0 G., globulin 5.8 G. (a-globulin 1.0 G. per 100 mls., (3 0.8 per 100 mls., y 4.0 G. per 100 mls. (normal 0.6-1.3)). Electrophoresis showed a marked monoclonal band in the slow gamma region with reduced a- and (3-globulins. Immunoglobulins-IgG greater than 3,000 mgms. per 100 mls. (diffusely

Addendum: Galli, M., Landi, G., Rastelli, D.L. and Scarlato, G. Myasthenia gravis with a monclonalgammopathy. Report of a case. J. Neurol. Sci., 1980, 45/1, 103-108. The authors report the fourth case of an elderly man with myasthenia and monclonal gammopathy.

raised). IgA 390 mgms. per 100 mls. (normal 59-505). IgM 366 mgms. per 100 mls. (monoclonal). The bone marrow showed an increase in the lymphocytes, but not in the plasma cells. A skeletal survey showed no evidence of myelomatosis, but Paget's disease of the clavicles and lumbar vertebrae.

A diagnosis of intrinsic asthma, rheumatoid arthritis, auto-immune haemolytic anaemia, systemic lupus erythematosus, Paget's disease of bone and IgM macroglobulinaemia was made.

Case 28   Male, aged 60 years.   Under treatment for rheumatoid arthritis for 25 years.   Recent onset of spontaneous bruising beneath the skin and bleeding from the nose and gums, occasional haemoptyses, increasing effort dyspnoea and oedema of the feet.   Examination showed severe rheumatoid deformities of the hands and wrists, ankles and feet with ankylosis of both shoulder joints and pitting oedema of the feet.   There was peripheral muscular wasting.   All tendon reflexes were absent. Numerous haemorrhages were present under the skin.   The spleen and liver were enlarged 2 fingers breadth.   A blood count showed Hb 12.6 G per 100 mls.   Marked rouleaux formation. Achlorhydria. Serum showed RF +++. ANF ++ and thyroglobulin auto-antibodies +. Plasma proteins— albumin 2.8 G per 100 mls., globulin 8.2 G per 100 mls. Electrophoresis showed a monoclonal M band in the gammaglobulin region and immunophoresis the presence of a high IgM content (440 mgms. per 100 mls). Sternal marrow biopsy showed numerous plasma cells to be present. Skeletal survey showed no evidence of myelomatosis. A diagnosis of rheumatoid art hritis and Waldenstrom's macroglobulinaemia was made.

Case 29   Male, aged 75 years.   His wife died one year previously of cancer of the breast.   For six years he had suffered from migrating arthritis of various joints of the limbs, particularly of the elbows. For the last year generalized lymphadeno-

pathy and spontaneous bruising had been present.   Examination showed rheumatoid arthritic deformity of the hands, wrists, elbows (which were partially ankylosed), knees, ankles and feet and generalized lymphadenopathy and splenomegaly. Many purpuric haemorrhages were seen. A blood count showed Hb 15.0 G per cent. E.S.R. 60 mm. per hour. Rouleaux formation. No Bence-Jones protein in the urine. No lupus erythematosus cells in the blood. Achlorhydria present. Plasma proteins; albumin 3.2 G per 100 mls., globulin 8.2 G per 100 mls. Serum contained RF +++, ANF ++ and thyroglobulin antibodies+ +. Serum electrophoresis confirmed the presence of an M band in the gammaglobulin region. The sternal marrow showed an excess of lymphocytes. Immunophoresis showed IgG 1,000 mgms. per 100 mls. IgA = 86 mgms. per 100 mls. IgM = 21 mgms. per 100 mls. and an abnormal immunoglobulin not in these fractions. Skeletal survey normal. Biopsy of one of the enlarged lymph nodes showed the changes commonly associated with Waldenstrom's macroglobulinaemia. A lymphogram showed multiple lymph node enlargement. A diagnosis of rheumatoid disease with paraproteinaemia was made.

In a f urther patient a man of 52 years developed swelling of the left ankle and right wrist.   The serum RF was strongly positive and the serum showed a monoclonal gamma globulin with a very high level of IgG (2,100 mgms. per 100 mls.).

Thus, *monoclonal paraproteinaemia* or *Waldenstrom's macroglobulinaemia and Bence-Jones proteinuria may develop in cases of collagen* disease or *"auto-immune" disease of various organs.* The monoclonal paraproteinaemia may be preceded by polyclonal hypergammaglobulinaemia. Macroglobulinaemia may be associated with a blood eosinophilia of up to 25 per cent (Osserman, 1971) and with thrombocytopenia (Wintrobe, 1967).

It has been shown above that a plasmacytosis and the appearance of immature plasma cells and lymph follicles in the bone marrow may be found in various chronic infections and in coHagen diseases. The plasma cells and lymphocytes produce antibodies in response to antigenic stimulation and their proliferation in the marrow in chronic infections appears to be so produced. In cases of *collagen-auto-immune diseases the same changes in the marrow and changes in the gammaglobulins may well be the result of chronic antigenic stimulation due to the presence of a chronic infective agent.*

Furthermore, chronic infections, which may produce the above changes in the gammaglobulins in the blood and changes in the bone marrow may eventually be complicated by the development of amyloidosis, the amyloid being derived from the immunoglobulins. Such a condition is not uncommon in cases of rheumatoid arthritis (12 per cent of the series reported by Gardner (1969)) and may also occur in cases of ulcerative colitis. *This again suggests the possibility that collagen-auto-immune diseases accompanied by a chronic antigenic stimulation are a result of an infection.* Apart from chronic infections and collagen-a uto-immune diseases paraproteinaemia and Waldenstrom's macroglobulinaemia may be found in association with certain malignant diseases, such as lymphoma, myelomatosis and certain cancers, which raises the question as to whether such a chronic antigenic stimulation is responsible for the development of certain malignancies.

II, xxxi) Collagen and auto-immune disease and cryoglobulinaemia

Cryoglobulins were formally thought to occur only rarely in the blood, but it is now known that cryoglobulins belonging to IgG or IgM classes or both are found in a variety of diseases (Meltzer and Franklin, 1966; Wintrobe, 1967; Wager - and Rasanen, 1970; Bonomo et al., 1970). They are commonly found in cases of para-

proteinaemia. They appear to represent circulating immune complexes and occur in:-

1) Certain infectious diseases, which include syphilis, leprosy, kala azar, mononucleosis (cytomegalic virus or infectious mononucleosis), pneumonia, subacute bacterial endocarditis, staphylococcal osteitis, streptococcal nephritis and septicaemia.

2) Cases of systemic lupus erythematosus, rheumatoid arthritis, dermatomyositis, scleroderma, polyarteritis, Sjogren's syndrome, polycythaemia, Raynaud's phenomena, certain liver diseases, including cirrhosis and lu poid hepatitis, asthma and coeliac disease (Doe et al., 1971).

3) Malignancies of the immunological system, including malignant myeloma, leukaemia, malignant lymphoma and primary macroglobulinaemia (Waldenstrom's).

Of 29 cases of cryoglobulinaemia studied by Meltzer and Franklin (1966) 17 suffered from systemic collagen diseases. The IgM component of the mixed cryoglobulins may be polyclonal or monoclonal. The latter is actually a subgroup of Waldenstrom's macroglobulinaemia. In a number of cases with monoclonal IgM components arthralgias occur. Of considerable interest is the fact that cryoglobulins often exhibit ANF and RF activity in high concentration, whether found associated with collagen-auto-immune disease or with malignancies of the immunological system. The occurrence of cryoglobulins in association with various infectious diseases and in association with collagen and auto-immune disease suggests that the latter may well be infective in aetiology. Their appearance also in malignant disease of the lymphoid system and their exhibition of RF and ANF activity in such cases is also suggestive that these diseases may have been produced by a chronic infection related to rheumatoid disease and comparable to leprosy or syphilis.

II, xxxii) Collagen diseases and immunoparesis

In the above cases collagen-auto-immune diseases have resulted in the development of excess of and abnormal gammaglobulins in the blood. In some cases of advanced rheumatoid disease there develops an increased incidence of *bacterial* infections of any kind, such as bronchiectiasis, lung abscess, pneumonia, bronchitis, urinary infections, suppurative arthritis, septicaemic endocarditis and abscesses in the skin, bone, muscle, etc. (Leading Article, Brit. med. J., 1972, ii, 549). This is very typical of hypogammaglobulinaemia. In some cases this tendency to bacterial infections may be associated with a fall in the levels of IgA and IgG to almost negligible amounts but the level of IgM is usually high. Occasionally this may be low also resulting in secondary hypogammaglobulinaemia and so-called immune paresis. This occurred in the following cases:-

Case 30 Male, aged 55 years. Grandmother suffered from severe rheumatoid arthritis. Past history not relevant. The patient gave a 10 years history of severe rheumatoid arthritis. At the onset E.S.R. was 60 mms. per hour and serum albumin 3.6 G. per cent, globulin 3.5 G. per cent. Later his disease was complicated by Felty's syndrome and a very large spleen with Hb 7.0 G. per cent, W.B.C. 2,300 per cu. mm. He was later subject to frequent chest and urinary infections. Now plasma proteins, albumin 3.4 G. per cent, globulin 1.8 G. per cent. Electrophoresis showed a virtual absence of *y* globulins, IgG 65 *p.G.*, IgA 20 p.G., IgM 30 p.G. per cent.

Case 31 Male, aged 61 years. Past history irrelevant. Ten years previous to admission acute onset of rheumatoid arthritis followed a year later by left-sided geniculate herpes zoster. At this time Hb found to be 10.2 G. per cent with a normocytic hypochromic anaemia. Serum proteins, albumin 4.2 G. per cent, globulins 3.8 G. per cent. Five years after the onset of the arthropathy he developed a deep vein thrombosis of the left leg followed by pulmonary embolism. Two years before admission he was found to have polycythaemia vera and then developed pyoderma with extensive gangrene of the skin. He began to run a persistent pyrexia, shivering and sweating. Examination showed very severe rheumatoid changes, bilateral suppurative olecranon bursitis, rheumatoid nodules and the left foot was swollen, hot and painful. He was found to have a staphylococcal infection of both olecranon bursae and osteomyelitis of the tarsus of the left foot. There was extensive scarring of the skin over the right abdomen and hip. Hb was 22 G. per cent. P.C.V. 62 per cent. Plasma proteins total 4.0 G. per cent, albumin 3.3 G. per cent, globulin 0.7 G. per cent. IgA 20 G., IgM 25 G., IgG=nil.

Thymoma, which appears to be associated with collagen or auto-immune disease, may also be associated with acquired 'hypogammaglobulinaemia, persisting after thymectomy (Peterson et al., 1965; Tan, 1974 b).

II, xxxiii) Congenital or primary acquired agammaglobulinaemia or hypogammaglobulinaemia and collagen and auto-immune diseases

These conditions are reviewed by Janeway (1967) and Gabrielson et al. (1969). In them the immunoglobulins of the blood, especially IgA and IgG, are deficient and plasma cells lacking in the bone marrow. In general the subjects response to viral infections is normal, but they are especially liable to infections with pyogenic and other organisms, including protozoa, e.g. giardia (Zetzel, 1971). About one-third of patients with either congenital or primary acquired disease suffer from an arthritis identical with rheumatoid arthritis, but with absence of RF in the blood. They are also liable to develop other collagen diseases, such as systemic lupus erythematosus, dermatomyositis, scleroderma, etc. or "auto-immune" phenomena affecting the red blood corpuscles (leading to auto-immune haemolytic anaemia), liver and kidney (for references see Good and Rotstein, 1960; Wolf, 1962; Bywaters and Ansell, 1969; Hobbs, 1970). Since such .Patients are not especially liable to virus diseases, such observations are strongly against a viral origin of collagen-auto-immune diseases. In about 20 per cent of cases of either congenital or primary acquired hypogammaglobulinaemia steatorrhoea may occur. In some a villous atrophy of the jejunal mucosa resembling or identical with adult coeliac disease has been observed (Sleisenger, 1967; Mawhinney and Tomkin, 1971) or ulcerative colitis (Jensen et al., 1970). Other organ specific "auto-immune" diseases, such as gastric mucosal atrophy, pernicious anaemia, myxoedema or diabetes mellitus have been described in this condition (Lewis and Brown, 1957; Crowder et al., 1959; Gibbs and Pryor, 1961; Larsson et al., 1961; Lee et al., 1964; Klayman and Brandberg, 1965; Comings, 1965; Hooft et al., 1969; Walker-Smith and Griger, 1969; Twomey et al., 1970; Tomkin et al., 1971) and auto-immune thyroiditis may also occur (Kuitunen et al., 1971). Primary acquired hypogammaglobulinaemia associated with myasthenia and thymoma was reported by Velve et al. (1966) and with thyroiditis, pernicious anaemia and possible dermatitis herpetiformis, myxoedema, achlorhydria and steatorrhoea by Webster (1973).

The relatives of cases of hypo- or agammaglobulinaemia often exhibit various signs of collagen disease (rheumatoid arthritis or systemic lupus erythematosus, polyarthritis) or "auto-immune" disease (see Fudenberg et al., 1962; Rotstein and Good, 1962; Bywaters and Ansell, 1969). RF and ANF or tests for systemic lupus erythematosus or hypogammaglobulinaemia may be found in the blood of parents and siblings. Tomkin et al. (1971) described a family in which 5 members from two generations had isolated IgA deficiency,

one of these had coeliac disease, one pernicious anaemia, one asthma, one eczema and one recurrent respiratory infections.

The absence of RF from the serum in cases of rheumatoid arthritis, dermatomyositis, etc., developing in the subjects of primary hypogammaglobulinaemia is an argument against the role of this factor in producing lesions. The liability of patients with the congenital disease to intercurrent infections not of viral aetiology and also to collagen and auto-immune diseases suggests *firstly that collagen and auto-immune diseases are of* infectious *origin and secondly that this infection is not viral in* nature. As regards primary acquired cases of agammaglobulinaemia another explanation of the liability to collagen and auto-immune diseases is possible. It has been mentioned above that cases of rheumatoid arthritis are liable to develop immune paresis. It may well be that in primary acquired cases of agammaglobulinaemia the immune paresis is merely a manifestation of the later appearing collagen and auto-immune disease.

II, xxxiv) Collagen and auto-immune disease and bony changes

a) Osteoporosis

In cases of rheumatoid arthritis generalized *osteoporosis* may occur, even without steroid therapy. Vertebral collapse or spontaneous fractures may occur. In other cases osteolysis and disappearance of bones, for example phalanges (Boyle and Buchanan, 1971) may be found. In children rheumatoid disease leads to disturbance of bone growth and periostitis (rheumatoid dwarfism).

b) Paget's disease of bone (osteitis deformans)

Paget's disease of bone is not usually generalized, but may be confined to one or only part of a bone. The periosteal changes are reminiscent of an inflammatory periostitis and consist of infiltration with lymphocytes and plasma cells like the

Addendum: Rheumatoid periostitis of calcaneus responds to drilling treatment. Cheu Boaxing and Li Zumou. Chinese Med. J. 1981, 94. 5. 288·290 Rheumatoid periostitis is well recognized.

Addendum: Adult onset hypogammaglobulinaemia may be associated with various autoimmune diseases, namely primary hypothyroidism and hyperthyroidism; atrophic gastritis with pernicious anaemia; vitiligo; alopecia areata; diabetes; Coombs·positive haemolytic anaemia; autoimmune neutropenia; idiopathic thrombocytopenia and coeliac disease. Relatives more commonly than normal subjects show organ-specific autoantibodies in their blood. Development of insulin-dependent diabetes in adult onset hypogammaglobulinaemia. Young. RJ. Duncan LJ. Paton L. Yap PL. Brit. med. J., 1981, 2.82, 1668.

changes associated with "auto-immune" diseases. The whole thickness of the bone is affected by an osteitis, hence the name 05teitis deformans. Paget himself likened the condition to syphilitic osteitis. Periods of local remission and exacerbation in the bony changes are common. The serum alkaline phosphatase and E.S.R. are often raised and in several of the author's cases an hypergammaglobulinaemia has been found, similar to that occurring in an infection. The condition may be accompanied by an eosinophilia in the blood (Whitby and Britton, 1950). It tends to occur in later life, is rare before the age of 40 years and uncommon before 55 years of age. Collin (1956) states that one in every 30 patients over the age of 40 years has Paget's disease in one or more bones. Schmorl reported it as present in 3 per cent of autopsies. With such a common condition it would naturally be found associated with many other diseases in many elderly subjects. Little is known of its aetiology, however. Its occurrence in only one or part of a single bone and often asymetrically and the general features of the condition rule out an endocrine disturbance, which would affect all bones symmetrically. Little attention seems to have been paid to its association in any given case with other diseases, which are usually dismissed as unrelated. Luxton (1957), however, noted the association of the disease with Hashimoto's thyroiditis in which he found Paget's disease present in 7 of 35 cases. Luxton (1968) in a personal communication reports that he had found Paget's disease in about 11 per cent of 120 cases of Hashimoto's thyroiditis. Paget's disease with myxoedema has been reported on numerous occasions (Aubert et al., 1966) and sometimes with permctous anaemia (Govindaraj et al., 1970) and with parapsoriasis (Benjeam et al., 1967). Dr. D. Doniach (personal communication) states that she could not find thyroid auto-antibodies more frequently in cases of Paget's disease than in controls. Paget's

disease with arthropathy was described by Perez Galdos et al. (1966). It was found in 16 (16 per cent) of the 100 cases of rheumatoid arthritis admitted to a geriatric unit recorded earlier. It was present in association with rheumatoid arthritis and other features of the spectrum of collagen-auto-immune disease in Case 12, where it was associated with polycyth aemia, rheumatoid arthritis and renal involvement with hypertension, and Case 27, in which rheumatoid arthritis was associated with auto-immune haemolytic anaemia, systemic lupus erythematosus, intrinsic asthma and macroglobulinaemia as well as Paget's disease. Paget's disease associated with scleroderma was described by Com:n:mdr et al. (1967) and with macroglobulinaemia by Osserman (1958) and Jaccottet and Ramel (1965).

To try to determine what diseases may be found in association with Paget's disease all successive cases of Paget's disea,se seen by the author over a period of several years were investigated for present or past clinical evidence of collagen or auto-immune d;sease, for the presence of a chlorhydria, by determining the F.B.I. and by seeking the presence of auto-antibodies in the serum. The brief details of these cases are as in Table V.

Of 57 cases in 16 only were there no clinical or histological evidence of pre-existing or present collagen or auto-immune disease. In one of these cases there was neither achlorhydria nor serological abnormality. In 5 of the others there was serological evidence of collagen or auto-immune disease and in 10 both achlorhydria and serological abnormalities. In the rest of the cases Paget's disease was associated with long-standing or recent collagen or a uto-immune disease of various types. Such observations suggest a *significant relationship between Paget's disease and various manifestations of collagen and auto-immune disease and that the form2r is part of the spectrum of these diseases.*

A remarkable case, (Case 32) a female,

— 84

Table V

Case	Sex	Age	Presentation	Associated collagen and auto-immune disease	Presence of benign or malignant tumour	Presence of achlorhydria	Serum auto-antibodies
V, 1	F	59	Aged 40 years onset of severe *rheumatoid arthritis*. Two years later *Sjogren's syndrome* and goitre due to *Hashimoto's thyroiditis*. Widespread Paget's disease.		Autopsy 4 different carcinomata (both ovaries, stomach, pancreas and gall bladder).	+	ANF RF Thyroid
V, 2	M	58	Enlargement of hands and feet due to acromegaly. Paget's disease of skull.	Ten years history of moderately severe *rheumatoid arthritis*	Eosinophil pituitary adenoma		RF Thyroid
V, 3	M	60	*Myxoedematous* coma. Paget's disease of skull and spine.		Right-sided cerebral meningioma	+	Thyroid Gastric parietal cell
V, 4	M	60	Acute epididymo-orchitis. Orchidectomy showed epididymitis and testes heavily infiltrated with lymphocytes, plasma cells and some eosinophils. Paget's disease of pelvis and femora.			+	RF ANF
V, 5	M	93	Epilepsy. Paget's disease of pelvis, spine and skull present.		Astrocytoma grade II of left hemisphere		ANF Thyroid
V, 6	F	80	Dyspepsia due to gastric ulcer. Paget's disease of skull, pelvis and right femur.			+	ANF Gastric parietal cell
V, 7	M	61	A case of cerebral thrombosis. Paget's disease of lumbar vertebrae.				
V, 8	F	75	Heart failure. Paget's disease of pelvis and femora.			+	ANF
V, 9	M	64	Melanoma of eye removed 10 years previously. Now respiratory symptoms. Found to have extensive Paget's disease.	*Hashimoto's thyroiditis*	Melanoma of left eye. Reticulosarcoma of thyroid and left lung		RF ANF Thyroid
V, 10	M	62	Dryness of eyes and mouth due to *Sjogren's syndrome*. Paget's disease of skull and pelvis.				RF

Table V (continued)

V. 11	F	55	*Psoriasis* since age of 20 years. Onset of *arthropathy* aged 44 years. Paget's disease discovered aged 55 years.		–	ANF disease Gastric parietal cell
V. 12	M	60	Left-sided cerebral tumour. Paget's found affecting skull, lumbar vertebrae and pelvis.	Cerebral astrocytoma Grade III		
V. 13	F	62	*Pernicious anaemia.* Extensive Paget's disease.		+	Gastric parietal cell
V. 14	M	60	Epigastric pain. Extensive Paget's disease.	Carcinoma of stomach	+	Gastric parietal cell
V. 15	F	66	*Myxoedema.* Paget's disease of lumbar spine.	Two years history of *rhinitis* and mild symptoms and signs of *rhematoid arthritis.*	+	ANF Thyroid Gastric parietal cell
V. 16	M	62	Ten years history of chronic bronchitis. Paget's disease of pelvis and spine.	Carcinoma of gall bladder	+	ANF
V. 17	F	75	Abdominal pain. Widespread Paget's disease.	Carcinoma of descending colon.	+	RF ANF
V. 18	F	58	Tiredness and backache. Paget's disease of lower spine.	Myxoedema.	+	Thyroid Gastric parietal cell
V. 19	F	82	Abdominal swelling. Paget's disease of tibiae and clavicles.	Severe *rheumatoid arthritis, Sjogren's syndrome* and *myxoedema*	+	ANF Thyroid
V. 20	F	68	Twenty years progressive *rheumatoid arthritis*. Eight years previously *thyrotoxicosis* and *pernicious anaemia* discovered. Presented with abdominal swelling Paget's disease of pelvis, skull and humeri.	Bilateral ovarian cysts, one a serous cystadenoma, the other a malignant papilliferous cyst	+	ANF Thyroid Gast ric parietal cell
V. 21	M	70	Case of *myxoedema.* Found to have extensive Paget's disease.		+	Thyroid Gastric parietal cell

86

Table V (continued)

No.	Sex	Age	Clinical	Clinical	Associated tumour		Antibodies
V, 22	F	65	Aged 29 years onset of *acute rheumatoid arthritis*. Some years later *thyotoxicosis*. Now moderate *rheumatoid arthritis* in peripheries. Paget's disease of tibiae.			−	ANF RF Thyroid
V, 23	F	78	Paget's disease of skull and pelvis.	Severe *rheumatoid arthritis* 12 years. *Diabetes* 8 years.	Large rodent ulcer removed aged 70 years	+	RF
V, 24	M	70	Swelling of left face. Widespread Paget's disease found.	Ankylosing spondylitis and *rheumatoid arthritis* for 10 years.	Carcinoma of left parotid		
V, 25	F	60	Husband has diabetes and Paget's disease with thyroid auto-antibodies in serum. His brother has Hashimoto's thyroiditis, myxoedema, diabetes and Paget's disease with thyroid auto-antibodies††. Patient has Paget's disease of skull.	Treatment for sero-negative , *rheumatoid arthritis* for 10 years	Carcinoma of ileocaecal region	+	ANF
V, 26	F	74	Spontaneous fracture of right femur. Paget's disease of pelvis and femur.			+	ANF
V, 27	M	89	Congestive cardiac failure. Paget's disease of pelvis and spine.		Carcinoma of prostate		ANF Thyroid
V, 28	F	75	Congestive heart failure. Paget's disease of tibiae and sacrum	Longstanding case of *rheumatoid arthritis*		+	ANF RF Gastric parietal cell
V, 29	M	66	Tumour of left lung proved to be a benign adenoma. Severe Paget's disease.	Moderately severe *rheumatoid arthritis* over previous 10 years.	Adenoma of bronchus		RF Gastric parietal cell
V. 30	F	77	Old case of duodenal ulcer presented with ischaemic heart disease. Paget's disease of skull and pelvis.	Moderate *rheumatoid arthritis* changes		+	ANF Gastric parietal cell
V. 31	F	67	Goitre. Euthyroid. Paget's disease of skull.	Old case of *rheumatoid arthritis*. *Hashimoto's thyroiditis*.			ANF Thyroid Gastric parietal cell

Table V (continued)

	Sex	Age	Clinical notes				Autoantibodies
V. 32	M	67	Non-smoker. Metastasis of carcinoma of the bronchus in right femur. Paget's disease of lumbar spine, pelvis and both femora.	*Hypothyroidism*	Carcinoma of bronchus	−	ANF Thyroid
V. 33	M	84	Congestive heart failure. Advanced Paget's disease.	*Thyrotoxicosis*		+	ANF Thyroid Gastric parietal cell
V. 34	F	90	Pneumonia. Extensive Paget's disease.			+	ANF
V. 35	M	86	Hiatus hernia. Paget's disease of both femora and left forearm.			+	RF Gastric parietal cell
V. 36	F	93	Congestive cardiac failure and carcinoma of head of the pancreas. Paget's disease of pelvis and lumbar spine.	Long-standing *rheumatoid arthritis*	Carcinoma of pancreas	+	ANF Gastric parietal cell
V, 37	F	70	Digestive disturbance found to be due to *atrophic gastritis*. Paget's disease of lumbar spine and skull.	Aged 43 years operation righ t-sided *cystic mastitis*. Aged 44 years **ditto** *left sided.*		+	
V, 38	M	74	Case of *ulcerative colitis*. Paget's disease of lumbar spine and femora.				
V. 39	F	39	Severe pain due to generalized Paget's disease.	*Myxoedema, Rheumatoid nodules.*	Multiple rodent ulcers on back and face.	+	
V. 40	F	78	One daughter suffered from myxoedema and one daughter from pernicious anaemia. Had long history of *rheumatoid arthritis*. Paget's disease of spine, pelvis and **right femur**	Developed *pernicious anaemia* and *myxoedema* aged 65 years.		+	ANF **dema** Thyroid Gastric parietal cell
V. 41	**M**	70	Severe symptoms of *ulcerative colitis*. Paget's disease of pelvis and femora.	Mild *rheumatoid arthritis*		+	
V. 42	F	64	Mid-dorsal pain. Paget's disease of pelvis and lumbar vertebrae	Mild *rheumatoid arthritis.*			Thyroid

Table V (continued)

V, 43	M	50	Signs of severe *myxoedema* and lumbar backache. Paget's disease of pelvis and lumbar spine. Brother has diabetes.	Found to have *Hashimoto's thyroiditis*			Thyroid in very high titre
V, 44	F	59	Signs of *thyrotoxicosis* and goitre. Paget's disease of lumbar vertebrae, pelvis, femora and clavicles.				Thyroid Gastric parietal cell
V, 45	F	70	Backache. Paget's disease of spine and pelvis.				Thyroid
V, 46	M	56	Aged 40 years developed mild *rheumatoid arthritis*. Aged 58 years Paget's disease of skull and spine.	Aged 55 years onset of *ulcerative colitis*.			RF
V, 47	M	48	Case of *chronic active hepatitis*. Found to have Paget's disease of pelvis.				Gastric parietal cell
V, 48	M	55	Effort dyspnoea due to *fibrosing alveolitis*. Paget's disease of skull and femora.	*Sjogren's syndrome*			ANF RF
V, 49	F	70	Onset of *rheumatoid arthritis* aged 55 years. Found to have extensive Paget's disease at 70 years.				ANF
V, 50	M	50	Ischaemic heart disease. Past history of duodenal ulcer, adenomatous colonic polyp and prostatic enlargement. Paget's disease of vertebrae.	*Diabetes*	Colonic polyp		RF Thyroid
V, 51	M	69	*Thyrotoxicosis*. Paget's disease of femora.	Twenty years history of *intrinsic asthma*			AIVF Gastric parietal cell
V, 52	M	84	A fracturEd femur with ext ensive Paget's disease.				ANF Gastric parietal cell
V, 53	F	71	Congestive heart failure and iron deficiency anaemia. Paget's disease of skull and pelvis.	*Atrophic gastritis*		+	Gastric parietal cell
V, 54	F	18	Paget's disease of pelvis	*Chronic cholecystitis* and gall stones		+	AIVF

Table V (continued)

V, 55	F	79	Mother and one sister died of carcinoma of stomach. One sister died of cancer of breast. Patient aged 43 years operation for *cystic mastitis* of right breast. Aged 44 years operation for *cystic mastitis* of left breast. Widespread Paget's disease.		+	ANF
V, 56	F	93	Severe *rheumatoid arthritic* change. *Diabetes* for 15 years. Rodent ulcer removed from nose 3 years ago. Widespread Paget's disease. *Myxoedema.*	Rodent ulcer	+	ANF Thyroid
V, 57	M	78	Concomitant seropositive *rheumatoid arthritis* and generalized Paget's disease developing over 12 years.		+	RF+ Thyroid+

aged 56 years, was under the author's care. Eleven years previously she developed acute rheumatoid arthritis for which she was under treatment for some years. Three years later she was found to have thyrotoxicosis, enlargement of the right lobe of the thyroid gland and enlarged lymph nodes above the right clavicle. Biopsy of the latter showed only reactive hyperplasia. Partial right-sided thyroidectomy was carried out at Edinburgh Royal Infirmary and histologically the removed thyroid contained large areas of lymphocytic infiltration, especially in the area of enlargement on the right side. The patient became euthyroid. The enlarged lymph nodes gradually regressed. From that time the activity of the rheumatoid process varied. When first seen by the author, she was complaining of pain and swelling of the *right* sterno-clavicular joint and she appeared acromegalic. X-rays showed the presence of an enlarged pituitary fossa presumably due to an eosinophilic adenoma and also of Paget's disease localized to the *right* clavicle. The serum contained ANF and thyroid auto-antibodies, but RF was absent. In this case there was a localization of the various manifestations to a field, that is one area of the right side of the neck affecting lymph nodes, the right side of the thyroid, the right sterno-clavicular joint and the right clavicle, strongly suggesting a relationship of the rheumatoid arthritis and thyroid changes to Paget's disease.

In passing of considerable interest is the association of Paget's disease with the development of benign or malignant extraosseus tumours in 20 cases in the above series. These include single or multiple rodent ulcers; eosinophilic pituitary adenoma in a skull involved by Paget's disease; bilateral ovarian cysts, one benign and one malignant; adenoma of the bronchus; carcinoma of the bronchus, head of the pancreas, prostate, gall bladder, descending colon, parotid gland, ileocaecal region; reticulosarcoma; malignant melanoma of the choroid and reticulosarcoma; and cerebral meningioma and cerebral astrocytoma beneath a region of skull affected by Paget's disease twice. In one case cancer of four different tissues was present (ovary, stomach, pancreas and gall bladder).

II, xxxv) Collagen and auto-immune diseases and the male genitalia

a) The testis and epididymis

The male genitalia, like all other tissues, may be involved in the generalized changes of collagen disease, for example in disseminated eosinophilic collagen disease. The angeitis associated with these diseases may affect the testis and epididymis and also the spermatic cord (Harvey, 1967). Rheumatoid disease may be complicated by an acute epididymo-orchitis (Riches, 1960), the affected organs being bacteriologically sterile and exhibiting lymphocytic and plasma cell infiltration and often germinal centres or they may show evidence of rheumatoid granulomata. Again, in cases of systemic sclerosis the testis may be involved (Talbott and Ferrandis, 1956). Mackay and Burnet (1963) describe auto-immune disease of the testis and epididymis and Martinazzi et al. (1968) also report this condition referring to it as granulomatous orchitis. A number of cases have been associated with diabetes.

b) Acute hydrocoele

Rheumatoid disease is responsible for inflammation of all serous surfaces, including pericardium, pleura, possibly peritoneum, synovial membranes of joints, tendons and bursae and it would, therefore, be expected at times to be responsible for similar inflammation in the tunica vaginalis. Again cases of acute epididymo-orchitis have been seen to be sometimes a manifestation of collagen disease and extension of the inflammation to the surface of this organ may be complicated by the development of a hydrocoele. In less severe inflammation of the epididymuis and testis it

would be expected that hydrocoele may appear without obvious cause. Indeed, the author found that the development of an hydrocoele is a not uncommon finding in cases of rheumatoid disease if specifically sought. The development of hydrocoele for no obvious reason may well be a manifestation of latent collagen disease.

c) Auto-immune disease and benign nodular hyperplasia of the prostate

Like every other tissue in the body the prostate may be involved in collagen disease, for example disseminated eosinophilic collagen disease or polyarteritis. Benign nodular hyperplasia of the prostate is said to occur in 45 per cent of Caucasian males over 40 years of age and its frequency to increase with age, so that by the age of 80 years a very high proportion of men exhibit the change. The changes are those of lymphocytic infiltration and of a mixture of epithelial and fibromuscular proliferation and cystic changes. The condition is largely confined to the middle lobe of the gland. Mackay and Burnet (1963) draw attention to the similarity of the changes to those which occur in the breast in cystic mastitis and in the thyroid in adenomatous goitre, which may follow lymphocytic thyroiditis. They regard the condition as an "auto-immune" disease. However, the predilection of the change to one part of the gland is against such a conception, as all parts of the gland would be expected to be involved equally if the condition was "auto-immune" in nature.

II, xxxvi) Collagen and auto-immune disease and the female genitalia

As with all other tissues in the female the genitalia, including the vagina, uterus, uterine tubes and ovaries and the peritoneum covering the ovaries may be involved in acute generalized collagen disease, such as systemic lupus erythematosus, disseminated eosinophilic collagen disease and especially by the polyarteritis of these conditions.

a) Collagen disease of the vagina

Mention has been made of the mucosal atrophy which may affect any other organ in cases of Sjogren's syndrome. Atrophic vulvo-vaginitis (vulvo-vaginitis sicca) (senile vaginitis) may develop as an atrophic condition of a mucous membrane in this condition and cause dyspareunia. The Plummer-Vinson syndrome may likewise be associated with kraurosis vulvae (Rhoads, 1940). In a personal case of dermatomyositis (Case 4) occurring in a woman of 36 years atrophic vaginitis developed at the age of 42 years. Atrophic vulvo-vaginitis thus appears to be a manifestation of collagen and auto-immune disease and may occur at an early age long before senility. The senile cases are essentially of the same nature.

b) Collagen and auto-immune disease of the ovaries

The ovaries may also be involved in cases of systemic sclerosis (Talbott and Ferrandis, 1956). Primary gonadal (ovarian) failure may also occur in association with rheumatoid arthritis, for example Cases 1 and 2, and especially in Still's disease and it may also be associated with various "auto-immune" diseases. Thus, delayed menarche or amenorrhoea due to ovarian causes may occur in cases of myxoedema, thyrotoxicosis and other thyroid or adrenal auto-immune disease (Irvine et al., 1968) and in cases of diabetes (Kase, 1971). Idiopathic adrenal atrophy associated with alopecia, vitiligo, premature menopause and ovarian atrophy was described by Irvine et al. (1969). In all these cases there may be lymphocytic infiltration of the ovaries preceding to fibrosis (cirrhosis of the ovary). Acanthosis nigricans can also be associated with primary hypogonadism (See under acanthosis). In some of the above cases autoantibodies tosteroid-containing cells (theca interna or granulosa cells) of the rabbit ovary can be demonstrated in the blood by immunofluorescent techniques (Irvine et al., 1968).

c) Collagen and auto-immune disease, uterine myomata (fibroids) and benign ovarian cysts

Uterine leiomyomata (myomata, fibroids, fibromyomata) are very common. They show a peak incidence at 40-50 years of age. It has been suggested that as many as 20-25 per cent of women beyond 35 years of age have such growths and that they are due to oestrogen stimulation, but this view lacks confirmation and there are many arguments against it (Evans, 1966). The tumours are usually multiple and vary in size. They may be cystic, contain fat cells or calcify. They frequently show areas of lymphocytic infiltration.

It seems that the peritoneum like the pleura and pericardium may perhaps be affected in cases of collagen disease. *Benign* ovarian cysts arise from the serosal mesothelium covering the ovary (Evans, 1966) nnd are, in fact, serous or pseudomucinous cystadenomata. It could be that they arise because of some disturbance of the serosa covering the ovary, such as may occur in collagen diseases. They occur most frequently between 20-50 years of age. Thirty per cent are bilateral. No reports in changes in the remaining ovarian tissue have been found in the literature on the tumours.

It seemed that an investigation of patients who had operations for fibroids or benign ovarian cysts for the presence of collagen and auto-immune disease might yield important information. Short et al. (1957) indeed noted the marked frequency of hysterectomies and ovariectomies (presumably for benign conditions) in their series of cases of rheumatoid arthritis as compared with normals. Langston et al. (1959) described a case with dermatomyositis, lymphocytic thyroiditis, thymic tumour, splenic hyperplasia and bilateral benign ovarian cysts.

In Case 2, cited already, the patient suffered from numerous manifestations of collagen and auto-immune disease. These included rheumatoid arthritis, Sjogren's syndrome, myxoedema, atrophic gastritis, diabetes, intrinsic asthma, primary gonadal failure, Paget's disease of bone and also fibroids, which would seem to fall into the spectrum of collagen and auto-immune disease. The author examined and investigated every patient presenting with a history of operation for fibroids or benign ovarian cysts of various types encountered in a general medical practice over a period of several years. As in the previous series, apart from a careful history and examination, each case was investigated by determining the serum P.B.I. and investigating for achlorhydria and the various serum auto-antibodies. Fibroids and benign ovarian cysts were frequently found together or occurred with short intervals between.

Brief clinical histories of all the patients observed in a general Medical Clinic over several years were as follows:-

Case VI, 1 (same as Case 5)	Female, aged 53 years. Nine years previously menorrhagia. Hysterectomy showed numerous fibroids. Operation followed by onset of acute *dermatomyositis*. Serum contained ANF and thyroid auto-antibodies. Treated with prednisolone, which 6 months later resulted in the development of a peptic ulcer for which partial gastrectomy was performed. This resulted in spontaneous cure of dermatomyositis. Well for 8 years and then developed malignant lymphoma. Achlorhydria present. ANF and thyroid auto-antibodies now absent.
Case VI, 2 (same as Case III, 2)	Female, aged 69 years. Aged 33 years onset of *rheumatoid arthritis* and under treatment for many years. Now burnt out. Aged 37 years removal of adenoma of the right side of the *thyroid*. Aged 37 years hysterectomy for fibroids. Aged 42 years two operations on right breast for removal of areas of *cystic mastitis* in lower inner and upper outer quadrants of breast respectively. Aged 44 years dyspareunia due to atrophic vaginitis. Now carcinoma of the stomach. Achlorhydria. All antibody tests negative.
Case VI, 3	Female, aged 44 years. Life-long psoriasis and recent moderately severe *arthropathy*. Aged 29 years myomectomy for fibroids. Aged 36 years hysterectomy. Now carcinoma of the gall-bladder.
Case VI, 4	Female, aged 74 years. Aged 39 years hysterectomy for fibroids. Now well-marked rheumatoid arthritic deformities and carcinoma of the right ovary. Serum showed thyroid auto-antibodies.
Case VI, 5	Female, aged 63 years. Severe *rheumatoid arthritis*. Found to have calcified fibroids and carcinoma of the left kidney. Serum showed RF +.
Case VI, 6	Female, aged 55 years. Para 3. Menopause aged 53 years. Now *atrophic vaginitis*, huge fibroids and adenocarcinoma of body of uterus with inflammatory mucosal reaction. Serum showed thyroid auto-antibodies.
Case VI, 7	Female, aged 71 years. *Psoriasis and arthropathy* since twenties. Five years ago onset of symptoms of insulinoma of pancreas. Post mortem showed fibroids, cortical adrenal adenoma and insulinoma.
Case VI, 8	Female, aged 64 years. Aged 34 years hysterectomy for fibroids. Aged 50 years thyroidectomy for *thyrotoxicosis*. Now Grade III cerebral astrocytoma. Achlorhydria. Serum contained RF and thyroid auto-antibodies.
Case VI, 9	Female, aged 95 years. Mild *rheumatoid arthritic* changes for years. Post mortem showed fibroids and carcinoma of uterine body. Serum showed RF and thyroid auto-antibodies.
Case VI, 10	Female, aged 51 years. Aged 49 years menorrhagia. Found to have fibroids. Menopause 18 months ago. Now mild *rheumatoid arthritis* and *thyrotoxicosis*.
Case VI, 11	Female, aged 56 years. Marked family history of rheumatoid arthritis and carcinoma of the stomach. Onset of severe *rheumatoid arthritis* aged 49 years with menorrhagia. Hysterectomy for *fibroids*. Now carcinoma of both ovaries. Serum showed RF.

Case VI, 12	Female, aged 63 years. Aged 35 years onset of patches of *melanoderma* of face and body. Aged 43 years hysterectomy for fibroids. Now *alopecia universalis* and *cystic mastitis*.
Case VI, 13 {same as Case II, 23)	Female, aged 60 years. *Intrinsic asthma* since teens. Aged 40 years fibroids. Hysterectomy performed. Developed gout. *Cystic mastitis* developed and after giving up steroids *acute rheumatoid arthirtis*. Serum showed ANF, thyroid an::l gastric parietal cell auto-antibodies.
Case VI, 14	Female, aged 43 years. Mother had rheumatoid arthritis, myxoedr.ma, Sjogren's syndrome, pernicious anaemia, osteo-arthritis of the hips and adhesive otitis. Patient had ruptured ovarian cysts aged 22 years. Aged 35 years ectopic pregna ncy and fibroids. Aged 43 years *rheumatoid arthritis*.
Case VI, 15	Female, aged *60* years. Operation for fibroids 4 years ago. Now develop<d *Hashimoto's thyroiditis*.
Case VI, 16	Female, aged 37 years. Hysterectomy for fibroids. Now acu te myxor.dema due to *Hashimoto's thyroiditis*. Serum showed thyroid auto.antibodies.
Case VI, 17	Female, aged 82 years. Severe *rheumatoid arthritis*. Fibroids operation aged 55 years. Serum showed RF and achlorhydria present.
Case VI, 18	Female, aged 37 years. Hysterectomy for fibroids aged 31 years. Now developed *ulcerative colitis*. Serum showed RF.
Case VI, 19	Female, aged 40 years. Operation for thyroid *adelwma* aged 16 years. Fibroids, aged 30 years. Diabetes for 4 years. Now return of *thyrotoxicosis*. Serum showed RF.
Case VI, 20	Female, aged 46 years. For 3 years "fibrositis" of neck and shoulders. Now fibroids and menorrhagia. X-rays showed *rheumatoid arthritis of cervical spine*. Serum showed RF and ANF.
Case VI, 21	Female, aged 64 years. Hysterectomy for fibroids aged 36 years. Ro::lmt ulcer of nose aged 40 years. Th yrotoxicosis aged 54 years. Onset of *rheumatoid arthritis* aged 56 years. Five years ago severe pyorrhoea. One year ago severe dryness of mouth and li ps wit h ulceration of lips and oral mucosa. Marked enlargement of submaxillary and sublingual salivary glands *(Sjogren-M ikulicz syndrome)*. Crusting and dryness of the nose *(atrophic rhiniis)*. Perceptive deafness with indrawing of the tympanic membrane *(adhesive otitis)* . Achlorhydria. Serum showed gastric parietal cell and thyroid auto-antibodies.
Case VI, 22	Female, aged 60 years. Operation for fibroids aged 48 years. Now *atrophic gastritis*, koilonychia and iron deficiency anaemia. Also mild *rheumatoid arthritis*. Serum showed RF. Achlorhydria present.
Case VI, 23 (same as C<tse IV, 11)	Female, aged 59 years. Severe *polycythaemia* for 10 years. Three years ago hysterectomy for fibroids with no effect on polycythaemia. Now mild *rheumatoid arthritis*. Serum showed thyroid and gastric parietal cell auto-antibodies. Achlorhydria present.
Case VI, 24	Female, aged 56 years. Mother (aged 49 years), father and aunt had *rheumatoid arthritis* and thyrotoxicosis. One cousin had *thyrotoxicosis*. Patient aged 45 years had removal of angioma which developed in lower lip. Aged 50 yea rs hysterectomy for fibroids. Now *myxoedema, Sjogren's syndrome* and *mild rheumatoid arthritis*. Seru m showed thyroid auto-antibodies and RF.
Case VI, 25	Female, aged 46 years. Sister died of reticulosis. Patient had *juvenile rheumatoid arthritis* aged 10-15 years. Hysterectomy for fibroids aged 31 years. Now developed l ymphosarcoma.
Case VI, 26	Female, aged 68 years. Aged 48 yea rs hysterectomy for fibroids. Aged 57 yea rs thyroidectomy for *thyroto cosis*. Now developed retroperitoneal sa rcoma.

Case VI, 27   Female, aged 75 years. Hysterectomy for fibroids aged 45 years. Ten years later severe *rheumatoid arthritis.* Now retroperitoneal sarcoma. Serum showed ANF and RF.

Case VI, 28
(same as
Case III, 16)   Female, aged 69 years. Menarche aged 17 years. Periods always scanty. Menopause aged 43 years. Aged 53 years hysterectomy for *fibroids* and removal of lumps in periphery of both breasts, which showed *cystic mastitis.* This was accompanied by moderately severe changes of *rheumatoid arthritis* in fingers, wrists, ankles and feet. Aged 60 years found to have *diabetes.* Aged 69 years onset of reticulosarcoma. Serum showed ANF, thyroid and gastric parietal cell auto-antibodies. Achlorhydria present.

Case VI, 29   Female, aged 42 years. Aged 38 years onset of joint pains and swelling affecting digits, *wrists,* elbows, ankles, feet and knees and soon after by menorrhagia. Aged 40 years hysterectomy for fibroids. Aged 42 years partial gastrectomy for primary Hodgkin's disease of stomach on lesser curvature; local lymph nodes affected. Serum showed RF and thyroid auto-antibodies. Achlorhydria.

Case VI, 30   Female, aged 66 years. Aged 50 years hysterectomy for fibroids. Sudden onset of abdominal pain and foot and abdominal swelling. Hepatomegaly present. Blood showed acute monocytic leukaemia. Liver function tests and liver biopsy showed *chronic active hepatitis.* Bone marrow confirmed acute monocytic leukaemia. Autopsy showed chronic active hepatitis and malignant hepatoma. Serum showed ANF, RF and thyroid auto-antibodies. Achlorhydria present.

Case VI, 31   Female, aged 44 years. Mother and mother's sister had severe rheumatoid arthritis. Patient had had *acanthosis nigricans* for *10* years. Aged 42 years hysterectomy for *fibroids.* Soon afterwards onset of recurrent swelling of submaxillary and sublingual salivary glands and dryness of eyes and mouth and later of *atrophic stomatitis, pharyngitis and angular stomatitis, pyorrhoea* and sudden loss of teeth; cervical lymph nodes enlarged and soon after arteritis in one finger leading to gangrene. Investigations showed *Sjögren-Mikulicz syndrome, chronic active hepatitis and chronic lymphatic leukaemia.* Serum showed RF, cold agglutinins and monoclonal paraproteinaemia.

Case VI, 32   Female, aged 51 years. Marked family history of rheumatoid arthritis. Patient had hysterectomy for fibroids aged 38 years. Aged 48 years onset of acute *rheumatoid arthritis.* Under treatment since that time. Now has carcinoma of the oesophagus. Serum showed ANF, RF and gastric parietal cell auto-antibodies. Achlorhydria present.

Case VI, 33   Female, aged 69 years. Aged 38 years hysterectomy for fibroids. Well-marked rheumatoid arthritis present for *10* years. *Atrophic gastritis* and later developed carcinoma of the stomach. Serum showed ANF and gastric parietal cells. Achlorhydria present.

Case VI, 34   Female, aged 75 years. Aged 52 years cholecystectomy for *chronic cholecystitis* and gall stones and hysterectomy for fibroids. Long history of treatment of *rheumatoid arthritis.* Developed atrophic gastritis and carcinoma of the stomach. Serum showed thyroid auto-antibodies and achlorhydria present.

Case VI, 35   Female, aged 76 years. Mother died of cancer, primary unknown. Patient non-smoker. Hysterectomy for fibroids aged 55 years. Aged 58 years *pernicious anaemia* discovered. Now has carcinoma of the bronchus. Serum showed RF, thyroid auto-antibodies and gastric parietal cell antibodies. Achlorhydria present.

Case VI, 36   Female, aged 59 years. Two sisters had fibroids at same time as the patient. She had *asthma* aged 40-53 years. Aged 43 years hysterectomy for fibroids. Asthma ceased. Fibrositis of neck for 12 years. Now has *thyrotoxicosis.*

Case VI, 37
(same as
Case II, 23)   Female, aged 39 years, Indian from Tanzania. In England 11 years. Eight years history of *chronic rhinitis, intrinsic asthma* and migraine and now *atrophic gastritis* and iron deficiency anaemia. Calcified fibroids present. Serum contained thyroid and gastric parietal cell auto-antibodies +. Achlorhydria present.

Case VI, 38	Female, aged 49 years. Aged 31 years myomectomy for *fibroids*. Aged 33 years onset of acute *rheumatoid arthritis*. Aged 42 years hysterectomy for further *fibroids*. Now ependymoma of the cervical cord.
Case VI, 39	Female, aged 58 years. Operation for *fibroids* aged 41 years. *Thyrotoxicosis* aged 43 years. *Idiopathic Addison's disease* aged 53 years. Now carcinoma of the bladder.
Case VI, 40	Female, aged 49 years. Hysterectomy for fibroids aged 38 years. Aged 42 years operation for *cystic mastitis*. Now carcinoma of the pyloric end of the stomach. Marked *rheumatoid arthritis* of the feet and *ichthyosis acquisita*. Achlorhydria and gastric parietal cell auto-antibodies were found in the semm.
case VI, 41	Female, aged 65 years. Aged 49 years bilateral carpal tunnel syndrome. Myxoedcma was diagnosed and given thyroid extract. Aged 54 years onset of severe *rheumatoid arthritis* and under treatment since. Now rheumatoid arthritis burnt out, but has severe deformities. Aged 63 years operation for bilateral benign ovarian cysts. Aged 62 years onset of acromegaly and pituitary fossa found enlarged due to eosinophilic pituitary adenoma. Hypertensive. *Paget's disease* of bone in skull, vertebrae and pelvis. Serum showed ANF and thyroid auto-antibodies. Achlorhydria present.
Case VI, 42	Female, aged 67 years. Aged 40 years operation for bilateral benign ovarian cysts. Mastectomy for *cystic mastitis* aged 42 years. Aged 52 years menopause. Now moderate progressive, but painless *rheumatoid arthritis* of hands and feet. Has hypertension and Parkinsonism. Serum showed ANF.
Case VI, 43	Female, aged 63 years. Bilateral ovarian cysts aged 31 years. Now has *thyrotoxicosis*. Serum showed thyroid auto-antibodies.
Case VI, 44	Female, aged 78 years, Left ovarian cyst. Lungs showed fibrosing alveolitis. Has *rheumatoid arthritis* of feet. Serum showed ANF. Achlorhydria present.
Case VI, 45	Female, aged 66 years. *Rheumatoid arthritis* and benign pseudomucinous cyst of ovary. Serum showed ANF.
Case VI, 46	Female, aged 35 years. Menarche aged 15 years. Aged 15 years *juvenile rheumatoid arthritis*. Periods irregular. She has two children, one still-born. Aged 33 years had cyst of right ovary. Aged 34 years endometriosis and removal of uterine fibroid. Now has *myxoedema* and carpal tunnel syndrome. Serum showed thyroid auto-antibodies.
Case VI, 47	Female, aged 43 years. Aged 28 years had operation for bilateral ovarian cysts. Now menopause and well-marked *rheumatoid arthritis*. Polycythaemia found. ANF and RF present.
Case VI, 48	Female, aged 72 years. Mother died of diabetes. Patient aged 57 years had operation for removal of large benign ovarian cyst and cervical polyp. For more than 5 years she had sero-positive painful peripheral *arthropathy* treated with aspirin and steroids. Now has acute lymphoblastic leukaemia with severe mouth ulceration, Serum showed RF. Achlorhydria present.
Case VI, 49	Female, aged 87 years. Operation for bilateral ovarian cysts aged 60 years. Now has chronic lymphatic leukaemia, marked *rheumatoid arthritic* deformities of hands, wrists and knees. Achlorhydria present.
Case VI, 50	Female, aged 60 years. Aged 42 years removal of bilateral benign ovarian cysts. Now well-marked *rheumatoid arthritis* in fingers and toes, *ichthyosis acquisita* and leio-myo-sarcoma of oesophagus. Serum showed RF and thyroid auto-antibodies.
Case VI, 51 (same as Case I, II)	Female, aged 57 years. Aged 45 years onset of *rheumatoid arthritis* affecting hands, feet and shoulders. Symptoms persisted. Aged 48 years cholecystectomy for chronic *cholecystitis* and gall stones. Aged 50 years removal of benign uterine polyp. Aged 55 years onset of *ulcerative colitis*. Aged 56 years laparotomy revealed bilateral ovarian tumours, the left a pseudomucinous cystadenoma, the right a

metastases from a malignant carcinoid of the ileum. Serum showed gastric parietal cell auto·antibodies. Achlorhydria present.

Case **VI,** 52   Female, aged 70 years. Iraqi. Very marked family history of carcinoma of the uterus, breast, etc. and of rheumatoid arthritis. Aged 45 years onset of severe *rheumatoid arthritis* affecting hands, elbows, neck, ankles and feet. Under continuous treatment since. Aged 50 years bilateral oophorectomy for benign cysts. Now polygonal cell carcinoma of one breast. Serum showed ANF and thyroid auto-antibodies. Achlorhydria present.

Case **VI,** 53   Female, aged 45 years. Indian from Calcutta. Aged 32 years in India operation for benign ovarian cyst. Fifteen months ago onset of *thyrotoxicosis* and thin nodule in !eft thyroid. Operation showed heavy lymphocytic infiltration of thyroid with lymphocytes and an area of papillary carcinoma. Now *rheumatoid arthritis* of knees and ankles. Serum showed RF.

Case **VI,** 54   Female, aged 68 years. Aged 48 years onset of *rheumatoid arthritis* with increasing disability in use of hands, feet, knees and elbows and severe bambooing of spine. Now widespread *Paget's disease* and bilateral ovarian cysts, one a serous cystadenoma, the other a papillary carcinoma. Serum showed ANF and thyroid auto-antibodies. Achlorhydria present.

Case **VI,** 55   Female, aged 49 years. Eight months ago had operation for bilateral ovarian cysts. Now has acute *rheumatoid arthritis.*

Case **VI,** 56   Female, aged 60 years. Aged 29 years operation for right ovarian cystadenoma. Follicular appendicitis found. Now *myxoedema, rheumatoid arthritis,* lipoma of right forearm, cervical spondylitis. Serum contained thyroid auto-antibodies.

Case **VI,** 57   Female, aged 65 years. Aged 53 years hysterectomy for fibroids and left benign ovarian cyst removed. Now *severe rheumatoid arthritis.* Serum showed ANF, RF and gastric parietal cell auto.antibodies. Achlorhydria present.

Case **VI,** 58   Female, aged 49 years. Operation for fibroids and benign ovarian cyst, followed soon after by *severe rheumatoid arthritis.* Serum showed RF and thyroid auto-antibodies.

Case **VI,** 59   Female, aged 55 years. Aged 35 years onset of *Raynaud's* phenomena. Aged 37 years operation for large fibroids and bilateral benign ovarian cysts. Aged 45 years onset of *rheumatoid arthritis* in hands, feet and temporo-mandibular joints. Serum showed RF and thyroid auto-antibodies.

Case **VI,** 60   Female, aged 62 years. Aged 37 years hysterectomy for fibroids and bilateral oophorectomy for benign cysts. Aged 50 years onset of Raynaud's phenomena. Serum showed ANF and blood lupus erythematous cells.

Case **VI,** 61   Female, aged 61 years. Aged 51 years hysterectomy for fibroids. Aged 57 years bilateral oophorectomy for benign ovarian cysts. Now mild *rheumatoid arthritis.* Serum showed RF. Achlorhydria present.

Case **VI,** 62   Female, aged 51 years. Fibroids diagnosed aged 33 years. *Diabetes* found agd 44 years. Hysterectomy and bilateral oophorectomy for bilateral benign ovarian cysts aged 46 years. Now mild *rheumatoid arthritis* and lumber spondylitis. Serum showed ANF.

Case **VI,** 63 (same as Case III, 18)   Female, aged 63 years. Husband died of carcinoma of the prostate and sarcoma of right upper arm. Her brother was a diabetic. Patient had *cystic mastitis* found at opera tion aged 24 years. Breasts nodular since that time. Aged 40 years hysterectomy for fibroids and one ovary removed for benign cyst. *Diabetic* for 2 years. Now has carcinoma of the breast. Serum showed ANF and gastric parietal cell auto-antibodies.

Case **VI,** 64   Female, aged 68 years. Mother died of pernicious anaemia and father died of cancer, site unknown. Patient aged 42 years had hystercdomy for fibroids. Aged

44 years thyroidectomy for *thyrotoxicosis*. Now moderate *rheumatoid arthritis* of hands and feet and carcinoma of both ovaries. Serum contained ANF, RF, thyroid auto-antibodies and gastric parietal cell auto-antibodies. Achlorhydria present.

Case VI, 65 — Female, aged 28 years. Aged 18 years operation for chronic appendicitis. Appendicular wall showed lymphocytic infiltration (follicular appendicitis). At operation cystic right ovary and fibroids found. Aged 26 years rapid onset of *Sjogren's syndrome*, crusting of the nose and fulminant *pyorrhoea* with falling out of the teeth. Chronic *active hepatitis* found at liver biopsy. Serum showed RF and ANF. Now cervical lymphadenopathy due to lymphosarcoma. Mass in nasopharynx of the same nature. RF and ANF disappeared from serum at onset of cancer.

Case VI, 66 (same as **Case III, 13**) — Female, aged 42 years. Onset of *thyrotoxicosis*. Followed in next 3 years by recurrent swellings in the breast and eventually a persistent mass in the lower outer quadrant of the left breast. Removed and shown to be *cystic mastitis*. Then followe:i menorrhagia and later urinary obstruction due to fibroids. Hysterectomy performed. Bilateral serous cysts of ovaries discovered. Serum showed ANF and thyroid auto-antibodies.

Case VI, 67 — Female, aged 64 years. One brother died of cerebral tumour, one cousin was a diabetic, one niece had diabetes. Patient at the age of 3U years had operation for fibroids and bilateral benign ovarian cysts. Aged 52 years developed *diabetes* and severe hypertension. Aged 61 years *auto-immune haemolytic anaemia*. Aged 63 years Kaposi's sarcoma with moderate *rheumatoid arthritic* changes.

Case VI, 68 — Female, aged 65 years. Aged 43 years hysterectomy for fibroids. Bilateral benign ovarian cysts also removed. Long history of rheumatic pains and marked *rheumatoid arthritic* deformity of hands. Now has chronic lymphatic leukaemia. Serum showed thyroid auto-antibodies.

Case VI, 69 (same as **Case I, 9**) — Female, aged 75 years. Aged 40 years hysterectomy for fibroids and benign left ovarian cystadenoma. Aged 46 years cholecystectomy for *chronic cholecystitis* and gall stones. Aged 65 years operation for carcinoma of the right breast. Six months before being seen acute *rheumatoid arthritis* and now malignant melanomatosis. Achlorhydria present.

Case VI, 70 — Female, aged 50 years. *Raynaud's phenomena* since twenties. Aged 40 years hysterectomy for fibroids and bilateral benign ovarian cysts. Now moderately severe *rheumatoid arthritis*. Serum showed RF.

Case VI, 71 (same as **Case I, 4**) — Female, aged 58 years. One brother died of cerebral glioma aged 47 years. One brother had carcinoma of the bronchus aged 65 years. Patient moderate smoker. Aged 31 years hysterectomy for fibroids. Aged 38 years left oophorectomy for benign serous cyst. Aged 42 years cholecystectomy for *chronic cholecystitis*. Aged 56 years removal of a lump in the left breast. Histologically this was *cystic mastitis*. Now has mild *rheumatoid arthritis* symptoms and changes and carcinoma of the bronchus. Serum showed RF. Achlorhydria present.

Thus, in all these successive cases in which operation for benign ovarian cysts of various types and/or fibroids had been undertaken in the past and which were encountered in a general medical practice, there was found to be evidence of collagen or auto-immune disease in some form preceding, associated with or following the development of these tumours. In many of the cases malignant disease or other tumours of various organs also developed.

It seems highly probable, therefore, that fibroids and benign ovarian cysts of various types are part of the spectrum of collagen and auto-immune diseases as they affect the myometrium of the uterus and the ovaries. The former would explain the areas of lymphocytic infiltration frequently found in fibroids. The latter could be the result of disease affecting the serosa covering the ovary.

Collagen diseases and ectopic pregnancies

Normal fertilization of the ovum discharged from the ruptured Graffian follicle is thought to occur near the ovary and on the peritoneal lining. The fertilized ovum then reaches the internal opening of th uterine tube and descends on the endometrium of the tube to become implanted in the endometrium of the body of the uterus. Ectopic pregnancies result from an interference with the descent of the fertilized ovum. The cause of most ectopic pregnancies is unknown. Certain factors are, however, known to favour their occurrence. They are:-

1) Congenital abnormalities of the female genitalia.

2) A previous history of salpingitis and oophoritis due to gonoccocal, pneumococcal and other infections, which cause fibrosis of the tubal fimbria and tubal and uterine mucosal lining, thus hindering the normal descent of the fertilized ovum.

3) The presence of fibroids. Fibroids are commonly associated with endometritis and uterine polyps. This endometritis may involve the mucosa of the tubes and thus interfere with the normal descent of the ovum.

Collagen diseases could well be concerned in some cases of ectopic pregnancy. This appeared to be so in the following cases:-

Case 33 Female, aged 57 years. Menarche aged 12 years. Periods normal. No history of venereal disease. Aged 31 years ectopic abdominal pregnancy. Aged 35 years tubal pregnancy. No normal pregnancies. Menopause aged 46 years. Aged 49 years onset of arthritis of left hip and later of generalized rheumatoid disease. Aged 52 years onset of Raynaud's phenomena. Now well-marked rheumatoid deformities, Sjogren's syndrome and atrophic rhinitis. Serum showed no auto-antibodies. Lupus erythematosus cells not found.

Case 34 Female, aged 72 years. Menarche aged 13 years. No history of venereal disease. Ectopic pregnancy aged 25 years followed by normal pregnancy and a further ectopic pregnancy at the age of 37 years. Menopause aged 50 years. Onset of rheumatoid arthritis aged 57 years and of myxoedema aged 69 years. Deep vein thrombosis of left leg aged 70 years. At present suffering from coronary thrombosis.

Case 35 Female, aged 43 years. Mother suffered from severe rheumatoid arthritis, Sjogren's syndrome, myxoedema, atrophic gastritis and adhesive otitis. Patient ·experienced ruptured ovarian cyst at the age of 22 years. At the age of 35 years she had an ectopic pregnancy and was found to have fibroids. At the age of 43 years developed symptoms of rheumatoid arthritis.

Fibroids appear to result from collagen diseases. Furthermore, involvement of the peritoneum in the neighbourhood of the ovaries and internal orifice of the uterine tubes in a chronic inflammatory process, such as that found in collagen diseases, might also interfere with the descent of the fertilized ovum and its entry into the peritoneal opening of the tubes. Thus, collagen and auto-immune disease could be an important cause of ectopia.

Chapter III

The nature of collagen and auto-immune disease

III, i) **Summary** of the pathological changes in the body in collagen and auto-immune diseases

In summary, from the above considera-, tions it is apparent that the various *"collagen" and "auto-immune" diseases, including rheumatoid arthritis, show every com-bination and gradation from one to the other. It seems that the various manifestations are those of one disease. Every tissue of the body may be affected or the brunt of the disease is born by only one or two organs. Arthropathy is but one manifestation of the spectrum and may be absent.* The most acute and generalized manifestations of the disease are found in cases of disseminated eosinophilic collagen disease when every tissue in the body is involved. In the less severe but still generalized cases of the disease the patient may complain of fatigue, anorexia, weight loss and oedemas. The histological changes are manifest by collections of lymphocytes, often accompanied by plasma cells and eosinophils and frequently by the formation of germinal centres in these collections. Such changes have been shown to result from infection or antigenic stimulation (see Willis, 1958). These changes may be followed by fibrosis. An arteritis is frequently found affecting vessels of various sizes and also venules. This consists of cuffing and infiltration of the walls of the vessels with the same lymphocytes and plasma cells. There is commonly an endarteritis of smaller vessels. A tendency to intravascular arterial clotting occurs. Granulomatous rheumatoid nodules may affect any tissue and show focal collections of lymphocytes often in relation to a patch of arteritis with a central necrotic area and occasinally giant cells. Their granulomatous structure resembles that of an infection. The joint capsules may or may not exhibit collections of lymphocytes with germinal centres and changes of the same nature may occur in all exocrine glands, including lacrimal, salivary and pancreatic glands, breasts and kidneys. In these secondary changes lead to disappearance of acinar cells, fibrosis of the organ and dilatation of the ducts often leading to cyst formation. Chronic pyelonephritis is common in rheumatoid disease. All the endocrine glands, including thyroid, parathyroid, adrenals and pituitary may be affected and their secretions fail. Diabetes is commod The pleura and lungs show similar cellular infiltration. In the latter this may occur in the alveolar walls or as nodular formations. There is usually an hypertrophy of all lymphoid tissue, including lymph nodes, tonsils, adenoids and that in the appendix and the Malphigian corpuscles of the spleen may be similarly affected. It shows the changes of reactive hyperplasia or chronic inflammation like that produced by an infection. Splenomegaly is common. The thymus may show similar involvement with hypertrophy and the formation of germinal centres, sometimes with tumour formation. The pericardium, myocardium and endocardium may all be affected. The peritoneum may be involved leading to peritoneal adhesions and possibly ectopic pregnancies. Synovial membranes not only of joints, but also·of bursae and tendon sheaths, may be affected. The interfibrillary tissues of the muscles and peripheral nerves and the coats of the eye may be involved and in the last-named small lesions like rheumatoid nodules may be found. The periosteum may be locally involved producing rheumatoid nodules, but various bones, either single or multiple, may show the changes of Paget's disease. The liver may exhibit the same collections of lymphocytes in the periportal spaces producing either active chronic hepatitis, biliary or postnecrotic cirrhosis. In addition, the submucosal tissues of all the hollow viscera may be infiltrated by the same cells leading to chronic inflammation with swelling and later this results in atrophic lesions of parts of the mucosae of the gastro-intestinal tract anywhere from the lips to the anus. The mucosa of the gall bladder may likewise be involved. The endometrium and vaginal mucosa may be similarly involved. Fibroids may develop in the uterus and cysts of various types in the ovary. The central nervous system may show dural involvement or perivascular collections of lymphocytes or vasculitis may be found in any part of the neuraxis. This results in neurological or psychotic disturbances. This is quite distinct from the specific lesions of systemic lupus erythematosus. The peripheral nerves may show changes due to arteritis of the vasae nervorum or infiltration of the nerve roots or of the nerves more distally by collections of lymphocytes or the nerves may be involved by rheumatoid nodules. The skin may exhibit various lesions. The dermis may show widespread involvement by infiltration with lymphocytes affecting the sweat and sebaceous glands resulting in a condition of ichthyosis acquisita or it may show the changes of scleroderma or the hair roots may be involved in part or whole, resulting in localized or generalized alopecia. The skin may also lose or gain pigment resulting in vitiligo and melanoderma or may be involved in other ways producing acanthosis nigricans, eczema, psoriasis, parapsoriasis, pemphigus or dermatitis herpetiformis. There may occur a stomatitis and gingivitis and fulminant pyorrhoea and dental caries. Allergic manifestations, such as intrinsic asthma, bronchitis, urticaria, angioneurotic oedema or rhinitis may appear. There may be allergic responses to various drugs. The respiratory mucosa, both upper and lower, exhibits chronic inflammatory changes and oedema or this be replaced by atrophic changes. There may be deafness of various types. Eosinophilia may be seen in the blood and may be extreme. The E.S.R. is usually raised. In other cases there is an auto-immune haemolytic anaemia or purpura of Henoch-Schonlein type. There may be a fall or rise in the number of the various cellular constituents of the blood. In some cases there is a general stimulation of haemopoiesis resulting in the condition of polycythaemia vera or in other cases a general depression of the bone marrow may be found producing pancytopenia. In the marrow there may be an increase or decrease in the plasma cells with a corresponding rise or fall in the level of the gammaglobulins of the blood. The latter, like auto-immune haemolytic anaemia, may precede the appearance of other clinical manifestations of disease by years. Damage to the bone marrow may lead to myelofibrosis. Various antibodies may be found in the serum whatever the manner of presentation of the collagen and auto-immune disease. These include ANF, RF, organ-specific antibodies and even a positive Wassermann reaction. These are associated with a diffuse hypergammaglobulinaemia and even a monoclonal paraproteinaemia and cryoglobulinaemia or the appearance of Waldenstrom's macroglobulinaemia. Sometimes patients present with only a single manifestation of the disease spectrum, such as pernicious anaemia, thyroid disease, diabetes or Addison's disease and only some or none of the many auto-antib dies appear in the serum. In other cases a person may appear to be completely healthy and yet auto-antibodies may be present in the serum.

Secondary disturbances may result from the above lesions. Thus, involvement of the kidney may lead to fibrosis and hypertension or, when it produces renal tubular acidosis, leads to nephrosclerosis and osteomalacia, while involvement of the heart or lungs with or without hypertension leads to heart failure and amyloidosis may be found. Gout may follow polycythaemia and various endocrine deficiency syndromes may appear.

On consideration of the protean manifestation of collagen and auto-immune diseases, which may involve every tissue in the body, one is immediately reminded of syphilis. In fact, syphilis may likewise involve every tissue of the body and may cause a polyarthritis like certain forms of rheumatoid arthritis (Short et al., 1957), while a positive Wassermann reaction may occur in some cases of rheumatoid arthritis or systemic lupus erythematosus. This similarity is seen in the vasculitis or arteritis, the endarteritic swelling, in the rheumatoid nodules which resemble small gummata, in the osteitis which constitutes Paget's disease (Which Paget himself compared to syphilitic osteitis) and in involvement of the lungs and liver comparable with syphilitic gummatous changes in these organs. Amyloidosis may be seen in cases of both syphilis and collagen and auto-immune disease. Syphilis may lead to alopecia, various skin rashes and depigmentation and to muscle changes and involvement of the peripheral nerves and central nervous system as does collagen and auto-immune disease. It also causes the appearance of many different antibodies in the serum or of hypergammaglobulinaemia, paraproteinaemia and cryoglobulinaemia. Leprosy likewise leads to vitiligo. Waldenstrom and others, indeed, state that, "if the spirochaete had not been discovered, syphilis could be taken to be an ideal model of an auto-immune disease. The variety of tissue reaction antibodies, the widespread lymphocytic tissue damage and the vasculitis are characteristic features". On such grounds it might be presumed that collagen and auto-immune diseases are due to an infection.

Of some interest are reports that rheumatoid arthritis and auto-immune diseases of all kinds, including coeliac disease and ulcerative colitis, are rare in Africans (Greenwood, 1968; McGill, 1971; Hutt and Templeton, 1971; Navis et al., 1971). Greenwood (1969 a, b, c) found that both rheumatoid arthritis and Still's disease do occur, however, in Western Nigerians as in Europeans and raised the possibility that some agent in the tropical environment, perhaps protozoal, determines a different response in a tropical African population from that seen in temperate climates among Caucasians.

III, ii) The role of auto-antibodies in collagen and auto-immune disease

Because various immune antibodies active against cell constituents or specific organs of the body are found in the blood in collagen diseases and in certain conditions, such as focal or diffuse thyroiditis, Sjogren's syndrome, atrophic gastritis and idiopathic adrenalitis, in recent years these diseases have been termed "auto-immune". When the idea of auto-immune diseases was first brought forward, many considered the changes in the tissues in the various diseases to be brought about as the result of the reaction of the auto-antibodies with the antigens of the various tissues. There are, however, many arguments against this. Thus,

1) "Auto-immune" disease, for example of the thyroid, may occur in the absence of demonstrable thyroid auto-antibodies in the blood, while auto-antibodies may occur in the blood in the absence of auto-immune disease of the organ against which they are directed. This is true of other organs.

2) In systemic lupus erythematosus the role of auto-antibodies in producing tissue damage is doubtful (Holborow, 1963).

There is no evidence that ANF is the cause of systemic lupus erythematosus (Anderson et al., 1967).

3) There is no evidence that the RF is the primary cause of the joint changes of rheumatoid arthritis (Anderson et al.. 1967). Injections of the factor do not lead to the development of arthritis. Not infrequently the factor is absent in typical cases of rheumatoid arthritis or it may only appear at a late stage of the disease.

4) Polyarthritis indistinguishable from rheumatoid arthritis and other collagen diseases occurs in a third of patients with agammaglobulinaemia in the absence of auto-antibodies and RF in the blood (Good and Rotstein, 1960). They are also liable to develop dermatomyositis and other collagen diseases and auto-immune phenomena affecting the red blood corpuscles, liver and kidney (Janeway, 1967) in the absence of auto-antibodies in the blood.

5) In cases of Hashimoto's thyroiditis and systemic lupus erythematosus the antibodies cross the placenta and reach the same titre in the foetus as in the mother, but produce no detectable effects in the baby (Beck and Rowell, 1963).

Most observers do not believe that circulating antibodies are responsible for tile lesions in collagen or auto-immune disease, as exemplified by the thyroid lesions in Hashimoto's thyroiditis, but some other factor damaging the gland, such as an infection, may be necessary to allow access of the antibodies to the antigen substrate (Reinlein and Navarro, 1967; Doniach and Roitt, 1968). Asherson (1965) in a review of auto-immune disease points out that no considerations rule out the possibility that the disease is started by a virus or some other unknown agent and that the damaging immune response is directed against a causal antigen or indeed that the immune disease is not an important part of the disease process. According to Anderson et al. (1967) in their extensive review auto-immune antibodies are not the cause of auto-immune disease, but auto-immune response is the cause of at least part of the inflammatory change in Hashimoto's thyroiditis and its variants. Auto-immunity is of aetiological importance in producing the lesions in as much as the lesions of Hashimoto's thyroiditis would be different in its absence. The role of the immune mechanism in producing some of the features of "auto-immune" disease is also shown by the frequently reported benefit in collagen disease resulting from the administration of immuno-suppressive drugs which are, however, only effective in diminishing, but not abolishing the manifestations of the disease.

Auto-antibodies in the diseases under consideration do not occur from damage to tissues as a result of liberation of cell products into the circulation. Surgical injury to tissues, for example thyroidectomy, usually results at most in a weak transient auto-immune response (Anderson et al., 1967), nor does local infection of the thyroid result in the appearance of auto-immune antibodies. Again, gastric surgery does not result in the appearance of gastric parietal cell auto-antibodies in the blood from damage to the stomach (Ashurst, 1968). A range of micro-organisms have antigens similar to mammalian tissues, for example E. coli, haemolytic streptococci, T. pallidum, malaria parasites, glandular fever, mycoplasma pneumoniae, Listeria monocytogenes and M. leprae, and cause auto-immune phenomena. It has, therefore, been suggested that infection with such an organism could result in the appearance of auto-antibodies which then damage certain tissues. Mustakallio et al. (1967) postulate that infection may play a part in triggering off auto-immune disease. Adams (1967) likewise states that "it is possible that infection may provoke the formation of auto-antibodies in individuals who are genetically capable of producig them".

Interesting light is thrown on the relationship of some features of the collagen diseases to immune responses of the body by certain clinical observations. Case 3 will be recalled. He was suffering from rheumatoid arthritis and was treated with camoquin to which he was sensitive. The condition then changed into one of systemic lupus erythematosus. It is well-known that cases of cancer or malignant lymphoma exhibit depression of immune mechanisms and tissue anergy (Aisenberg, 1964; Hughes and Mackay, 1965; Watkins, 1973). These disturbances disappear with successful treatment of the malignancy. Alexander and Fairley (1968) report that in reticuloses, especially those involving lymphocytes and plasma cells and to a lesser extent in other reticuloses and carcinomata, circulating antibody formation is impaired. Talal and Bunim (1964) describe three cases of Sjogren's syndrome which developed malignant lymphoma. In one of these the RF and organ-specific tissue antibodies disappeared from the blood as reticulum cell sarcoma developed. Nilsen et al. (1967) describe the case of a 51 year old woman who suffered from systemic lupus erythematosus for 10 years before she developed Hodgkin's disease. All clinical and laboratory signs of systemic lupus erythematosus disappeared with the onset of Hodgkin's disease and none were found at autopsy. Fernandez-Herlihy and Kott (1967) report the case of a boy of 5 years who suffered from migrating arthralgias, butterfly rash, fever and haematuria due to systemic lupus erythematosus. At the age of 15 years he developed lymphosarcoma. With this all the laboratory tests for lupus erythematosus became negative and the rash disappeared. Szegedi et al. (1968) describe two cases. In the first the thyroid was removed for thyrotoxicosis. Two years later she developed dermatomyositis. Lupus erythematosus cells, ANF and RF were present in the blood. Five years later Hodgkin's disease developed and all signs of dermatomyositis and the blood changes disappeared. In the second case joint pains and erythema multiforme appeared. Lupus erythematosus cells and RF were found in

the blood. Three years later Hodgkin's disease developed and with it the blood changes and rash disappeared. Klingmuller and Vorleander (1965) also describe two patients with systemic lupus erythematosus who developed Hodgkin's disease. In both the skin lesions and blood changes of lupus erythematosus and RF and the joint swellings disappeared with the onset of Hodgkin's disease. In one case with successful treatment of the Hodgkin's disease with radiotherapy they reappeared. Schmidt and Gebhardt (1969) also describe a case of discoid lupus erythematosus which developed Hodgkin's disease and then the skin lesions healed. Again, in cases of rheumatoid arthritis which develop myelomatosis, in which immunoparesis may exist, a number of observers have found that the arthropathy disappears (Wegelius et al., 1970). Furthermore, the manifestations of rheumatoid arthritis may in part be relieved by immunosuppressive drugs (Harris et al., 1971).

This evidence suggests that many manifestations of systemic lupus erythematosus and dermatomyositis are *in part* hyperergic and disappear if a decrease or absence of fixed cell and circulating antibodies occurs. Even if an auto-immune mechanism were accepted as being responsible for producing the organ changes in "auto-immune" disease in their entirety, the question of the origin of the auto-antibodies in the blood in these diseases still remains. Since a range of micro-organisms have antigens similar to mammalian tissues, it is, therefore, postulated that an infection with such an organism may be the primary disturbance in auto-immune diseases.

III, iii)   The infective aetiology of collagen and auto-immune disease

For many years rheumatoid arthritis was considered to be an infection (Hollander et al., 1960; see Robinson, 1967), but with the advent of the concept of auto-immunity

-104-

this idea lost favour. Such a view has recently been revived (Leading Article, Lancet, 1970, 2, 303). It is supported by many observations.

1) The pyrexia, anorexia, weight loss, oedemas, raised E.S.R. and hypergammaglobulinaemia seen in cases of collagen diseases are typical of a chronic infection.

2) In the form of the disease characterized as disseminated eosinophilic collagen disease as described above, the features are typical of an infection and especially of a parasite.

3) An infective cause of Sjogren's syndrome, a manifestation of rheumatoid arthritis and other collagen or auto-immune diseases, has been suggested by many writers, including Shearn (1971), who also compared the manifestations of Sjogren's syndrome with syphilis. Again the suggestion of an infection or external cause for Hashimoto's thyroiditis has been made frequently (Furszyfer et al., 1970).

4) The lymphadenopathy with its chronic inflammatory changes or reactive hyperplasia, splenomegaly and granulomata found in collagen and auto-immune disease are typical of an infection.

5) The lymphocyte collections with follicles and germ cell centres seen in the lesions of collagen and auto-immune disease are typical of infections (see Willis, 1958), particularly protozoal.

6) Hypochromic normocytic anaemias, acute haemolytic anaemias, neutrophil leucocytosis or leucopenia, lymphocytic or lymphopenia and thrombocytopenia, which may all occur in association with collagen and auto-immune diseases, are often due to infections (Dacie, 1962; Young, 1967; Wintrobe, 1967).

7) Plasmacytosis and lymphoid follicles of the bone marrow may occur in chronic infections, such as tuberculosis and syphilis, as well as in collagen diseases (Evans, 1966; Osserman, 1971).

8) It has been shown above that paraproteinaemia and cryoglobulinaemia, which may be manifestations of collagen and auto-immune diseases, are also produced by chronic infections, such as malaria, syphilis and osteomyelitis (Osserman, 1971), and treatment of the underlying infection may cause the paraproteinaemia to disappear (Fran!.;ois et al., 1966).

9) Amyloidosis, which may occur in cases of collagen disease, may also complicate chronic infections.

10) The eosinophilia and allergic manifestations which may occur in collagen and auto-immune diseases are suggestive of infection with some parasite.

11) The villous atrophy of the small intestine seen in cases of coeliac disease may be produced by infections and especially by worm and protozoal infestation.

12) Rhetimatoid factor (RF) is a gammaglobulin with a sedimentation co-effici-ent of 19S and belongs to the class of macroglobulins in the serum. It probably exists in loose combination with several molecules of the 7S variety. RF is an antibody. The antigenic stimulus is unknown. It occurs in the IgM. fraction, . RF may be found in the blood, albeit in low concentration, in many infections, including subacute bacterial endocarditis, infective hepatitis, pulmonary tuberculosis, syphilis, leprosy, etc. (Anderson et al., 1967; Mustakallio et al., 1967; Ball, 1969; Doniach and Roitt, 1969). In these diseases arthritis is not a feature and successful treatment of the underlying disease causes the RF to disappear from the blood. Not only the RF, but also ANF, a positive Wassermann reaction and thyroid auto-antibodies and lupus erythematosus cells may also be present in the sera of a high proportion of cases of leprosy (Cathcart et al., 1961; Bonomo et al., 1963, 1965). In these cases again RF and other auto-antibodies and lupus erythematosus cells in the blood appear as a response to infection, suggesting a similar mechanism in .the collagen and auto-immune diseases.

As well as in collagen diseases RF occurs, however, in *high concentration* in *chronic infections with any pro-tozoon, in-*

eluding *malaria, trypanosomiasis, kala azar, visceral leishmaniasis and amoebiasis.* M-antiglobulins (RF-like globulin) occur in a high titre in the blood in infections with certain protozoa in Africans in Central Africa in the absence of rheumatoid arthritis. These include trypanosomiasis and malaria (Van Tongeren, 1962, 1966; Housa and Allison, 1966) and in cases of kala-azar and visceral leishmaniasis (Ball, 1969), in all of which conditions there may be a blood eosinophilia. Adenyi-Jones (1967) found that in Nigerians the serum contains a RF-like macroglobulin in 91 per cent of rural adults and 39 per cent of infants, while this is absent from the umbilical cord blood, indicating exposure to antigen. He related the findings to malarial infection. Shaper et al. (1968) report that in the immigrant and indiginous population of Uganda there are found a high titre of malarial antibody and high levels of IgM, RF and circulating auto-antibodies to heart, thyroid and gastric parietal cells. The levels of the latter and RF were related to that of the malarial antibody titre. This immunological syndrome was related to malarial infection. These blood changes Glso gradually disappear on treatment with anti-protozoal drugs.

Taken together such observations make it impossible to believe that collagen and auto-immune diseases are anything other than infective in aetiology. The cumulative evidence suggests that there is some profound immunological stimulus in these diseases to sustain the high level of RF for so long a period. The nature of this stimulus is unknown, but much of the evidence points to the possibility of some parasitic, possibly protozoal, infection. The appearance of RF, ANF and auto-antibodies and lupus erythematosus cells in the blood would be an antibody response to this infection. After the establishment of this infection immune responses then play a part in determining the exact type of collagen or auto-immune disease which develops and reactions between auto-antibodies

and tissue antigens determine in part the extent of damage to any particular tissue, such as the thyroid gland. Even if the brunt of the disease is borne by one tissue, the disease is generalized.

III, iv) Localization of rheumatoid lesions in regions of irritation and trauma

Burrows (1932) in an interesting book pointed out that the lesions of generalized bacterial and virus diseases tend to become localized in areas of trauma and chronic irritation where the organisms collect. This applies to T. pallidum, M. leprae, M. tuberculosis, B. typhosum, pneumococci, streptococci and viruses, such as those of measles, vaccmta and varicella, and tumour-producing viruses in animals. It has been mentioned above that rheumatoid nodules (granulomata) and bursitis tend to localize in regions of pressure, such as on the bridge of the nose from the pressure of spectacles. This probably explains their tendency to occur around the elbows, where they are found over the pressure points.

In certain "auto-immune" skin diseases it is well known that injury or chronic irritation may lead to the appearance of the skin lesion in this area (Kohner's phenomenon). Caplan's syndrome is an interesting manifestation of this phenomenon and Caplan described pneumoconiosis in coal miners suffering from rheumatoid arthritis. A similar change may occur in asbestos workers and gold and chalk miners (Gardner, 1972). The mildly irritant effects of dust are apparently sufficient to make the lungs a major focus of rheumatoid involvement. These observations indicate the generalized nature of the disease and suggests a particulate or organismal causation.

III, v) Precipitating factors of collagen and auto-immune diseases

The various collagen and auto-immune diseases may be precipitated or recur as a result of the operation of certain known factors. Thus, the onset or recurrence of latent rheumatoid arthritis may be precipitated by acute illnesses, such as tonsillitis or exanthemata, or by emotional shock or occur about the time of the menopause. Dermatomyositis may be precipitated by many different factors, which include drugs, intercurrent infections and operations (Winkelmann et al., 1968). In Case 5 hysterectomy for fibroids was followed immediately by the onset of acute dermato-myositis. Systemic lupus erythematosus may be precipitated by local infections, emotion or physical stress, exposure to sunlight and by the administration of certain drugs, such as gold, isoniazid, procain amide, anticonvulsants, antibiotics or hydralazine (Leading Article, Brit. med. J. 1970, 1, 192). An operation may likewise precipitate the development of systemic lupus erythematosus as was well exemplified by Case XX, 30. This woman had a thyroidectomy for thyrotoxicosis at the age of 31 years, cystic mastitis at the age of 34 years and at the age of 58 years developed lumps in both breasts, one of which was due to cystic mastitis and the other due to carcinoma. Prior to operation there were numerous lupus erythematosus cells in the blood and the serum contained RF and ANF in high concentration and thyroid auto-antibodies. Immediately after bilateral mastectomy she developed acute and severe polyarthropathy. Tonsillitis or pharyngitis or emotional disturbances are well-known to predispose to thyrotoxicosis and emotional factors may appear to precipitate the appearance of ulcerative colitis.

In all the above conditions it seems very probable that latent disease already exists in many subjects and the above factors precipitate the onset of obvious manifestations. In so far as collagen and auto-immune diseases are often familial some genetic factor must control the response

to the infection.

III, vi) Systemic lupus erythematosus syndrome and collagen diseases caused by drugs

Mention has been made of the fact that certain drugs, such as hydantoins, procaine amide, isoniazid, hydralazine and certain antibiotics, may cause the appearance of the systemic lupus erythematosus syndrome. This may consist merely of the presence of lupus erythematosus cells in the blood or the fullblown syndrome of fever, polyarthritis, polyserositis, haematological changes, eosinophilia and pulmonary infiltration. Grob and Herold (1972) record benign lymphadenopathy and periarteritis occurring following the administration of hydantoins. Sorrell et al. (1971) describe a depression of immunological function in patients treated with phenytoin sodium. Grob and Herold also found that hydantoins may cause lowering or disappearance of IgA and lowering of β CIA levels in the serum and depression of skin reactions to antigens. Hence, there is a depression of both humoral and cellular immunity as a result of hydantoin administration. It would seem, therefore, that at any rate in the case of hydantoins, the occurrence of the manifestations of collagen disease, such as systemic lupus erythematosus, arthropathy, periarteritis and benign lymphadenopathy following administration of certain drugs could be explained as due to depression of resistance to a latent infection, which causes collagen diseases.

III, vii) Sarcoidosis and collagen and auto-immune disease

Sarcoid reactions in the tissues occur as a response to many substances. In contrast the aetiology of the generalized disease, sarcoidosis, however, remains obscure, but it is now generally accepted as a single disorder (Siltzbach, 1971). Efforts to implicate various infective agents have met with little success, but most authorities regard the condition as a chronic infection. It is a systemic granulomatous disease of variable course, which may undergo spontaneous remission. Almost any organ of the body may be affected by the inflammatory process. There may be fever and sweating. There are secondary immunological abnormalities with partial failure of cellular immunity (Siltzbach, 1971) and an *increased susceptibility to certain infections.* Thus, there may be superimposed tuberculosis. In addition, the manifestations of collagen and auto-immune disease may develop in the course of the illness as exemplified by a polyarthropathy identical with that occurring in rheumatoid arthritis, hyper-splenism, Hashimoto's thyroiditis, myxoedema, hyperthyroidism, Addison's disease, fibrosing alveolitis (Scadding, 1969; Goldsmith, 1970; Karlish and MacGregor, 1970; Leppard, 1971), asthma, granulomatous arteritis, pancreatitis, fibroids and adenomyosis of the uterus with eosinophilia (Bottcher, 1959), alopecia (Maycock et al., 1963), hyperglobulinaemia, cryoglobulinaemia, the presence of RF and of thyroid adrenal and gastric parietal cell auto-antibodies in the blood in a high proportion of cases, blood eosinophilia (Maycock et al., 1963) and of plasma cells in the bone marrow (Osserman, 1959). These changes are essentially those of collagen and auto-immune disease. They occur as a complication of a disease in which there is a partial failure of immunity me<::hanisms and this could be interpreted as favouring the infective nature of collagen and auto-immune diseases.

III, viii) The incidence of collagen and auto-immune diseases and auto-antibodies in the blood with age

Rheumatoid disease may be found at birth and as Still's disease occurs from about the age of 6 months to 16 years. About 3 per cent of the population in this country are said to suffer from rheumatoid arthritis sufficiently severely to require treatment (Hart, 1970). However, a surprisingly high proportion of cases of rheumatoid arthritis in a population survey in this country have never sought medical advice (Duthie, 1969). A large number of individuals have intermittent mild episodes of arthritis, not permanently disabling and for which they may not seek medical aid. Five per cent of males and seven per cent of females over 15 years of age give a past history of polyarthritis. The prevalence of rheumatoid arthritis over 15 years of age was reported as 2.1 per cent in males and 5.2 per cent in females, increasing with age and reaching 6 per cent in males over 75 years of age and 16 per cent in females aged 65-75 years of age. The incidence is much the same in seven countries of northern Europe, but the disease is rare in Central Africa and India. In older subjects in this country typical painless rheumatoid arthritic deformities of the hands, hallux valgus and overlapping toes and rheumatoid changes in the cervical spine are seen frequently, though no advice has been sought for them. RF is usually absent from the serum. However, about 25 per cent of cases of otherwise classical rheumatoid arthritis never show RF or ANF *in* their sera. Against this must be set the fact that many subjects without evidence of collagen or auto-immune disease nevertheless show RF or ANF in the sera, presumably evidence of latent infection with an organism causing the disease, that is assuming that other infectious causes for these serological changes are excluded. Heimer et al. (1963) found that RF occurs in the serum of about 45 per cent of persons over the age of 65 years.

Likewise, the incidence of manifest Hashimoto's thyroiditis and focal thyroiditis increases with age (Gardner, 1968; Furszyter et al., 1970). Both conditions may exist with or without the presence of thyroid auto-antibodies, while thyroid auto-antibodies may be found in the blood in the absence of thyroid disease. Fowler et al. (1970) state that thyroid auto-antibodies may be detected in about 10 per cent of the population of this country, while Assem et al. (1965) claim that the serum of more than half the normal adult population contains antibody against thyroglobulin. Doniach and Raitt (1969) record the incidence of thyroglobulin antibodies in normal subjects in relation to age and sex. They describe a gradual increase in incidence with age and a threefold increase in females over males up to 60 years of age. This may reach 16 per cent In the older a,ge group. The mean incidence of microsomal and colloid fluorescent thyroid antibodies is 3.7 per cent in males and 5.6 per cent in females. Whittingham et al. (1971) found the incidence of thyroglobulin antibodies in controls increased with age from 5 per cent below the age of 40 to 10 per cent between 41 and 60 and 30 per cent over 60 years. RF and thyroid auto-antibodies are often present together in elderly subjects (Sachse and Poser, 1961).

In a similar manner the incidence of atrophic gastritis, achlorhydria and pernicious anaemia increases with age. Howitz and Schwartz (1971) state that achlorhydria in the absence of carcinoma of the stomach is almost always due to atrophic gastritis. Atrophic gastritis and achlorhydria are very common over 50 years of age. According to ·Bloomfield and Polland (1933) and Vanzant et al. (1932) achlorhydria is found in apparently healthy subjects increasing with age. From 20-39 years it is found in 3 per cent of males and 7 per cent of females. From 40-59 years it is found in 13 per cent of males and 17 per cent of females and from 60 years upwards in 27 per cent of males and 25 per cent of females. In Finland 28 per cent of the "normal" population have atrophic gastritis (Leading Article, Brit. med. J., 1972, ii, 309). Baron and Lennard-Janes (1971) likewise found atrophic gastritis so frequent with increasing age that it is often considered an aging process. The

frequency with which gastric parietal cell antibodies are found in the blood likewise increases with age. Kravetz et al. (1967) found gastric parietal cell antibodies in 2-19 per cent of healthy persons increasing with age.

About 12-14 per cent of the population are diabetics. The incidence increases with age. Over the age of 70 years in this country as many as 50 per cent of the population are diabetics (see Sonksen, 1972). Similar findings are reported from the United States of America.

As regards cystic mastitis the inc'dence in "normal" breasts is very high and varies from 28-33 per cent at autopsy (see Evans, 1966), increasing with age. In other subjects it appears that from 1-3 per cent show the changes of Paget's disease of bone, the incidence increasing with age. It has been stated that 20-25 per cent of women beyond 35 years of age have uterine fibroids (see Evans, 1966). One per cent of the population are stated to exhibit vitiligo in the skin (Lerner, 1967). Moreover rheumatoid infection may exist and produce paraproteinaemia and the presence of non-specific or organ specific antibodies up to perhaps 50 years before signs of disease show themselves. One per cent of the total population of this country and 3 per cent of those over 70 years of age are found with paraproteinaemia, but without symptoms (Hall n. 1963; Hobbs, 1966). Again the incidence of Waldenstrom's macroglobulinaemia and of amyloidosis (senile amyloidosif>) a manifestation of chronic antigenic stimulation, gradually increases with age.

If it is assumed that the presence of RF, ANF and thyroid and gast ric parietal cell antibodies, of paraproteinaemia in the blood and the development of various collagen and auto-immune diseases is due to a single infective cause, then it must be that *evident or latent infection with the causative organism is present in a high proportion of subjects, increasing with* age. Moreover, such latent infection may be present for many years before signs of the disease process appears (Ward and Reinhard, 1971). Infection, thus, occurs at any time of life and presumably repeated infections may occur. Many of the *collagen and auto-immune diseases*, for example, rheumatoid arthritis, atrophic gastritis and lymphocytic thyroiditis, are so common in old age, as to *constitute part of the aging process*.

III, ix) The lack of effect of antibiotics on rheumatoid disease

The possible aetiological factors and pathogenesis of rheumatoid arthritis have been reviewed by Gardner (1972). They include infections with mycoplasmas, bacterial "L" forms, diphtheroids, protozoa and metazoa, viruses, immunological changes, lysosomes, collagen injury and vascular injury. No conclusions were reached. One difficulty has been the chronicity of the disease which has been ascribed by Glynn to a persistent immunological response. Gardner states "There is no evidence that ...... organisms, such as protozoa, are capable of initiating rheumatoid arthritis. However, less attention has been paid to the immunological characteristics of agents, such as leishmania, in this context than is desirable. It is always salutary to compare a rheumatoid granuloma with the skin lesions of onchocerciasis". Most workers have sought the cause of the disease in the joint tissues, which seems ridiculous in a generalized disease.

Neither antibiotics, which act on bacteria and mycoplasma, antituberculous drugs, such as streptomycin, PAS and INAH, nor antispirochaetal drugs, such as penicillin and its derivatives, have any beneficial effect on rheumatoid arthritis or other collagen or auto-immune diseases. This indicates that neither bacteria, for example diphtheroids, mycoplasma, spirochaetes or acid fast bacilli, are the cause of these conditions. Furthermore there is no evidence that viruses are the cause of collagen diseases (see Klippel et al., 1973). However, gold salts may have a beneficial effect on rheumatoid diseases and systemic lupus erythematosus. These substances have been shown to affect certain bacteria adversely, for example B. tuberculosis and haemolytic streptococcus, and can be effective in syphilis and this could point to an organismal cause for rheumatoid disease.

III, x) Congenital agammaglobulinaemia and collagen and auto-immune disease

In cases of congenital agammaglobulinaemia it has been mentioned above that there exists a special liability to bacterial and protozoal infections, but *not to virus diseases*. It has been seen that these patients are especially liable to develop collagen or auto-immune diseases, a 'finding strongly against a viral cause for such diseases. Thus, the evidence suggests an infective, but not a bacterial or virus aetiology of collagen and auto-immune disease and considerable evidence to suggest the possibility of a protozoal causation, a suggestion borne out by the effects of antiprotozoal drugs on collagen diseases.

III, xi) Collagen and auto-immune disease and antiprotozoal drugs

It has been seen that RF in the serum found in a high proportion of cases of collagen disease is typical of chronic protozoal infections. A high proportion of "collagen" diseases (70-80 per cent) respond, albeit sometimes slowly, to various antiprotozoal drugs. These include the 4-aminoquinolines, chloroquine, hydrochloroquine (plaquenil), amodiaquin (camoquin), but also daraprim (pyramethamine) and mepacrine (Page, 1951; Bagnell, 1957; Fuld, 1960; Hollander et al., 1960; Soderstrom et al., 1961). Sjogren's syndrome may likewise be relieved by these drugs (Heaton, 1963). A case of dermatomyo-

Addendum: Schweiger F. (International Medical News, October 1st. 1980) stated at a meeting of the Royal College of Physicians and Surgeons of Canada that the aetiology of RA is unlikely to be associated with the genetic marker HLA–DRw3 or 4 or with virus infection.

sitis responding to 4-aminoquinolines was reported by the author (Wyburn-Mason, 1964). These drugs are unique in their effect on the collagen diseases in that, unlike other anti-rheumatic drugs, they result in *complete reversal of all the phenomena of the* disease. They cause joint swelling and tenderness to disappear with improvement in joint function, improvement or normalization of the laboratory tests, a lowering of blood sedimentation rate, improvement of the serum electrophoretic pattern and in particular the rheumatoid serum factor disappears (Michette and Vauslippe, 1959; Schiegl and Anders, 1959; Vorlaender, 1960; Baumer, 1961; Propert et al., 1961). Such observations could be explained if the various collagen diseases resulted from infection with a protozoon.

Part II
The possible limax amoebae aetiology of
"collagen" and "auto-immune" disease

Your Notes

Your Notes

Chapter IV

Amoebic infection in man

The vast majority of amoebae are free-living organisms and only a comparatively small number are truly parasitic and adapted to their hosts in such a way that a free extra-corporeal existence does not occur. Many of the free-living non-parasitic forms are able to produce protective cysts of a resistant nature to enable them to withstand desiccation. Such encysted forms are frequently eaten accidentally by human beings or animals, and are thought to pass unharmed through the intestinal canal. After escape from the body in the dejecta they may find themselves in an environment which is favourable for further development. The amoebae emerge from the cysts and by active multiplication increase enormously in numbers in a comparatively short time. In the case of true parasites the only forms which survive outside the body are as a rule the encysted forms, which remain quite passive and unchanged till they are ingested by another host. The unencysted stages are present in the freshly passed stool, and show a degeneration which becomes more marked as the interval since their escape from the body increases. In contrast, the small free-living non-parasitic forms which are thought to pass through the alimentary canal in the encysted state are at the height of their free-living existence some time after the escape of the cysts from the body. Such forms are known as coprozoic amoebae or Amoebae limax.

There are many species of limax amoebae which are difficult to identify on account of their resemblance to one another. They differ in their method of nuclear division, character of the cysts and other details.

Classification of amoebae is difficult and different authorities use different methods. Thus, some confusion exists about Vahlkampfia, Hartmanellids and Acanthamoebae, all three terms being used for the same organism. Some have been shown to be the amoebic phase of a flagellated organism. Others appear to be true amoebae having no flagellate stage. Small free-living amoebae can be found in almost any sample of surface soil taken anywhere in the world and their cysts are often present in the air and in contaminated or tap water. Among many genera so found are the two common ones, Hartmanella (Acanthamoeba) and Naegleria. Species of Hartmanella are frequently found in stale faeces or on agar plate cultures made from dirty water, faeces or other material or merely develop on an agar plate exposed to the air for a while. Hartmanella (Acanthamoebae) may also contaminate tissue cultures (Armstrong and Pereira, 1967). They can also be recovered from the nasopharynx, throat and bronchus of many patients (Armstrong and Periera, 1967). Amoebae of the genus Vahlkampfia may also be found in the faeces and have been cultivated from liver abscess pus and tap water. All these organisms are characterized by cysts possessing pores in their walls (see Wenyon, 1926). Such cysts must, therefore, be continually ingested or inhaled by man and animals from his enviroment and *every human being* or *animal must be continually infected and reinfected during life.* Some of these organisms are found in the intestines of lizards and frogs and are parasitic on the gills of fish or on oysters, hydra, etc. (Wenyon,

1926). Whether these limax organisms are pathogenic to higher animals remains to be seen and evidence for this will now be examined.

Singh and Das (1970) revised the classification of small amoebae and found that, while metronidazole (flagyl) kills E. histolytica, it has little or no effect on Naegleria aerobia (Hartmanella culbertsoni). Emetine, entobex, chloroquine and camoquin were ineffective against the latter organism in mice. Hawkins (1973) reports on the inhibitory effect on growth and division of various strains of large free-living amoebae of various substances. The amoebae were A. proteus, discoides and dabia. She reported that Actinomycin D, phenanthridinium compounds, mitomycin C, cycloheximide, streptomycin, metronidazole (Flagyl), emetine and the 4-aminoquinolines. chloroquine and antrycide have such an inhibitory effect.

a) Entamoeba histolytica infections

The condition of human amoebiasis due to E. histolytica infection is considered by Marsden (1971). This author emphasizes how entamoeba may be *mistaken for macrophages in* tissues *and counting chambers.* Doxiades (1962) likewise stressed the same point. Strains of E. histolytica vary in their pathogenicity, which is increased by passage. Amoebiasis is found in all parts of the world and perhaps one per cent of the world population are infected. Infection occurs by ingesting free-living cysts. Chloroquine, plaquenil, dehydro-emetine, flagyl and Naxogin (Erba) ' kill the organism. While the organisms chiefly affect the large bowel, they can, if sought for, be found in many other tissues (Doxiades, 1962). Like other amoebae they are killed by a solution of bile salts in the same concentration as is found in the small intestine. This probably explain why amoebic dysentery does not affect this part of the gut. The organism is *often a commensal* in the bowel and possibly associated bacteria play a part in determining the pathogenicity of a strain

of entamoeba histolytica as well as the host's resistance. A rise in corticosteroid level in the blood and, thus, also stress, appears to increase the invasiveness of the organisms and hence severe amoebic disease often occurs in pregnancy. Sex hormone levels in the blood also appear to influence the development of lesions.

The blood may occasionally exhibit eosinophilia and sometimes contains RF in chronic cases. Spread appears to occur from the bowel via the portal vein. The liver may show lymphocytic infiltration of the portal tracts like that which occurs in cases of rheumatoid disease. In many cases of colonic or hepatic lesions due to E. histolytica infection various other bodily disturbances have been reported (see Wilmot, 1962). These include joint manifestations identical with rheumatoid arthritis (Rappaport et al., 1951; Rinehart, 1952; D'Antoni, 1952; Shookhoff, 1967), urticaria (Rappaport et al., 1951; Radke, 1952), fever, night sweats, migraine, headaches, cephalgia, rashes (Radke), fibrositis, backache, fatigue, nervousness and psychoneurotic symptoms (D'Antoni). The diarrhoea, E. histolytica in the faeces and the associated symptoms have disappeared with anti-amoebic drug treatment. Such associated symptoms were, therefore, attributed to E. histolytica invasion in such cases. In the absence of evidence of E. histolytica infection extracolonic and extrahepatic conditions of the same type as those found in cases of amoebiasis, such as psychoneurosis, rheumatoid arthritis, urticaria, headaches and fibrositis of the neck have thus also been attributed to E. histolytica infection. Thus, Rinehart (1952) found that 92 per cent of 101 patients with rheumatoid arthritis and 87 per cent of 15 cases of "rheumatoid spondylitis", who apparently had E. histolytica in their faeces in the absence of bowel symptoms, showed marked improvement in their symptoms on treatment with anti-amoebic drugs and he argued that rheumatoid arthritis was due to E. histolytica in-

Arthritis and arthralgia associated with toxocaral infestation. Williams D, Roy S. Brit. med. J., 1981 283, 192, The authors report cases of toxocaral infection with transient arthropathy and also arthritis and arthralgia with various filarial infestations cured by diethyl-carbamazine.

fection. However, Wilmot (1962), Elsdon-Dew (1972) and others argue strongly against such conclusions, pointing out that in the absence of bowel symptoms the presence of E. histolytica in the stools may be as a commensal or the amoeba could be wrongly identified. The fact remains that in the absence of evidence of bowel or liver disturbance or E. histolytica in the stools, headaches, cephalgia, fibrositis of the neck, urticaria, rheumatoid arthritis and psychoneurosis have frequently been reported as disappearing with anti-amoebic drug treatment.

' b) Infections with free-living amoebae

Until recently free-living amoebae have not been known to be pathogenic for animals, though they re "parasitic" on fungi and yeasts. Culbertson et al. (1959) in experimental infections of mice and monkeys with Acanthamoebae showed that the organism was pathogenic and concluded that infections can occur spontaneously in animals. Mice were infected following intranasal inoculation producing lesions in the olfactory bulbs, and pulmonary granulomata. Intracerebral, intraspinal, intravenous or intramuscular injections in monkeys also caused lesions, particularly a lymphocytic choriomeningitis. Abscesses developed in some cases and contained amoebae. The organism migrated in the tissues and there was a notable *invasion of the veins* and dissemination to all organs. There was a considerable tendency to *migration about the* blood vessels. *A most notable feature in the affected animals was that the amoebae often could not be demonstrated in the tissues after a short while and this was due to the histological similarity* to *degenerated mononuclear cells in ordinary preparations.* The organisms developed by mitosis and in culture often appeared *joined together after division by intracellular septa* somewhat reminiscent of an organoid arrange-**nt.** The rounded amoebae measured about 30 Jl in diameter. The cytoplasm g ves a positive periodic-acid Schiff (PAS)

stain. The trophozoites were soluble in bile and bile salts. The cysts and precysts in tissue cultures formed clusters looking like groups of yeast cells. (This solubility of trophozoites in bile salts is also a feature of almost all amoebae)

Culbertson et al. (1972) investigated the effects of subcutaneous injections of Naegleria aerobia on guinea pigs. They found they produced a different effect from that occurring in mice. N. aerobia proved to be uniquely virulent after subcutaneous injections and caused death by general invasion without involvement of the central nervous system. The typical lesion was a grey indurated area of muscle and subcutaneous fat underlying an area of either normal, reddened, or in a few cases, ulcerated skin overlying the site of injection. The regional lymph nodes of the inguinal, pelvic and abdominal groups were enlarged when the injection was made in the hind quarter. The *spleen* was enlarged, and the *liver* showed grey discrete subperitoneal areas, which were also visible on the cut surface of the liver. The brain showed no gross lesions. The kidney occasionally showed small grey areas in the cortex and in a few animals small nodules of greyish thickening were present in the wall of the small intestine.

At the site of the injection there was a mixture of acute abscess, fat necrosis, fibrous tissue proliferation and colonies of amoebae in the fat and often clustered around arteries and veins. The vessels were usually thrombosed and showed marked intimal proliferation with amoebae in the lumen of the vessel as well as in the vessel wall. In some instances the layers of the vessel walls were separated and interspersed with eosinophils and neutrophils in a manner reminiscent of "periarteritis nodosa" in man.

In the early stages the lymph nodes showed amoebae among the proliferating lymphocytes and reticulum cells with focal collections of neutrophils and sparsely scattered eosinophils. The acute picture

−117−

gradually changed to a granulomatous reaction, with *some lymphocytes and plasma cells and intense reticulum* cell *proliferation and multi-nucleated cell formation.*

The skin overlying the site of injection was ulcerated in some cases, but the dermis showed a rather nonspecific inflammatory reaction with no amoebae demonstrable, possibly because the examination was made in a relatively late stage of the local infection. No *specific* histologic *changes which would suggest that the amoebae had caused them* were *identified,* other than an occasional clump of amoebae associated with an acute neutrophilic reaction. The authors remarked that the *amoebic aetiology of the lesion would probably not be discovered by the casual observer,* because the amoebae often stain lJOOrly with routine methods. Such a l sion, therefore, would seem to merit no special attention were it to be present in a human tissue specimen, since the amoebae would probably be mistaken for faint-staining leucocytes, and thus, the cause might easily be regarded as a non-specific bacterial infection. No cystic forms were identified in any lesions in his study and it is presumed that N. aerobia does not form cysts in such circumstances.

The *liver* was the site of a large number of amoebic lesions, usually *grouped about the portal triads* and varying from a clump of amoebae in a sinusoid without cellular response about them to large areas of necrosis, often in association with severe vascular lesions and even invasion of the bile ducts. In a few instances focal lesions were found in the small intestine. These lesions caused tumour-like thickening of the intestinal wall with mucosal destruction from beneath by swarms of infiltrating amoebae and in the same lesion amoebae penetrating into the smooth muscle, pushing muscle cells apart and emerging beneath and perforating the peritoneal layers. Nodular granulomatous lesions appeared throughout the *lungs.*

There were a few amoebae seen in the glomerular capillaries and in the pelvis of the kidney of several animals there was severe *pyelitis with marked inflammation.* In the inflamed *renal pelvis amoebae* were *difficult* to demonstrate. The suggestion is made that careful attention to the possibility of amoebic infection in man is justified when urinary tract infections are being studied.

Stress must be laid on the similarity of the lesions to those of collagen and auto-immune disease (peri-) arteritis, periphlebitis, lymph node, liver and kidney changes, especially the pyelitis, the presence in the lymph nodes of cells like the Reed-Sternberg giant cells of Hodgkin's disease and the difficulty in identifying the amoebae in the tissues. The authors remark that the *proliferation of these amoebae and their effect on the host* (guinea pig) are *reminiscent of the invasion of* a *host animal by a malignant tumour.*

Apley et al. (1970) and Carter (1972) reviewed the condition of primary amoebic meningo-encephalitis in man, which is due to infection with a species of Naegleria, commonly found in water pools. Apley et al. state that up to the time of their report some 44 cases had been described from North America, Australia, New Zealand and Czechoslovakia and they reported two certain and a third possible case in this country. By 1972 Jager and Stamm (1972) state that more than 60 cases had then been described. The organism enters through the nose. The cases present with signs of haemorrhagic meningitis, especially affecting the base of the brain, oedemas and often splenomegaly and hepatomegaly and the amoebae can be found in the C.S.F., where they show only very slow movement. The amoebae may also be found in the lungs, spleen and heart blood. *The authors stress that the amoebae are easily mistaken for polymorphs* or *lymphocytes in ordinary counting* chambers or *in* sections, especially if only a few are present. Hoare, in a discussion which followed Carter's paper, recalled that in the first

Addendum: Species of free-living amoebae may be non-pathogenic or pathogenic to different animals including man. Addendum: Elsdon-Dew, R. (Lancet, 1979, i , 1038) points out that pathogenic Entamoeba histolytica produce cytotoxins, toxins and specific iso-enzymes and that the body produces serum antibode s to the pathogenic type. The same may be true of some species of free-living amoebae.

reported cases the Naegleria had been misidentified as Iodamoeba, stressing the difficulties of identification. Infection appears to occur intranasally and through the cribriform plate from contaminated soil or bathing in inland lakes or polluted pools. Carter (1972) considered that most cases were due to a new organism, Naegleria fowleri. Anderson and Jamieson (1972) found these free-living amoebae in surface soil and a domestic water supply in South Australia. They grow more commonly at body temperature and in culture may show a biflagellate form and can be killed by boile salts present in the concentration found in the small intestine. Clotrimazole (Bayer) is both amoebistatic and amoebicidal (Jamieson and Anderson, 1974).

Armstrong and Pereira (1967) recovered similar amoebae from the nasopharynx, throat and bronchus in patients, usually young, with fever and respiratory symptoms and again emphasized that this *organism can be easily overlooked* and, indeed, it had been *mistaken for a virus!* Subjects develop transient complement-fixing antibodies to the organism in the serum after the illness and these gradually disappear. The organism is not an uncommon infection.

Jager and Stamm (1972) described a case of multiple brain ab cesses which contained a free-living amoeba, probably a species of Hartmanella, in a patient with long-standing Hodgkin's disease of the lung. The organism was identified by immunofluorescent te hniques using antisera prepared against E. histolytica and several species of Naegleria and Hartmanella. They were not sought in the growth. Scattered small blood vessels in the brain contained recent thrombi. Occasionally blood vessel walls were oedematous and infiltrated with granulocytes. Amoebae tended to cluster round the vessels and occasionally small vessel lumina appeared plugged by amoebae. No amoebae were found in the lungs. Jager and Stamm stressed that *amoebae are difficult* to see *in brain*

sections and very much more so *in other organs.* Stamm (1972) has speculated on the possibility that Hartmanella may produce more chronic conditions than acute meningo-encephalitis in man, either in the central nervous system or elsewhere. He remarks that, if amoebic meningo-encephalitis has been missed for years, how much more likely it is that a low grade infection with few amoebae would ·have been missed.

Amoebic infection of the eye with a free-living amoeba, probably Acanthamoeba polyphaga, has recently been described by Nagington et al. (1974).

Naegleria exhibit thermotropism when occurring naturally and have been reported in the thermal discharge water of electric power stations in Florida, but not in lakes not receiving thermal discharges (Willaert a nd Stevens, 1976) . In Australia they have also been found to occur in warm tributaries of larger streams, but not in the main stream into which the warm tributaries run. Wellings et al. (1977), however, could not confirm the findings of Willaert and Stevens and found Naegleria in fresh water lakes. They suggest that other factors probably host related play a greater role in the development of infection than does the mere presence of the organism in the water.

c) Amoeba chromatosa

Ely et al. (1922), Kofoid and Swezy (1922) and Kofoid et al. (1922) described an amoeba in the bone marrow in cases of rheumatoid arthritis. This appeared to have a different type of mitosis from human cells and probably had six chromosomes, unlike the 46 of human cells. It could be grown in cultures on which the effects of drugs were tried. Subsequent work by Twort (1930) and Schreiner and Mattick (1924) failed to verify that this was E. histolytica as postulated, though its nature was never elucidated. Furthermore, Craig and Faust (1957) state that *amoebae have been demonstrated in practically* every soft *tissue of the body.* Again, Hartmanella has been cultured from a liver

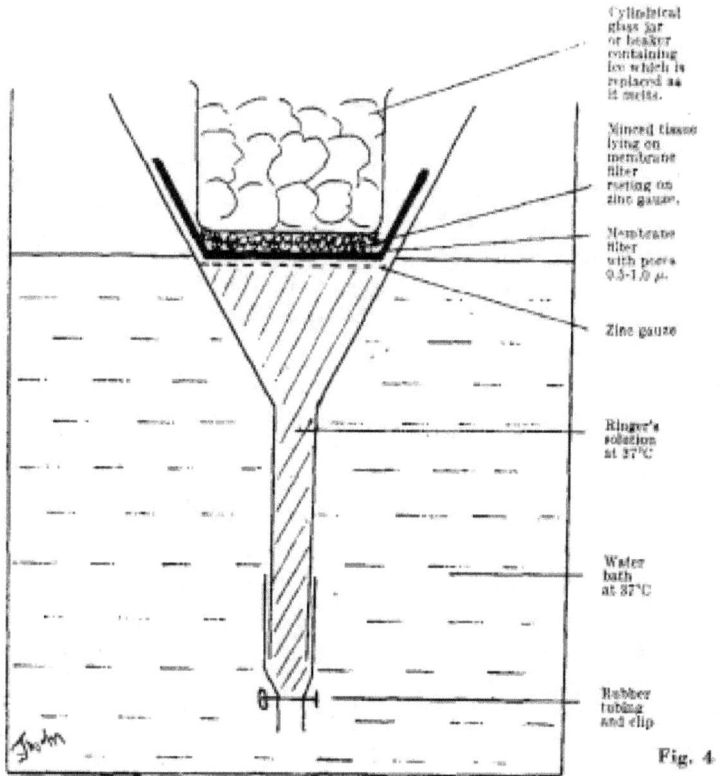

Fig. 4 Drawing of apparatus used to enable migration of organism to take place under thermotropic influences.
(Reproduced from "A New Protozoon", courtesy of Henry Kimpton, London).

The labels on the figure read:

Cylindrical glass jar or beaker containing ice which is replaced as it melts.

Minced tissue lying on membrane filter resting on zinc gauze.

Membrane filter with pores 0.5-1.0 μ.

Zinc gauze

Ringer's solution at 37°C

Water bath at 37°C

Rubber tubing and clip

Fig. 4

abscess in man (see Wenyon, 1926). The author (Wyburn-Mason, 1964) described the isolation of a small amoeba, named by him as Amoeba chromatosa, from the body tissues of man and certain animals in certain clinical conditions described below. This was done by utilizing the property of thermotropism possessed by many parasites of warm-blooded animals and by Naegleria. Thermotropism is the attraction of such organisms to an environment at body temperature from one below this.

An apparatus (Fig. 4) was devised in which minced fresh human or animal tissue could be exposed to a temperature gradient between 0° and 37°C. Across a stainless steel funnel was placed a perforated zinc diaphragm anchored about half way down. To the stem of the funnel was attached a piece of rubber tubing, which was closed by a metal clip or Spencer-Wells forceps. The funnel was filled with Ringer's solution to reach to just above the zinc diaphragm. On the diaphragm was placed a 15 cms. diameter "Oxoid" membrane filter with pores of 0.5 – 1.0 μ in diameter and turned up at the edges. On the membrane was placed a layer of the minced unfixed tissue obtained at autopsy, biopsy or operation. This was spread out to a thickness of about 0.5 cms. On top of this tissue was placed a glass jar or

— 120 —

beaker with a diameter almost as great as that of the zinc diaphragm. This was filled with ice, which thus cooled the underlying tissue. The funnel was placed in a water bath maintained at 37°C, the level of the water in the bath reaching to the level of the zinc diaphragm. This heated up the Ringer's solution in the funnel in contact with the tissue to the same blood temperature. The whole operation was usually carried out in sterile conditions, the apparatus having been sterilized before use and to the Ringer's solution was added 20 units of penicillin and 40 \lnits of streptomycin per ml.

The temperature gradient established above was maintained for 1-2 hours, the ice being replaced as it melted and the water bath temperature maintained with a thermostat. Originally at the end of this period the Ringer's solution was run off into a centrifuge tube and centrifuged at 250 revolutions per minute for 15 minutes. The supernatant fluid was then run off except for a ml or so. The latter was then gently agitated round the bottom of the tube and then transferred to a slide where what appeared to be small amoebae were found. These, however, bad been killed by the centrifuging and could not be cultured. If centrifuging was avoided and the Ringer's solution was replaced by "amoeba saline" as described by Page (1967 a) and this was later run off, it was found to contain a small living amoeba, which could be cultured on agar by methods used for free-living amoebae (Page, 1967 a, b), including inoculation of Noble agar plates carpeted with a live strain of Escherichia coli.

The organism was isolated —

1) From all the tissues of all cases of collagen and auto-immune diseases examined, including cases of rheumatoid arthritis, systemic lupus erythematosus, lymphocytic thyroid lesions, salivary glands affected by' Sjogren's syndrome, etc. In these cases it was found not only in the region of the affected joints, muscles,

thyroid and salivary glands, but also in the spleen, lymph nodes and central nervous system, and, in fact, in all apparently normal tissues.[1][2][0]

2) From all body tissues in all cases of human leukaemia and lymphoma examined.

3) From all of a large number of human and animal malignant tumours examined, when it occurred in large numbers in the tumour itself, but in lesser numbers in all the unaffected tissues of the body.

4) From all aborted material exhibiting congenital growth anomalies examined and in many normal placentae.

5) From hypertrophied tonsils and adenoids removed at operation.

6) From the normal tissues in many healthy subjects killed in accidents.

7) From human and mammalian faecal material.

8) From uncooked beef, mutton and pork.

9) From unsterilized milk and eggs.

10) From some specimens of surface soil.

11) From certain plant tumours growing at the site where the stem passes through the soil.

It was not found in laboratory mice and rat cancers. The isolation of the organism from various tissues and cancers by this method was confirmed by Dr. Magda Uhrinova working at the Bratislava Oncological Institute and by Dr. W.J. Overstreet, III, working in the Biology Department of Vanderbilt University, U.S.A. (personal communication).

The organism was difficult to classify. "Rein n'est plus difficile, en effect, de determiner une amibe" (Dandeard, 1910). Preliminary identification was made by examination of wet preparations of trophozoites and cysts. The normal size of the trophozoites is from 25 p. to 30 p. in diameter (Fig. 5). It is obvious that they are able to pass through a fine-mesh filter and thus are contractile. The P.A.S. stain showed a well-marked positive reaction in the cytoplasm. When recovered from the

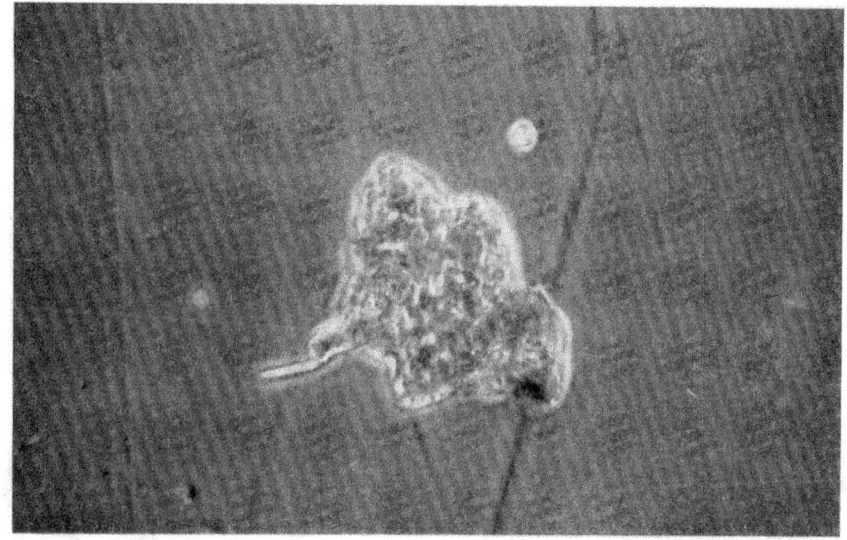

Fig. 5

Fig. 5 Photograph of a limax amoeba which emigrated from the malignant tissue in a case of carcinoma of the bronchus (unstained). (X 1500). Note single spike-like pseudopodium, typical of many species of Nacgleria.

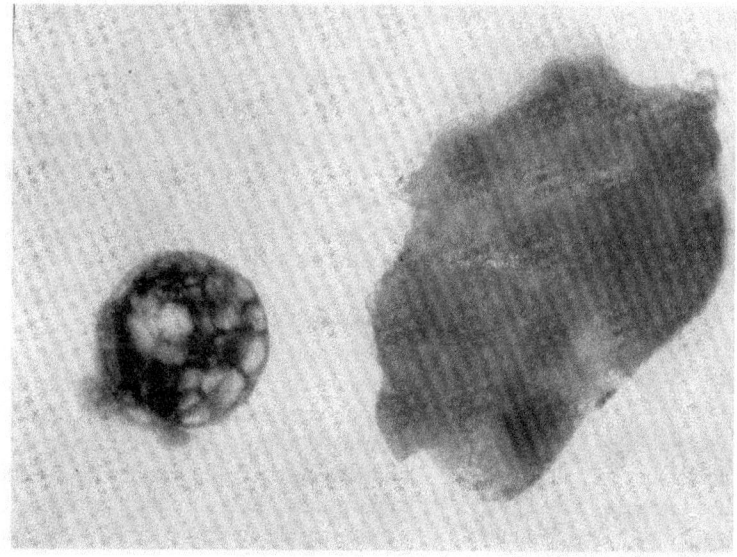

Fig. 6

Fig. 6 A cyst of a limax amoeba beside a trophozoite heavily pigmented as recovered from human malignant tissue. The pigmentation is presumably due to phagocytosis of debris from the minced-up tumour tissue (unstained). (X 2000). Compare with Fig. 1 in Jager and Stamm (1972).

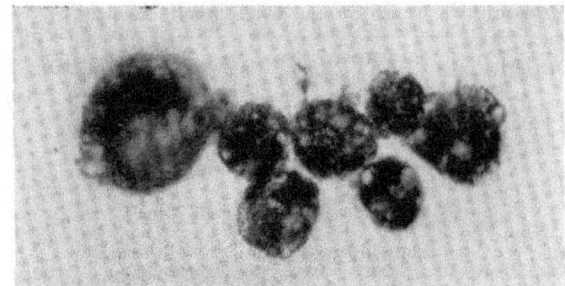

Fig. 7

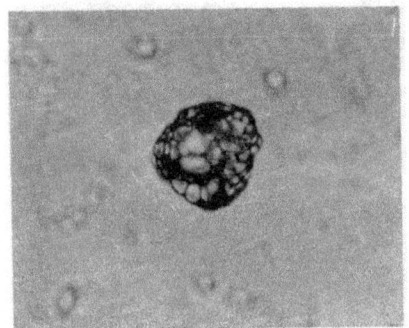

Fig. 8

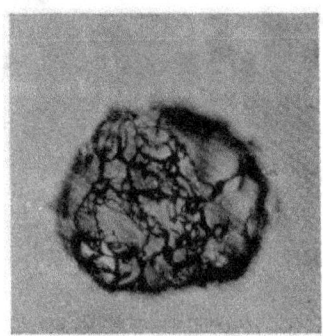

Fig. 9

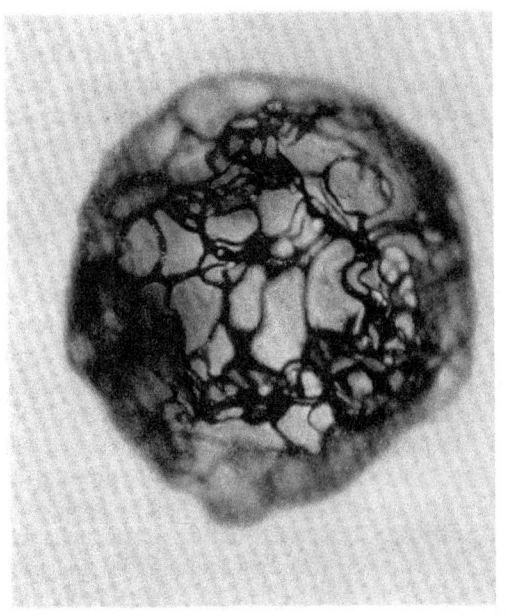

Fig. 10

Fig. 710 Cyts of lirnax amoebae formed after migration from malignant tumours
under the inAuence of thermot ropism
(unstained). Fig. 7 shows simultaneous
cyst formation from a duster of trophozoites (X950) Fig. 8 (X 1000). Fig. 9
(X 2000) and Fig. 10 (X 4000). The
cysts have pore3 in their walls giving a
reticulated appearance. Compare with
Fig. 1 in Jager :Ind Stam m (1972).

Comparison of organism with representative Naegleria and Hartmanella strain&

	Naegleria fowlri	Acanthamoeba castellanii	Isolated organisms
Trophozoites:—			
Shape	llmax mainly	rounded mainly	llmax mainly
Size	22X7p	7.2-37p mainly 18.1p	25-30p
Pseudopodis	single lobose	lobose and spike-like	single lobose or spike-like
Contractile vacuoles	1-6	1	1-12(14)
Rate of movement	rapid up to 66p/mm.	very slow	rapid up to 60p/mm.
Cysts:			
Size	9p	9-27p	9-30,u brown or black
Nuclei	0-1		not visible
Type of wall	smooth surface	rinkled and polygonal fenestrated	polygonal and fenestrated
Encystment			
a) *in vitro*	moaerate	readily and in large numbers	readily
b) in tissues	none	frequent	none
Biflagellate forms in distilled water	occur	none	occur

tissues, it is often dark brown or red in appearance, evidently due to the ingestion of damaged material from the minced tissues from which it was recovered. The trophozoites have limax, i.e. slug-like, features with single lobose pseudopodia (Fig. 5) 1-12 (14) contractile vacuoles and rate of movement of up to 60 p./mm. per minute. The cysts are 30 p. in diameter, spherical, dark brown or black in colour with a fenestrated wall (Figs. 6-10). No nuclei are visible. Encystment does not occur in the tissues but moderate numbers are found in vitro. Biflagellate forms occur in distilled water. Many forms closely resemble those of the smaller Acanthamoeba (Hartmanellae) and Naegleria described by Page (1967 b), but the trophozoites do not exhibit the thorn-like processes or acanthopodia of the Acanthamoebae. Since 1964 further work has shown that the trophozoites of the amoebae, like those of acanthamoeba (Culbertson et aL, 1959) and

Naegleria fowleri (Carter, 1972), are readily soluble in bile salts of the same concentration as is found in the gut and in one per cent deoxycholate. It had already been found that the trophozoites were destroyed by 4-aminoquinolines and by copper ions in extreme dilution (Wyburn-Mason, 1964). Since the organisms can be isolated from human and animal faeces by the above method, they are, in fact, coprazoic amoebae. The features of the trophozoites and particularly of the cysts of the organism (Figs. 6-10) with large pores in their walls seem identical with those of various species of limax amoebae, especially of Hartmanella and Naegleria, including the Hartmanella photographed by Jager and Stamm (1972) present in cerebral abscesses in a case of Hodgkin's disease. Naegleria, unlike Hartmanella infections, are not characterized by the presence of cysts in the affected tissues and in the lesions from which the organism was induced to migrate no amoebic cysts are visible. This and the general features of the trophozoites with single spike-like pseudopodia suggest that the organisms may, in fact, be species of Naegleria (see below) other than N. fowleri. Since the amoebae migrate under the influence of thermotropism, it would be naive to think that they would not invade the tissues once within the body, upper gastro-intestinal tract or lungs and exposed to body temperature. The question as to whether they are pathogenic must be considered.

The author isolated the amoeba from the tbyroid gland removed in a case of Hashmoto's thyroiditis and from metastatic lesions of a case of carcinoma of the bronchus. No amoebae could be seen in ordinary sections stained by haematoxylin and eosin. Air Vice-Marshall W.P. Stamm at the Amoebiasis Research Unit, Royal Free Hospital, London, kindly stained ordinary paraffin sections of these tissues by an indirect immunofluorescent antibody technique using rabbit antisera prepared against various species of amoebae as described by Parelkar et al. (1971). He reported (personal communication) that the tissues showed immunofluorescence of some cells in these sections with the antiserum against Naegleria aerobia (Culbertsoni) (HB-1 strain), but not with any other of the amoebic antisera used. This suggests that Naegleria amoebae are perhaps present in these tissues. However, he was still not able to identify cells in the sections as amoebae using ordinary stains. This finding is again in accord with the probability that the organisms are species of Naegleria. Possibly further investigation may show that other species of free-living amoebae than Naegleria may occur in tissues. The general term, limax amoebae, for these infections will, therefore, be used in the following pages.

Dr. Alfons Weber of Erding, Bavaria, Germany recently showed the author a technique he has developed. He anchors fresh specimens of human tumours by

means of wire to a cork fixed in the top of a centrifuge tube. The rest of the tube is filled with Ringer's solution and the tube slowly centrifuged. A sediment consisting of cells and debris forms at the bottom of the tube. This is removed and examined unstained on a slide. Most of the sediment consists of dead tumour cells and is featureless, but in addition there are also seen large mobile cells which are characterized by 10-14 vacuoles forming and reforming continuously and appear typical of the amoeba described above.

Reasons for failing to identify limax amoebae in the tissues.

The question arises as to why the amoeba has not been seen in histological sections of lesions in collagen and auto-immune diseases and in tumours. In this regard attention has been drawn by many authors, including those mentioned above, to the fact that in infections with Acanthamoeba or Naegleria the organism can often not be seen in the tissues. They stain poorly by routine stains and look like poorly staining leucocytes (Culbertson et al., 1959, 1972). Kudo (1954) also emphasizes that amoebae appear identical in sections with mononuclear macrophages. Apley et al. (1970) showed that amoebae are easily mistaken for polymorpbs or lymphocytes or for macrophages in tissue and counting chambers. Both give positive P.A.S. tests. Doxiades (1962) and Marsden (1971) stessed the same point in cases of infection with E. histolytica.

Conclusion

Man and other animals are continually exposed to infection and re-infection by various species and strains of free-living limax amoebae and indeed these may be found in the faeces and in the nasopharynx and bronchi. In all parts of the world they form part of our environment. Experimentally in animals they induce changes like those of collagen and auto-immune disease and are characterized by vasculitis, myositis, hepatitis, pyelitis and splenomegaly. They can often not be seen in the

Addendum: A leading Article, Brit. med. J., 1978, ii, 379, emphasizes false-positive identification of entamoeba histolytica in mistake for leucocytes in sections or vice versa failure to diagnose amoebiasis by clinicians of laboratories to regard amoebae as leucocytes. Identification requires skill and diligence. Amoebae are easily missed in routine histological sections and requires immunofluorescent techniques by an expert.

tissues of such animals. Such animals show lymphadenopathy with an appearance like that of human Hodgkin's disease or a state like that of advanced malignant disease. These organisms may also be recovered from all the tissues of cases of collagen and auto-immune diseases and from human and many animal tumours and may also occur in the tissues of apparently healthy individuals. They cannot be identified in ordinary histological sections, but can be demonstrated by immunofluorescent methods. The trophozoites of these organisms are killed or inhibited by , 4-aminoquinolines, copper ions in low concentration and by bile salts in the concentration occurring in the small intestine. Clotrimazole (Bayer) is amoebistatic and amoebicidal against Naegleria fowleri. As flagellates free-living amoebae would be expected to be killed by pentamidine. Anti-amoebic drugs may improve various conditions which may or may not occur in association with E. histolytica infection.

Reference has already been made above to the finding of so-called free-living amoebae in any of the tissues of apparently healthy subjects by the method employing thermotropism described above. Cursons, R.T.M., et al. (Lancet, 1977, ii, 875) point out that pathogenic free-living amoebae of the genera Naegleria and Acantha-moeba are readily isolated from nasal and throat cavities, chlorinated swimming and potable waters, soil, sewage, thermal pools, and temperate lakes and rivers, yet disease is rare. They tested 200 sera from healthy New Zealanders for antibodies against free-living amoebae by the indirect fluorescent-antibody test and found antibodies in ALL of the undiluted sera. Titres ranged from neat to 1/120 for pathogenic and non-pathogenic Naegleria and from neat to 1/80 for pathogenic and non-pathogenic Acanthamoeba. The authors refer to similar findings by others. THESE OBSERVATIONS SHOW CONCLUSIVELY THAT EVERY HUMAN BEING (AND PROBABLY ANIMALS ALSO) HAVE BEEN OR ARE PRESENTLY INFECTED WITH ACANTHAMOEBA AND/OR NAEGLERIA, THOUGH THESE MAY NOT HAVE BEEN OBSERVED IN THE TISSUES. THUS ALL HUMANS CONTAIN FOREIGN ANTIGENS IN THEIR PLASMA AND TISSUES. THE DISCOVERY THAT FREE-LIVING PROTOZOA ARE NOT PURELY NON-PATHOGENIC, BUT ARE ABLE TO INFECT MAN AND ANIMALS "HAS REVOLUTIONIZED THE VERY CONCEPT OF PARASITOLOGY" (Leading Article; Lancet, 1977, 2, 1165).

Addendum: As pointed out by Pasteur, Koch and others any organism introduced into the body tends to collect in areas of trauma, inflammation or tumours. This applies to amoebae.
Addendum: Entamoeba histolytica produces cytotoxins, toxins and specific iso-enzymes (Elsdon-Dew, R., Lancet 1979, i, 1038-9). It appears that the invasive strains of Entamoeba histolytica produce the enzyme phosphoglucomutase which the non-invasive or non-pathogenic type does not (Leading Article, Pathogenic Entamoeba Histolytica, Lancet 1979, i, 303). Cursons R. (Personal Communication, 1979) states that both pathogenic and non-pathogenic types of Acanthamoeba and Naegleria produce phospholipase 2, the pathogenic species producing more of this enzyme. Phosphlipase 2 and its derivatives, lysophospholipase 2 and free fatty acids are extremely inflammatory compounds. The first named has also been found in trypanosomes and suggested as the cause of the inflammation in this disease.

Chapter V

Evidence for the protozoal causation of
collagen and auto-immune diseases

Contrary to Gardner's (1972) statement, quoted above, on the lack of evidence that a protozoon might initiate the changes of rheumatoid arthritis, there ·is much to suggest that a protozoal infection might be liesponsible. In the foregoing pages numerous references have been made to the possibility that various features of collagen and auto-immune diseases might be explained if the disease was caused by infection with a protozoon in subjects sensitive to this. Among these are:-

1) The author found limax amoebae migrated from all the tissues of all cases of collagen and auto-immune diseases in which it was sought (see above).

2) The high blood eosinophilia occurring in various manifestations of collagen and auto-immune diseases, which in cases of disseminated eosinophilic collagen disease may be extreme. An almost identical condition results from parasitic disease, such as ascariasis, trichiniasis, larva migrans and tropical eosinophilia. This suggests that collagen and auto-immune disease might be due to a protozoal or metazoal infection.

3) Rheumatoid factor may occur in high concentration in the blood of the same order as in rheumatoid disease in chronic infections with many protozoa, such as cases of African trypanosomiasis, malaria, Kala-azar, visceral leishmaniasis and amoebiasis. This occurs in the absence of evidence of arthropathy and subjects may be symptomless.

4) The manifestations of collagen disease may be completely reversed by various antiprotozoal drugs, including 4-amino-quinolines (chloroquine), daraprim and mepacrine.

5) If a patient with rheumatoid arthritis develops hepatic jaundice from any cause, this commonly results in a remission in the arthritic symptoms (Hench, 1949; Short et al., 1957: Kornreich et al., 1971). Experimental work has shown that this is independent of adrenal cortical function and that bile has no effect on inflammation. Hench showed that the jaundice capable of causing such remission was obstructive or hepatic in type, but not haemolytic, and that transfusion of icteric serum will produce a remission of the arthritic symptoms. This applied also to psoriatic arthropathy, asthma and hayfever. It was seen above that deconjugated bile salts lyse the trophozoite forms of certain amoebae. This raises the possibility that the effect of obstructive jaundice on cases of rheumatoid arthritis might be due to the appearance of bile salts in the circulation with their lytic effect on amoebae.

6) In the protozoal disease. amoebiasis histolytica, an arthritis almost identical with that occurring in rheumatoid arthritis may be observed and an eosinophilia may occasionally occur in the blood (Shookhoff, 1967) as in cases of rheumatoid disease and the enteritis does not affect the small intestine where bile salts are present.

7) Goobar (1977) describes 66 children in Argentina with intestinal Giardia lamblia, who developed a rheumatoid syndrome affecting especially the knees intermittently, but also ankles, tarsal joints. shoulders and elbows and pains in the hands and legs. gastrointestinal and allergic symptoms and occasional low fever. The E.S.R.

was raised and serum RF positive in some cases. Non-specific changes were present in the sy novia. Treatment with the anti-protozoal drugs quinacrine (atebrine) or met ronidazole for 10 days freed the stools of parasites and the joint symptoms disappeared in over 90 per cent of cases.

8) Again, cases of polymyositis like those forming part of the collagen and auto-immune disease group, but due to the protozoon, toxoplasma, have been reported by Rowland and Greer (1961) and Chandar et a!. (1968).

9) Protozoal infection ma y lead to mal-a bsorption and villous atrophy of the small intestine (see above) like that seen in collagen and auto-immune diseases.

The above considerations suggest that the limax amoebae found in all the collagen and auto-immune diseases may well be the aetiological agent of these conditions and that anti-protozoal drugs help by their action on these organisms.

It seemed necessary to try the effects of various other antiprotozoal drugs on cases of rheumatoid disease or of various localized manifestations of this. The substances investigated were 4-aminoquinolines (chloroquine, hydroxychloroquine (plaquenil), amodiaquine (camoquin)); copper sulphate, a most potent anti-protozoal substance; bile salts (dehydrocholine), which are effective in killing the trophozoites of many amoebae in the concentration found in the small intestine; clotrimazole (canesten): and tinidazole. All of these were actually shown experimentally to kill limax amoebae. In addition other antiprotozoal drugs were also investigated. They included suramin, pentamidine, dehydro-emetine (DHE or mebadin), metronidiazole (flagyl) or nitrimidazole (naxogin (Erba)), phanquone (entobex) and diloxanide (furamide).

The 4-aminoquinolines were given by mouth in a dose of 200 and 400 mgms. daily reduced after a month to 200 mgms. twice weekly, care being taken to examine the eyes at intervals to gua rd against keratitis or macular changes. Copper salts were administered in the pharmaceutical dose of 25 mgms. of copper sulphate in aqua chloroformi by mouth three t-imes daily. This may produce vomiting and/or diarrhoea and the dose have to be decreased to 10 mgms. three times daily. Only a small amount of the metal is absorbed, however, and no other side effects are observed even when taken over several months. Deconjugated bile salts as dehydrocholin were given in the pharmaceutical dose of 500-1000 mgms. three times a day by mouth. They may produce mild colic. This may be prevented by simultaneous administration of a kaolin mixture. Pentamidine was at first given by intramuscular injection into the buttock in doses of 200 mgms. daily for 10 days. The course was repeated twice with intervals of 7 days between. This substance is liable to produce local necrosis or abscess formation. Pentamidine can be given by mouth, but its absorption is uncertain. Moreover, it may produce nausea, vomiting and diarrhoea. However, many patients tolerate it by this route. Capsules containing 200 mgms. were especially made and a dose of 200 mgms. twice daily to 400 mgms. three times daily by mouth were tried in various combinations. Clotrimazole was administered by mouth in doses of 100 mg/kg daily over several months. Suramin was given by intravenous injection of 0.05 G in 10 mls. of water and after this every 4 days I G was injected until 10 G had been given. :rhe course was repeated once after 4 months. Dehydro-emetine (DHE) was given by intramuscular injection in doses of 60 mgms. daily for 10 days and repeated after 7 days, or 60 mgms. three times daily by mouth for 7-12 days repeated after an interval of 10 days, Before commencing treatment E.C.G's were taken and repeated before each successive injection. Metronidazole (flagyl) was given in doses of 4{)()-600 mgms. three times daily by mouth and nitrimidazole (naxogin) in doses of 75 mgms. three times daily. Phanquone (entobex) was given in doses of 100 mgms. twice daily by mouth for 7 days, repeated at intervals of a week. Diloxanide (furamide) was given in doses of 500 mgms. three times daily for 10 days and repeated once. Tinidazole was administered in increasing doses of one tablet (500 mgms.) weekly rising to four tablets in a single dose per week.

In this regard a synthetic organic copper compound, Cuprimyl (8, hydroxyquinolin e-his (dimethylamine sulphate)), containing no ionic copper and resembling an antiprotozoal drug, was used in the treatment of rheumatoid arthritis (see Cuprimyl, 1950) on the grounds that metallic compounds other than gold might help the disease. Variable results were reported, but improvement was noted especially in cases of less than a years duration.

Reference has been made above to the disappearance of symptoms, such as arthropathy, urticaria, cephalgia, headache, migraine, nervousness and psychoneurotic manifestations occurring in association with infection with E. histolytica, as a result of treatment with anti-amoebic drugs. In addition there are many reports of the disappearance of such symptoms occuring in the absence of evidence of invasive lesions of E. histolytica as a result of treatment with anti-amoebic drugs (Rinehart, 1952; D'Antoni, 1952; Wilmot, 1962). Doubt, however, has been expressed as to their relationship to E. histolytica infection, though the effect of such drugs on the symptoms appears proven.

The various substances tested above were tried on cases of rheumatoid arthritis of varying severity, systemic lupus erythematosus, dermatomyositis and other manifestations of collagen and auto-immune disease and observations made on the clinical condition, oedema, morning stiffness, E.S.R., plasma proteins, RF, ANF and organ-specific antibodies in the serum. No attempt at a double-blind trial was made as it became obvious fairly early or even

the day after commencing treatment whether beneficial effect was obtained and furthermore the symptomatic improvement was associated with improvement or disappearance of the abnormal blood changes, indicating that the drug was effective and improvement not due to suggestion. No beneficial effect was obtained from flagyl, naxogin, entobex, suramin or furamide in the doses used. However, Abd-Rabbo et al. (1972), using a derivative of nitro-imidazole (naxogin), BT 985 Merck A.G. which is active against amoebae, giardia and trichomonas, obtained dramaticaHy beneficial effects in one case of systemic lupus erythematosus and nine of ten cases of rheumatoid disease. The drug was given in doses of 250 mgms. daily for 14-39 days and the cases followed up for months. Improvement was complete in 2-3 weeks. This drug is an imidazole derivative like clotrimazole and tinidazole. The effect of the other substances will now be considered.

The results of treatment of cases of collagen and auto-immune diseases with antiprotozoal drugs.

These will be considered as follows:–

I. The results of treatment of cases of rheumatoid arthritis and systemic lupus erythematosus with antiprotozoal drugs.

   A. The effects of compounds shown experimenta!Jy to kill limax amoebae.
      a) 4-aminoquinolines.
      b) Copper sulphate. '
      c) Bile salts.
      d) Clotrimazole.
      e) Levamisole.
      f) Tinidazole
   B. The effects of other antipr6t'tizoal' drugs.
      a) Pentamidine.
      b) Dehydroemetine.
      c) Diodoquin.

II. The results of treatment of cases of dermatomyositis with antiprotozoal drugs.

III. The effect of antiprotozoal drugs in Sjogren's syndrome and auto-immune parotitis.
   a) Chloroquine.
   b) Pentamidine.
   c) Copper sulphate.
   d) Bile salts.
   e) Clotrimazole.

IV. The effects of antiprotozoal drugs on cases of thyrotoxicosis.
   a) 4-aminoquinolines.
   b) Pentamidine.
   c) Copper sulphate.
   d) Bile salts.

V. The effects of antiprotozoal drugs on cases of "endocrine exophthalmos".

VI. The effects of antiprotozoal drugs on intrinsic asthma and urticaria.

VII. The effect of antiprotozoal drugs on Schonlein-Henoch's purpura.

VIII. The effect of antiprotozoal drugs on cases of atrophic gastritis with or without pernicious anaemia.

IX. The effect of antiprotozoal drugs on cases of ulcerative colitis.
   a) Chloroquine.
   b) Clotrimazole.

X. The treatment of idiopathic Addison's disease with antiprotozoal drugs.

XI. The effects of antiprotozoal drugs on chronic skin lesions of rheumatoid disease.

XII. The effects of antiprotozoal drugs on leucoderma and melanoderma.

XIII. The effects of antiprotozoal drugs on chronic rheumatoid liver disease.

XIV. The effect of antiprotozoal drugs on cases of Paget's disease.

XV. The effect of antiprotozoal drugs on diabetes mellitus.

XVI. The effects of antiprotozoal drugs on cases of migraine.

XVII. The effects of antiprotozoal drugs on cases of myasthenia gravis.

I. The results of treatment of cases of active rheumatoid arthritis and systemic lupus erythematosus with antiprotozoal drugs

A. The effects of compounds shown experimentally to kill limax amoebae.

a) 4-aminoquinolines (chloroquine, hydroxychloroquine and amodiaquine). These have already been described above.

b) Copper sulphate

As far as could be ascertained from textbooks of pharmacology this substance produces no ill-effects on long continued administration apart from nausea, vomiting and diarrhoea. However, because of this it is not possible to give amounts which raise the level of the serum copper content appreciably. The effect of this substance was tried in doses of 25-50 mgms. three times daily on 57 cases of early or moderately severe active rheumatoid arthritis, one case of systemic lupus erythematosus and one of psoriatic arthropathy. Treatment was continued for up to twelve months. Most of these had already been treated by the usual anti-rheumatoid drugs and in these cases the previous treatment was continued and the copper sulphate was given in addition. One of the cases of rheumatoid disease had been successfully treated for carcinoma of the thyroid gland. In one case the treatment had to be abandoned as the patient was unable to take the copper sulphate by mouth. In 3 of the cases the first effect of treatment was to cause exaggeration of the joint pains and swelling resembling an Herxheimer reaction. In 2 cases there was no symptomatic improvement. In the cases of psoriatic arthropathy there was a mild improvement in the joint stiffness, but the psoriasis was unchanged. In all the other cases of active rheumatoid arthritis and the one case of systemic lupus erythematosus there was a rapid and usually dramatic response to treatment beginning within 24-48 hours.

In the cases in which there was an

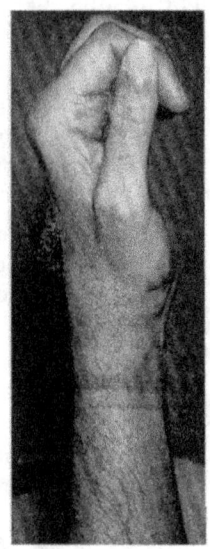 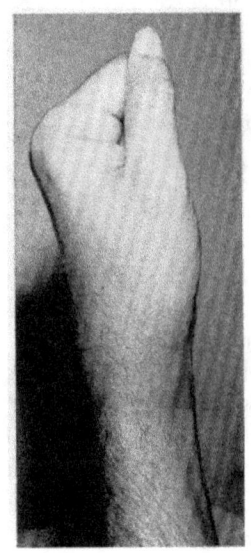

Fig. 11-A   Fig. 11-B

Fig. 11 Male, aged 33 years. Five years hiswry of sero-positive rheumatoid disease showing hand "A" before and "B" onr week after beginning treatment with copper sulphate (Case 36). Note disappearance of joint and hand swelling and return of ability w flex digits.

Herxheimer effect the exaggeration in the symptoms passed off rapidly and improvement then occurred. The joint swelling, oedema and pain ceased within 24 hours. Movements became freer and morning stiffness less. Improvement continued for about 3 months. The E.S.R. fell. The albumin-globulin ratio returned to normal. The RF disappeared from the serum after 6 months. The effects were similar to those of pentamidine (see below). In the case of systemic lupus erythematosus improvement began slowly. This patient had been subject to the development of hard, painful nodules in the pulps of the fingers and in the substance of the lower lip. These continually came and went every 3–4 days. The administration of copper sulphate caused this manifestation to cease as the first beneficial effect and this was followed by improvement in the pain and swelling of the joints, fall in the E.S.R. to normal and the reversal of the albumin-globulin ratio disappeared. Lupus erythematosus

cells vanished from the blood within two weeks. Symptoms, however, tend to recur a variable time after discontinuance of the treatment. *Copper salts like chloroquine usually reverse all the manifestations of active rheumatoid disease.* Examples of such cases are as follows:-

Case 36 Male aged 42 years, Kenyan Indian, who came to England 9 months previously. Five years history of pain, swe!Hng and stiffness of the wrists, fingers, shoulders, hips, temporomandibular joints and aching of the lower dorsal spine. The joints were especially stiff in the morning and the symptoms were accompanied by sweating and headaches. Examination showed hotness, swelling and stiffness of the wrists, fingers, ankles, and feet. He was unable to get the fingers into the palms or to move the wrist joints more than a few degrees. Temperature was 99.4°F. The serum showed RF strongly positive. E.S.R. was 5 mms. per hour. Hb was 101 per cent. W.B.C. 6,900 per

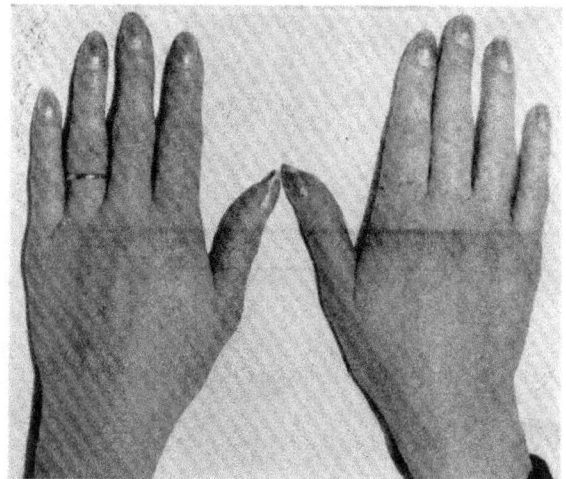

Fig. 12-A

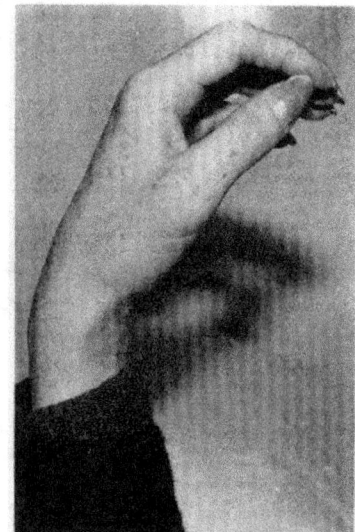

Fig. 12-B

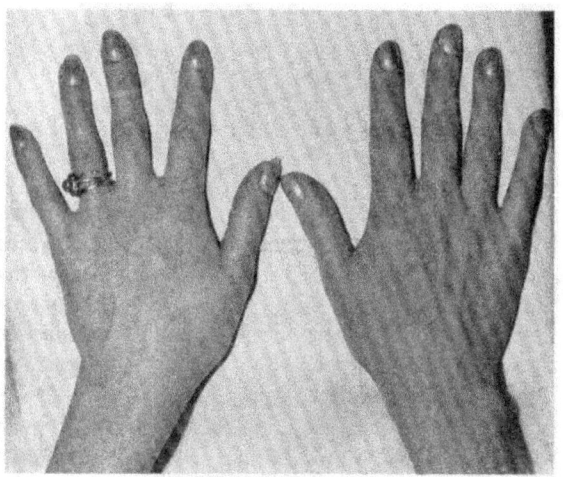

Fig. 12-C

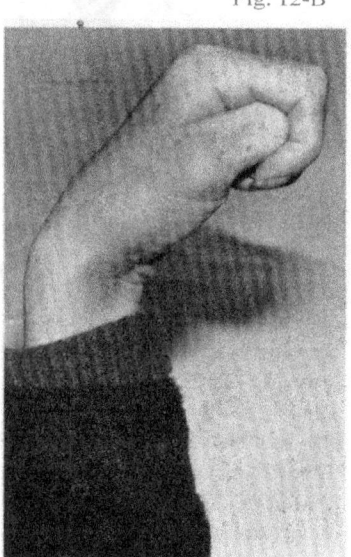

Fjg. 12-D

Fig..12 Female, aged 29 year. Three years seroposlltve rheumatoid di case. '·A·· shows appearance of har.ds and "B" attempts to make a fist before and "C" and "ŋ·· the corrc sponding appearances after 4 days treat ment \\'ith copper sul pha te (Case 37).

cu. mm. He was treated with copper sul phate 50 mgms. t.d.s. and rapid improve ment in the swelling and pain and mobility of the joints followed. Within 10 days all symptoms had disappeared. Treatment conti nued for 4 weeks. He was then dis charged to be followed as a n out- patient without treatment and has remained well during six months (Fig. 11).

Case 37 Female. aged 32 years. Two years history of joint pains and swelling of the hands and feet, wrists, elbows,

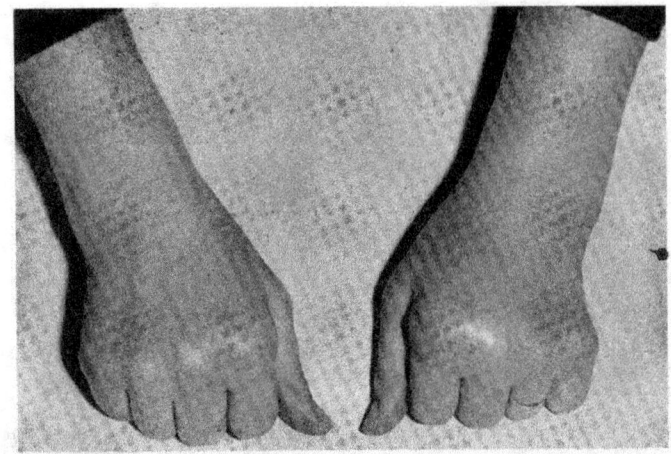

Fig. 13-A

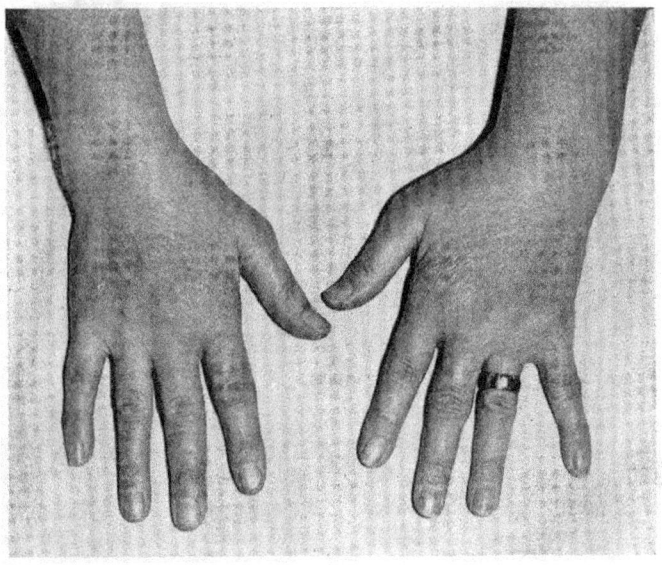

Fig. 13-B

Fig. 13 Female, aged 31 years. Seropositive rheumatoid disease showing "A" acute swelling of knuckles before and "B" one week after being treated with copper sulphate (Case 38).

shoulders and knees accompanied by morning stiffness. Three weeks previously there had occurred a severe exacerbation of her symptoms. Examination showed typical rheumatoid arthritic swelling of the affected joints with inability to flex the fingers. The patient was obviously in severe pain. The temperature was 100.4°F. Hb was 69 per cent. W.B.C. 9,100 per cu. mm., 80 per cent polymorphs. Serum alkaline phosphatase 25 KA units per 100 mls. E.S.R. 48 mms. per hour. Serum albumin 3.0, globulin 3.1 G per 100 mls. RF negative. She was treated with copper

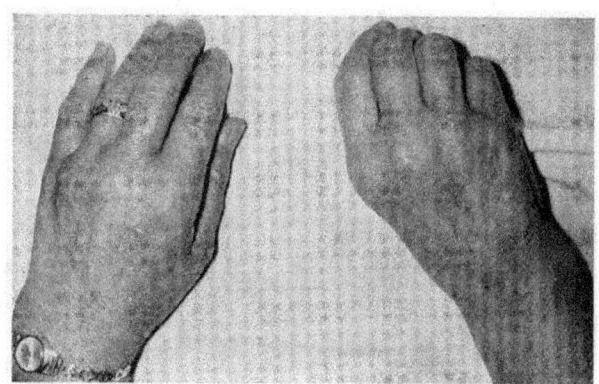

Fig. 14-A

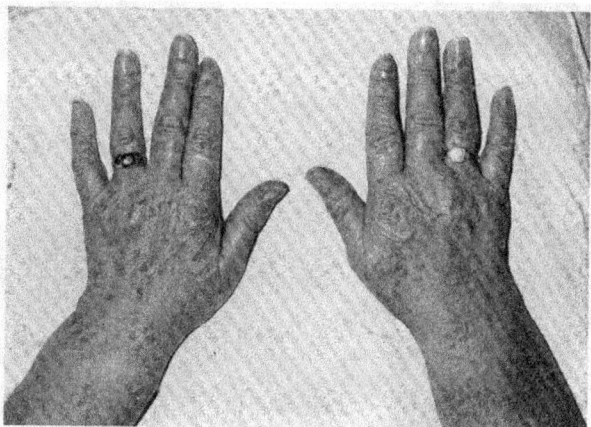

Fig. 14-D

sulphate 25 mgms. t.d.s. After 7 days all the symptoms and signs had disappeared. The treatment was continued for another five weeks. Six weeks later the E.S.R. was 18 mms. per hour. Hb 86 per cent. Serum albumin 3.6, globulin 2.8 G per 100 mls. She was followed for 12 months without treatment and with no recurrence of symptoms. RF was negative in the blood one year after commencing treatment (Fig. 12).

Case 38 Female, aged 39 years. She gave a 12 years history typical of rheumatoid arthritis affecting chiefly the hands. E.S.R. was 90 mms. per hour. Serum RF was weakly positive. W.B.C. were normal. She was treated with copper sulphate 50 mgms. t.d.s. with immediate improvement in the pain and swelling of the hands, which disappeared for 6 weeks. However, in spite of continued treatment she had a mild return of pain and swelling of the knuckles of the right hand lasting a week or so and then disappearing again (Fig 13).

The finding that copper administration may relieve the manifestations of active rheumatoid disease recalls the folk treatment of rheumatoid arthritis in India and neighbouring countries, where the disease is treated by filling copper vessels with water and allowing them to stand overnight. The patient drinks the contents of the vessel in the morning and sufferers report considerable benefit from continued treatment by this method.

There is a widespread belief that copper

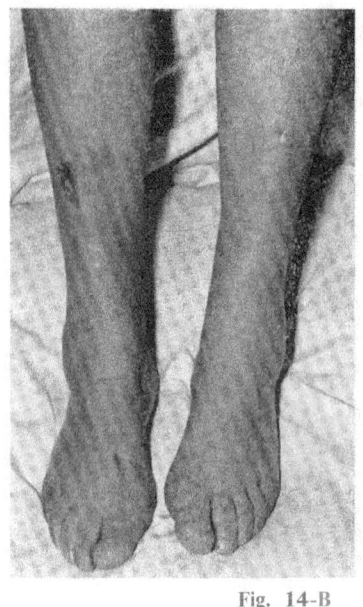

Fig. 14-B

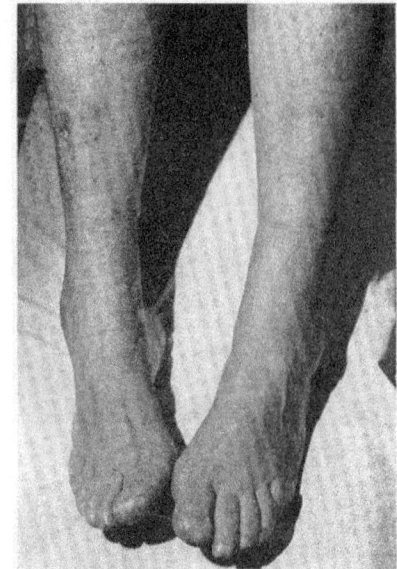

Fig. 14-E

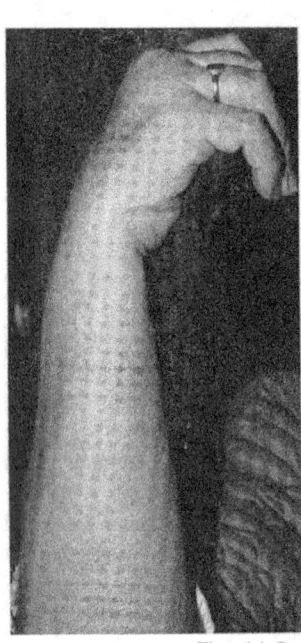

Fig. 14-C

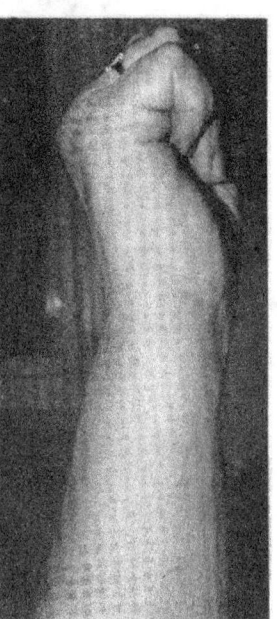

Fig. 14-F

Fig. 14 Female, aged 49 years. Five years history of sero-positive rheumatoid disease showing appearance of "A" hands and "B" feet and "C" an attempt to flex fully the fingers before and "D", "E" and "F" the corresponding states 8 days after commencing treatment with copper sulphate.

— 135 —

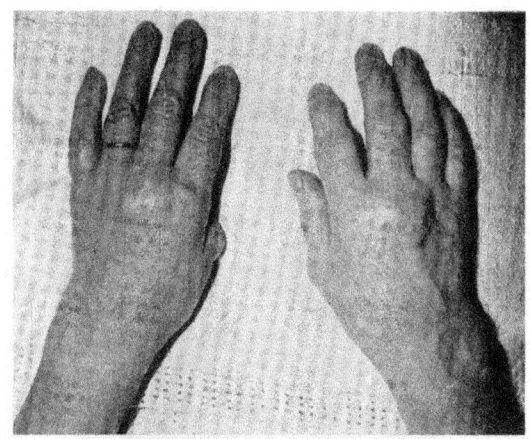

Fig. 15-A

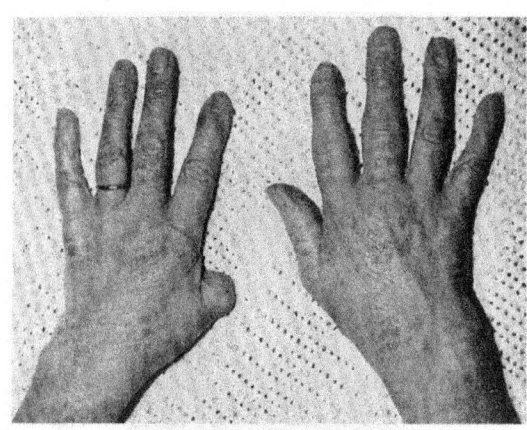

Fig. 15 Female, aged 46 years. Six years history of seroposi tive rheumatoid disease. Appearances of hands "A" before and "B" 8 days after commencing treatment with copper sulphatr. Note disappearance of joint swelling.

Fig. 15-B

bracelets help rheumatoid arthritis, a view disbelieved by rheumatologists. Walker and Keats (1976) showed that the metal of copper bracelets is soluble in sweat and absorbed through the skin and the copper dissolves in physiological saline, but not in distilled water. They showed in a controlled trial of copper bracelets in cases of rheumatoid arthritis that the bracelets relieved symptoms, whereas control "fake" bracelets did not do so. Minute amounts of copper were absorbed from the bracelets.

c) Bile Salts

Hench (1949) described relief of symptoms in cases of active rheumatoid arthritis by administering deconjugated bile salts. In the author's investigations de-conjugated bile salts were administered in a dose of 500-1,000 mgms. three times daily by mouth. These are normally excreted rapidly by the liver, but some rise in the blood level must occur as they have a rapid effect on cases of rheumatoid arthritis. Treatment was carried out in 60 cases of active rheumatoid disease. In twelve no benefit was obtained. In the other 48 cases the results were identical or closely resembled those obtained with copper sulphate. Copper sulphate is often e cctive when bile salts are not. However, bile salts are much more easily tolerated than copper salts. The patient only complains of occasional looseness of the bowels. When first administered bile salts not infrequently produce a temporary ex-

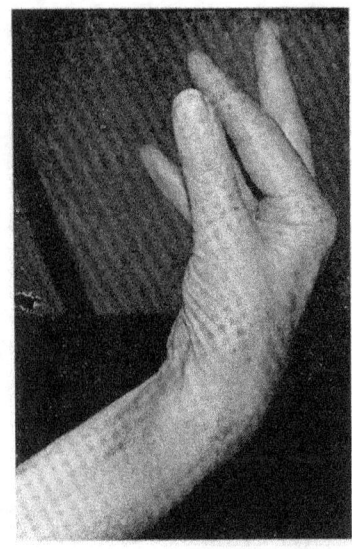
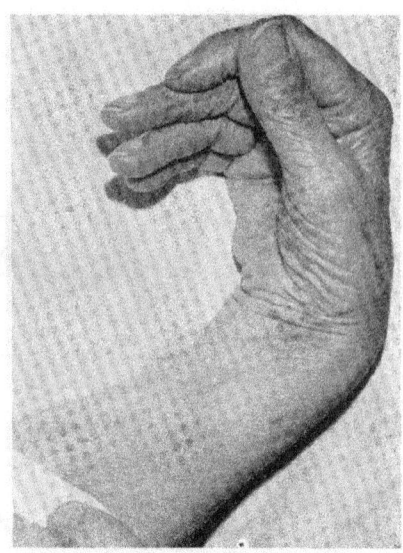

Fig. 16·A   Fig. 16-B

Fig. 16 Female, aged 56 years. Six years history of rheumatoid disease. "A" shows attempts to grip and flex wrist
before and "B" the same one week after beginning treatment
with bile salts (Case 39).

aggeration of the symptoms of rheumatoid disease with increased morning stiffness of the affected parts and increased pain and swelling in the joints lasting several days and suggesting that the substance is affecting the causative organism of the disease and results in an Herxheimer reaction. The substance is successful in relieving the symptoms of the disease in about 6Q-70 per cent of cases. In chronic cases it often works slowly and its effects may be manifested by sudden giving way of adhesions around the affected joints.

An example is the following case:–

Case 39 Female, aged 56 years. Onset with right-sided carpal tunnel syndrome aged 43 years. At the time the E.S.R. was 37 mms. per hour and Hb 80 per cent with a normal W.B.C. She gradually developed aching and swelling of the fingers and toes and both wrists and at the age of 50 years the RF in the serum was strongly positive. P.B.I.= 6.2 /G per 100 mls. An operation for division of the right flexor retinaculum of the wrist was carried out at the age of 52 years with complete relief of the symptoms of carpal tunnel compression. For the last six years she had been under various treatments for active rheumatoid arthritis, which, however, gradually progressed, the E.S.R. being raised slightly to 30 or more mm. per hour. Serum RF was now positive. Treatment included prednisolone, butazolidine, aspirin, chloroquine, indocid in various combinations, but the condition of the joints, especially of the metacarpophalangeal joints continued to trouble her. Treatment was continued as before. She was then given dehydrocholin 750 mgms. three times a day with rapid improvement in the joint swelling.Treatment was continued for 3 months at the end of which time she was quite symptomless and showed no abnormal physical signs. The E.S.R. was now 9 mm. per hour. One year later she was still symptomless and the RF had now become negative (Fig. 16).

Addendum: Bruusgaard, A. and Andersen, R.B., Lancet. 1976, 1, 700. reported that the administration of chenodeoxycholic acid chemically closely related to deoxycholic acid, 750-1000 mgm. daily for 3-11 weeks to 16 patients with rheumatoid arthritis caused initial exaggeration of the joint and general condition, sometimes rather severe, and accompanied by fever. This was followed by obvious remission in the disease and fall in the ESR.

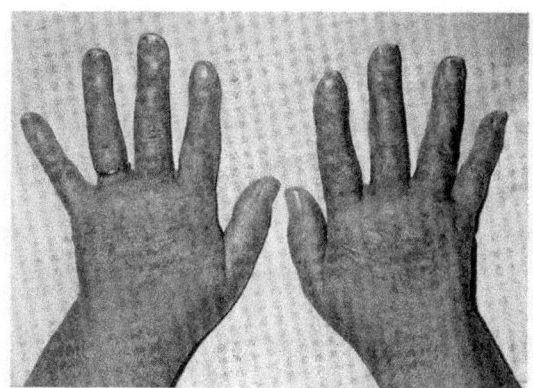

Fig. 17·A

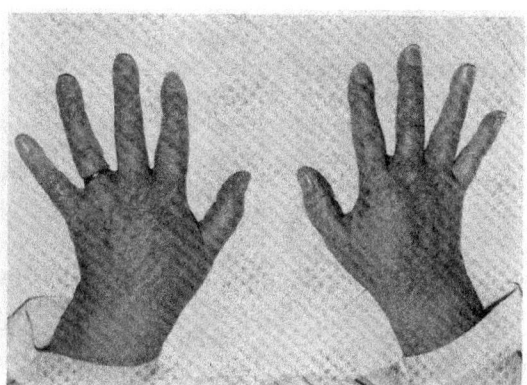

Fig. 17·B

Fig. 17   Female, aged 53 years.   Four years history of rheumatoid disease.   "A" shows hands before and "B" 6 days after
treatment with bile salts.

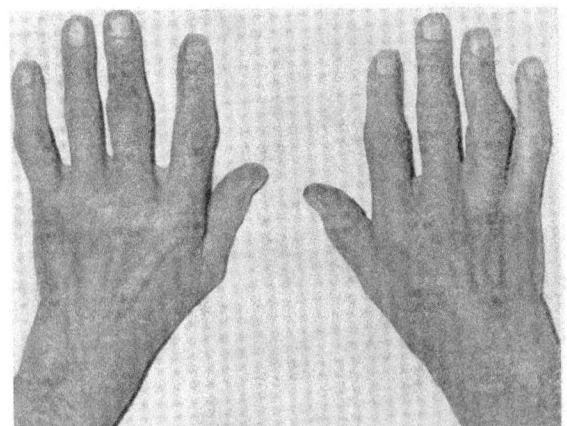

Fig. 18-A

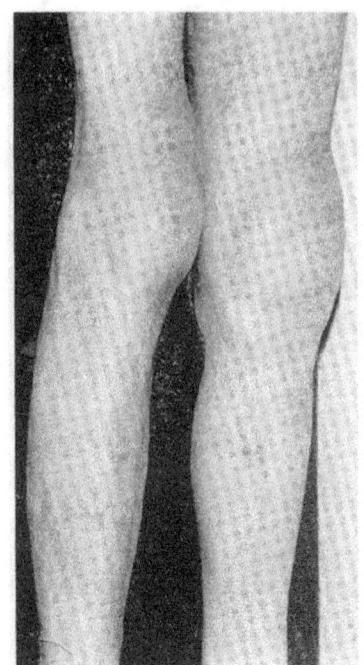

Fig. 18-B

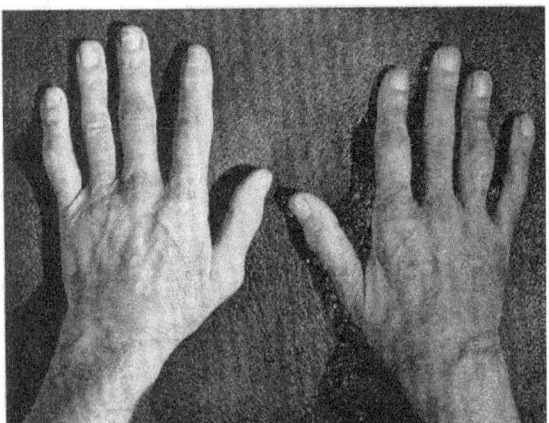

Fig. 18-C

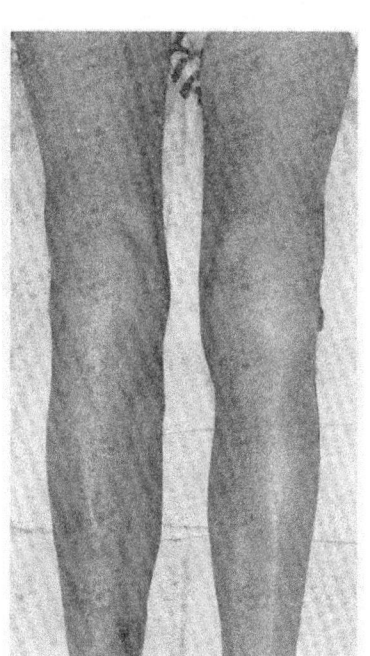

Fig. 18-D

Fig. 18   Male, aged 42 years. Two years history of
rheumatoid disease. ANF positive, sho,ving "A"
hands and "B" knees before and "C" hands and "D"
knees after 10 days treatment with bile salts.

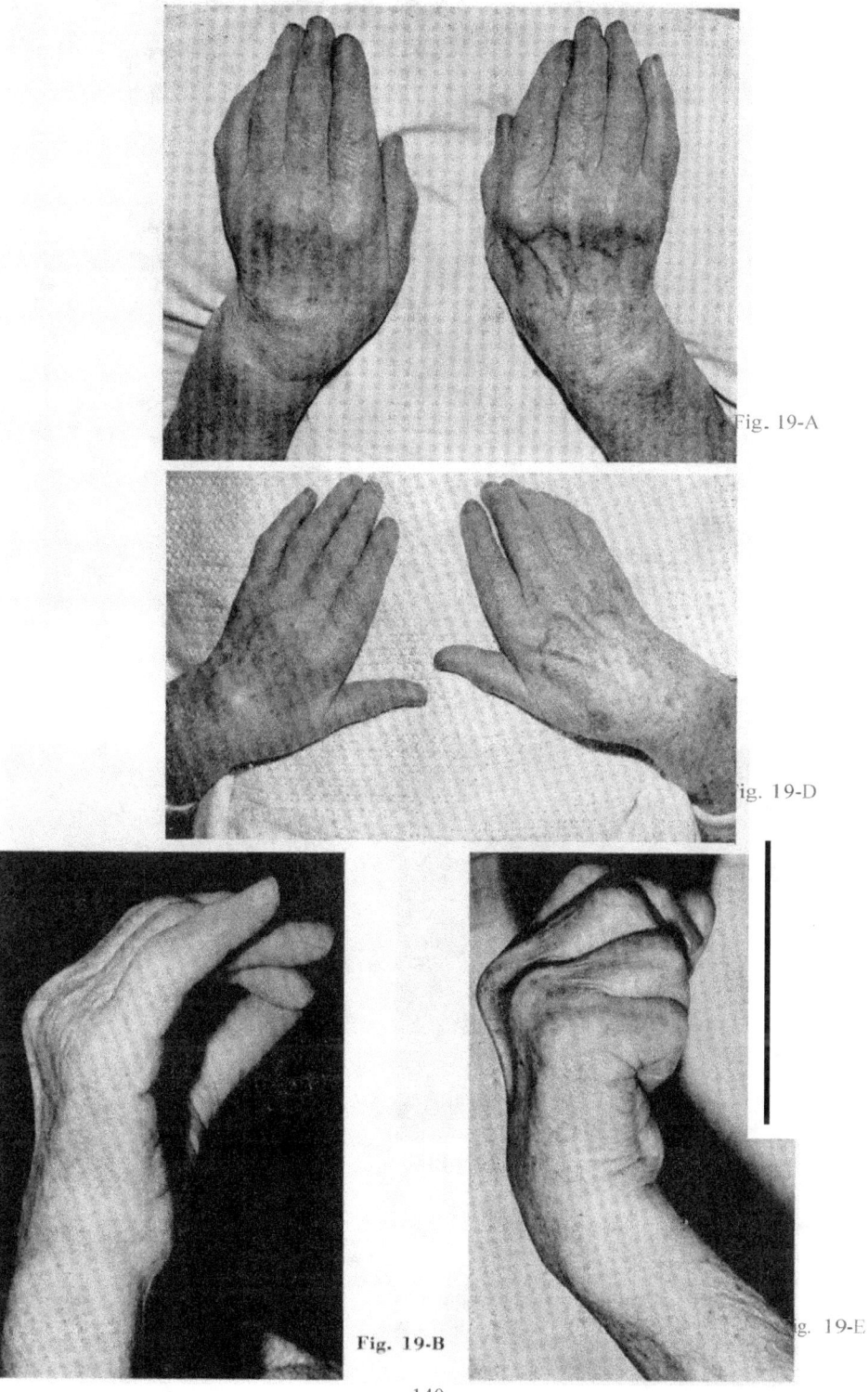

Fig. 19-A

Fig. 19-D

Fig. 19-B

Fig. 19-E

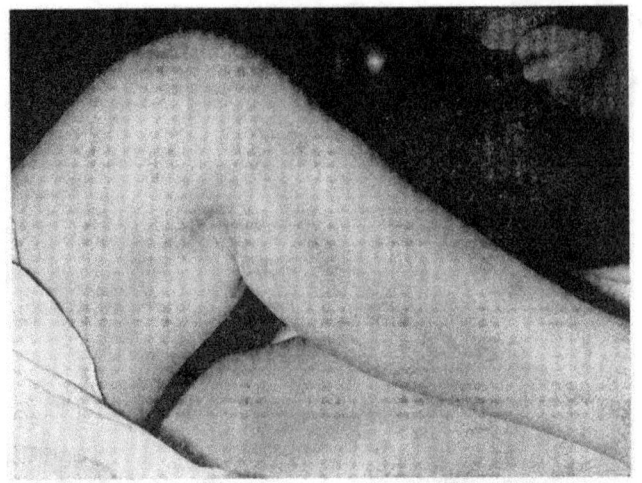

Fig. 19-C

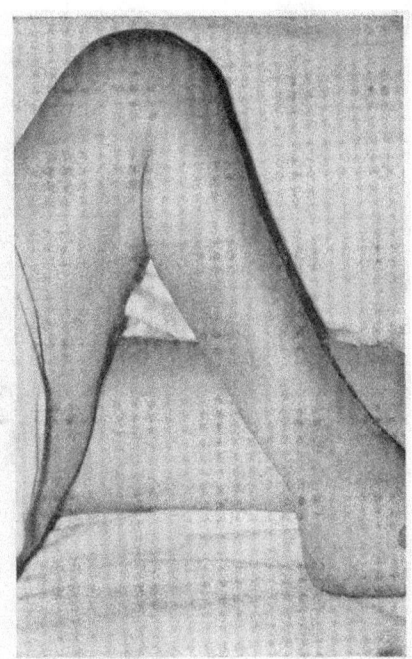

Fig. 19-F

Fig. 19 Male, aged 56 year. Five years history of seropositive rheumatoid disease. "A" shows swelling of hands and
wrists. "B" an attempt to make a fist. "C" the limit of flexion
of the right knee before treatment, "D", "E" and "F" show
the same 8 days after treatment with bile salts.

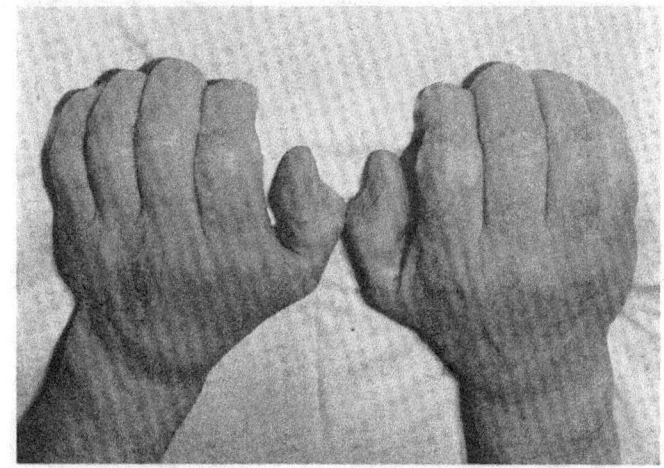

Fig. 20-A

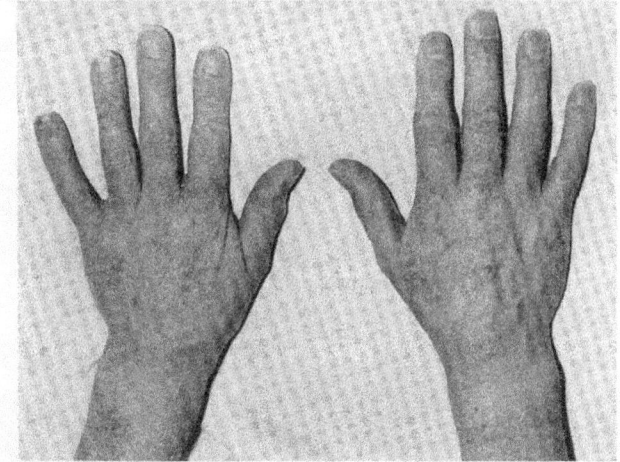

Fig. 20-D

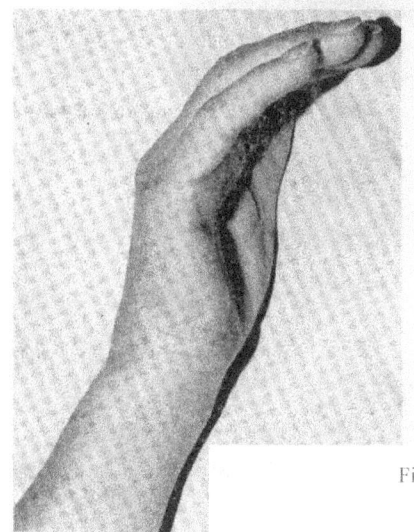

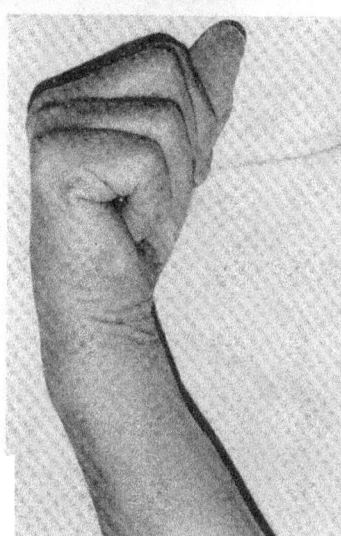

Fig. 20-B

Fig. 20-E

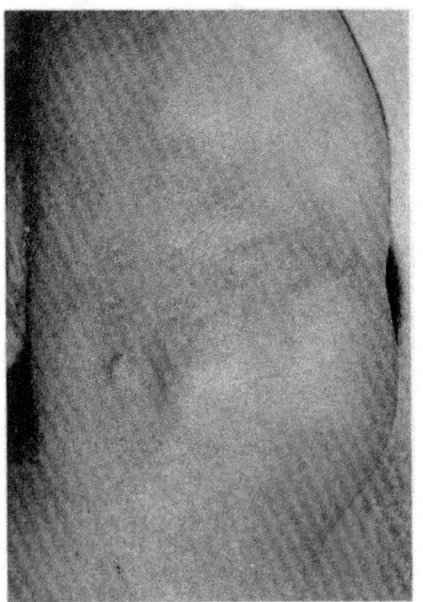
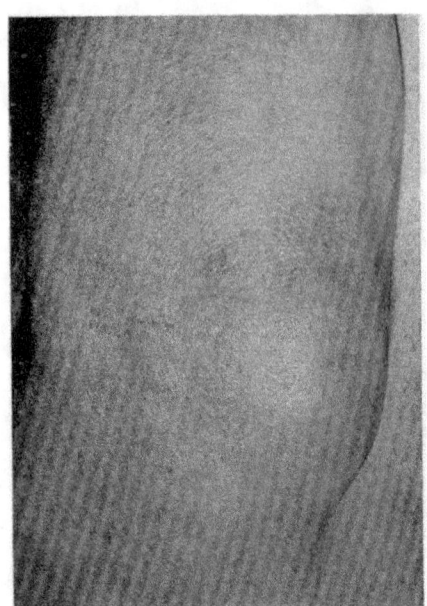

Fig. 20-C   **Fig. 20-F**

Fig. 20 Male, aged 52 years. Two years history of seropositive rh<'uma toid disease, showing "A" back of hands, "B" attempts to make a fist and "C" rheumatoid nodules about the right knee before treatment and "D" hands, "E" ability to make a fit and "F" disappearance of rheumatoid nodule after 2 weeks treatment with bile salts.

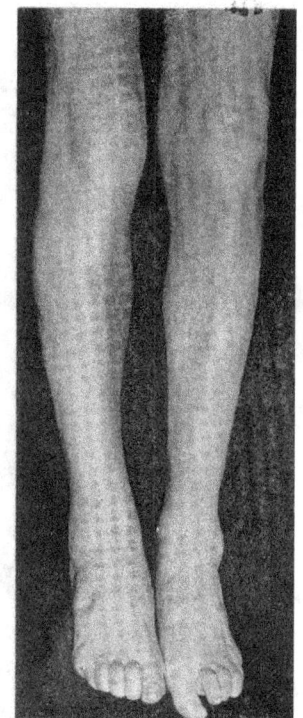

Fig. 21-A

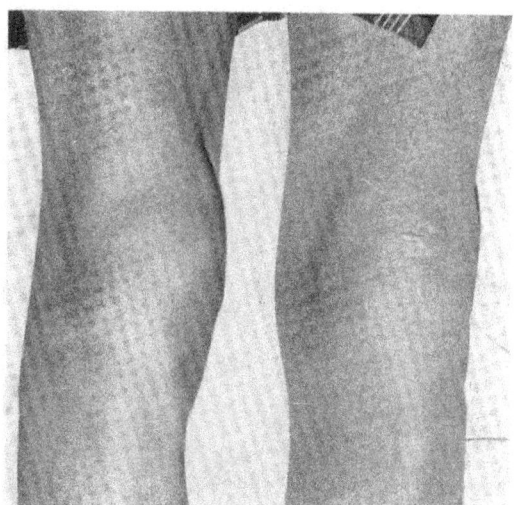

Fig. 21-B

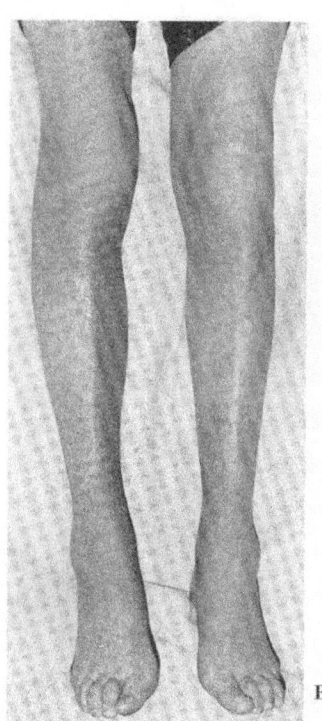

Fig. 21-D

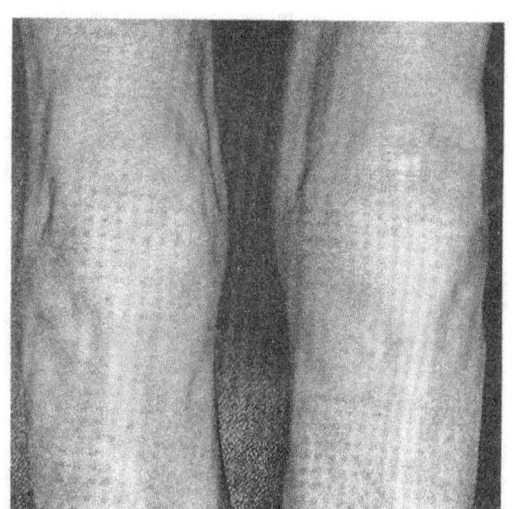

Fig. 21-E

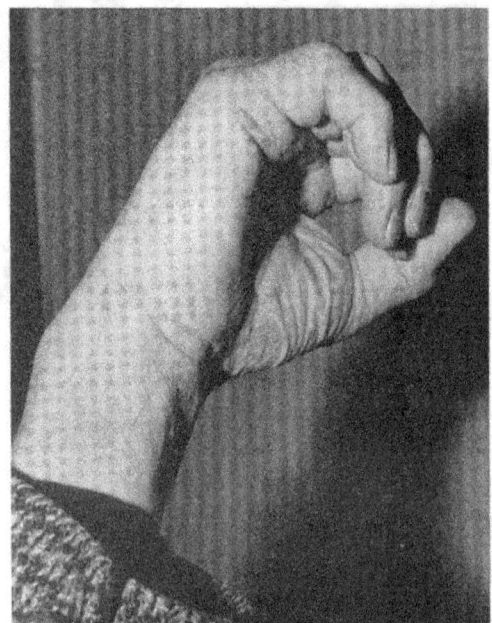

Fig. 21-C

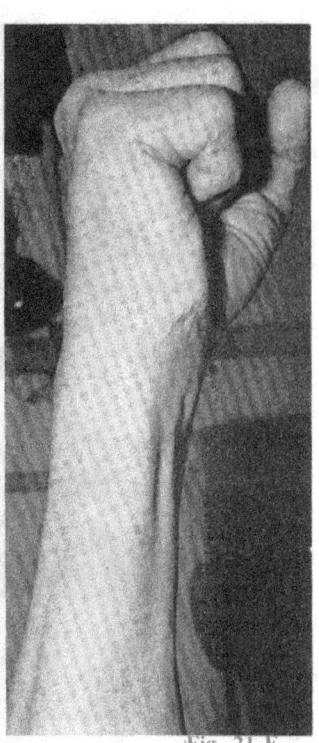

:Fig. 21-F

Fig. 21 Male. aged 58 years. Seropositive subacute rheumatoid disease of 3 years duration accompanied by pitting oedema
of the feet "A", swelling of the knees "B", inability to make
a fist "C", "D", 'E' and "F" show the effects of treatment with
bile salts for 6 days. Note disappearance of oedema and joint
swelling.

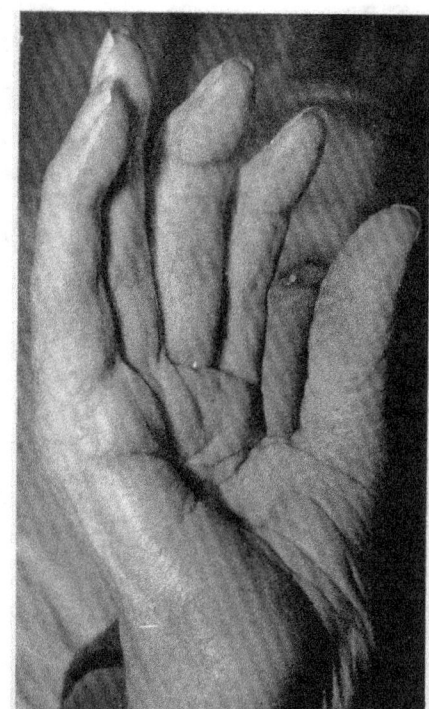

Fig. 22-A

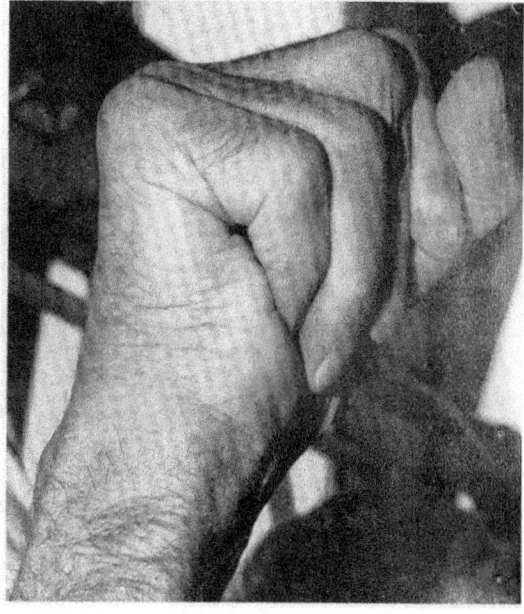

Fig. 22-B

Fig. 22 Male. aged 55 yrars. Six year hi tory of chronic rheumatoid disease showing "A" attempts to make a fist before and "B"' after treatment "ith bile salts.

— 146 —

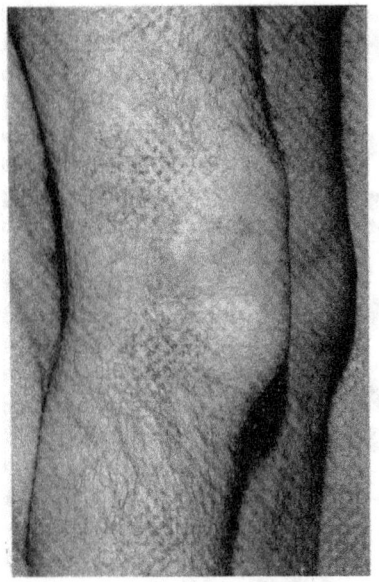

Fig. 23·A

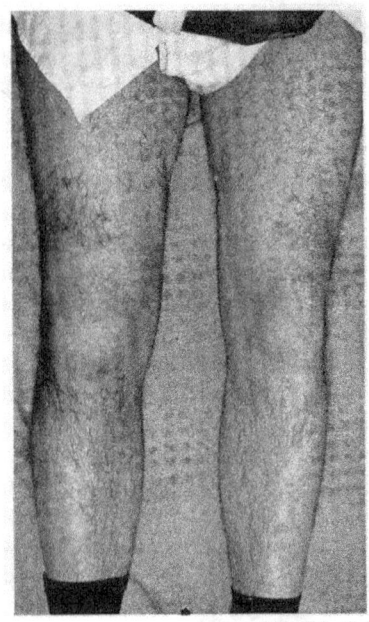

Fil-(23- C

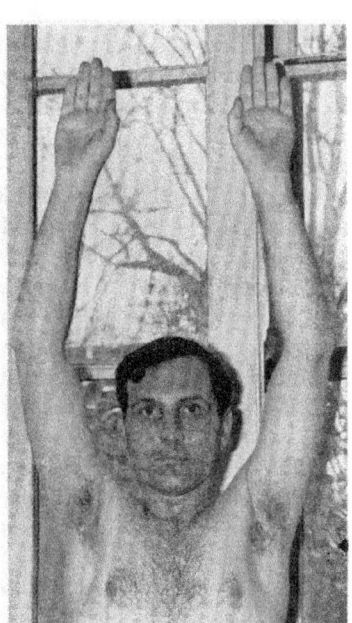

Fig. 23-D

Fig. 23·B

Fig. 23   Male, aged 30 years.   Four years history of seropositive rheumatoid disease, affecting knees, hands, feet and shoulder-
rs.   "A" shows swelling of knees before and "B" the inability
to abduct the upper arm more than a right angle before treatment with bile salts.   "C" shows disappearance of swelling of
knees and "D" the normal shoulder joint movements and absence of pain after 5 days treatment.

— 147 —

d) Clotrimazole

Clotrimazole (Bayer Pharmaceuticals) is a tritylimidazole derivative, and thus chemically related to BT 985 Merck A.G., the nitroimidazole derivative found so effective against S.L.E. and rheumatoid disease (Abd-Rabbo et al., 1972). It is an antimycotic agent with a broad spectrum. It is fungistatic against candida, crypto-coccus, nocardia spp.; madurella spp.; dermatophytes, blastomycetes, chromomycytes as well as certain moulds, aspergillus and certain gram positive organisms. It is also active against certain protozoa, such as histoplasma and flagellates (tricho-monas). It is amoebistatic and amoebici-dal in different concentrations against the free-Jiving amoeba, Naegleria fowleri (Jamieson and Anderson, 1974). In view of the latter observation it seemed that trial of the drug in cases of rheumatoid disease was indicated. This formed part of a pilot study authorized by the Committee on the Safety of Drugs to be published elsewhere (Wyburn-Mason, 1976). The effect of clotrimazole in doses of 100 mgms. per kilogram per day in 3-4 divided doses taken immediately after meals with milk were tried in 12 cases of early active rheumatoid disease. They were hospitaliz-ed, but not confined to bed. No other drugs were given or, if they ·had been, these were discontinued. The response was dra-matic in all cases and closely resembled the effects of copper and bile salts. Bayer Pharmaceuticals report that the drug may cause nausea, vomiting and diarrhoea in some cases. In few of the author's cases of rheumatoid disease did this prove a problem. It was found that usually within 24 hours the pain, joint swelling and stiff-ness began to subside. In one case this was complete in 3 days. In the other cases disappearance of symptoms was complete in 2-4 weeks. In cases of longer duration, though all evidence of active di-sease disappeared rapidly, some evidence of permanent inactive disease persisted. In one case bilateral olecranon bursitis re-solved. In every case the drug caused an increase in the E.S.R., a slight fall in the red blood count and haemoglobin content of the blood after about 7-10 days. This was associated with a transient blood eosinophilia in 5 of the 12 cases. In two cases at this time there developed slight transient painful lymphadenopathy and in three cases an itchy generalized erythema-tous rash lasting about a week. This was accompanied by a transient recurrence of the joint swelling. *These reactions resem-bled an Herxheimer reaction and suggest* the *drug was destroying an organism sensi-tive to the drug.* Afterwards the E.S.R. fell to normal and the blood returned to normal after about 4--5 weeks. It was found that administration of the drug had to be continued for about 8 weeks before it could be left off without a return of symptoms. The cases were followed up for two years after this without return of symptoms. At this time retesting of the serum for RF and auto-antibodies showed that these had now disappeared completely.

Examples of such cases are as follows:–

Case 40 Male, aged 47 years. A Sikh carpenter. Nothing of significance in the past history. He gave a nine months his-tory of pain and severe restriction of movement of wrists, fingers and ankles making it impossible for him to continue work. He also complained of swelling and pain of the olecranon bursae. He had been unable to work for six months. He had previously been treated with distal-gesic without benefit. *Examination.* Heat, marked swelling, redness, pain and severe restriction of movements of fingers; wrists and ankles with swelling of the feet and enormous swelling and tenderness of the olecranon bursae. He was unable to make a fist on either side (Fig. 24).

Investigations Blood count W.B.C. 9,000 per cu. mm., R.B.C. 4.53 mill. per cu. mm. Hb 12.2 grams per 100 mi. Differ-ential white count normal. E.S.R. 50 mm. per hour. No lupus erythematous cells seen. Serum albumin, 3.2 G. per 100 ml.

globulin, 4.1 G. per 100 ml. Liver function tests; normal. Free hydrochloric acid present. Gastric parietal cell antibodies positive. ANF negative, RF negative. Thyroid antibodies negative. He was given clotrimazole 100 mgms. per kilo daily. Within 3 days the pain and swelling of the joints began to disappear. After one week he developed an itching erythematous rash over the whole trunk and the blood eosinophil count rose to 9 per cent of 5,400 W.B.C. per cu. mm. with the E.S.R. increased to 72 mm. per hour. The drug was continued, the rash and eosinophilia disappearing after a week and after a month the E.S.R. had fallen to 6 mm. per hour. By this time all pain and stiffness of joints and swelling of the feet had disappeared and all movements had returned to normal, (Fig. 24), but there still remained some painless thickening of the metacarpophalangeal and ankle joints. The olecranon bursitis had disappeared completely after 3 weeks. Treatment was continued for 8 weeks and then stopped without return of symptoms. He returnd to his work without recurrence of symptoms. Retesting his blood six months after commencing treatment showed the gastric parietal cell auto-antibodies had now disappeared.

Case 41 Male, aged 52 years. Engineer. Sixteen years previously he had suffered from a duodenal ulcer and 20 years previously he had thrombophlebitis in both legs, which cleared up completely. Three months prior to hospital admission he had suffered from "rheumatic" pains in the neck and one month later aching and swelling of the ankles, knees, elbows, wrists and fingers. The joints were especially stiff on waking and he sweated especially in his sleep. *Examination.* There was swelling of both wrist joints, which were hot and their movements restricted. Both ankles were likewise hot, swollen with restricted movements and there was marked pitting oedema of the dorsum of the feet (Fig. 25). He was treated prior

to admission with distalgesic and indocid tablets without benefit.

Investigations Blood count 5.29 mill. R.B.C. per cu. mm., Hb 15.2 G. W.B.C. 6,500 per cu. mm. 60% polymorphs. E.S.R. 34 mm. per hour. Plasma proteins, albumin; 3.6 G. per 100 mi., globulin; 2.9 G. per 100 mi. Bilirubin 1 mgm. per 100 mi. Alkaline phosphatase 7.5 KA units per 100 ml. Thymol turbidity 2 units per 100 mi. Lupus erythematous cells not seen. RF negative.

He was treated with 100 mgms. per kilo. body weight of clotrimazole with dramatic effect. All manifestations of arthritis and the oedema had disappeared within 3 days (Fig. 25). Four days after beginning treatment the E.S.R. rose to 47 mm. per hour and the Hb had fallen to 13.6 Grams per 100ml. and the W.B.C. to 4,970 per cu. mm. He was discharged from hospital after two weeks symptomless and followed as an out-patient. Three weeks after beginning treatment he developed erythema nodosum (thought to be an allergic phenomenon) on his legs. This disappeared after a week. One month after beginning treatment he returned to work. At this time he was symptomless and the liver function tests and E.S.R. had returned to normal.

Case 42 Female, aged 53 years. Eighteen months previously she had developed tenosinovitis of the flexor tendons of the right hand. At this time the RA latex fixation test was positive >1 in 20. She was treated with phenylbutazone and the symptoms disappeared over the course of the next six months. On admission she gave a two months history of painful swelling of both wrists and of generalized morning stiffness. She had been treated with phenylbutazone without relief. *Examination.* The only positive findings were pain. heat, welling and restricted movement of both wrist joints (Fig. 26).

Investi&"ations Blood count R.B.C. 4.19 mill. per cu. mm., Hb 11.8 G. per 100 mls., W.B.C. 15,500 per cu. mm., 80 per cent

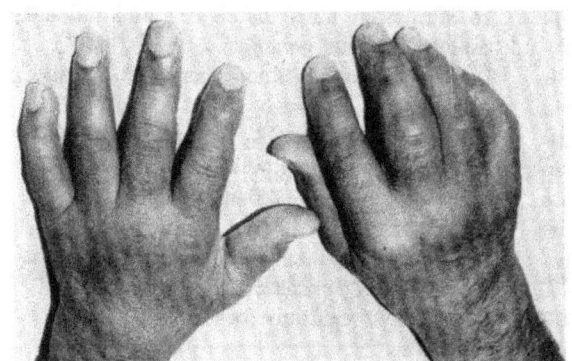

Fig. 24-A

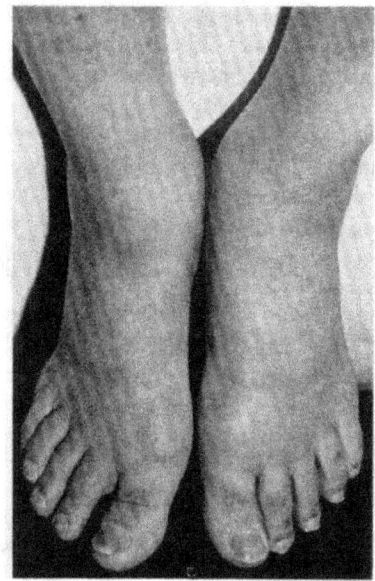

Fig. 24-B

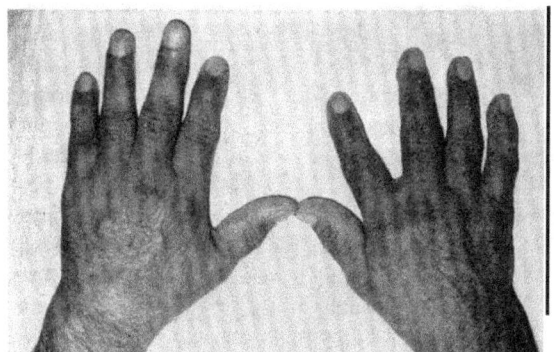

Fig. 24-A ₁

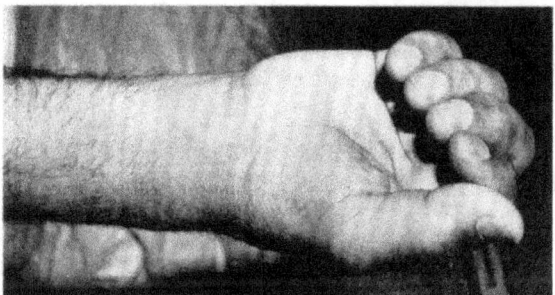

Fig. 24-C

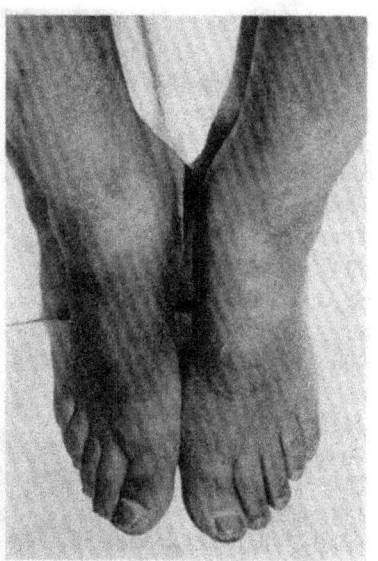

Fig. 24-B.

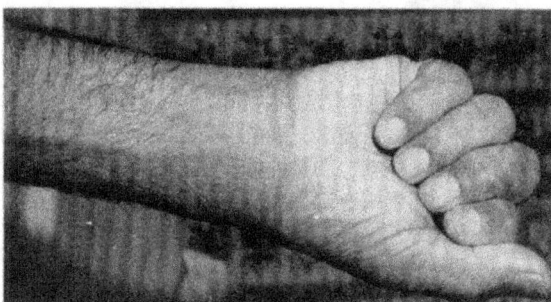

fig. 24-C.

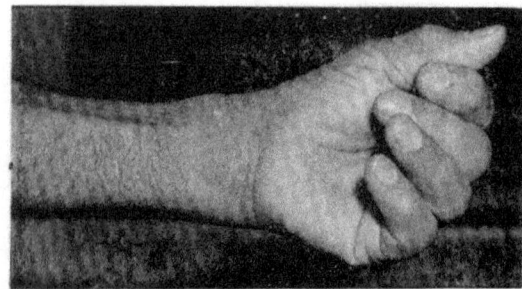

Fig. 24-D

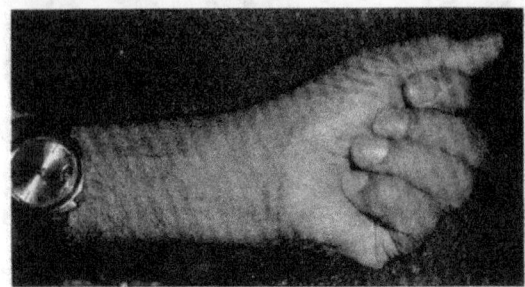

Fig. 24-D.

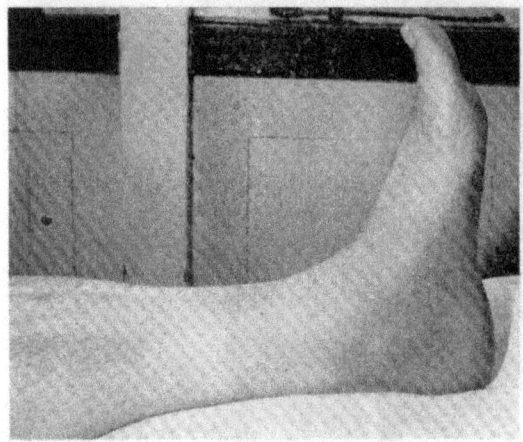

Fig. 24-E

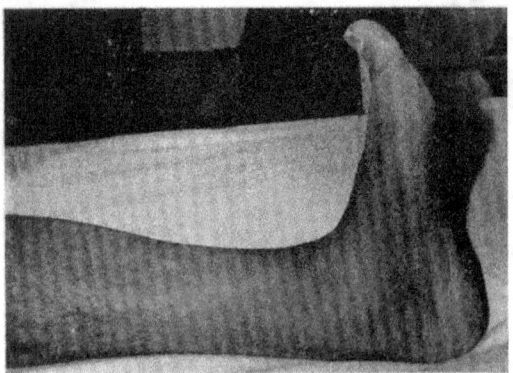

Fig. 24-E,

Fig. 24 Case 40. Male, aged 47 years. A case of seropositive rheumatoid arthritis affecting the wrists, fingers and ankles showing appearances of hands A. feet and ankles B. attempts to make a fist C and D and attempts at dorsiflexion of the left ankle and foot E, and the same one month later AI, BI, CI, DI and EI after treatment with clotrimazole. Note the disappearance of the joint swelling and the return of movements to normal.

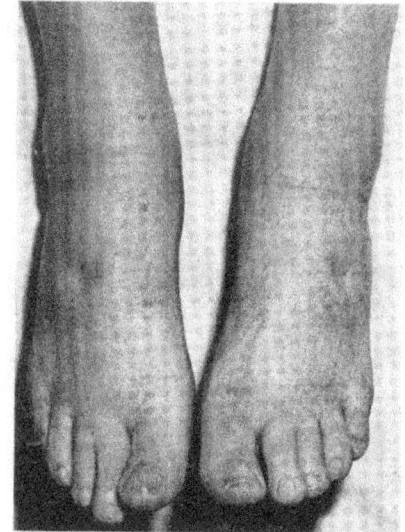
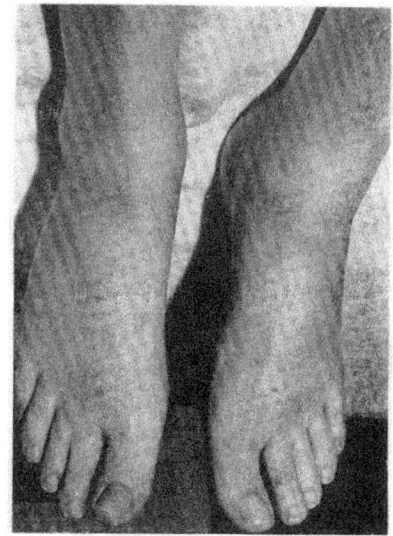

Fig. 25-A   Fig. 25-A

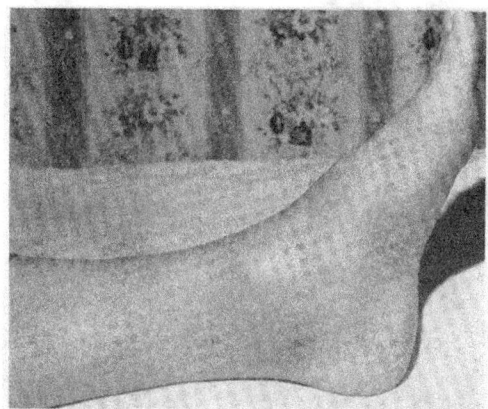

Fig. 25-8

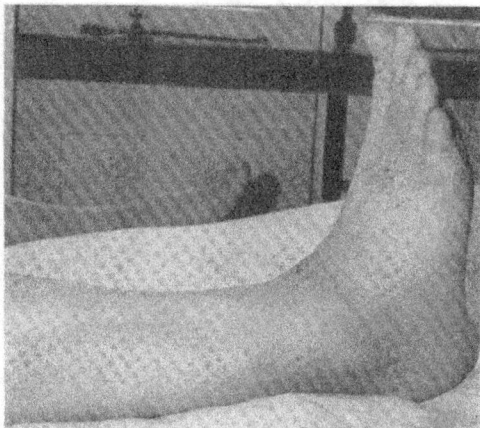

Fig. 25-8₁

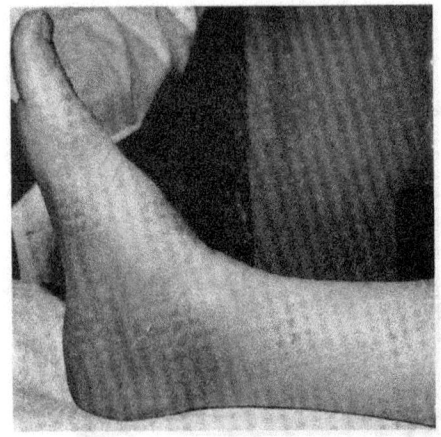

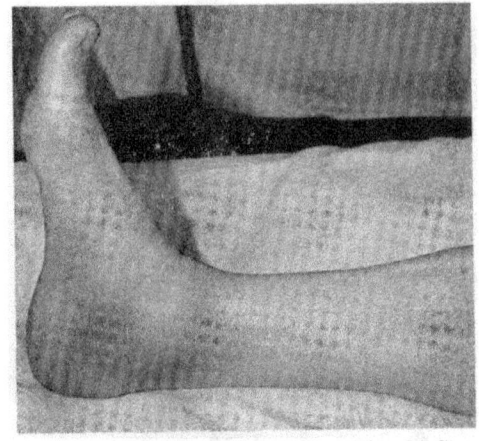

Fig. 25-C   Fig. 25-Cl

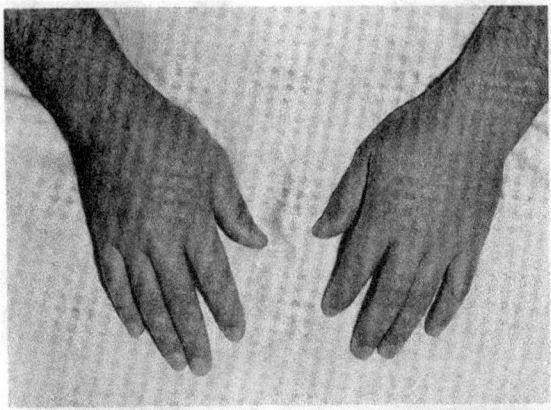

Fig. 25-D

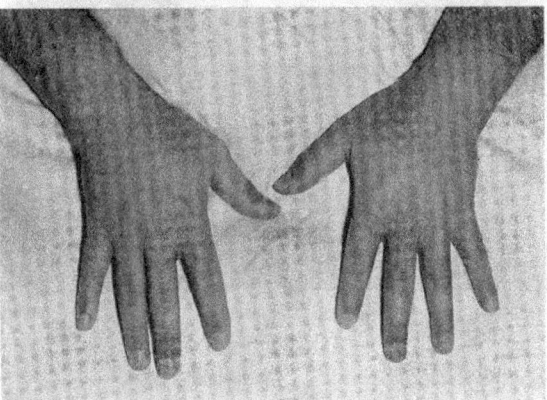

Fig. 25-Dl

Fig. 25   Case 41.   Male, aged 52 years.   A case of seropositive rheumatoid arthritis of one month duration affecting ankles, knees, elbows, wrists and fingers with marked pitting oedema of the feet, showing A appearances of feet and ankles active attempts at dorsiflexion of the right and left ankles B and C and appearance of hand D and the same Al, Bl, Cl and Dl after 3 days treatment with clotrimazole. Note the disappearance of the oedema and joint swelling and the improvement in the degree of movement of the joints.

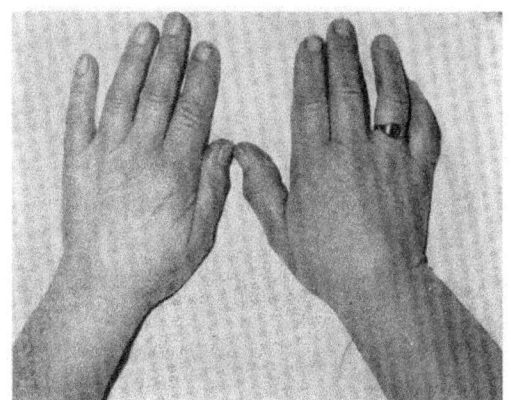
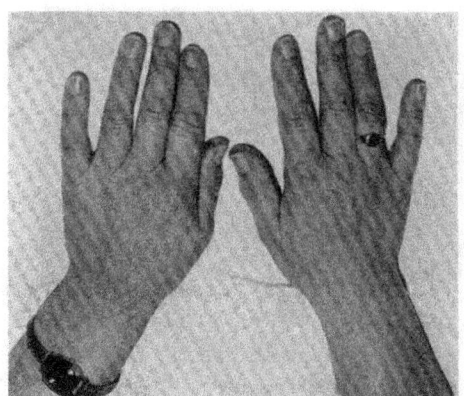

Fig. 26-A   Fig. 26-A,

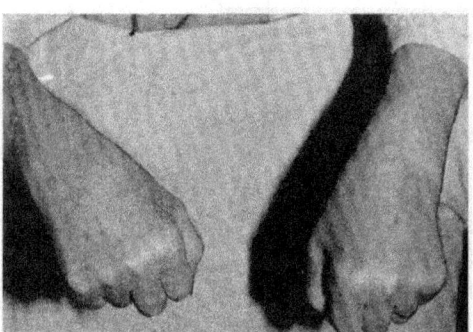
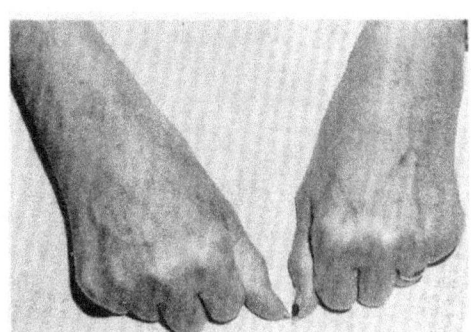

Fig. 26-B   Fig. 26-B,

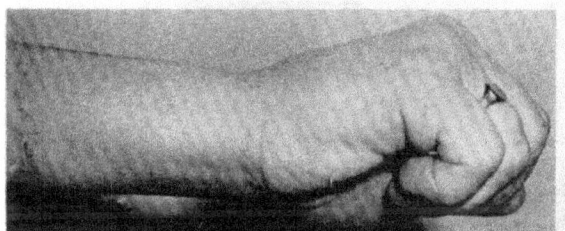
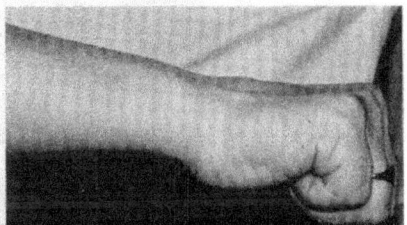

Fig. 26-C   Fig. 26-C,

Fig. 26   Case 42.   Femal r. aged 53 year with an 18 months
history of eropositive rheuma toid art hritis affecting the wrist
and hands howing A and B appea rance of the hands and C
an attempt to make a fist with the rig ht hand and the sam<
a week after brginning t reatment with clotri mazole Al , Bl and
Cl. / ote the di appea rance of the swelling and the improvement in the drgree of joint movement.

—154—

polymorphs, 20 per cent lymphocytes. E.S.R. 34 mms. in one hour. Blood RF negative. ANF negative. Thyroid auto-antibodies and gastric parietal cell auto-antibodies positive. Liver function tests normal. Serum albumin 3.9 G. per cent., globulin 3.3 G. per cent.

She was treated with clotrimazole 100 mgms. per kilo daily. Within 24 hours the pain, swelling and heat of the joints had disappeared (Fig. 26) and a week after commencing treatment the W.B.C. was now 5,600 per cu. mm. and the E.S.R. had fallen to 6 mms. per hour. She was discharged from hospital; but ran out of tablets and within 4 days mild symptoms reappeared until she recommenced taking the drug, when they again rapidly disappeared. She remained free of symptoms over the next six months while taking the drug. After stopping the drug there was no return of symptoms. After nine months the auto-antibodies had disappeared from the blood.

Case 43 Female, aged 67 years. Menarche aged 14 years. Periods always scanty with long intervals between them. S'he had suffered from psoriasis and attacks of urticaria since her teens and had a period suffering from iron deficiency anaemia. She was diagnosed as a case of myxoedema at the age of 50 years for which she was treated with !-thyroxin 6 years before. She had suffered pain and swelling of the wrists and elbows since the menopause at the age of 48 years and for which she had received from her general practitioner prednisolone 5 mgms. t.d.s. *Examination.* No evidence of anaemia or of myxoedema. There was marked pain, swelling, heat and limitation of movement of both wrists and elbows (Fig. 27).

Investi&"ations Liver function tests normal. Plasma albumin, 3.0 G. per 100 ml., globulin, 2.6 G. per 100 ml., R.B.C. 3.77 mill. per cu. mm., Hb 12.1 G. per 100 ml., W.B.C. 5,500 per cu. mm., 64 per cent polymorphs, 35 per cent lymphocytes. E.S.R. 35 mms. per hour. No achlorhydria. Rose

Waaler and RA latex tests negative. ANF, gastric parietal cell antibodies, thyroid antibodies negative. Folate concentration 3.2 mgms. per mi. Vitamin B,. concentration 290 *p.p.G.* per mi.

She was weaned off prednisolone and after a week without treatment, was given clotrimazole 100 mgms. per kilo. daily in divided doses. After 3 days the pain, swelling and hotness of the wrists had disappeared (Fig. 27) and after 5 days she noticed some swelling of the lymph nodes in the neck, which were slightly tender. After a week the W.B.C. had fallen to 4,200 cells per cu. mm. of which 10 per cent were eosinophils. The E.S.R. had risen to 50 mms. per hour. There was no change in the liver function test or plasma protein levels. The lymph node swelling rapidly disappeared. At the end of 3 weeks the E.S.R. had fallen to normal. She continued treatment for 6 months. There was no return of symptoms 3 months after discontinuing treatment.

Case 44 Male, aged 65 years. Suffered from asthma and eczema from the ages of 11 to 35 years. He gave a four months history of pain, swelling, hotness and restriction of movement and morning stiffness in the hands, elbows, shoulders, knees and ankles. *Examination* showed considerable swelling, · tenderness and restricted movements of hands, knees and ankles which were warm to the touch (Fig. 28).

Investigations Blood count 4.37 mill. R.B.C. per cu. mm., Hb 12.7 G. per 100 mls., W.B.C. 16,500 per cu. mm., polymorphs 79 per cent., lymphocytes 21 per cent., E.S.R. 53 mm. per hour. Serum uric acid 3.8 mgms. per 100 mls. Albumin 3.7 G. per 100 m!s., globulin 3.7 G. per 100 mls. Rose Waaler test positive. RA latex test positive. ANF, thyroid auto-antibodies, gastric parietal cell auto-antibodies all negative. Liver function tests normal.

He was treated with soluble aspirin 600 mgms. 4 hourly and butazolidine 200 mgms. t.d.s. without benefit. Then clotrimazole 100 mgms. per kilo. (i.e. 2 G. six hourly)

with milk was substituted. Within 24 hours there was marked improvement in swelling and pain in joints and this continued for another 24 hours. Then the swelling reappeared and the pain became more intense for a further two days after which time all the joint symptoms :capzdly disappeared within four days (Fig. 28). This exaggeration of symptoms coincided with the appearance *oi* itching of the sl{in and rise in E.S.R. to 68 mms. per hour. There was no change in the liver function tests. He was discharged from hospital after two weeks taking clotrimazole and watched as an out-patient. He remained completely symptomless for two weeks and then ran out of tablets and within 3 days his symptoms reappeared with less severity. Treatment was recommenced and all the symptoms again disappeared rapidly. At the end of a further 4 weeks the E.S.R. had fallen to 7 mms. per hour and the plasma proteins were now albumin, 4.2 G. per 100 mi., globulin, 2.9 G. per 100 mi. Treatment was stopped after 6 weeks and he remained symptomless for the next 6 months at the end of which time the RF had disappeared from the blood.

After the initial twelve cases the drug has now been used in a total of some 80 active cases, including a number of children and several cases of systemic lu pus erythematosus. In these a different procedure was adopted. Except when the patients were running a high fever they were not confined to bed or hospitalized, though twice weekly blood investigat lons were carried out, including full blood counts, blood urea and E.S.R. estimations and liver function and urine tests for blood. However the patients previous treatment was continued. In almost all cases the same results as those recorded by Wyburn-Mason (1976) were obtained, namely a rapid disappearance in all signs of active disease. With this the previous treatment was stopped and steroids tapered off without return of symptoms. In adults it was

found that a dose of only 2.0-2.5 G. per day was necessary and with this dosage nausea, vomiting and diarrhoea did not occur. Herxheimer reactions with temporary increased swelling, heat, pain and restricted movement of the joints occurred in 6 cases. In 3 cases a severe toxic reaction developed in which there occurred a pyrexia of 102-4°F, drenching sweats, malaise, headache and a severe increase in the joint symptoms which necessitated abandonment of the treatment. In the other cases treatment was continued for 10 weeks and the patients have been followed up for varying periods of up to 15 months without return of evidence of active disease. One case had mild temporary haematuria. The treatment has, of course, no effect on joints in which bony and cartilaginous changes have occurred. However, in cases in which joint movements ar restricted by bony and fibrous adhesions only and when rheumatoid nodules are present these gradually disappear and normal joint movements return. In cases of systemic lupus erythematosus similar results have been obtained.

In children the effects are perhaps more dramatic than in adults. Ten such cases have been treated in ages varying from 5 to 18 years. All were receiving steroids in varying doses with stunting of growth and typical Cushingoid appearance. Clotrimazole was given in doses of 0.5-1.0 G. per day according to weight. The steroids were continued. In one case, a girl of 5 years, a doctor's daughter, the child had been running a temperature of 104-5°F' for 3 months and was taking 80 mgms. of prednisolone per 24 hours without controlling the joint swelling and pain, sweating or pyrexia. She was given 0.5 G. of Clotrimazole a day and her temperature fell to normal in 12 hours with disappearance of all her symptoms. The steroids were rapidly cut down and then stopped and the patient continued on Clotrimazole for 12 weeks without return of symptoms when this was stopped. She is still under

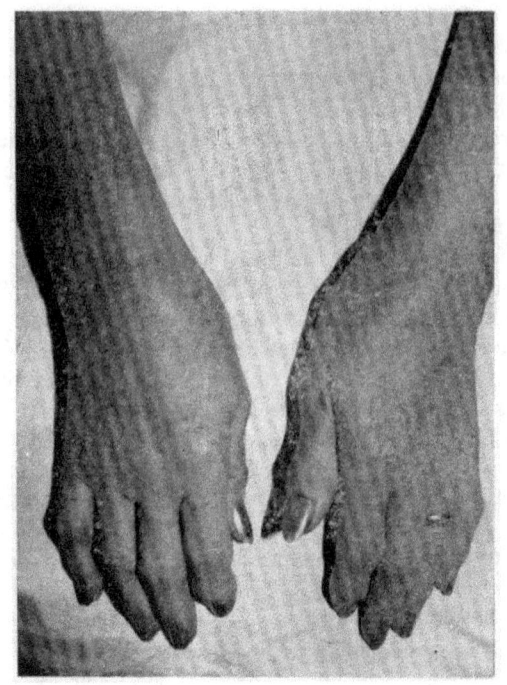

Fig. 27-A

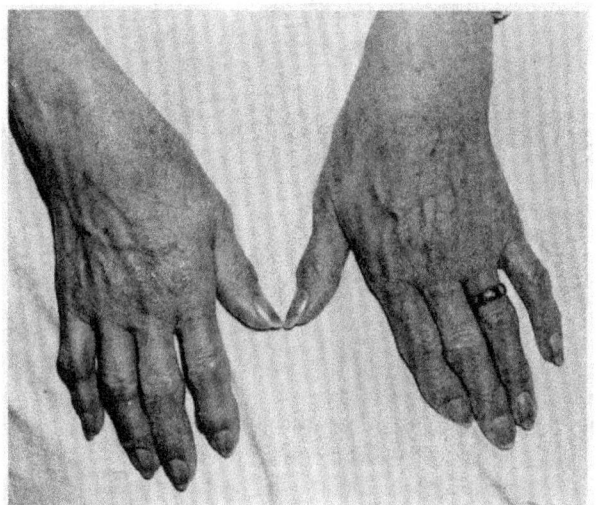

Fig. 27-B

Fig. 27 Case 43. Appearance of wrists and finger before, A, and five days after beginning treatment with clotrimazole, B.

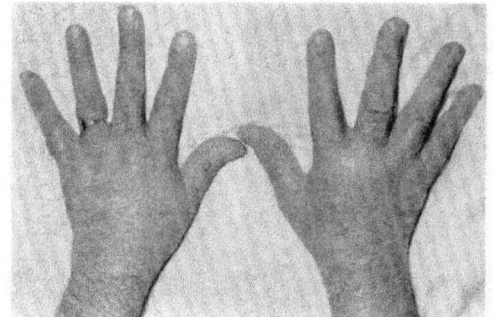
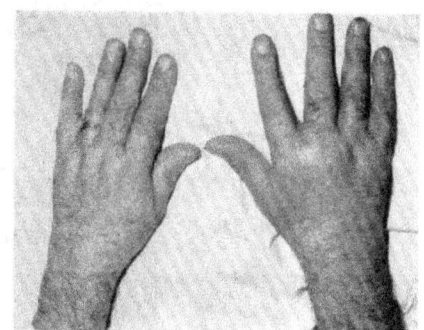

Fig. 28-A   Fig. 28-A .

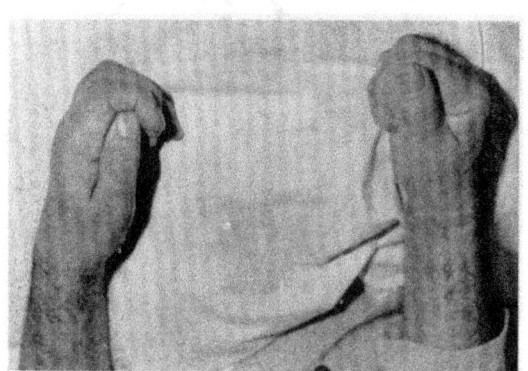
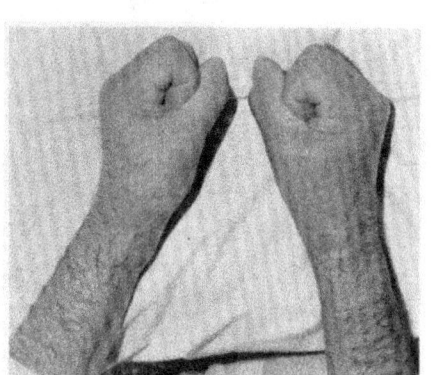

Fig. 28-B   *Fig*. 28-B.

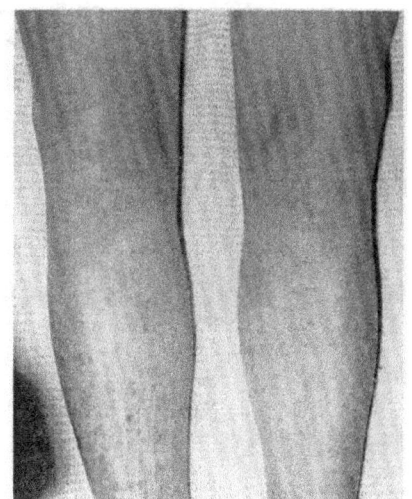
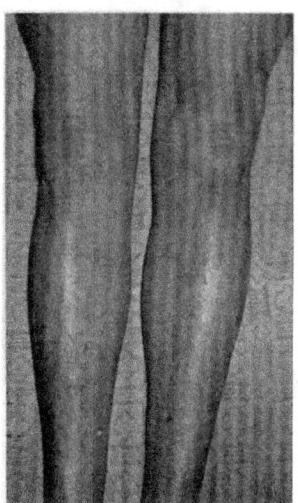

Fig. 28-C   Fig. 28-C.

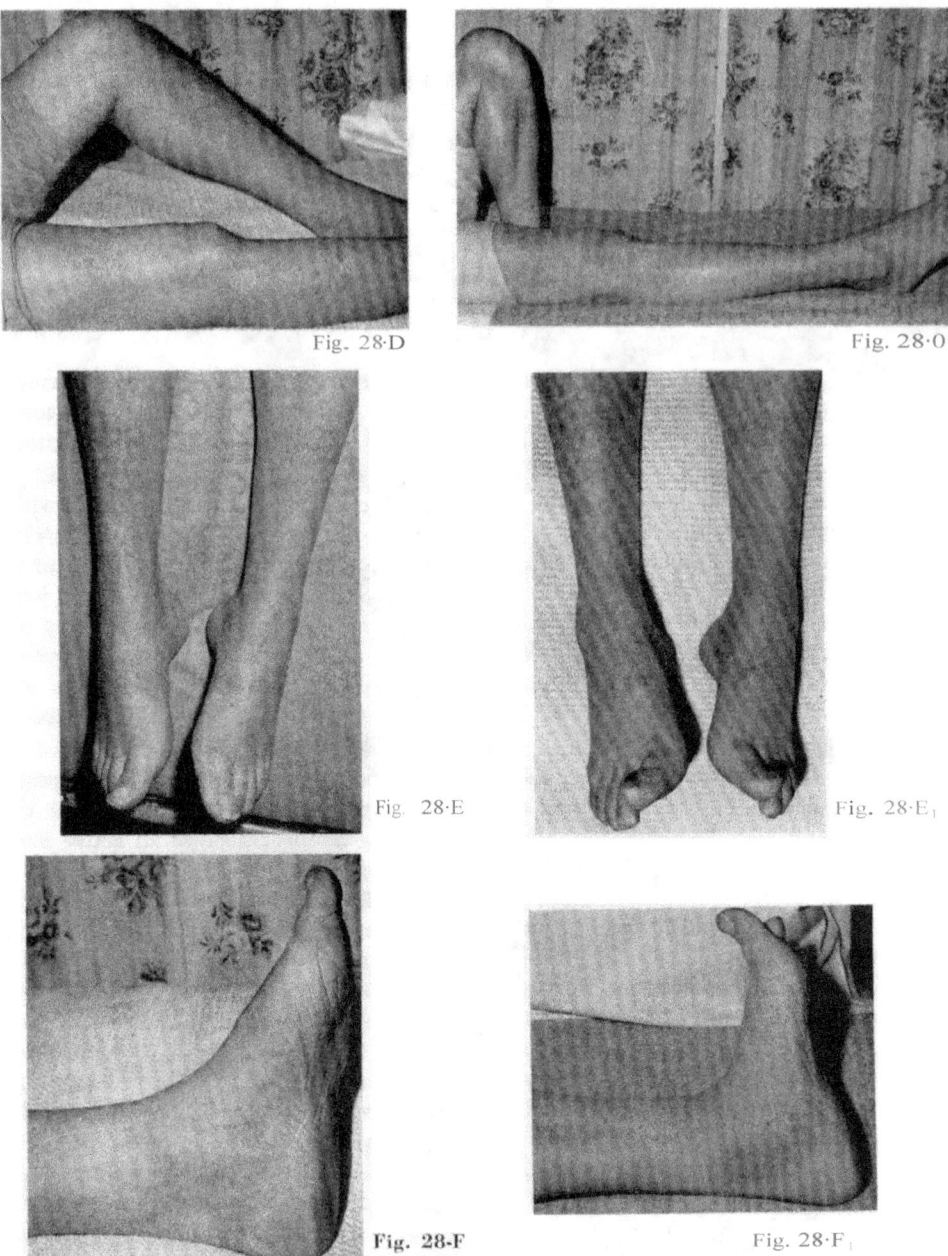

Fig. 28·D

Fig. 28·O₁

Fig. 28·E

Fig. 28·E₁

Fig. 28-F

Fig. 28·F₁

Fig. 28 Case 44. Male, aged 65 years. Four months history of acute seropositive rheumatoid arthritis affecting the hands, elbow, shoulders, knees and ankles, showing A appearance of hands, B attempts at making a fist, C appearance of knees, D attempts at flexion of the left knee, E appearance of feet and F anempts at dorsiflexion of the left ankle and big toe with the corresponding appearances 5 days later. Al-Fl, after treatment with clotrimazole. Note the disappearance of joint swelling and the improvement in joint movements.

observation. Another boy of 5 years old began the disease at the age of one year. He had been taking 15 mgms. of predniso-lone for 2 years and was 8.5 kilograms overweight and 10 ems. under height for his age and very lethargic. Administra-tion of Clotrimazole 0.5 G. per 24 hours produced an immediate dramatic change in the child's vivacity. The steroids were tapered off and the Clotrimazole continued for 10 weeks. A month later his weight was normal for his height and he had grown 6 ems. in a month. He remains well after a further 4 months without treat-ment. Similar results were obtained with the other children.

Communications from various parts of the world from patients treated by this method by their doctors have confirmed the above findings.

Similar results have been obtained in 12 cases of ankylosing spondylitis with relief of pain, breaking down of adhesions and improved spinal involvement.

e) Levamisole

Levamisole like Clotrimazole is an imida-zole compound and has been used as an anthelmintic and also possesses antiproto-zoal activity. It has been claimed as affect-ing immune responses (Schuermans, 1975), though this has been denied by Flannery et al. (1975) and Kay and Karlin (1975). Schuermans treated six patients with ac-tive rheumatoid disease who had respond-ed poorly to anti-inflammatory or analges-ic drugs with levamisole and this resulted in striking improvement in pain, joint swelling and range of movement within a week. The rheumatoid factor became nega-tive in three patients.

f) Tinidazole

Attention has been drawn above to the fact that antiprotozoal substances contain-ing imidazole groups are effective in rheu-matoid disease. Tinidazole is an imidazole derivative closely related to metronidazole, but also containing a sulphone group in a side chain. It is *purely an antiprotozoal substance*, being active in vitro and in vivo against different species of protozoon, in-cluding trichomonas, amoebae, giardia, emeria tenella and histomonas, but is inac-tive against trypanosomes or plasmodia berghei in mice. It is made in tablets of 500 mgms. It is highly effective in doses of 2-3 tablets a day for a week in the treatment of amoebiasis and trichomonas infection. Tinidazole has the advantage that it is slowly excreted and can be used successfully in the treatment of both trichomonas and entamoeba infections in a single dose of 2 G. In such cases it causes no adverse reactions whatsoever and no exaggeration of the symptoms. When given to cases of rheumatoid ar-thritis in this dose it usually causes within 12-36 hours a violent Herxheimer reaction with an exaggeration, often severe, of the inflammatory changes in the affected joints and often also of others previously un-affected with sweating, headache, pyrexia and general malaise lasting 2-7 days with minor symptoms lasting several weeks. When repeated after two weeks this reac-tion lessens progressively with repeated doses and then in early cases there is a complete disappearance of all active mani-festations of the disease with gradual fall in E.S.R., rise in the blood count and dis-appearance of RF from the serum. In one long-standing case with involvement of the knees previous aspiration of fluid from both knees had yielded only clear, slightly yellow fluid. Treatment with tinidazole 2 G in single doses every two weeks caused an immediate painful hot swelling of both knees with recurrence of free fluid after a month. Both joints were aspirated and produced a large amount of bacteriologi-cally sterile intensely green, thick pus. This resulted in marked relief of pain, hot-ness and swelling of the knee joints. Two weeks later the administration of 500 mgms. of tinidazole caused within a few hours a temporary recurrence in the heat and pain of the knee joints lasting 24 hours. *These findings using a purely an-tiprotozoal drug which in other diseases causes no* such *response show conclusively that the drug has caused the death of an organism within or in the neighbourhood of the affected joints and this is not a bacterium, but presumably a protozoon.* These results caused such large doses of the drug to be abandonGd and afterwards the drug was given in doses of 500 mgms. once every one or two weeks gradually increasing the dose. This smaller dose often caused minor exaggerations of the symptoms and no further drug was given until the exaggeration had died down. After a few doses the exaggeration of sympto.ns disappeared but the drug was continued for up to 10 weeks in doses 500 mg:ns. or more twice weekl y. The response was a disappearance o⁷ all evidence of activity of rheumatoid disease. but, of course, no regeneration of the destroyed bone or cartilage.

B. The effects of other antiprotozoal drugs

a) Pentamidine

Treatment with this drug as described above was tried in 11 cases of early active rheumatoid arthritis without permanent joint changes and 2 cases of systemic lupus erythematosus. Some of them had had previous treatment which, however, was not controlling the disease, and in this case this was continued unchanged. All cases exhibited pain, swelling and restricted movements of joints, morning stiffness, raised E.S.R., RF and/or ANF in the serum and in some cases thyroid and/or gastric parietal cell auto-antibodies. Some showed lupus eryt hematosus cells in the blood in va rying numbers. The albumin-globulin ro.tio was reversed. Anaemia of some degree was present. In one case both Hashimoto's thy roiditis and Sjogren's syndrome were also present and in another Sjogren's syndrome only. Several of the patients were unable to stand or walk beca use of the arthropathy. In some cases injections of the drug caused a short-lived pyrexia, which disappeared after the injections were stopped. The cases were followed for from 1--4 years.

In every case there was a rapid disappearance of oedema, pain and joint swelling and this began within a few hours of the commencement of treatment and was complete within a few days *resembling the affect of an antibiotic* in cases *of bacterial disease.* Patients unable to walk could do so again within 3–6 days. In two cases associated lymphadenopathy disappeared within 6 days of commen cing treatment. The pyrexia disappeared within 3--4 days. The E.S.R. and albumin-81obulin ratio returned to normal withi n 3-6 weeks. If lupus erythematosus cells werpre3ent in the blood, they disappeared within 2-3 weeks. The patients rapidly ga ined weight and became symptomless. The RF, ANF and organ-specific auto-antibodies may gradually disappear from the serum in a bout 12 months. Tn one case after a single course of pentamidine all symptoms disappeared within 48 hours, but returned 2 months later. In more chronic cases with contractures and permanent articular changes it would not be expected that such changes could be reversed, but a surprizing improvement in the pain, swelling and mobility of the joints may be observed. In two cases rheumatoid nodules d:sappea red in the course of three months. In one of the cases associated with goitre due to Hashimoto's thyroiditis and with Sjogren's syndrome present for a year the goitre and dryness of the mouth and eyes disappeared in 8 weeks and the thyroid auto-antibodies had disappeared from the serum 6 months after beginning treatment.

In t he follow up period patients usually remained well for at least a year, after which time joint symptoms may begin to return and they may again be improved by a further course of pentamid ine treatment. For reasons of space the details of each case are not given, but several cases of interest are described.

Case 45 Male, aged 38 years. At the age of 27 years he woke one morning with

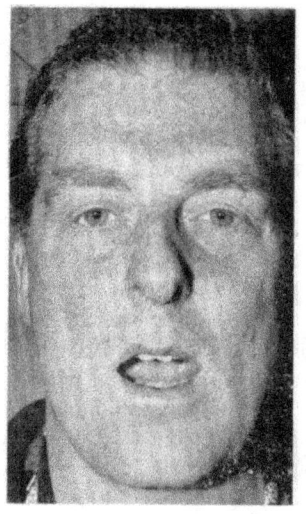

Fig. 29-A

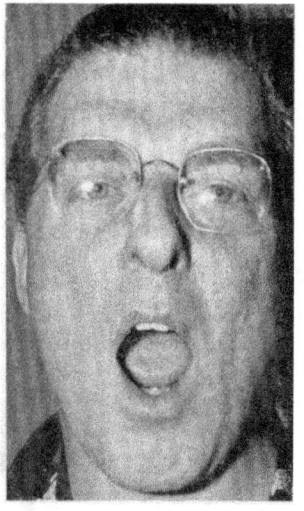

Fig. 29-B

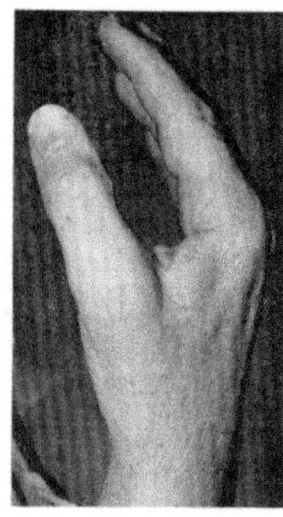

Fig. 29-D

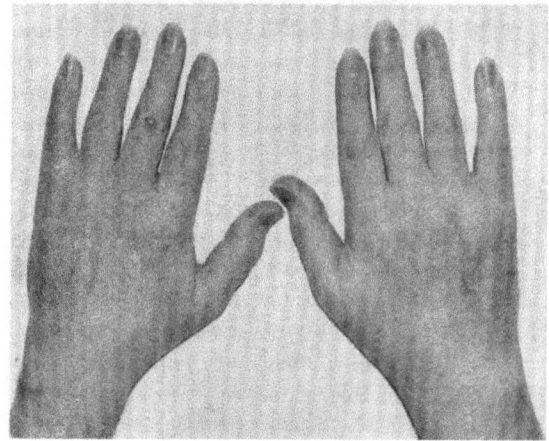

Fig. 29-C

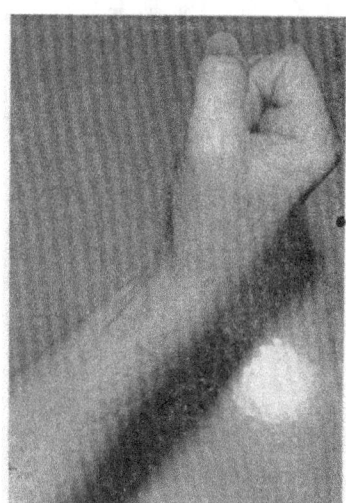

Fig. 29-E

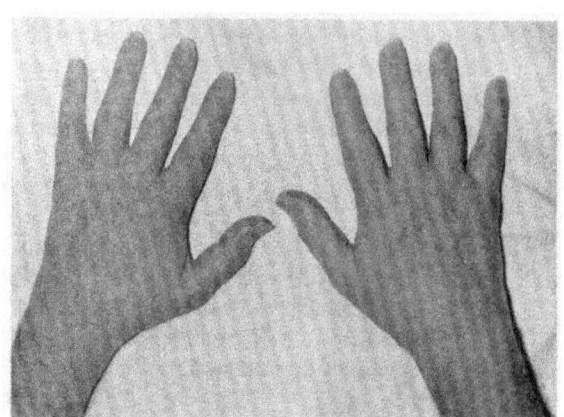

Fig. 29-F

Fig. 29 Male, aged 40 years. Fifteen years history of seropositive rheumatoid disease with systemic lupus erythematosus affecting all joints, including temporomandibular. Photographs taken before showing "A" restriction of gape, "B" attempts at closure of fingers and "C" swelling of the knuckles. "D". "E" and "F" show the corresponding appearances one week after commencing treatment with pentamidine (Case 45).

his shoulders fixed. This eased during the course of the day, but returned on most mornings and two months later he developed painful, swollen and fixed wrists with severe morning stiffness. These symptoms persisted and shortly afterwards the knees, ankles and feet became swollen and extremely painful. At this time the serum DAT was positive 1 in 128. Two years after the onset X-rays showed erosion of the cartilaginous surfaces of the bones of the wrist joints. He had been treated with aspirin, chloroquine, prednisolone and indomethacin in various combinations and had been taking prednisolone in the last 7 years. For the last 2 years he had noticed small fluid-filled blisters forming in various parts of the body, which burst and disappeared and for 6 months recurrent tender swellings in the pulps of the thumb and fingers. These would last several days and disappear. Similar changes occurred in the lower lip. In the last year he had been unable to open his mouth fully because of severe pain in the temporomandibular joints and had had to live off pappy food taken through a straw. For the last 18 months he had noticed swellings aver the tips of the elbows and restriction of movements and pain in the neck. There had been a severe increase in symptoms wer the last year. Examination showed a inan looking much older than his years and in considerable pain. His gape was markedly diminished preventing the entrance of a spoon into his mouth. There was considerable tenderness over the temporomandibular joints and swelling of the parotid glands on both sides. The movements of the head on the trunk were markedly limited and painful and there was severe tenderness on pressure over the sides of the neck. All movements of the shoulder joints were grossly restricted and painful. The wrists were fixed and swollen. The hands were markedly swollen and the digits swollen and fixed in a few degrees of flexion. The hips and knees were unaffected. but the ankles and feet markedly swollen and tender. He was unable to move the ankle joints and mid-tarsal joints and the movements of the toe joints were markedly restricted.

Both olecranon bursae were severely swollen and tender and there was a row of rheumatoid nodules along the posterior surface of the radii on both sides. X-rays showed ankylosed wrists and carpal bones. The blood contained very large numbers of lupus erythematosus cells. The latex fixation test was weakly positive and the Rose-Waaler test negative. The ANF was positive. E.S.R. 55 mms. in 1 hour. Hb 14 G. per cen . W.B.C. 4,600 per cu. mm.

He was treated with injections of pentami dine 200 mgms. daily as outlined above and all other treatment stopped. The effect was dramatic. After 2 days all pain had disappeared and the swelling of the hands, feet and parotid glands was no longer present. The gape had now returned to normal and movements of the affected joints was markedly improved. In 4 days he was able to make a fist and the nodules in the lip and the pulps of the digits ceased to appear. He was now able to walk about and after a fortnight he was symptomless except for the ankylosis of the wrist joints (Fig. 29) . At the end of 6 weeks the lupus erythematosus cells had disappeared from the blood. He was followed up over 4 years. At the end of 2 years he had a mild recurrence of symptoms in the fingers. This was, however, controlled by prednisolone, 5 mgms. daily, on which he has continued throughout this time.

Case 46 Male, aged 52 years. One year history of pain, stiffness and swelling of the right knee, the toes of both feet and of the fingers and wrists. The symptoms were worse on waking. Examination showed the presence of hot, painful, swellings of the joints of the fingers and thumbs, of the right knee which contained free fluid and of the ankles, feet and toes. Investigations showed Hb 94 per cent, E.S.R. 52 mm. per hour., a few lupus erythematosus cells were present in the blood, the

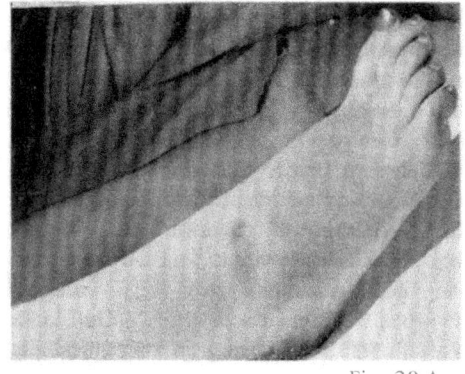

Fig. 30-A

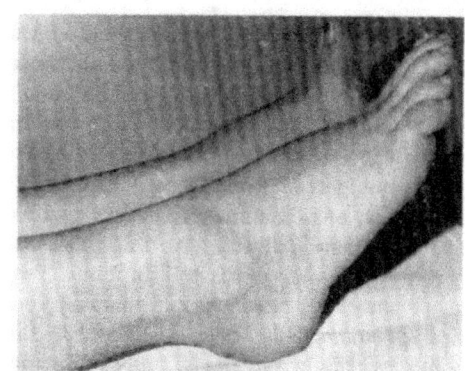

Fig. 30-0

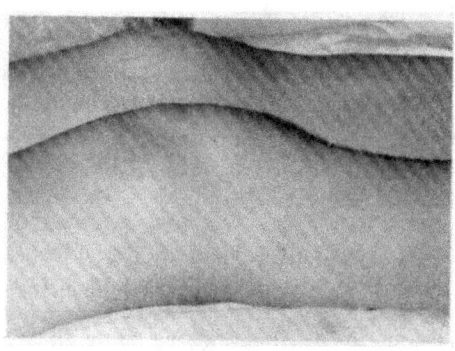

Fig. 30-B

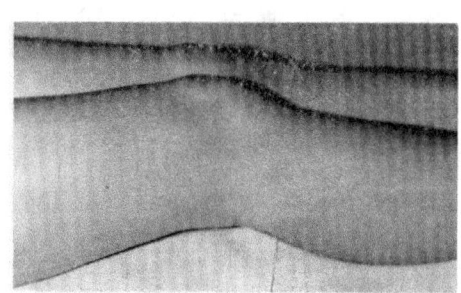

Fig. 30-E

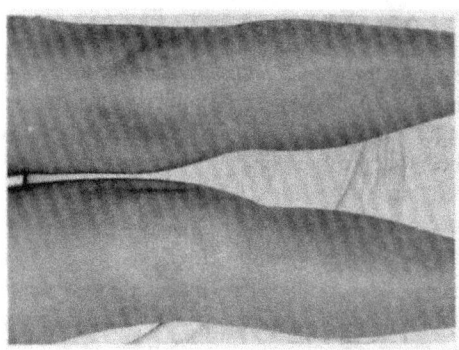

Fig. 30-C

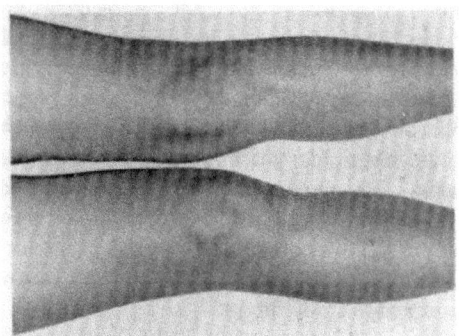

Fig. 30-F

Fig. 30 Female, aged 29 year . Acute eropositive rheumatoid di ea e affecting knees, ankle , neck, hands and trmporomandibu lar joints with oedema of the feet as shown in "A", "B" and "C". "D'., "E" and "F" tak rn 3 days after commrnrr mrnt of trratment with pentamidin e (Case 47). Note di sap pra rance of pitting oedema and joint swelling.

Rose-Waaler test was positive 1 in 512 and the RA latex fixation test positive greater than 1 in 64. An X-ray showed some minor changes in some of the small joints of the fingers. Serum albumin 3.7, globulin 3.8 G. per 100 mi. ANF weakly positive, thyroid and gastric parietal cell auto-antibodies negative. He was treated with four courses of injections of pentamidine. All his symptoms began to improve within 36 hours and relief was complete in 5 days. Two months after beginning treatment the E.S.R. had fallen to 11 mms. per hour. He remained symptomless during the next two years. After a year all the tests for serum antibodies were negative.

Case 47 Female, aged 29 years. Four months previously she developed painful blisters over both feet and two months later the right foot became painful and swollen followed 2-3 days later by pain and swelling of the left knee, the right temporomandibular joint and the right elbow. She felt ill and sweated profusely, especially at night. She then developed stiffness, pain and restricted movements in the neck, pain on attempted movement of the left shoulder and then severe pain and swelling of the right knee. Examination showed she was pale and sweating. The temperature was 99.2°F. There was tenderness and swelling of the right temporo-mandibular joint, severe pain on attempted passive movement of the head on the neck and gross restriction of all head movements. The left shoulder was markedly painful on attempted movement. The right wrist and hand were swollen and hot and no active movement was possible. Both knees were swollen, hot and could not be fully extended. Movement was extremely painful. The right foot was hot and oedematous and all movements impossible. She was unable to stand or walk. Blood count showed Hb 69 per cent., W.B.C. 9,400 per cu. mm., E.S.R. 48 per hour, Rose-Waaler and latex fixation test negative, and ANF positive in the

serum. Thyroid and gastric auto-antibodies were absent from the serum. PBI 5.2 p.G. per cent. A few lupus erythematosus cells were observed in the blood. She was given one course of pentamidine injections with dramatic improvement. In 3 days the oedema of the right foot had disappeared and the pain in the temporo-mandibular joint had gone. In one week the pain on neck movement had disappeared and the sweUing of the knee had subsided (Fig. 30). In 2 weeks all symptoms had regressed. The blood count now showed Hb 84 per cent with E.S.R. of 5 mms. per hour. Six weeks after commencing treatment the ANF disappeared from the serum. She has been followed for 12 months and has remained completely symptomless.

Case 48 Female, aged 77 years. Eight years previously she developed pain and swelling of the feet and ankles, later affecting the knees. After 4 years the pain and swelling involved the fingers and wrists and later the elbows and shoulders became stiff and painful so that she was unable to feed herself owing to weakness and restricted movement of the hands. Walking became so difficult that for the last six months she had been confined to bed. Over the last year she had noticed dryness of the mouth and her eyes felt dry and pricked and no tears formed, even wh· n crying. A goitre had been present for about 18 months.

Examination showed a very thin, pale old lady with obvious dryness of the mouth. The skin of the hands was thin and shiny. The hands exhibited marked contractures with ulnar deviation of the fingers. The thumbs and fingers could not be moved voluntarily and gripping was impossible. Movements of the elbows and shoulders was mark edly restricted and painful. Rheumatoid nodules were present on the fingers and elbows. Hip movements were normal. The knees were markedly swollen and hot and could not be extended fully. The feet showed marked swelling and oedema with severe restriction of an-

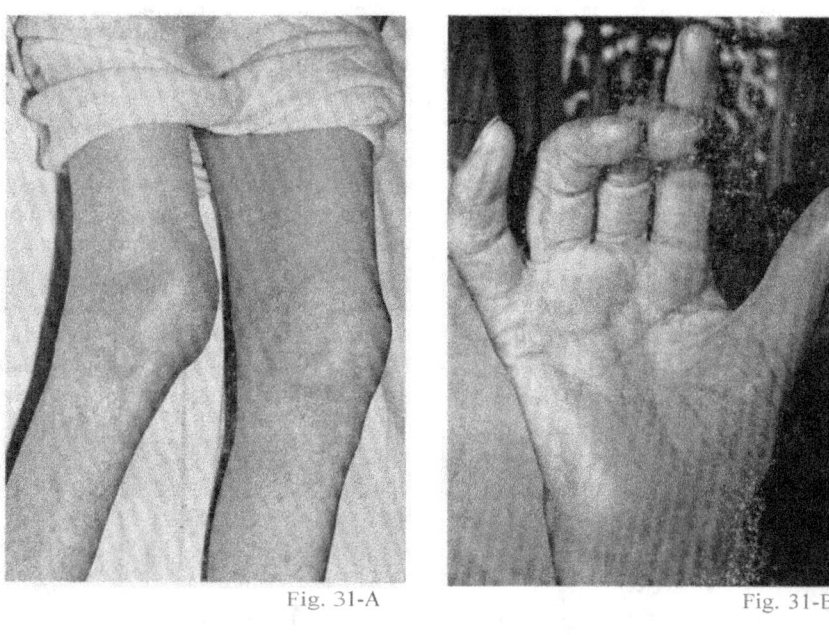

Fig. 31-A   Fig. 31-B

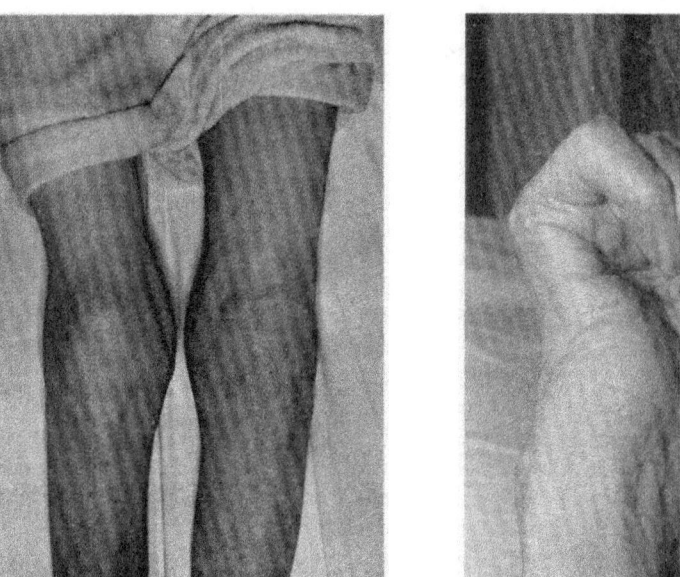

Fig. 31-C   Fig. 31-D

Fig. 31 Female, aged 72 years. Long-standing seropositive
rheumatoid disease with Sjogren's syndrome, showing inability
to extend and swelling of knees and inability to make a fist.
"A" and "B". After 9 days treatment with pentamidine the
improvement is seen in "C" and "D" (Case 48).

kle and toe movements. The lacrimal and parotid glands were not enlarged. The thyroid gland was diffusely enlarged and hard. X-rays showed severe rheumatoid lesions in the hands and wrists and slightly in the toes. Schirmer's test for the lacrimal secretions showed practically complete absence of tears as compared with the normal control. There was no lacrimation on exposure to onions. The serum Rose-Waaler test was positive 1 in 512. Latex fixation test was positive greater than 1 in 20, ANF was positive. Thyroid auto-antibodies and gastric parietal cell auto-antibodies were absent. Hb 69 per cent, W.B.C. 5,400 per cu. mm., E.S.R. 27 mms. in 1 hour, direct Coombs test positive, plasma albumin 3.8 G., globulin 2.8 G. per cent, P.B.I. 4.2 *p.G.* per 100 mls. Lupus erythematosus cells absent from the blood. Drill biopsy of the thyroid gland showed that the structure of the follicles was preserved, but the whole biopsy tissue was heavily infiltrated with lymphocytes and plasma cells and occasional macrophages. A number of lymphoid follicles were present. She was treated with two courses of pentamidine injections with one week interval between. There was a rapid improvement in her condition. The swelling and pain of the knees and the movements of the fingers, wrists, ankles and feet rapidly improved, though the finger deviation persisted (Fig. 31). She was able to feed herself and comb her hair, etc. During the next month the contractures of the flexors of the knee joints disappeared, so that they could be fully extended and the elbows could also be fully extended. She was able to move her toes and ankles and at the end of three weeks could walk unaided, though the deformity of the feet persisted. The rheumatoid nodules over the elbows disappeared in six weeks. After a month the salivary and lacrimal secretions returned to normal as evidenced by Schirmer's test and the ability to shed tears when exposed to onions. The dryness of the mouth also

ceased. The thyroid swelling disappeared over the course of 12 weeks during which time she gained 14 lbs. in weight. At the end of 9 months a blood count showed Hb 92 per cent, E.S.R. 11 mms. per hour, Coombs test negative. The ANF was now absent from the plasma and the Rose-Waaler and latex fixation tests had become negative. After a further 6 months the thyroid auto-antibodies had disappeared from the serum and she was again running her house. She has been followed for three years and her improvement has been maintained.

Case 49 Male, aged 52 years. His illness began at the age of 17 years with aching and stiffness across the shoulders and affecting the shoulder joints. Symptoms gradually spread to involve the hands, which at the age of 23 years, became deformed. There has been a gradual progression of symptoms. At the age of 26 years he attended another hospital and was given gold injections, which did not help and produced dermatitis. Owing to the deformity and stiffness of his hands he became largely helpless. In the previous three years before being seen the knee joints, ankles and feet had became stiff, swollen and creaked on movement and the hips were occasionally painful. The neck had become stiff and movements were restricted, accompanied by a grating sensation. One month previous to hospital attendance he had a tooth extracted and this was followed by severe bleeding from the socket and repeated epistaxis. He had become markedly short of breath.

Examination showed a temperature of 100.2°F, marked pallor and purpura of the forearms, shins and buccal mucosa. There was gross rheumatoid deformity of the hands with ulnar deviation and he was unable to close the fingers or grip. The elbow joints were normal. Both shoulder joints were completely ankylosed. Head movements were markedly restricted. The wrists could not be extended and only 20 degrees of flexion was possible. The fin-

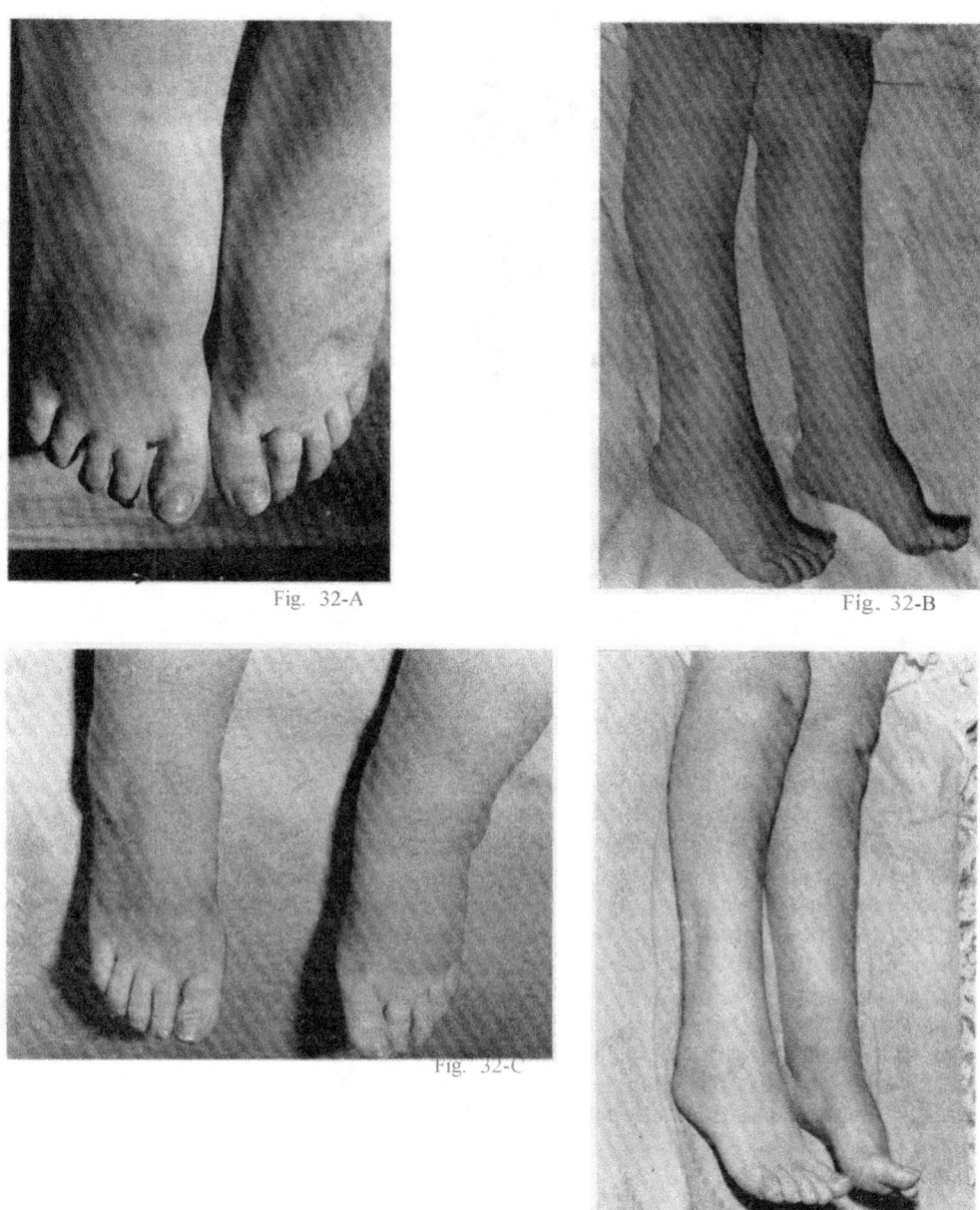

Fig. 32-A

Fig. 32-B

Fig. 32-C

Fig. 32-D

Fig. 32 Female, aged 50 years, suffering from rheumawid
disease and systemic lupus erytiH'matosus, showinO<'drma of
feet and swelling of knees before "A" and "B" and the disappearance of these 4 days after beginning treatment with
pentamidine "C" and "D" (Case 50).

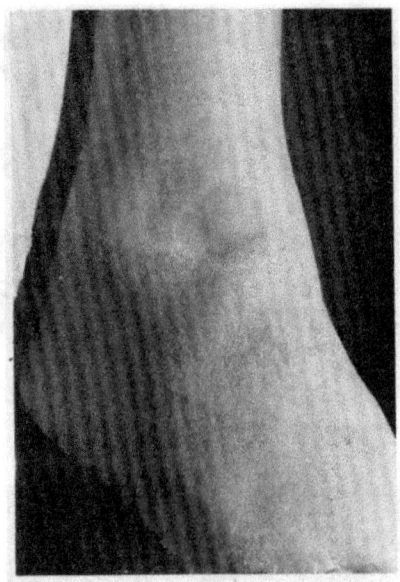
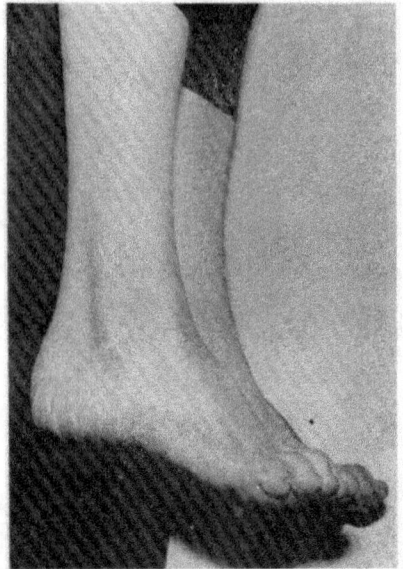

Fig. 33-A   Fig. 33-B

Fig. 33   Male, aged 29 year with acute eroposllJ VC rheumatoid disease accompanied by severe pitting ordema of the feet
and ankles. "A" before and "B" 3 days after commencing
treatment with pentamidine. Tote disappearance of oedema.

gers were flexed at the metacarpo-phalan-
geal joints and the fingers flail-like. Lumbar spinal movements were normal. The
hip joints were normal. The knees were
swollen with considerable restriction of
movement and crepitus. The ankles were
not swollen, but they exhibited crepitus.
The mid-tarsal joints were fixed. The toes
were deformed, deviated outwards and
pulled upwards. He was unable to walk.
The liver was not enlarged. The spleen
was enlarged four fingers breadth below
the costal margin. There was no lymphadenopathy. A blood count showed Hb 26
per cent, W.B.C. 1,500 per cu. mm., platelets
30,000 per cu. mm., E.S.R. 85 mms. per
hour. Sternal bone marrow showed an
excess of plasma cells and a depression of
all forms of haemopoiesis. No lupus erythematosus cells were seen in the blood.
The Rose-Waaler test was positive 1 in
1,024 and the latex fixation test positive
greater than 1 in 20. Plasma albumin 3.9.

globulin 5.0 G. per cent. Thyroid and
gastric auto-antibodies were absent from
the serum. A diagnosis of *Felty's syndrome* was made.

He was transfused with 3 pints of blood
after which the purpura disappeared and
the blood count showed Hb 48 per cent,
W.B.C. 2,000 per cu. mm., platelets 80,000
per cu. mm. He was treated with 3 courses
of pentamidine over the next 6 weeks. At
the end of this time the spleen was no
longer palpable and the blood Hb had risen
to 64 per cent, W.B.C. 3,000 per cu. mm.,
and platelets to 200,000 per cu. mm. The
E.S.R. was 30 mm. in 1 hour. The swelling
of the knee joints had disappeared and the
feet felt much freer. Some movement had
returned to the terminal joints. The stiffness and restricted movements of the shoulders and neck naturally, however, remained unchanged. He gained 16 pounds (6
kilograms) in weight. At the end of 4
months the blood count showed Hb 98 per

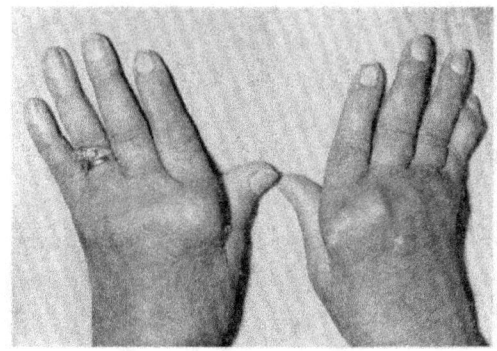
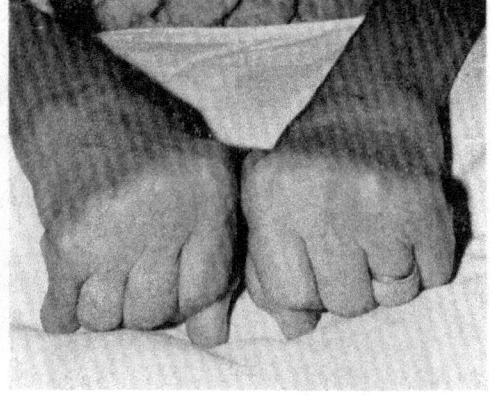

Fig. 34-A

Fig. 34-B

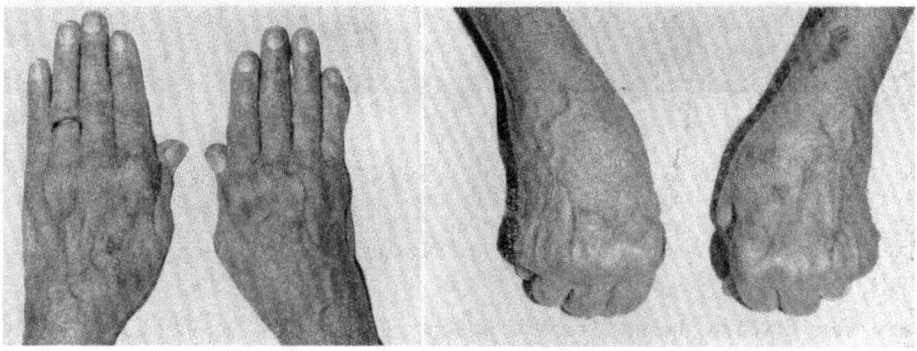

Fig. 34-C

Fig. 34-D

Fig. 34 Female, aged 62 years. Advanced case of seropositive rheumatoid joint disease. "A" and "B" before treatment and "C" and "D" one week after beginning treatment with pentamidine.

cent, E.S.R. 12 mms. per hour, plasma albumin 4.2 G. per cent, globulin 2.3 G. per cent. He has remained unchanged for the last two years without treatment. At the end of 16 months the Rose-Waaler and latex fixation tests had become negative.

Case 50 Female, aged 50 years. Admitted to hospital with vague joint pains and oedema of the feet. No other abnormal physical signs were elicited. The blood count and E.S.R. were normal. The serum

ANF positive 1 in 200, RF positive. Lupus erythematosus cells in blood. Adrenal auto-antibodies were present. She was treated with two courses of pentamidine injections. All her symptoms disappeared within 24 hours. Twelve months later the patient remained symptomless. ANF and adrenal auto-antibodies were absent from the serum. The patient was lost from follow-up (Fig. 32).

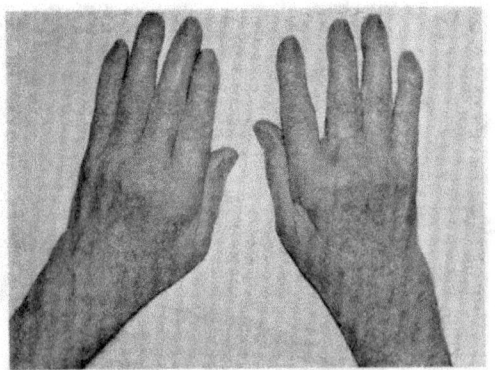

Fig. 35-A

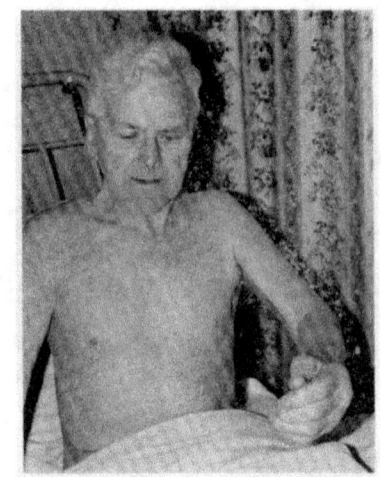

Fig. 35-B

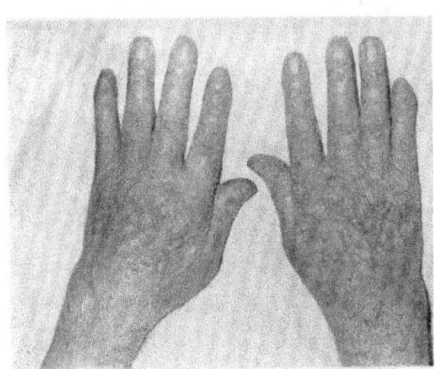

Fig. 35-C

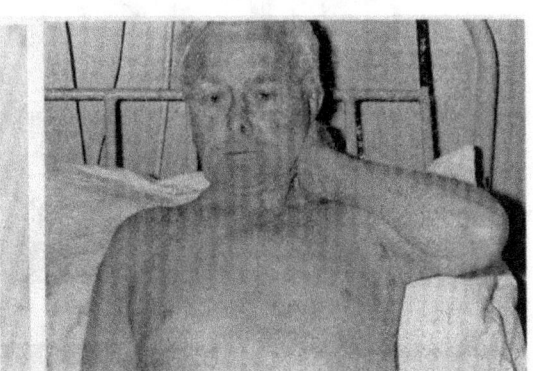

Fig. 35-D

Fig. 35 Malr. aged 68 years. Long-standing seropositive rheumatoid disease with Sjogren's syndrome with pecial involvement of the left shouldrr joint causing pain and inability to raise th(left arm above the position scrn at "B" and with affrction of thr hands as in "A". Six days after lwginning treatment with pentamidine the patient could raise the left arm to touch the back of his neck without pain or restriction and the "elling of the hands had diminishrd "C" and "D".

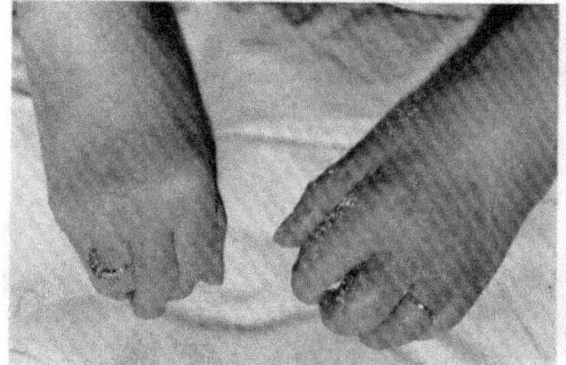

Fig. 36-A

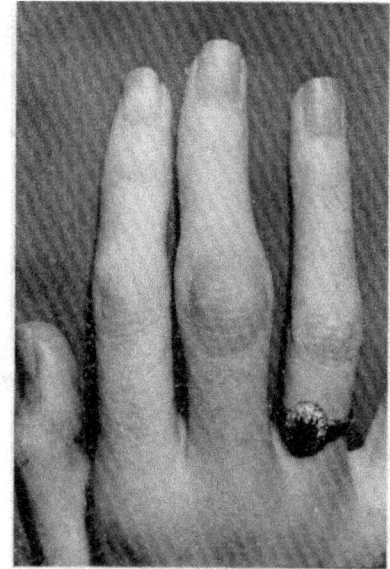

Fig. 37-A

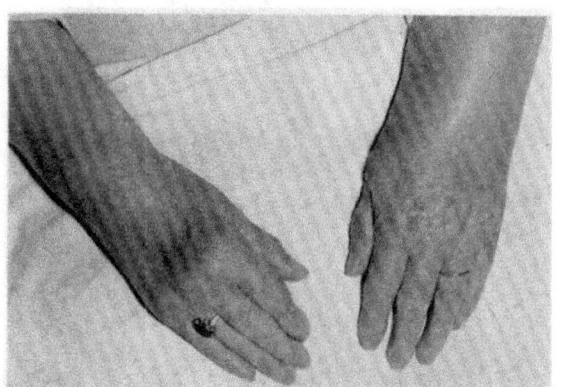

Fig. 36-8

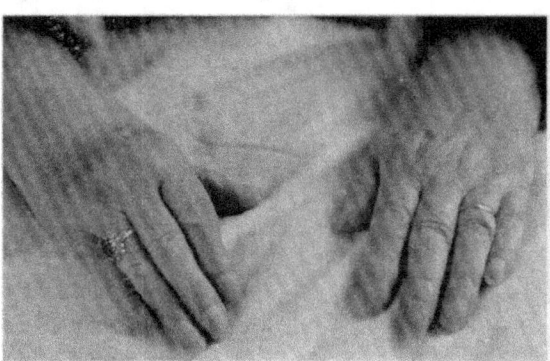

Fig. 36-C

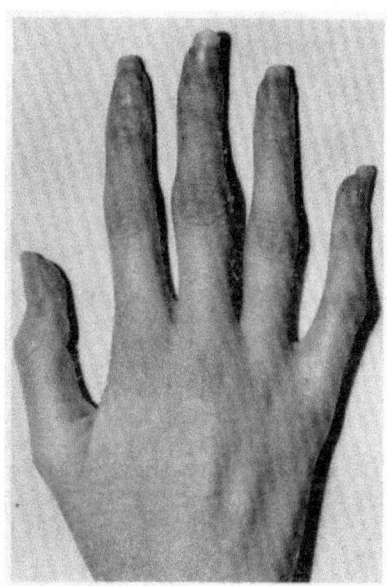

Fig. 37-8

Fig. 36 Femalr, aged 66)'Cars. Long-standing rheumatOid di rase ho"ing appearance "A"' and "B" before and "C"' 5 days artcr beginning treatmrnt with pentamidine.

Fig. 37 Fema le, agrd 21 vrars. Fou r year histor) or seropoitivr rheumatoid disease. Appearances or righ t ha nd "A"' berore a nd "B" 6 days after begin- ning trea tment "ith pentamidine. ote di appra rance or joint wel ling.

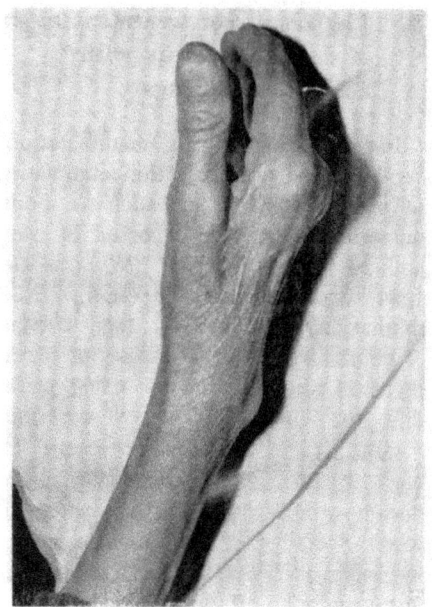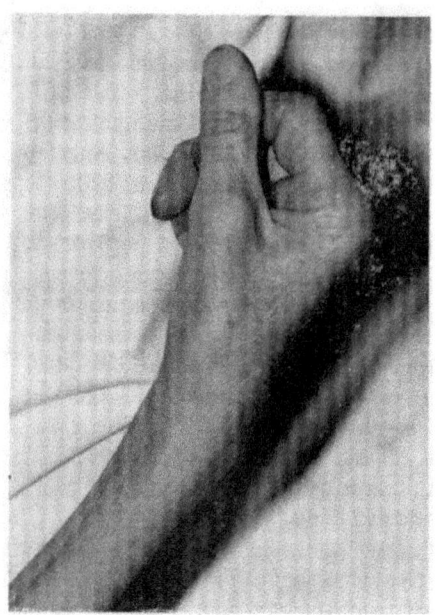

Fig. 3U·A   Fig. 38·8

Fig. 38 Female, aged 72 ear . Long-standing rheuma toid
disea\e. Posi tion or riht ha nd in exerting maximal eⅡorⅠ to
grip "A.. *before* and "B" 8 da y arter beginni ng treat ment
with prntamidinr.

b) **Dehydroemetine (mebadin)**

The mode of administration of this drug
has been described above. Its effect on
early cases of rheumatoid & rthritis was
tried in 8 cases. Th e patien ts were all
early cases of the disease with joint swelling and morning stiffness and RF present
in t he serum. The E.S.R. was raised in
each case. No previous treatment for the
disease had been given. The patients were
hospita lized, but not treated by bed rest.
The results of treat m ent were essentia lly
similar to, but less dramatic than those
obtained with the administration of pentamidine in 6 of the 8 cases. In 2 cases
treatment had to be stopped owing to
changes in the E.C.G. a ppearing. In the
others the joint swelling, pain and stiffness

grad ua!ly disappeared and the E.S.R. returned to norma l within 12 weeks. The
patients were followed up for a year or
more a nd three of t hem had no return of
symptoms, wh ile the other three had some
ret urn of joint pain and swell i ng within
this period, the E.S.R. again rising. Dr.
J.B. Todd of Los Angeles informs me (personal commun ication, 1975) t hat he had
two cases of advanced rheu matoid a rthritis wit h amoeba histolytica in f ection which
he treated with emeti ne h ydrochloride
against the l atter a nd both cases suff ered
severe acute exacerbation of the rheumatoid arthrit is, suggesti ng the drug was
acting on the causative orga nism of the
latter.

—173 —

c) Diodoquin

Diodoquin is an anti-amoebic drug as well as being effective against other protozoa. A recent personal communication (1975) from Dr. J.B. Todd of Los Angeles who had been in charge of an arthritis clinic in the Orthopaedic Hospital in that city for twenty years informed me that he had been successful in some cases in curing the disease by the administration of this drug. A further personal communication from Dr. Robert Bingham of Riverside, California (1975) informed me that in about one third of his cases of active rheumatoid disease he had been successful in obtaining remission of symptoms with this antiprotozoal drug.

Herxheimer reactions in rheumatoid disease treated with antiprotozoal drugs

When using copper sulphate, bile salts, clotrimazole or tinidazole in the treatment of active rheumatoid disease it was found that not uncommonly the first effects of these substances was to cause a transient increased pain and swelling of the affected joints and lymph node swelling resembling an Herxheimer reaction. These observations point to the presence in the affected regions of an organism sensitive to these substances.

The effects of antiamoebic drugs on ankylosing spondylitis

The effects of copper salts, deconjugated bile salts and clotrimazole were tried on twenty one cases of ankylosing spondylitis in various stages of the disease. The results were similar with all three substances. There is a rapid improvement in the extent of cervical movements and a gradual reappearance of some degree of movement of the rest of the spine. This is accompanied by lessening or disappearance of pain and in the course of the next months of breaking down of adhesions in the spine which may occur with a sudden snapping noise and increase in the degree of movements. There is a considerable feeling of well-being during and following treatment.

II. The results of treatment of cases of dermatomyositis with antiprotozoal drugs

Improvement in this manifestation of "collagen" disease on the administration of antiprotozoal drugs, such as 4-amino-quinolines, has been reported by various authors. The author (Wyburn-Mason, 1964) described a severe case which was dramatically relieved by such treatment. A similar response in a case of dermatomyositis was obtained by using pentamidine injections. This is now described.

Case 51 Female, aged 34 years. Two years prior to being seen she suddenly developed a pyrexial illness in which there were severe generalized muscle pain and weakness, swelling of the eyelids and an erythematous and irritating rash of the face, arms, legs and upper chest. This was accompanied by photophobia and the eyes became reddened and the eyelids swollen. The muscle weakness became so severe that there was complete paralysis of the lower limbs and almost complete paralysis of the upper. Breathing became difficult and she was unable to raise her head from the pillow. She was admitted to the National Hospital, Queen Square, where biopsies of skin and muscle were carried out. The former showed a non-specific dermatitis with infiltration of the corium with areas of lymphocytes and plasma cells and some eosinophils and some increase in macrophages. The muscle biopsy showed that the interfascicular connective tissue was oedematous and invaded by increased numbers of macrophages, lymphocytes and plasma cells and some eosinophils, especially round the blood vessels. Slight fragmentation and swelling of the muscle fibres was present. A diagnosis of dermatomyositis was made and she was discharged taking prednisolone 10 mgms. t.d.s. without any change in her condition. She remained at home for eighteen months, lying in bed in a darkened room because of the photophobia and unable to do anything for herself, completely paralysed in the lower limbs and neck muscles and only able to move her arms to a limited extent at the shoulders.

Examination She had a temperature of 99.4°F, photophobia, marked oedema of the eyelids with reddening of the conjunctivae, a violaceous erythematous rash of the forearms, face, neck, chest, shins and around the joints. Complete paralysis of the lower limbs at all joints with absent tendon reflexes was present. The muscles were tender on pressure. Almost complete paralysis of the upper limbs except for weak movements at the shoulder joints was present with absent tendon reflexes. She was unable to raise the head from the pillow. There was slight swelling of the peripheral joints of the fingers and feet. There was no lymphadenopathy or splenomegaly. E.M.G.; action potentials of short duration, polyphasic and reduced in size. No reduction in the number of motor unit discharges on attempted voluntary contraction. Blood count showed Hb 95 per cent, W.B.C. 11,500 per cu. mm., eosinophils 10 per cent; E.S.R. 80 mms. per hour; serum transaminase within normal limits; no lupus erythematosus cells; Rose-Waaler test positive 1 in 56, latex fixation test negative. Plasma albumin 2.4 G. per cent, globulin 3.8 G. per cent. ANF positive. She was treated with two courses of 10 injections of pentamidine, with a week's rest between and the prednisolone tapered off. From then on she made a steady and even dramatic improvement beginning within 3 days. The swelling of the eyelids and joints rapidly disappeared and the erythematous rash and photophobia subsided in 7-10 days. The temperature settled on the third day. A fortnight after beginning treatment she was able to raise her head from the bed and was beginning to move her limbs. In 6 weeks she was able to sit up in bed. Intensive massage and active exercises were commenced. In 10 weeks she was able to sit out of bed and in 12 weeks she

could walk unaided. In the course of the next two months she returned to almost normal activity, the only abnormal finding being a waddling gait, which has persisted over the next four years of observation. Twelve months after beginning treatment the E.S.R. had fallen to 20 mm. per hour, the ANF was absent from the serum, the Rose-Waaler test was negative and the latex fixation weakly positive. Plasma albumin 4.2 G. per cent, globulin 2.6 G. per cent. The investigations were repeated 18 months after commencing treatment and showed normal muscle action potentials. The E.S.R. was now 11 mm. per hour. The Rose-Waaler and latex tests were negative, W.B.C. 7,200 eosinophils 2 per cent, ANF negative. She now runs her own home in a normal manner and walks several miles, taking part in normal activities.

III. The effect of antiprotozoal drugs on Sjogren's syndrome and "auto-immune parotitis"

a) Chloroquine

Sjogren's syndrome has been seen to be a manifestation of rheumatoid disease and as such would be expected to be helped by 4-aminoquinolines. As mentioned already, Heaton (1963) found chloroquine helpful in improving the lacrimal and salivary secretions in cases of Sjogren's syndrome. Reference has been made to the fact that Sjogren-Mikulicz's syndrome may be preceded by recurrent painless swelling of the salivary glands, sometimes unilaterally, constituting so-called "auto-immune parotitis", in which condition there are frequently found either RF, ANF or organ specific auto-antibodies in the serum. The author treated a number of cases of this condition with chloroquine.

Case 52 Male, aged 33 years. The patient gave a 15 months history of recurrent swelling of the right parotid salivary gland extending to the right side of the neck and only slightly painful. The attacks lasted up to 8 weeks and his present attack had occurred 3 weeks previously. On examination there was marked non-tender swelling of the right parotid salivary gland and of the lymph nodes below the angle of the jaw. The blood count and E.S.R. were normal. The RF was present in moderate dilution in the serum, but other auto-antibody tests were negative. The attack subsided spontaneously within a week of first being seen, but recurred again two months later. He was treated with chloroquine (ICI) 250 mgms. dililY for 15 months and followed up for a further 3 years. The parotid and lymph node swelling died down within 3 days of commencing treatment and did not recur during this period. The RF had disappeared from the serum at the end of 15 months.

Case 53   Male, aged 49 years. His wife died of polyarteritis nodosa 10 years previously. The patient had suffered from constant rhinitis for years. Six months previous to being seen he developed moderate swelling and slight pain in the left parotid salivary gland with some enlargement of the cervical lymph nodes below this. The swelling came and went on several occasions and on first being seen there was also a less marked swelling of the right parotid gland. The E.S.R. was 30 mms. per hour and the blood contained thyroid auto-antibodies in high titre. He was given chloroquine (ICI) 250 mgms. daily for a year. The salivary gland and lymph node swelling disappeared within 3 days and did not return during the next <! years. His rhinitis cleared completely. After a year the serum thyroid auto-antibodies had disappeared.

Case 54   Female, aged 15 years. One brother had suffered from coeliac disease from the age of 5 years and a sister developed it at the age of 21 years. Her grandfather suffered from severe rheumatoid arthritis. She gave a two years history of recurrent painful swelling and morning stiffness of the left big toe, left knee and

left wrist and for the same time had suffered from recurrent painless swelling of the left parotid gland and on one occasion of the right. She had bad 7 attacks in all, each lasting about 2 weeks. On examination the left parotid salivary gland and the submaxillary and sublingual glands were markedly swollen, but not tender and there were enlarged lymph nodes below the angle of the jaw on that side. There was crepitus in both knees wit h slight free fluid, but the other joints showed no abnormality. The blood showed Hb 11.0 grams per cent, E.S.R. 32 mms. per hour. RF strongly positive, ANF +, submandibular gland auto-antibodies positive, smooth muscle auto-antibodies negative in the blood. She was treated with chloroquine (ICI) 250 mgms. daily for a year with immediate cessation of the salivary gland swelling and the arthropathy, which has not recurred over two years. The RF and ANF in the blood had disappeared at the end of this time.

b) Pentamidine

It was shown above that i n cases of *Sjogren's syndrome* associated with rheumatoid arthritis t he administration of *pentamidine* may be effective in restoring the lacrimal and salivary secretions, if the manifestations of Sjogren's syndrome are comparatively recent in onset. This has now been observed in 7 such cases. In 3 cases of Sjogren's syndrome with a comparatively recent onset and unassociated with rheumatoid arthritis treatment with pentamidine by mouth was tried and was successful.

Case 55   Female, aged 49 years. Her husband suffered from Hashimoto's thyroiditis with myxoedema and arthropathy. The patient gave a 2 years history of dryness of the mouth and eyes, which itched and in which she had a gritty feeling. The eyelids were puffy and she was subject to recurrent blepharitis. In addition she had pains in the shoulders and neck. There was a past history of acute rheumatoid arthritis at the age of 19 years which settled after treatment. Examination showed swollen and red eyelids and the signs of blepharitis. There wus comple loss of tears. Schirmer's test being positive on both sides. There was Rose Bengal staining of the cornea. The mouth was extremely dry. There was no clinical evidence of arthropathy. The E.S.R. was 32 mms. per hour. The serum P.B.I. was normal at 5.0 p.G per 100 mi. The plasma protein content of both albumin and globulin was 3.5 G per 100 mi. All non-specific and organ specific auto-antibodies were absent from the serum.

Owing to continued blepharitis epilation of the lashes was carried out without improvement. She was later given pentamidine 200 mgms. t.d.s. by mouth for 6 weeks. Within 3 weeks there was a dramatic improvement in the dryness of both eyes and mouth. Salivation returned to normal. The eyes began to water again and after 6 weeks the blepharitis had cleared. Schirmer's test became negative and after 3 months the Rose Bengal staining disappeared.

Case 56 Female, aged 63 years. Thirty years previously she developed myxoedema for which she had been treated ever since. For the last 6 years she suffered minor joint pains and swelling particularly of the hands, shoulders and knees. For the last 2 years she had suffered from dryness oi the mouth and eyes and had been diagnosed as a case of Sjogren's syndrome at the Royal Eye Hospital, Moorfields with positive Schirmer's tests and Rose Bengal staining of the cornea on both sides. While taking L-thyroxin, th- P.B.I. was 6.6 MG per 100 mls. Hb 12.8 G per 100 mls. E.S.R. 15 mms. per hour. Gastric parietal cell auto-antibodies strongly positive in the serum. RF, ANF and thyroid auto-antibodies negative. While under investigation, she developed thrombophlebitis of the veins of the left leg. She was treated with pentamidine 400 mgms. b.d. by mouth for 6 weeks. Within 3 weeks all her symptoms had disappeared and 2 months after

beginning treatment Schirmer's test had become negative. After 6 months the gastric parietal cell auto-autibodies were no longer present in the serum. She had been followed for 18 months without return of symptoms.

c) Copper sulphate

The effect of *copper sulphate* administration on cases of Sjogren's syndrome was investigated in 4 cases of recent onset. In all these cases there was a dramatic disappearance of the dryness of the mouth and eyes. A brief description of these cases follows.

Case 57 (Case VI, 31 or X, 23). Female, aged 44 years. Her mother, her mother's sister and the patient's own sister all suffered from rheumatoid arthritis. Three years previously the patient had suddenly lost all her teeth and in addition had begun to suffer from joint pains and swelling. She had fibroids removed by myomectomy at the age of 37 years. Her periods ceased 2 years previously to first being seen. She stated that some 15 months before she began to get bouts of recurrent "influenza", which consisted of cough with slight sputum, general aching, headaches, pyrexia and sweating, particularly during sleep. The temperature would reach 100°F and she noticed that her throat, nose and mouth were becoming increasingly dry. A blood count at this time showed W.B.C. were 3,200 per cu. mm., 73 per cent being lymphocytes and 5 per cent eosinophils. Some atypical lymphocytes were present. From the onset of these symptoms she began to lose weight, which amounted to 20 lbs. (8 kilograms). She became anorexic and had periods of vomiting, the food appearing to stick in the chest when she swallowed. Her eyes felt dry and pricked. She also stated that for the last 7–8 years she had dark pigmentation of the skin behind the knees, in the axillae and on the side of the neck and recurrent swelling of the cervical lymph nodes. On examination the patient was thin, edentulous, the nasal mucosa was dry and the mucosa of the mouth and tongue dry, red and sore. She was unable to open the mouth fully because of arthritis of the temporo-mandibular joints. There was painful enlargement of the lymph nodes on both sides of the neck, but no peripheral arthropathy. The eyes were dry and red and Schirmer's test was positive on both sides. The changes of acanthosis nigricans were present in the flexures of arms and legs and on the sides of the neck. The tip of the right middle finger was tender, black, cold and gangrenous. Ulcerative and angular stomatitis was present. X-ray of the chest showed old calcified tuberculosis. A barium meal and follow through were normal. Liver function tests showed alkaline phosphatase 35 K.A. units per 100 ml. Thymol turbidity test 9 units. E.S.R. 30 mms. per hour. Hb 12.4 G per 100 mls. W.B.C. 4,400 per cu. mm., 60 per cent lymphocytes with 4 per cent atypical cells and 10 per cent monocytes. Albumin 3.5 G, globulin 5.7 G per 100 mls. Lupus erythematosus cells not present. Bone marrow showed relative eosinophilia and the changes of chronic lymphatic leukaemia. P.B.I. 7.5 II-G per 100 mls. RF positive in serum. Electrophoresis revealed a diffuse increase in the gammaglobulins. Cold agglutinins present in the serum. Liver biopsy showed the changes of chronic active hepatitis. A further blood count showed up to 10 per cent of eosinophil cells and the typical changes of chronic lymphatic leukaemia. Tests for toxoplasmosis and cytomegalic virus were negative. Immunophoresis showed increased IgG, IgM and IgA consistent with a leukaemia. RF was positive in serum. ANF, thyroid and gastric parietal cell auto-antibodies negative. A diagnosis of Sjogren's syndrome, acanthosis nigricans, arteritis, fibroids, chronic active hepatitis and chronic lymphatic leukaemia was made. She was treated with copper sulphate 25 mgms. t.d.s. for two months with rapid improvement in her symptoms. The pains in the joints, the dryness of the mouth and eyes and the swelling of the

cervical lymph nodes rapidly improved. After two months the Hb had risen to 96 per cent and the abnormal lymphocytes disappeared from the peripheral blood. The white blood cell count showed 3,900 per cu. mm., 40 per cent being neutrophils and 54 per cent lymphocytes. Five per cent were eosinophils. The E.S.R. fell to 12 mms. per hour. The serum albumin was 4.2 G and the globulin 2.9 G per 100 mls. The liver function tests returned to normal. She has remained symptomless since that time over a year and the gangrenous lesion of the right middle finger has healed.

d) Bile salts

The effect of bile acid administration was tried on several cases of Sjögren's syndrome.

Case 58 Female, aged 37 years. Her daughter suffered from hay-fever and an aunt from rheumatoid arthritis and allergic rashes. Her son was born with ecchondromata of the hands and knees (multiple exostoses). She suffered from nettle rash as a child and hay-fever since the age of 16 years. She had also suffered from symptoms of multiple sclerosis extending back 14 years. For the last 4 years she was subject to recurrent redness and ulcers on the right eye and more recently to recurrent painless swelling of both parotid salivary glands and of dryness of the mouth. Examination showed extreme dryness of the mouth and Schirmer's test was positive on the right eye only. The parotid glands were swollen, but not tender. RF was positive in the blood. There were multiple slightly enlarged nodes on the right side of the neck and bilateral hallux valgus and over-riding of the other toes. Mild evidence of multiple sclerosis was present. She was treated with dehydrocholin 500 mgms. t.d.s. This produced a most curious sensation. She felt detached, had difficulty in focusing her eyes and the legs and arms tingled. She took the tablets for only two weeks because of these symptoms, which took a week to wear off, but after this time the dryness of the mouth had disappeared, but Schirmer's test was still positive on the right side. She has remained in this state over the last six months.

Case VI,21 Female, aged 64 years. Her mother and a sister suffered from rheumatoid arthritis. At the age of 37 years she had a hysterectomy for fibroids. At the age of 40 years she had a rodent ulcer removed from the nose and at 55 years was treated for thyrotoxicosis. She gave a seven years history of rheumatoid arthritis and six months of dryness of the mouth and eyes with frequent ulcers in the mouth and lumps in th substance of the lips. The nasal mucosa was dry and crusted. Examination showed the lips and mouth were dry, the submandibular and sublingual salivary glands were enlarged, Schirmer's test was positive on both eyes. RF was present in the serum, which also contain0d thyroid and gastric parietal cell auto-antibodies. A diagnosis of rheumatoid arthritis, Sjogren's syndrome, fibroids, thyrotoxicosis and rodent ulcer was made. She was treated for two months with dehydrocholin 500 mgms. t.d.s. with rapid disappearance of dryness of the mouth and eyes and considerable improvement in the joint pains and stiffness. After 18 months her symptoms had not returned.

Case VI, 65 or VII, 59 Female, aged 28 years. She gave a six years history of recurrent sore throat, nasal blockage and for a year had complained of severe dryness of the mouth and soreness of the tongue. Three months previously most of her teeth became loose and fell out. Her knees and hands felt stiff on waking in the morning. At the age of 18 years she had had an operation for follicular appendicitis and a large cyst on the right ovary.

Examination Nasal mucosa dry and crusted. She was edentulous. The :mouth and tongue were very dry and red, the mucosa thinned and angular stomatitis present. The cervical lymph nodes were enlarged. Schirmer's test was positive on

both sides. Chest X-ray was normal. A blood count showed Hb 12.2 G per cent. E.S.R. 42 mms. per hour. W.B.C. 14,600 per cu. mm., neutrophils 73 per cent, lymphocytes 19 per cent, serum albumin 3.7 G, globulin 6.0 G per cent. Liver function tests serum bilirubin >1 unit; thymol turbidity 10 units, alkaline phosphatase 7.5 K.A. units per 100 mls. RF positive, ANF positive (speckled to 1 in 270) in serum. No lupus erythematosus cells present. Gastric parietal cell auto-antibodies negative. Thyroid cytoplasmic fluorescent antibodies positive. Liver biopsy showed chronic active hepatitis. Biopsy of a cervical lymph node $=$ lymphosarcoma. Treated with copper sulphate 50 mgms. t.d.s. for one month during which time all symptoms of Sjogren's syndrome disappeared. Schirmer's test became negative and the lymphadenopathy disappeared. She was followed over 6 months during which time she remained symptomless and the E.S.R. fell to normal. The serum albumin and globulin became equal and the blood count returned to normal.

e) Clotrimazole

This has similar effects to other antiamoebic drugs. In a male of 48 years disease began six years previously with pain in the left shoulder and seropositive arthropathy soon became generalized, especially involving the knees. He then developed Sjogren's syndrome with atrophic rhinitis, a large right parotid swelling, atrophic tracheo-bronchitis with recurrent bronchopneumonia attacks. He had been treated with cortisone and gold injections and radio-active yttrium injections into both knee joints. He was markedly dyspnoeic and had to use artificial tears. He was unable to close his fingers and his mid-tarsal joints were fixed. RF was strongly positive in the blood. He was treated with clotrimazole 1 G daily for 7 weeks. The effect was remarkable. In 10 days the tears and saliva returned, the right parotid swelling disappeared, he was no longer dyspnoeic and his cough disap-

Addendum: The beneficial effect of jaundice and bile salts and their derivatives in rheumatoid patients has been confirmed by Sullivan SN. The effect of jaundice on rheumatoid arthritis. J. Rheumatol 1980, 7. 417-418 and Famaey J-P J. Rheumatol 1981 8 181.

peared. In one month his feet became mobile and all joint pain ceased. He is still under observation.

IV. The effects of antiprotozoal drugs on cases of thyroiditis

a) 4-aminoquinolines

Ito et al. (1968) found that in cases of chronic thyroiditis chloroquine caused regression of the goitre and diminished the thyroid auto-antibody titre in the serum. The effect of 4-aminoquinolines on cases of Hashimoto's thyroiditis or of thyrotoxicosis associated with the presence of thyroid or other auto-antibodies in the serum was investigated by the author in a number of cases. In 4 cases of thyrotoxicosis in which thyroid auto-antibodies of some kind were present in the serum chloroquine (ICI) 250 mgms. daily was administered for a year. At the end of this time the auto-antibodies in the serum had disappeared in each case. In 5 cases of myxoedema thyroid auto-antibodies were present in very high concentration in the serum suggestive of the existence of Hashimoto's thyroiditis. In one case this was associated with rheumatoid arthritis, in another with intrinsic asthma and in a third with Paget's disease and diabetes. In yet another case gastric parietal cell auto-antibodies were present in the serum. After rendering the patients euthyroid by the administration of L-thyroxin the patients were treated with chloroquine or camoquin 200 mgms., daily. The effect of this was to cause the thyroid or gastric parietal cell auto-antibodies to disappear from the serum within 18 months. In the case associated with intrinsic asthma the latter disappeared and in that with Paget's disease the bone pain ceased and the serum alkaline phosphatase fell. The effect of chloroquine on a case of Hashimoto's thyroiditis is illustrated by the following case:--

Case II, 2 (III, 14)   Female, aged 26

years. She suffered from severe hayfever and asthma as a child and these still occurred, but with less frequency. Four years previously, while living in California, there was an acute onset of myxoedema associated with swelling of the thyroid gland and at the same time she developed an area of cystic mastitis in the left breast, which was removed surgically. Investigations at that time showed a serum P.B.I. of 1.1 ,G per cent. She was treated with L-thyroxin, which rendered her euthyroid, but from time to time she continued to have feelings of pressure in the neck and difficulty in swallowing. Examination showed a diffusely enlarged thyroid gland, but she was otherwise clinically normal. The serum showed a thyroglobulin tanned R.B.C. agglutination titre of 1 in 250,000, thyroid C.F.T. 1 in 32 and thyroid cytoplasmic auto-antibodies were positive. The L-thyroxin was omitted for 6 weeks by which time the serum P.B.I. had fallen to 1.2 ,G per 100 mls. She was then treated with chloroquine (ICI) 250 mgms. daily over the next 2 years. The asthmatic attacks ceased immediately and the thyroid swelling disappeared over the next two months. The thyroid auto-antibodies disappeared from the serum within the next 24 months, at the end of which time the serum P.B.I. in the absence of L-thyroxin administration was now 5.1 ,G per 100 mls., that is chloroquine had rendered her euthyroid, the goitre had disappeared and her asthma had ceased.

b) Pentamidine

The effect of the administration of pentamidine to cases of Hashimoto's thyroiditis and myxoedema was investigated in several cases. In Case 70, described below, in which hypothyroidism, due to Hashimoto's thyroiditis and idiopathic Addison's disease were present, treatment with pentamidine caused the hypothyroidism and various serum antibodies to disappear. There were three other cases of Hashimoto's thyroiditis and one of myxoedema following Hashimoto's thyroiditis.

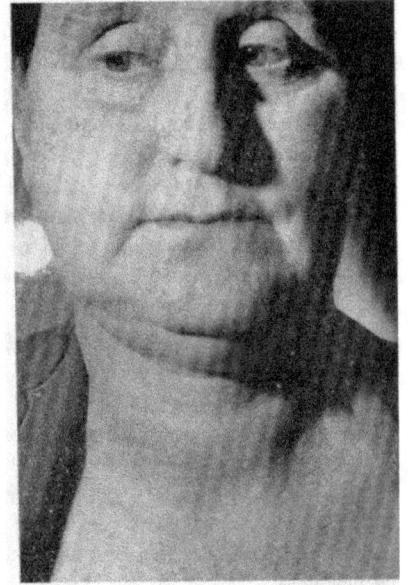
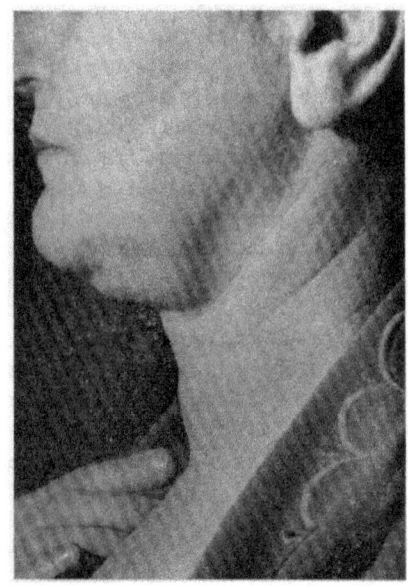

Fig. 39-A

Fig. 39-B

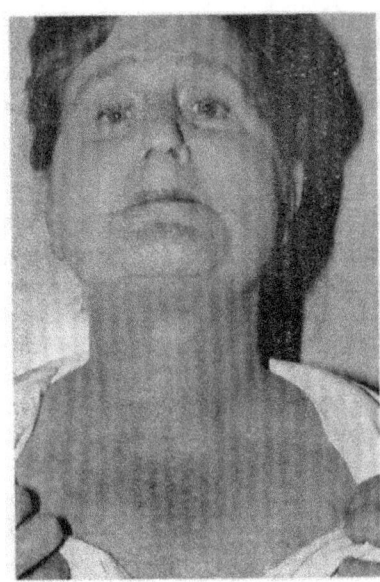
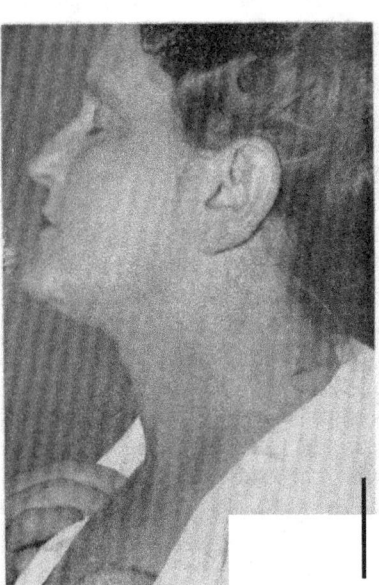

Fig. 39-C

Fig. 39-D

Fig. 39 Female, aged 55 years. Mildly hypothyroid due to Hashimoto's thyroiditis. Appearances of neck were then as at "A" and "B". Treated with two courses of pentamidine, each lasting four weeks. She had become euthyroid after 6 months, when appearances of neck were as at "C" and "D". Note disappearance of thyroid swelling (Case 59).

Case 59 Female, aged 55 years. Marked family history of rheumatoid arthritis. Patient gave a thirty years history of joint pains and stiffness on waking and for the last year of spontaneous bruising. Examination showed numerous subcutaneous bruises, and mild rheumatoid changes in the peripheral joints. The thyroid gland was diffusely enlarged and hard. Blood investigation showed a haemoglobin of 12.7 G per 100 mls., W.B.C. 18,500 per cu. mm., 90 per cent being granulocytes, platelets 1,079,000 per cu. mm., ANF negative, RF negative, thyroglobulin tanned R.B.C. agglutination titre 1 in 250,000, thyroid C.F.T. 1 in 64, thyroid cytoplasmic fluorescent antibodies +, gastric parietal cell auto-antibodies negative, F.B.I. 1.1 *p.G* per 100 mls., sternal marrow biopsy showed increased activity of the granulocyte series and of megakaryocytes. A diagnosis of myxoedema, thrombocytaemia and probably Hashimoto's thyroiditis was made. She was treated with pentamidine 200 mgms. t.d.s. by mouth for 4 weeks. Within 3 weeks the thyroid swelling had disappeared (Fig. 39) and in *2* months the haemoglobin had reached 14.0 G per 100 mls. The W.B.C. was 7,200 per cu. mm. and the platelet count was 492,000 per cu. mm. The E.S.R. had returned to normal. The spontaneous bruising had ceased and the joint pains and swelling had disappeared. The course of pentamidine was repeated after an interval of a month and after 12 months the thyroid auto-antibody tests in the serum had become negative. She was now euthyroid.

Case 60 Female, aged 56 years. The menopause had occurred at the age of 46 years. She gave a 3 months history of painless swelling of the thyroid gland, tiredness, gain in weight, hot flushes and pain and swelling of the left knee. Examination showed a blood pressure of 200/110 mms. The thyroid was generally enlarged and firm. Mild crepitus in the left knee joint. X-rays showed no evidence of pressure on the oesophagus by the en-

larged thyroid gland and moderate cardiac enlargement. F.B.I. 3.6 P-G per 100 mls. Serum showed thyroglobulin tanned R.B.C. agglutination titre 1 in 250,000. Thyroid C.F.T. 1 in 32, thyroid cytoplasmic fluorescent auto-antibodies ++. ANF negative, RF negative. Gastric parietal cell auto-antibodies negative. She was treated with pentamidine 400 mgms. b.d. for one month. This was repeated after a months rest. The pain and swelling of the knee joint rapidly disappeared and the swelling of the thyroid was no longer visible after 3 months. Eighteen months after the commencement of treatment the thyroid auto-antibodies had disappeared from the serum.

Case 61 Female, aged 47 years. Seventeen years previously she developed a diffuse painless swelling of the thyroid gland which continued to increase in size, especially on the right side and began to cause difficulty in swallowing. The B.M.R. was found to be -16. Partial thyroidectomy was performed and the histology of the removed gland S'howed the typical changes of Hashimoto's thyroiditis. She was now complaining of gain in weight, swelling of the feet, falling of hair and sensitivity to cold. Examination showed a markedly dry skin and mouth, a typical myxoedematous appearance; the pulse rate was 78 per minute. F.B.I. 1.4 *P-G* per 100 mls., blood cholesterol 515 mgms. per 100 mls., RF negative, thyroglobulin tanned R.B.C. agglutination titre less than 1 in 5, thyroid C.F.T. + greater than 1 in 16, thyroid colloid immunofluorescent cytoplasmic antibodies +, ANF negative, gastric parietal cell immunofluorescent test negative, E.S.R. 38 mms. per hour, Hb 10.4 G per 100 mls. She was treated with !-thyroxin and became euthyroid within 6 weeks. The auto-antibody tests were then repeated and the results were the same as previously. She was then treated with pentamidine intramuscularly with two courses as described above. After nine months the thyroid auto-tmtibody tests had become negative.

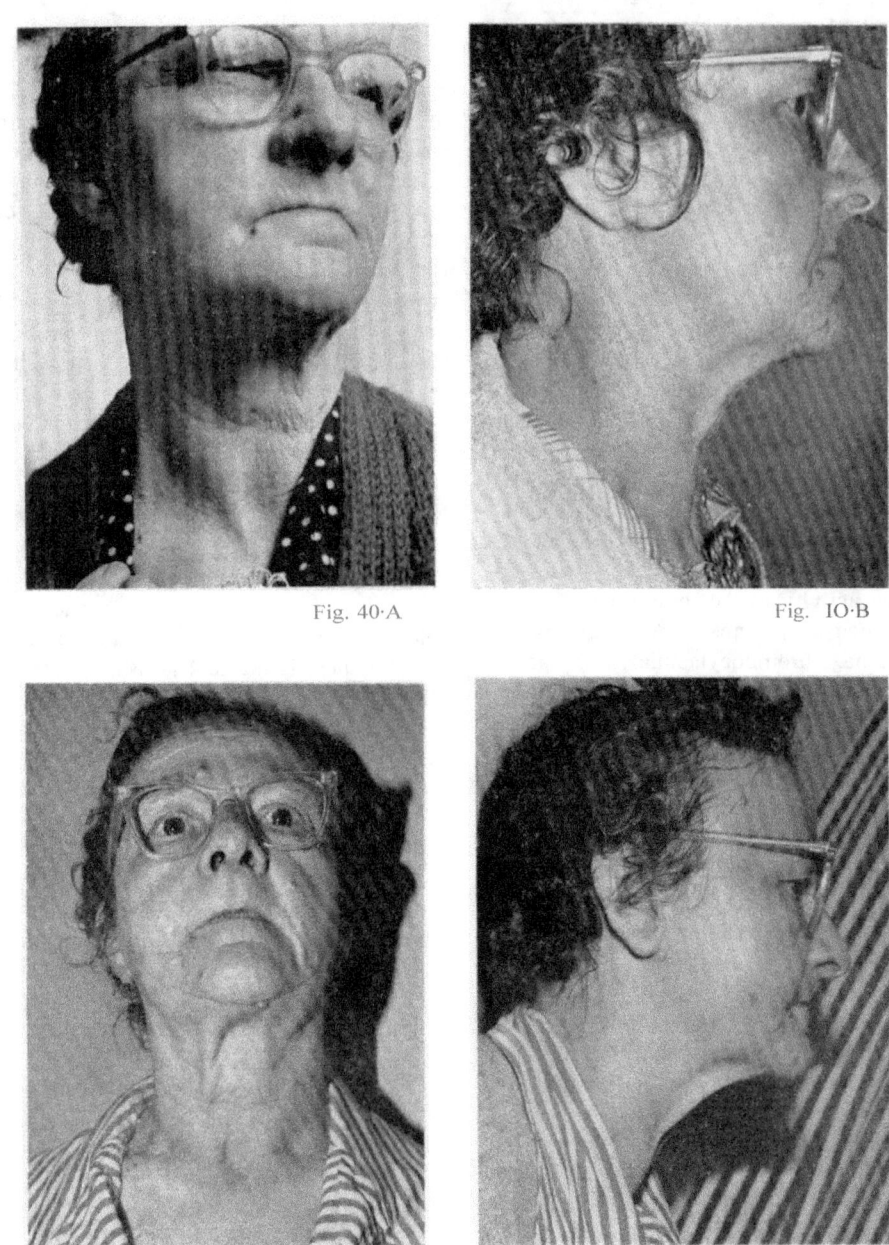

Fig. 40·A

Fig. IO·B

Fig. 40·C

fig. IO·D

Fig. 40 Female aged 68)Ca rs. Hashimoto' thyroiditis "ith rheumatoid disease. Appea rance of thyroid bef ore treatment at "A" and "B" and after 2 months treatment with copper ulphate at "C" and "D". Note di<appearance of thyroid gland swelling.

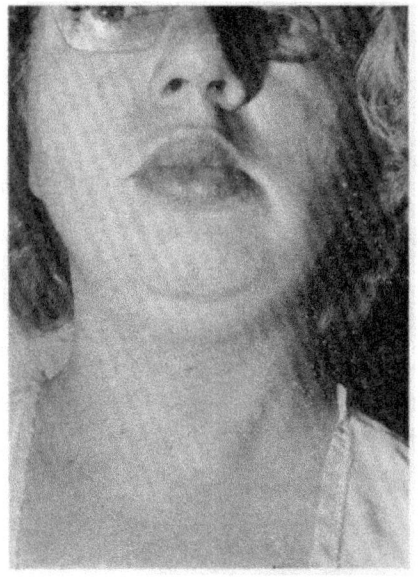

Fig. 41-A

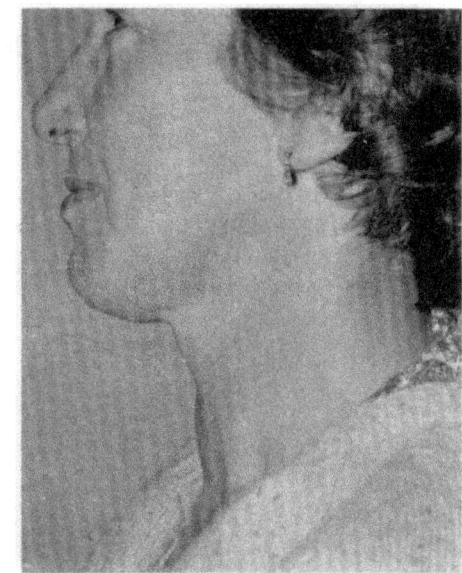

Fig. 42-A

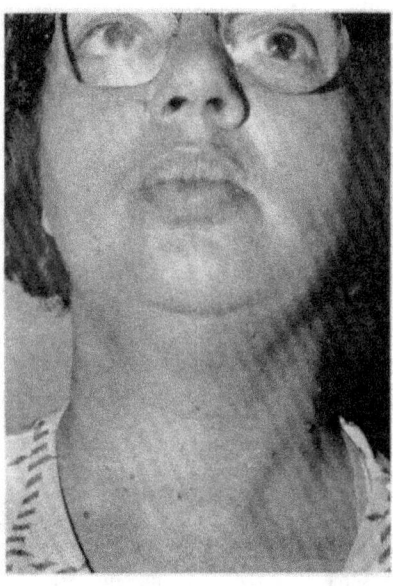

Fig. 41-B

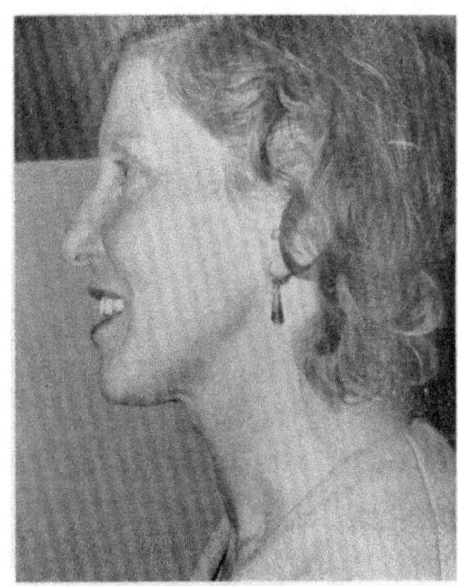

Fig. 42-B

Fig. 41 Female, aged 32 years. Hashimoto's thyroiditis. "A" before and "B" two months after treatment with bile salts, showing disappearance of swelling of the thyroid gland.

Fig. 42 Female, aged 32 years. Euthyroid. Hashimoto"s thyroiditis of one years duration. "A" before and "B" after treatment with bile salts for 2 months showing disappearance of thyroid gland welling.

Case 62 Female, aged 72 years. Admitted to hospital in myxoedematous coma. P.B.I. was found to be 1.2 μG per 100 mls. Serum thyroid cytoplasmic fluorescent auto-antibodies positive. Thyroglobulin tanned R.B.C. agglutination titre 1 in 2,500, thyroid C.F.T. 1 in 64, RF, ANF, gastric parietal cell auto-antibodies alb negative. E.S.R. 26 mms. per hour. She was treated with !-thyroxin 0.1 mgms. t.d.s. and became euthyroid. She was then given pentamidine 400 mgms. b.d. by mouth and this was repeated after one months rest. After a year the thyroid auto-antibody tests had now become negative. She remained well two years later.

c) Copper sulphate

The administration of copper sulphate to cases of Hashimoto's thyroiditis was tried in 3 cases. It resulted in a rapid decrease in the size of the thyroid gland and the disappearance of the swelling. This occurred within 3-4 weeks and the thyroid auto-antibodies were found to have disappeared from the blood in all 3 cases a year after beginning treatment (Fig. 40).

d) Bile salts

The effect of bile salts is exactly similar to that of copper sulphate administration. It was tried in 4 cases (Figs. 41 and 42).

V. The effects of antiprotozoal drugs on cases of "endocrine ex;ophthalmos"

Harden et al. (1967) reported that metronidazole (flagyl) 400 mgms. t.d.s. produces an appreciable reduction in the exophthalmos and resolution of the ophthalmoplegia in cases of exophthalmic ophthalmoplegia. The treatment had no effect on thyroid function. The author (Wyburn-Mason, 1964) reported a similar effect from the administration of chloroquine in cases of endocrine exophthalmos. Three cases are now reported showing the effect of 4-aminoquinolines on endocrine exophthalmos.

Case 63 Female, aged 55 years. Onset of moderately severe thyrotoxicosis with bilateral exophthalmos and lid-lag, slight iron deficiency anaemia and achlorhydria. She was treated with neomercazole over 4 years with complete disappearance of the thyrotoxicosis, including the ocular disturbances. The treatment was then stopped. She was kept under observation without treatment and 11 years after the onset of the thyrotoxicosis she developed a left-sided exophthalmos with lid-lag. Investigations at that time showed that she was euthyroid. The serum contained thyroid tanned R.B.C. agglutination antibodies to a titre of 1 in 250. She was treated with chloroquine (ICI) 250 mgms. daily. The ocular disturbances disappeared within 6 months and after a year the thyroid auto-antibodies could not be found in the serum (Fig. 43).

Case III, 15 Female aged 31 years. Seven months history of prominence and lid-lag affecting the right eye only. Examination showed a palpable thyroid, but the serum P.B.I. was within normal limits. There were no signs of thyrotoxicosis and RF and thyroid auto-antibodies were absent from the serum. She was given chloroquine (ICI) 250 mgms. daily for 8 months, after which the eye abnormalities had disappeared (Fig. 44). It was then noticed that she had developed cystic fibrosis of the left breast confirmed by biopsy.

CasII, 2 Female, aged 65 years. A long history of intrinsic asthma and for 2 years of myxoedema, for which she had received treatment with !-thyroxin. For the last 4 years she also suffered from a severe anxiety state and had spent 4 years in a mental hospital. On examination, apart from some tachycardia, the only abnormal finding was a left-sided exophthalmos. The serum P.B.I. was within normal limits and thyroid auto-antibodies were absent from the serum. She was treated with chloroquine (ICI) 250 mgms. daily for 2 months only, at the end of which time the exophthalmos had disappeared (Fig 45).

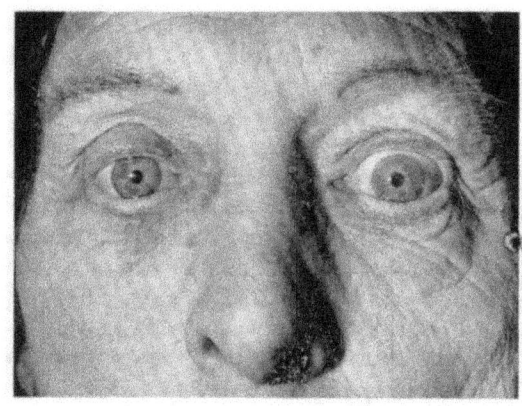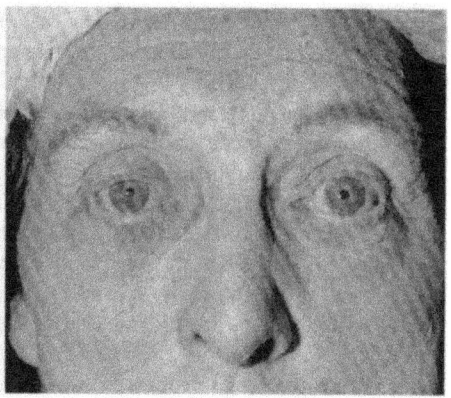

Fig. 43-A   Fig. 43-0

Fig. 4.3 F;malr, aged 55 years. Ek"en years pr'viowly he
was treatrd for thyrotoxicosis with exophthalmo< and lid-lag
with cariJimazoi(' over 4 yrars. B<came euthyroid and ocular
manifestations disappea red. Remained well for II years, then
return of left-sided exophthalmo and lid-lag, though she ri'-
mairwd euthyroid "A". Treated with chloroquine with
di appC"ara nce of ocular di\turbance within 3 months. "B"
(Casr 63).

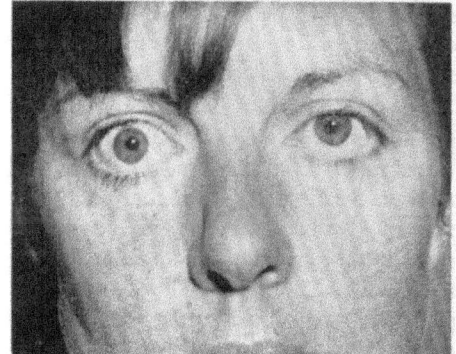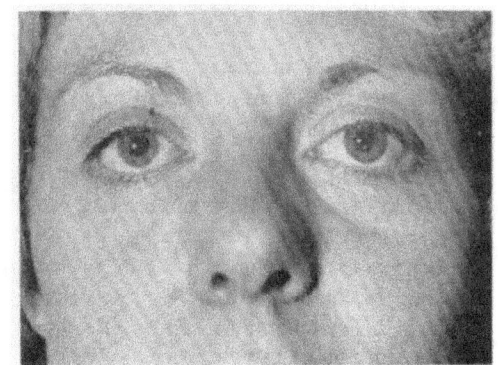

Fig. 44-A   Fig. 44-B

Fig. 44. Female, aged 31 years. Euthyroid. Right-sided ex-
ophthalmoand lid-lag with widening of the   palpebral fissure
as seen at "A". Treated with chloroquine \ith di<appea rance
of ocular disturb:mces at end of 3 months, "B" (Case III, 15).

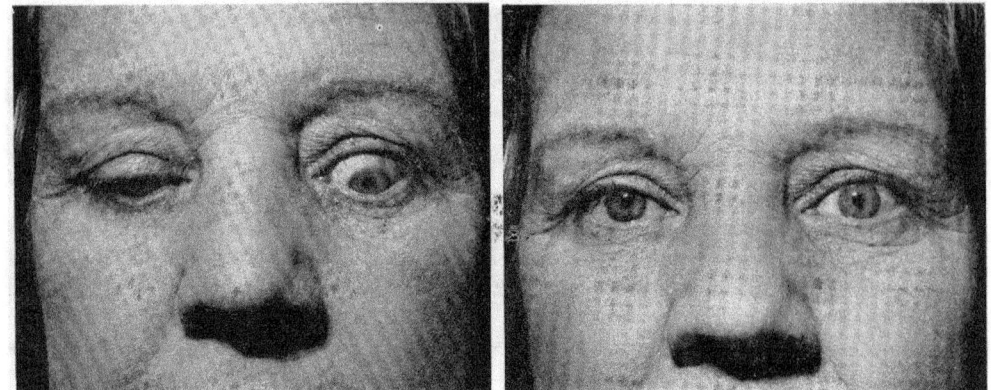

Fig. 45-A   Fig. 45-B

Fig. 45   Female, aged 40 years.   Euthyroid.   Left-sided propto·
sis and lid-lag as seen at "A".   After treatment with chloroquine
for 6 months the eye disturbances had disappeared as at "B"
(Case   II, 2).

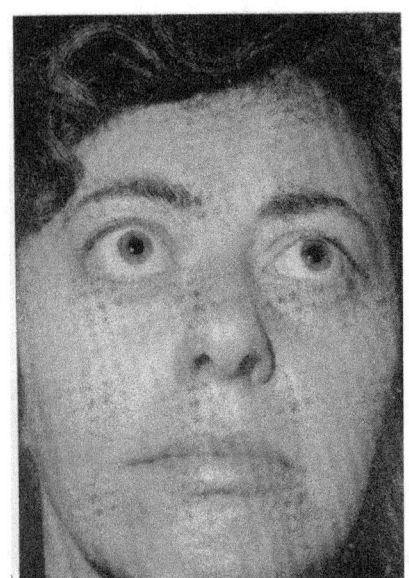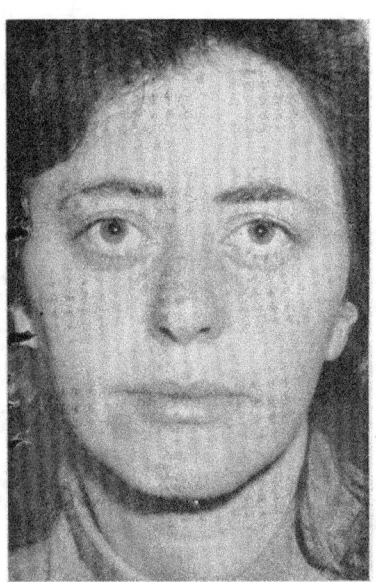

Fig. 46-A   Fig. 46-B

Fig. 46   Female, aged 30 years.   Suffering from thyrotoxicosis
with proptosis and lid-lag.   The eye signs persisted after being
rendered euthyroid with carbimazole.   Appearances then as at
"A".   Treated with copper sulphate for 2 weeks when eye
disturbances disappeared as at "B" (Case 64).

The most effective treatment of endo-crine exophthalmos is by the use of *copper sulphate* in the usual dose. This was used in 4 cases. Examples are the following:–

Case 64 Female, aged 30 years. Onset of thyrotoxicosis with bilateral exophthalmos more marked on the right side. Rendered euthyroid with neomercazole 10 mgm.s t.d.s., but eye changes persisted. Treated with copper sulphate 25 mgms. t.d.s. with marked regression of the exophthalmos (Fig. 46).

Case 65 Female, aged 77 years. A known diabetic for 15 years with the disease reasonably controlled by diet, morning injections of soluble insulin 20 units and protamine zinc insulin 10 units. She had noticed a gradually increasing prominence of the right eye over two years. *Examination.* An obese old lady. Blood pressure 180/90. All the tendon reflexes were unobtainable. There was frequent passage of 2 per cent glucose in the urine. T4I 4.4 *p*G per 100 ml. Blood urea 26 mgms. per cent. Hb 15.2 G per 100 mls. Random blood sugar 145 mgms. per 100 mls. The serum contained no auto-anti-bodies. On admission to hospital she was put on a normal diet, eating what she liked. The insulin injections were stopped and she was treated with copper sulphate 25 mgms. t.d.s. Next day the glycosuria and hyperglycaemia had disappeared and remained absent during the next 6 weeks while copper sulphate was administered. Within 10 days the proptosis of the right eye had disappeared (Fig. 47). She was discharged on this treatment and followed as an out-patient without return of glycosuria or proptosis during the next 3 months.

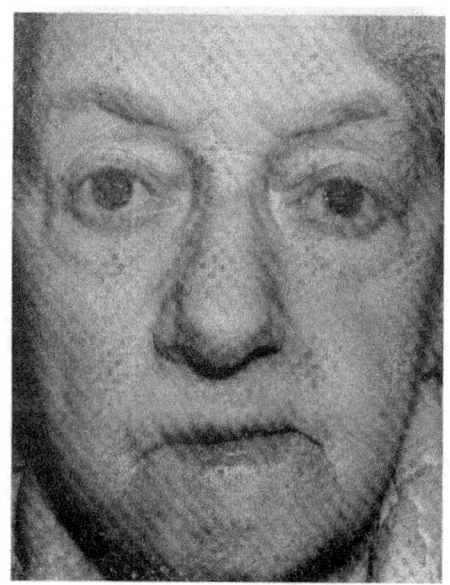

Fig. 47-A

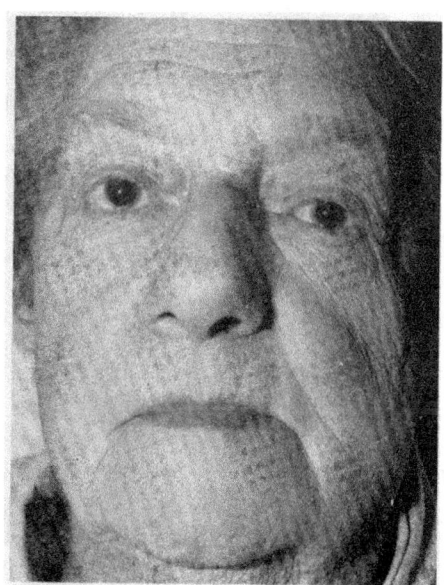

Fig. 47-B

Fig. 47 Female, aged 77 years. Euthyroid. Suffering from diabetes and right-sided exophthalmos as shown at "A". After 2 weeks treatment with copper sulphate both the diabetes and exophthalmos disappeared as at "B" (Case 65).

VI. The effects of antiprotozoal drugs on intrinsic asthma and urticaria

Sidi and Reinberg (1960) found the anti-protozoal 4-aminoquinolines very effective in the treatment of urticaria and angioneurotic oedema arising from no obvious cause. Reference has also already been made to the frequent reports of relief of urticaria by various anti-amoebic drugs. Hench (1949) found that urticaria is relieved by bile salts administration.

Edgeskjold et al. (1977) point out that in both intrinsic and extrinsic asthma as compared with controls there is a high incidence of IgG-RF, IgM-RF and IgA-RF, though the latex fixation and Rose-Waaler tests were negative.

In the "Clinical Review" on the use of chloroquine published by Imperial Chemical Industries in 1961 are cited a number of references to the successful use of both chloroquine and mepacrine in cases of asthma. Kimura et al. (1964) and the author (Wyburn-Mason, 1964) both report frequent beneficial and often dramatic results in the treatment of intrinsic asthma with 4-aminoquinolines. The author's experience since 1964 in cases of intrinsic asthma has been similarly favourable in a proportion of cases. Often response is immediate and patients may be kept free from attacks almost compfetely over long eriods. This may continue long after discontinuance of treatment. Moreover, intrinsic asthma is not infrequently associated with a chronic rhinitis and this also may be greatly benefitted by the administration of these drugs. An example of the beneficial effect of chloroquine on asthma was Case II, 2 (III, 14), in which both asthma and Hashimoto's thyroiditis were cured by this drug.

Copper sulphate or bile salts likewise may have the most beneficial effect on some cases of intrinsic asthma, especially if associated with evidence of collagen and auto-immune disease. Hench (1949) reported the beneficial effects of bile salts on cases of asthma. These effects may be seen in the following cases:—

Case 66 Male, aged 13 years. Family and past history irrelevant. Onset of severe asthma and rhinitis 18 months previously. This had been treated by various methods by his doctor. Between severe attacks he was never free of wheezing. His tonsils and adenoids had been removed 6 months previously without improvement. Examination showed severe nasal engorgement and generalized rhonchi in the chest. A blood count was normal. E.S.R. :1ormal. Skin tests showed no definite sensitivities. X-ray of chest normal. Plasma proteins normal. He was treated with copper sulphate 25 mgms. t.d.s. over the next 6 months without any side effects and with the most dramatic response. His asthma and rhinitis ceased immediately and 6 months later he was sufficiently well to be Victor Ludorum in his school sports. He has remained perfectly well over the next 12 months.

Case II, 23 or VI, 13 Female, aged 58 years. Hysterectomy for fibroids aged 35 years, shortly before which she developed intrinsic asthma. For the last 15 years she had taken daily prednisolone as a prophylactic. In spite of this, when emotionally upset or when she developed a cold, the attacks of asthma would reappear. **If** she attempted to stop taking the steroid, the attacks soon returned. She was treated by copper sulphate 25 mgms. t.d.s. for a month, during which she had no attacks of asthma. She was then weaned off the steroid and had had no return of asthma during the last 18 months.

Case II, 16 Female, aged 48 years. Onset of intrinsic asthma and thyrotoxicosis simultaneously 6 years previously. The thyrotoxicosis was cured by antithyroid drugs, but the asthma persisted. All investigations as to the aetiology of the asthma were unfruitful and skin tests were unhelpful. FEV1 =' 1.6 litres. She was treated with copper sulphate 25 mgms. t.d.s. for 6 weeks with immediate cessation of the asthma. After stopping the copper sulphate the asthma did not return during the next six months. FEVI now 2.2 litres.

Case 67 Male, aged 60 years. Very severe intrinsic asthma since the age of 42 years with gradual onset of persistent chronic bronchitis and severe cough and dyspnoea. At first this was relieved in part by the administration of steroids, which, however, had to be discontinued owing to the development of steroid myopathy. He was relieved only in part by other anti-asthmatic drugs. FEVI = 1.3 litres. These were continued and he was then also given copper sulphate 25 mgms. t.d.s. This resulted in a dramatic response with marked improvement in both the dyspnoea and expectoration. FEVI now 2.0 litres. He has continued to take this substance for five months and the benefit has been maintained.

In three other cases of intrinsic asthma unassociated with rheumatoid disease or auto-immune disease only partial or temporary relief was obtained by the use of copper sulphate or dehydrocholine.

VII. The effect of dehydrocholine on Schonlein-Henoch's purpura

Case 68 Female, aged 17 years, Pakistani. Two brothers and her mother had suffered from asthma and allergy to various drugs, including penicillin. Patient was admitted to hospital with a 10 week history of purpuric rash all over the body occurring in crops with joint pains, abdominal discomfort and loose motions. Apart from generalized purpuric spots all over the body no other abnormality could be made out. All investigations of the blood proved negative. No improvement was obtained with steroids. She was treated with dehydrocholine 500 mgms. t.d.s. over 2 weeks. The purpura ceased after about 3 days and disappeared completely. It did not recur over the next year.

VIII. The effect of antiprotozoal drugs on cases of atrophic gastritis with or without pernicious anaemia

The effects of chloroquine on one case of atrophic gastritis and two cases of pernicious anaemia and of pentamidine on two cases of atrophic gastritis with pernicious anaemia were investigated. In the case of atrophic gastritis thyroid cytoplasmic fluorescent auto-antibodies and complement fixation tests were both positive. Treatment with chloroquine (ICI) 250 mgms. daily for a year had no effect on the achlorhydria, though the auto-antibodies had disappeared from the blood two years later. In two cases of atrophic gastritis associated with pernicious anaemia gastric parietal cell auto-antibodies were present and in one thyroid cytoplasmic fluorescent auto-antibodies were also found. The administration of chloroquine for a year caused the disappearance of the auto-antibodies from the blood, but no change in the achlorhydria.

In two cases of atrophic gastritis associated with pernicious anaemia treated with pentamidine by daily injections of 200 mgms. daily for 10 days followed after a month by 200 mgms. twice daily for 6 weeks both the gastric parietal cell immunofluorescent antibodies, the intrinsic factor auto-antibodies and in one case the thyroid auto-antibodies disappeared from the serum when tested two years later, but achlorhydria persisted.

IX. The effect of antiprotozoal drugs on cases of ulcerative colitis

In severe and fulminating cases of ulcerative colitis 4-aminoquinolines do not appear to have any beneficial effect when added to treatment with steroids and salazopyrin. However, in mild and moderately severe cases the administration of 4-aminoquinolines not infrequently results

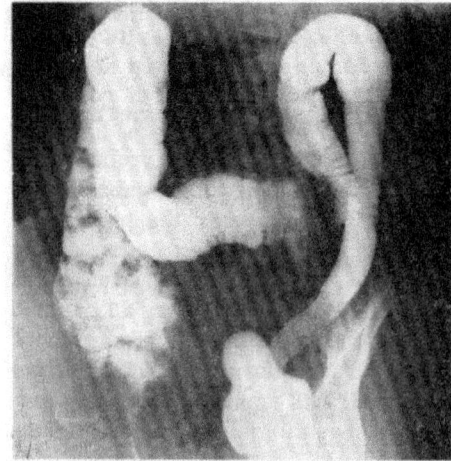

Fig. 48-A

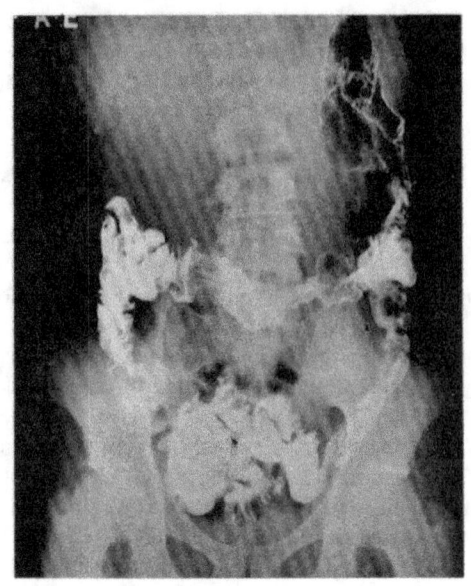

Fig. 48-B

Fig. 48 Male, aged 21 years. Symptom of ulcerative colitis for 2 years. Barium enema appearances before "A" and 18 month after treatment with chloroquine "B", where abnormalities of descending colon have disappeared (Case G9)

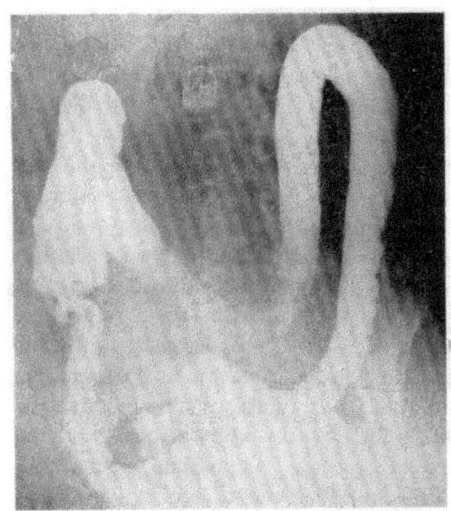

Fig. 49-A

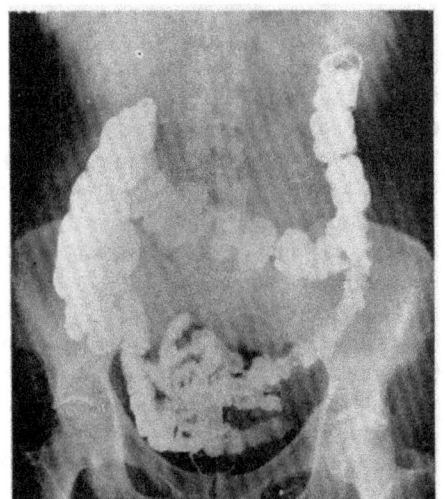

Fig. 49-B

Fig. 49 Female, aged 50 years. Moderately severe ulcerative colitis. Barium enema at onset of disease showing typical appearances "A" and "B" after one year treatment with chloroquine. The abnormalities have disappeared (Case 70).

in an immediate disappearance of symptoms, return of the E.S.R. to normal and disappearance of associated anaemia. Eventually complete cure may be obtained and the radiological appearance in the colon may return to normal. Such a case was reported by the author (Wyburn-Mason, 1964). In addition the following cases have been treated with 4-amino-quinolines.

Case 69 Male, aged 21 years. Eighteen months history of diarrhoea occurring every half hour accompanied by slime and blood in the stools and by some vague abdominal pain. These symptoms occurred in bouts lasting 6-8 weeks. Investigations showed the stools contained no ova, cysts or parasites. Sigmoidoscopy showed the typical appearance of ulcerative colitis affecting the sigmoid colon and rectum and a barium enema showed well-marked changes of ulcerative colitis affecting the left hemicolon. The faeces contained blood. The faecal fats were normaL The blood Hb was 11.5 G per 100 mls. The glucose tolerance test was normal. The E.S.R. was normal. The serum iron was 137 $_0$G per 100 mls. He was treated with camoqu!n 200 mgms. daily for 6 months. His symptoms disappeared immediately he started the drug and did not recur when this was stopped. A repeat barium enema 2 yean; after the first showed a completely normal appearance of the colon (Fig. 48).

Case 70 Female, aged 50 years. Two months previously sudden onset of abdominal pain with severe diarrhoea and the passage of slime and blood. Examination showed evidence of some anaemia and tenderness over the ascending and transverse colon. E.S.R. 47 mms. per hour. Hb 10.2 grams per cent. A barium enema showed marked changes of ulcerative colitis in the terminal ileum and ascending and transverse colon, the left hemicolon appearing normal. Sigmoidoscopy was normaL She was treated with chloroquine (ICI) 250 mgms. daily for a year. Her symptoms disappeared almost immediately.

The blood count and E.S.R. had returned to normal after 5 months and after 2 years a repeat barium enema showed no abnormality. There was no return of symptoms in the next 5 years (Fig. 49).

Case 71 Female, aged 37 years. Aged 31 years hysterectomy for fibroids. Recent onset of diarrhoea with the passage of blood and slime and of irritation of the anal skin. A barium enema, blood count and E.S.R. estimation were all normal. Sigmoidoscopy showed the typical changes of ulcerative colitis affecting the rectum and sigmoid with granulating areas of congestion and much slime with loss of mucosal pattern. She was treated with chloroquine (ICI) 250 mgms. daily. All her symptoms cleared within a week. Treatment was continued for 6 months. There had been no return over 4 years. A repeat barium enema was refused.

Case 72 Male, aged 59 years. Onset of symptoms of ulcerative colitis two years previously. A barium enema showed the typical changes of ulcerative colitis affecting the descending colon and the rectum. The diagnosis was confirmed by sigmoidoscopy. A blood count and E.S.R. were normal. He was treated with chloroquine (ICI) 250 mgms. daily. All his symptoms disappeared within 2 weeks and did not return during the next 18 months, though treatment was stopped after 6 months. The barium enema appearances returned to normal (Fig. 50).

Case 73 Female, aged 78 years. Suffered from well-marked rheumatoid arthritis over the last 15 years. For 2 years she complained of severe diarrhoea with the passage of blood and slime. Examination showed the changes of rheumatoid arthritis and tenderness over the transverse and descending colon. A barium enema confirmed the existence of ulcerative colitis affecting the transverse and descending colon. Sigmoidoscopy normaL Blood Hb 13.0 G per cent. E.S.R. normal. RF and ANF negative. P.B.I. 6.9 p.G per 100 ml. She was given chloroquine (ICI) 250 mgms.

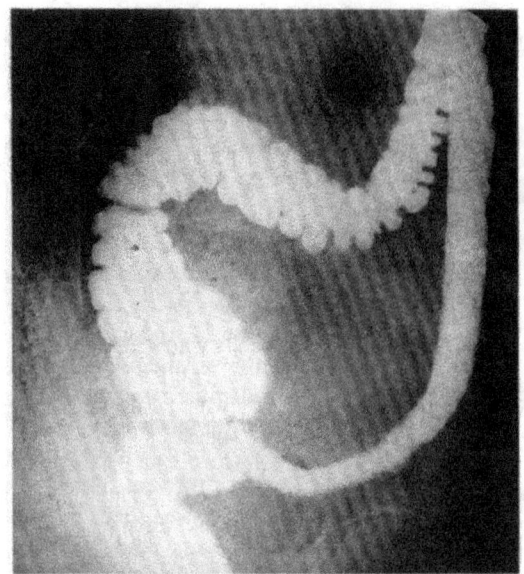

Fig. 50-A

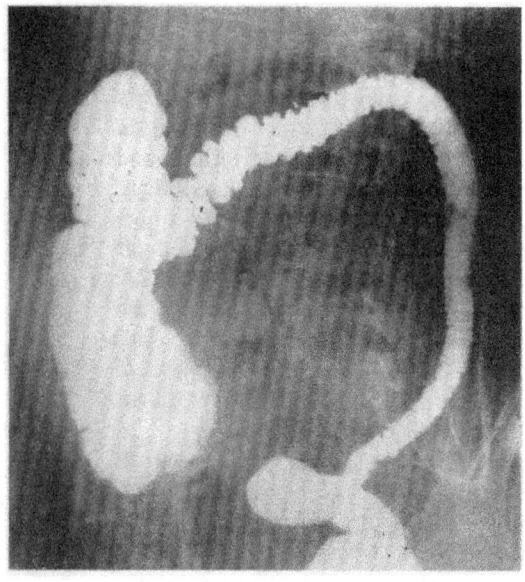

Fig. 50-B

Fig. 50 Male, aged 59 years. Two year history of ulcerative coliti affecting de cending colon. Barium enema before, "A", and "B" 18 months after con tin uo us trea tm en t with chloroquine howing return to normal appea rances (Case 72).

daily for a year with complete control of her symptoms, which did not return over the next 3 years in spite of stopping the chloroquine.

The effect of copper sulphate in cases 'Of ulcerative colitis is shown in the following case:-

Case 74 Male, aged 15 years at onset of severe and fulminant ulcerative colitis with toxic megacolon and abdominal pain. At the onset control of symptoms was obtained by 15 mgms. of prednisolone t.d.s. and salazopyrin, reduced to prednisolone 10 mgms. t.d.s. and salazopyrin 2 tablets t.d.s. The addition of chloroquine 250 mgms. daily to these medicaments had little effect on the symptoms. He was kept under this regime for the next 3 years. Attempts were made to reduce the dosage of steroids and salazopyrin during this period, but this resulted in recurrence of diarrhoea. Eventually he was treated with copper sulphate 50 mgms. t.d.s. with a rapid disappearance of the irregularly occurring colicky pains. The salazopyrin was then stopped while the steroids and copper sulphate were continued and there was no return of symptoms. After a further month the steroids were tapered off while the copper sulphate was continued for a period of 4 months during which the patient remained well. The copper sulphate was then stopped and the patient remained symptomless without treatment over the next two years.

Another patient, a Pakistani, aged 26 years, from Kenya developed acute ulcerative colitis affecting the whole colon over two months. He was having 8-10 bloody fluid stools a day. The diagnosis was confirmed by sigmoidoscopy and by barium enema examination. The blood E.S.R. was 108 mms. per hour and the blood haemoglobin 7.8 G per cent. He was treated with copper sulphate 25 mgms. three times daily with rapid improvement in his condition. After 6 weeks he was having only two normal stools a day and his E.S.R. had fallen to 16 mms. per hour and the

blood haemoglobin had risen to 13.4 G per cent.

Not only may chloroquine and copper sulphate benefit cases of ulcerative colitis, but also clotrimazole. This was shown by the following cases.

Case 75 Male, aged 30 years, Pakistani, who had lived in this country for 6 years. Six months history of blood and mucus in the stools, diarrhoea with the passage of fluid stools up to 12 times a day and in the last 3 months of abdominal pains and loss of a considerable amount oweight. Examination. His temperature was 100 F. There was evident loss of considerable amount of weight. He was thin, dehydrated and the tongue was dry and furred. There were tenderness and resistance in the left side of the abdomen. Rectal examination was normal except for blood on the examining finger. Blood count showed Hb 37 per cent. E.S.R. 46 mms. per hour. W.B.C. 14,300 per cu. mm. Serum albumin 3.1 G/100 ml., globulin 3.1 G/100 mi., serum iron 23 .uG/100 mi. The stools did not contain Entamoeba histolytica. RF, ANF and auto-antibodies were absent from the serum. Sigmoidoscopy and biopsy of the colon indicated the changes of ulcerative colitis. A straight X-ray of the abdomen showed lack of haustration in the transverse and sigmoid colon consistent with ulcerative colitis. An attempt at a barium enema confirmed loss of haustration in the sigmoid colon and fluid levels in the pelvis, probably in the small bowel due to ileus. The patient was feeling extremely ill and was unable to retain the barium. The barium which did enter the rectum and sigmoid colon revealed marked ulceration of the mucosa consistent with a severe ulcerative colitis, though it was impossible to estimate its extent. The patient was given blood transfusions and slowly responded to salazopyrin and isogel, his temperature beginning to settle, but he again deteriorated and his blood haemoglobin again fell to 46 per cent and he was therefore given prednisolone 5 mgms. t.d.s. in

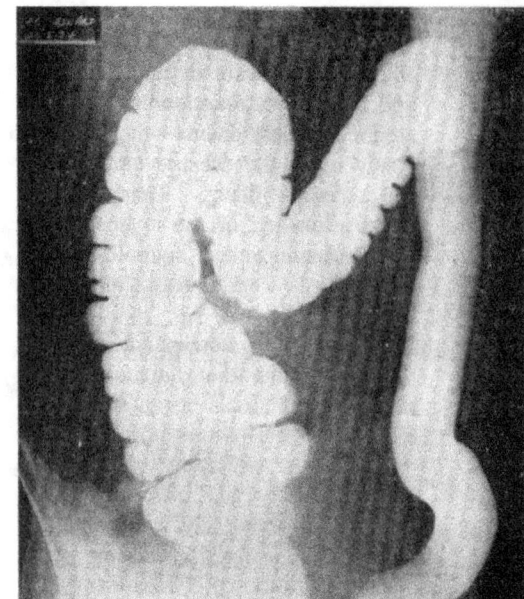

Fig. 51-A

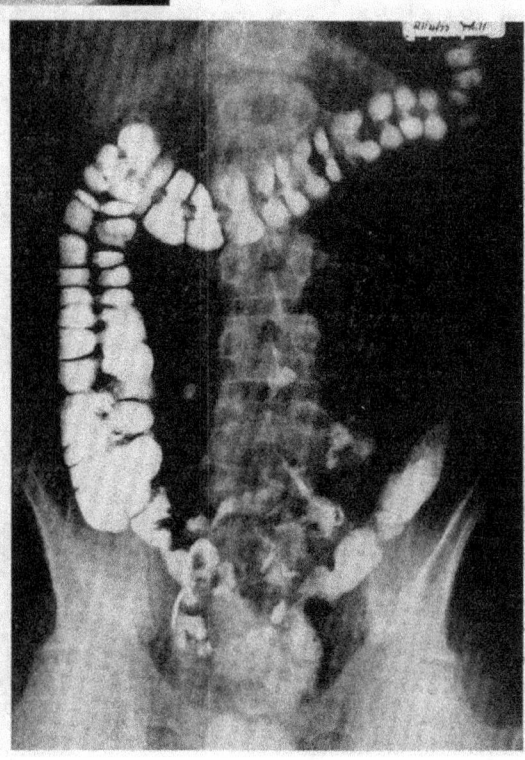

Fig. 51-B

Fig. 51 Case 76. Male, aged 35 years. A 10 years history of ulcerative colitis showing barium enema appearance before A and 2 months after continuous treatment with clotrimazole. B. Note the return of haustration in B.

addition. His temperature failed to settle completely though the diarrhoea was reduced to 3 motions a day with occasional blood and mucus in the stools. The blood count continued to show an Hb content of around 50 per cent and E.S.R. persisted in the region of 50 mms. per hour. He remained in this condition for a month. He was then given copper sulphate 25 mgms. t.d.s. in addition to salazopyrin 10 mgms. q.d.s. and prednisolone E.C. 5 mgms. t.d.s. Within a few days the motions became formed and blood and mucus disappeared and he began to eat and gain weight. His temperature settled within 10 days and the abdominal pain ceased. Within a month his motions had returned to normal, occurring once a day. The salazopyrin was then stopped and the prednisolone tapered off over the course of 2 weeks. He remained symptomless. Five months later the blood count showed 5.06 million R.B.C. per cu. mm., Hb 12.9 gm. per 100 ml. E.S.R. 5 mms. per hour, serum albumin 4.6 G/100 mi., globulin 3.0 G/100 ml. The copper sulphate was then stopped. He remained symptomless over the next 4 months at the end of which time the diarrhoea with the passage of blood and mucus returned. He had 5 fluid motions a day. He was then treated with clotrimazole 1 G t.d.s. Within 3 days the diarrhoea had ceased and the blood and mucus disappeared. His appetite improved and he began to gain weight. The symptoms did not return in the next 6 months while under treatment and at the end of this time he had gained 15 lbs. in weight. His blood E.S.R. was now normal.

Case 76   Male, aged 35 years. He gave a ten year history of the passage of blood and mucus per rectum, abdominal pain and diarrhoea six times a day. *Examination.* He was thin. The tongue was furred. There was generalized abdominal tenderness.. Rectal examination showed blood on the examining glove. Sigmoidoscopy was normal. Blood count R.B.C. 5.19 million R.B.C. per cu. mm. Hb 15.0 G/100 ml.

E.S.R. 3 mms. per hour. Serum albumin 4.4 G/100 ml, globulin 2.5 G/100 ml. Stools contained no cysts or amoebae. RF, ANF and organ auto-antibodies absent from serum. Barium enema-the barium flowed freely up to the caecum and refluxed into the terminal ileum. There was loss of haustration and of the mucosal pattern in the descending and sigmoid colon. The appearances were those of ulcerative colitis (Fig. 51).

He was given clotrimazole 1 G t.d.s. and within 2 days the diarrhoea, blood and mucus in the stools began to lessen. In a week the stools were nonnal, once daily only and the abdominal pain had ceased. He was discharged from hospital within two weeks completely symptomless taking clotrimazole and followed for six months without return of symptoms. A repeat barium enema showed no abnormality six months later when treatment was stopped (Fig. 51).

Case '77   Female, aged 48 years. She gave a 10 year history of diarrhoea six times daily with the passage of mucus and blood and over the last six months painful swelling of both wrists, especially the left, and of both knees, especially the right, and loss of weight and appetite. *Examination* showed a thin woman with some generalized abdominal tenderness, heat and severe swelling of both wrists and knee joints with free fluid in the right knee joint.

Investigations Blood count Hb 7.2 G/100 ml. (50 per cent). E.S.R. 46 mm. per hour. Serum proteins, albumin 2.3 G/100 mls., globulin 4.2 G/100 mls. X-rays of the wrists and knees N.A.D. RF, ANF and organ specific auto-antibodies absent from serum. A barium meal showed loss of haustration and mucosal pattern throughout t'he colon. Sigmoidoscopy and biopsy showed ulceration of a friable bleeding mucosa and histological changes consistent with the diagnosis of ulcerative colitis.

She was treated with clotrimazole 1 G t.d.s. Within three days the pain and swelling of the joints was much less. At the end of a week it had disappeared completely and the diarrhoea began to lessen. Blood and mucus had disappeared from the stools. At the end of a month the patient was completely symptomless. Treatment was continued for six months at the end of which time she had gained 5 kilogram::; in weight and she now tended to be constipated. The E.S.R. was now 5 mms. per hour. The blood count showed Hb 14.2 G/100 ml. Serum albumin was 4.2 G/100 ml., globulin 2.8 G/100 ml.

Thus, it seems that various drugs active against limax amoebae cause a disappearance of all the manifestations of ulcerative colitis, including the arthropathy.

X. The treatment of idiopathic Addison's disease with antiprotozoal drugs

Two cases of idiopathic Addison's disease were treated.

Case 78   Female, aged 46 years. Rapid onset of Addison's disease which was treated in the usual way with fludrocortisone and hydrocortisone. At the onset the blood showed an eosinophilia of 16 per cent of 7,800 W.B.C. The serum contained thyroid cytoplasmic fluorescent auto-antibodies, but no auto-antibodies to adrenal cortical cells, RF or ANF. . Treatment with chloroquine (ICI) 250 mgms. daily for a year resulted in the disappearance of the thyroid auto-antibodies from the serum.

Case 79   Male, aged 30 years. Onset of acute Addison's disease with nausea, vomiting and generalized weakness preceded for 5 years by darkening of the skin of the face and accompanied by some enlargement of the cervical lymph nodes. The blood pressure was 85/50 mms. and there was the typical increase in pigmentation around the waist, in the axillae and inside the mouth. The E.S.R. was raised. Blood P.B.I. was 1.4 p.G per 100 mls. A fractional test meal showed free hydrochloric acid. Plasma cortisol levels were less than 1 p.G per 100 mls. The serum contained a mod-

erately high titre of thyroid auto-antibodies and a very high titre of gastric parietal cell and adrenal cytoplasmic auto-antibodies. The serum vitamin B12 and folic acid levels were within normal limits. He was treated with L-thyroxin 0.1 mgms. b.d., fludrocortisone 0.1 G daily, hydrocortisone 20 mgms. twice daily with rapid disappearance of the symptoms. The E.S.R., however, remained raised to 30 mms. per hour. He was treated with pentamidine 200 mgms. intramuscularly daily for 10 injections and then 200 mgms. t.d.s. by mouth at intervals of one month for a month at a time for three courses. A year later he began to put on weight rapidly and he developed a Cushingoid appearance. On retesting after 18 months all auto-antibodie had disappeared from the blood. The P.B.I. was then found to be 9.6 flG per 100 mls. The L-thyroxin administration was stopped. After 6 weeks it was found to be 4.6 JLG per 100 mls. The hydrocortisone and fludrocortisone were then tapered down over six weeks. He was followed for three months and showed no return of symptoms of Addison's disease. A repeat plasma cortisol now showed a level of 12.6 JLG per 100 mls. at 12 p.m., so that the treatment with pentamidine appeared to have cured the thyroid and adrenal lesions.

XI. The effects of antiprotozoal drugs on chronic skin lesions of rheumatoid disease

Light sensitivity eruptions may respond favourably to atebrine (mepacrine) and chloroquine (Knox et al., 1954; Whisnant et al., 1963). Quinacrine and chloroquine may also be helpful in cases of lupus erythematosus and pemphigus (Whisnant et al.) and seborrhoeic dermatitis and psoriasis may also respond favourably to mepacrine, chloroquine or iodochlorohydroxyquinoline, an anti-amoebic drug (Ingram, 1964).

Hyperkeratoses of the skin occur with

increasing age. They appear especially in exposed areas. It was found that when patients with other diseases and who also had hyperkeratoses were treated with bile salts over 3-4 weeks the hyperkeratotic lesions fell off and disappeared. They did not recur when the treatment was stopped.

XII. The effects of antiprotozoal drugs on leucoderma and melanoderma

Banerjee and Choudhury (1965) found that the administration of the antiprotozoal drug, mepacrine, to cases of vitiligo result-ed in fading or marked improvement in the depigmentation of the skin. In one of the author's cases of vitiligo the serum con-tained thyroid auto-antibodies and admin-istration of chloroquine (ICI) 250 mgms. daily for 18 months resulted in a gradual disappearance of the depigmented areas on the skin of the neck and wrists and dis-appearance of the auto-antibodies from the serum. In a second case assochted with pernicious anaemia, achlorhydria and the presence of gastric parietal cell and in-trinsic factor auto-antibodies in the serum oral administration of pentamidine 200 mgms. t.d.s. for a month repeated after a months rest resulted after 18 months in a marked fading of the depigmented areas and disappearance of the auto-antibodies from the serum. The achlorhydria, how-ever, persisted.

XIII. The effects of antiprotozoal drugs on chronic rheumatoid liver disease

At the 4th. International Congress of Gastro-enterology held in Copenhagen in 1970 Doxiades rep rted that chloroquine, 500 mgms. daily causes improvement both clinically and as shown by laboratory tests and liver biopsy in chronic parenchymal diseases of the liver and to be superior to the results obtained by treatment with

corticosteroids and diuretics. Doxiades et al. (1971) likewise found that 70 per cent of patients suffering from chronic active hepatitis showed satisfactory clinical and laboratory improvement on administration of chloroquine. In Case X, 20 (page 303) a female of 61 years, suffering from myx-oedema, chronic active hepatitis, mild rheu-matoid deformities of the hands, atrophic gastritis, achlorhydria and chronic lympha-tic leukaemia, the serum contained ANF and a high titre of gastric parieta l cell auto-antibodies. Treatment with chloroquine (ICI) 250 mgms. daily caused a return to normal in the liver function tests.

In Case VI, 65 or VII 59 (page 294) suffering from Sjogren's syndrome and chronic active hepatitis, the administration of copper sulphate also restored liver func-tion tests to normal.

XIV. The effect of antiprotozoal drugs on cases of Paget's disease

In six cases of thyroid disease associated with Paget's disease of bone observed by the author the bone disease caused back pain. In ten cases of Paget's disease of bone the author found that the administra-tion of chloroquine in the usual doses re-sulted in a rapid improvement in the bony pain and a fall in the serum alkaline phos-phatase and E.S.R. while the drug was being taken, but the pain and the blood changes tended to recur sometime after cessation of administration of the drug. An example is the following case:-

Case 80 Female, aged 76 years. Paget's disease of the spine. Serum alkaline phos-phatase 31.5 K.A. units, E.S.R. 44 mm. per hour, serum proteins albumin 3.1, globulin 4.2 mgms. per 100 mls. Thyroid cytoplasm fluorescent auto-antibodies present. Treat-ed with chloroquine (ICI) 250 mgms. daily. One month later E.S.R. 21 mms. per hour, Alkaline phosphatase 18 units per 100 mls. Relief of backache occurred immediately on taking the drug.

In another case of extensive Paget's disease oral pentamidine was found to have a similar effect both on the pain and on the alkaline phosphatase levels and E.S.R.

Case 81 Female, aged 72 years. Rodent ulcer removed from forehead 6 years previously. Now very widespread Paget's disease of bone. Serum alkaline phosphatase 80 K.A. units per 100 mls. E.S.R. 38 mms. per hour. Treated with camoquin 200 mgms. daily with much relief of pain and 2 months later serum alkaline phosphatase 40 K.A. units per 100 mls. E.S.R. 14 mms. per hour. She was later treated with flagyl without any obvious effect and later still with a course of intramuscular pentamidine 200 mgms. daily for 10 days and this was repeated after 10 days rest. This resulted in relief of pain and a fall in the serum alkaline phosphatase from 48 to 26 K.A. units per 100 mls. and of the E.S.R. from 48 to 26 mms. per hour.

The most dramatic effect, however, occurred in one case using copper sulphate.

Case 82 Female, aged 76 years. Past history of renal calculi, hypertension and cystic mastitis. Paget's disease was discovered 2 years previously and was associated with various aches and pains. The disease affected the skull, right scapula, pelvis and lumbar vertebrae. Serum RF and gastric parietal cell antibodies negative. Thyroid auto-antibodies negative, ANF absent. Achlorhydria present. Serum alkaline phosphatase 39.6 K.A. units per 100 mi. E.S.R. 80 mms. per hour. Treated with copper sulphate 25 mgms. t.d.s. with dramatic results. "I feel marvellous and young again. My back pains have disappeared, I can walk without a stick now and have no rheumatism and I enjoy food again". Six weeks after beginning treatment the alkaline phosphatase level in the blood had fallen to 26 K.A. units per 100 mls. and the E.S.R. was 28 mms. per hour and remained at this level during the next six months.

Copper sulphate, dehydrocholine and clotrimazole may also cause relief of bone pain and fall in the serum alkaline phosphatase and E.S.R. in cases of Paget's disease as shown in the following case.

Case 83 Female, aged 76 years. When first seen she was complaining of severe pain in all regions of the spine.

Examination showed a well preserved woman with no evident abnormality.

Investigations X-rays, however, showed Paget's disease of the skull, lumbar and dorsal vertebrae, pelvis, right scapula and acromion process and the upper one-third of both femora. The blood count showed no abnormality. E.S.R. was 15 mm. per hour. The serum proteins were normal. Serum alkaline phosphatase 37.1 K.A. units. RF, ANF and organ specific auto-antibodies were absent from the serum.

Treatment She was treated with chloroquine 200 mgms. daily with marked relief of the pain after several weeks. Treatment was continued for 18 months during which time the serum alkaline phosphatase fell to 25.6 K.A. units. Treatment was then discontinued owing to the risk of eye complications of chloroquine and a year later the pain in the back had increased considerably, the serum alkaline phosphatase having risen to 31-5 K.A. units. She was given copper sulphate 25 mgm. t.d.s. which also rapidly relieved her pain and resulted in the serum alkaline phosphatase falling to 21.5 K.A. units. After 2 months this was stopped. Four months later the pain again became severe and the serum alkaline phosphatase rose to 30 K.A. units. She was then given dehydrocholine 750 mms. t.d.s. for 2 months with an almost miraculous effect on the pain and a fall in the serum alkaline phosphatase level to 11 K.A. units. She stated she felt rejuvenated and remained well for about a year, when the pain returned and became so severe as to require morphine to relieve it. The serum alkaline phosphatase was now 41 K.A. units. Treatment with clotrimazole 100 mgms./kilo was begun and within 2 weeks the pain had lessened considerably and within 4 weeks had disappeared completely. The serum alkaline phosphatase fell to 12 K.A. units. Unfortunately liver function tests began to show abnormalities and treatment had to be dis-<:ontinued, though she remained pain-free during the next 4 months at the end of which time the serum alkaline phosphatase was 16 K.A. units.

XV. The effect of antiprotozoal compounds on diabetes mellitus

In cases of mild diabetes me!Jitus controlled by diet and oral hypoglycaemic agents the administration of chloroquine over a period may sometimes result in the disappearance of the dia betes and also of any auto-antibodies present in the seru m. This was observed on five occasions.

Case 84 Female, aged 65 years. Her mother, sister and brother all suffered from diabetes. She herself had developed rheumatoid arthritis at the age of 53 years and had been a diabetic for 5 years. The latter was controlled by diet and by diabinese 250 mgms. b.d. and dibotin 25 mgms. b.d. Exa mination showed moderately severe rheumatoid arthritis, but no evidence of active inflammation in the joints. The tendon reflexes were absent. The serum contained ANF and the thyroglobulin tanned R.B.C. agglutination titre was 1 in 256. Rheumatoid factor and gastric parietal cell auto-antibodies were absent from the serum. The diabetes was not completely controlled on the treatment given and a random blood sugar estimation showed a level of 150 mgms. per cent. A glucose tolerance test was typically diabetic. She was treated with chloroquine (ICI) 250 mgms. daily over 9 months. At the end of this time ANF and thyroid auto-antibodies could not be demonstrated in the serum and the patient began to suffer attacks of hypoglycaemia. No sugar was demonstrable at any time in the urine at this stage. Treatment with diabinese and dibotin was

therefore discontinued and the patient was allowed to take a normal diet. A repeat glucose tolerance test was normal. Observation over the course of the next six months showed no return of glycosuria and random blood suga r estimation showed a level of 120 mgms. per cent.

Case 85 Female, aged 60 years. She gave a 5 year history of diabetes with mild arthritic symptoms. This was controlled with diet and diabinese 400 mgms. daily. Thyroid auto-antibodies were present in the serum. She was treated wit h chloroquine (ICI) 250 mgms. daily for a year, at the end of which time the diabinese was topped and she reverted to a normal diet. She then showed only occasional mild glycosuria. Random blood sugar estimation was now within normal limits. The thyroid auto-antibodies had disappeared from the serum.

Case 86 Male, aged 65 yea rs. A mild diabetic for 6 years treated with diet and 40 units of insulin daily. Control of the diabetes with tablets had been found to be impossible. He was treated with chloroquine (ICI) 250 mgms. f or 18 months and it was found necessary to reduce the dose of insulin owing to the appearance of hypoglycaemic attacks and finally he was able to control the diabetes with diabinese 250 mgms. b.d.

case 8'7 Male, aged 55 years. He had suffered from Paget's disease of bone and myxoedema for 5 years and t hen developed diabetes necessitating dietary control and the administration of soluble insulin 20 and protamine zinc insulin 24 units daily. He was given chloroquine (ICI) 250 mgms. daily for 19 months and during the course of this time the dosage of insulin had to be progressively reduced because of hypoglycaemic attacks. Eventually insulin injections were stopped and the diabetes was now able to be controlled by dietary means alone. This has continued for the next two years.

The most dramatic effect of antiprotozoal agents on diabetes mellitus is seen, however, using *copper sulphate* or *dehydrocholine*. Mention has already been made above of a case of diabetes with unilateral exophthalmos (Case 65), both of which disappeared rapidly on the administration of copper sulphate. Numerous other cases of this effect on diabetes have been observed.

Case 88 Male, aged 47 years, Pakistani. He came to this country from Karachi ten years previously. For 6 years he had noticed progressive vitiligo which began on the face and now involved most of the body, so that he appeared to be white skinned. He had suffered from gout for 5 years and in the last 9 months from polyuria with some loss of weight. The left side of his nose had been obstructed for 13 years and he had an operation for chronic appendicitis some 4 years ago. *Examination* showed very widespread vitiligo, absent tendon reflexes in the lower limbs, a blood pressure of 170/90 mms. and the urine at ail times contained more than 2 per cent of glucose. A chest X-ray was normal. The serum albumin and globulin were both 3.9 Grams per cent. Hb 15.8 per 100 mls. E.S.R. 15 mms. Random blood sugar 205 mgms. per 100 mls. A glucose tolerance test was typically diabetic. Serum uric acid 9.6 mgms. per 100 mls. Serum lipaemic. All auto-antibodies absent from serum. He was given copper sulphate 50 mgms. t.d.s. and allopurinol 100 mgms. t.d.s., but was not put on a diet. Next day the urine was sugar-free and remained so without other treatment throughout the day. A random blood sugar estimation showed 126 mgms. per 100 mls. After one month the administration of copper sulphate was stopped. The glucose tolerance test was now normal. He was followed for 3 months without return of symptoms or glycosuria, but 4 months later symptoms had returned and the urine now contained sugar again.

case 89 Female, aged 81 years. A long-standing case of myxoedema for which she had been under treatment for 10 years.

She had been short of breath on exertion and her feet had tended to swell for the last 2 months. She was admitted to hospital because she fainted while out shopping. On examination there were well marked changes of burnt-out rheumatoid arthritis. The skin was dry, the hair scanty and the pulse rate only 60 per minute. The blood pressure was 170/90 mms. The tendon reflexes were all present. The urine contained more than 2 per cent of sugar throughout the day. A random blood sugar showed 250 mgms. per cent. A glucose tolerance test was diabetic. A blood count showed Hb of 14.6 G per cent. T4 I =3.7 JJ.G per 100 mls. She was given copper sulphate 50 mgms. t.d.s., but no diet and L-thyroxin was increased to 0.1 mgms. b.d. Next day the urine was sugar-free and remained so for the next month while she was taking copper sulphate. This was then withdrawn and she remained sugar free without treatment over the next two months. A repeat glucose tolerance test was now normal.

Case 90 Female, aged 61 years. Admitted to hospital because of pruritus vulvae, dryness of the mouth, polyuria and weight loss. On examination blood pressure was 170/90 mms. The ankle jerks were abs:mt, but otherwise there were no abnormal physical signs. The urine contained more than 2 per cent of sugar at all times and a random blood sugar gave a reading of 210 mgms. per 100 mls. A glucose tolerance test was typically diabetic. The E.S.R. was 20 mms. per hour. The Hb was 122 per cent. An E.C.G. was normal. She was given copper sulphate 50 mgms. t.d.s. without dietary restriction. Sugar disappeared from the urine completely in 24 hours and the pruritus ceased at the same time. She was kept on the treatment for 3 weeks, during which the urine remained sugar-free and the blood sugar fell *to* 90-130 mgms. A glucose tolerance test was now normal. The copper sulphate was then stopped, after which she began to show 1/4 per cent of sugar irregularly in

-201

the urine. This was easily controlled with diet alone for the next six months.

Case 91 Female, aged 70 years. Diabetic for 9 years taking 26 units of insulin daily. Admitted to hospital because of an attack of acute bronchitis. She was found to have 2:1 heart block, a blood pressure of 180/90 mms. and an aortic ejection murmur. The temperature was 100.5"F. There were signs of acute bronchitis. The ankle jerks were absent. Blood Hb 75 per cent. Random blood sugar 390 mgms. per 100 mls. T4 4.4 $_{J.IG}$ per 100 mls. The bronchitis was treated with antibiotics, after which she was given copper sulphate 25 mgms. t.d.s. The glucosuria disappeare!d in 48 hours. The insulin administration was then stopped and she was allowed a normal diet. T•re was no glycosuria during the next 4·' weeks of her hospital stay and at the end of this time a random blood sugar gave a reading of 125 mgms. per cent. The glucose tolerance test was now normal. She was discharged from hospital without any treatment and 6 weeks later seen again. At that time she was showing irregular glycosuria of 1/4 per cent. She is still under observation.

Case 92 Male, aged 70 years. Diabetes for 5 years controlled by diet and 10 units of P.Z. and 10 units of soluble insulin. For the last 3 months he had noticed left foot-drop, and was found to have no knee and ankle jerks. Copper sulphate 25 mgms. t.d.s. was given. Two weeks later the tendon reflexes had returned and the foot-drop had disappeared. He developed hypo-glycaemic attacks and insulin had to be withdrawn. He was discharged without treatment after 6 weeks. A glucose tolerance test was now normal. The glycosuria, but not the neurological disturbancreappeared 3 months later.

Case 93 Female, aged 62 years. Indian from Punjab. Known diabetic for 8 years and on treatment with oral diabetic tablets. She gave a 2 weeks history of weakness and tiredness and tingling and numbness in both hands and feet, headaches and diz-

ziness. On examination the positive findings were a patch of vitiligo on the right thigh, pallor and absent knee and ankle jerks. The E.S.R. was 37 mms. in 1 hour. Liver function tests and plasma proteins were normal and the fasting blood sugar 257 mgms. per cent, rising in the glucose tolerance test to 460 mgms. with 2 per cent of sugar in the urine after 2 hours. She was treated with a 1,600 calorie diabetic diet and this had no effect on the glycosuria. She was then given dehydrocholine 500 mgms. t.d.s. and within 48 hours the glycosuria had disappeared and a random blood sugar had fallen to normal. The weakness disappeared. She was kept on this regime for a month and discharged without treatment apart from dietary restriction. A glucose tolerance test was now normal. At the end of this time she was again passing sugar and was treated with diabinese and dibotin.

Case 9<1 Female, aged 73 years. A year previously she noticed increasing shortness of breath and was found to be suffering from fibrosing alveolitis and later myxoedema. She was treated with prednisolone with some improvement in her dyspnoea, but after a year became thirsty and lost weight and was found to have diabetes mellitus with continual passage of 2 per cent of sugar in the urine. A random blood sugar at 10 a.m. was 230 mgms. per cent. The glucose tolerance test was diabetic. Serum RF was negative. Achlorhydria was present. L.F.T. normal. Serum albumin and globulin both 3.3 grams per cent. Blood count and E.S.R. normal. ANF positive. Gastric parietal cell auto-antibodies negative. Thyroglybulin tanned R.B.C. agglutination titre 1 in 25,000. Thyroid C.F.T. positive. She was rendered euthyroid with !-thyroxin. The steroids were continued as before. She was then given dehydrocholine 500 mgms. t.d.s. with immediate disappearance of thirst, polyuria and glycosuria. The blood sugar fell to normal levels. This lasted for a month after the discontinuance of the dehydrocholine.

It must be emphasized that occasional cases of mild diabetes fail to respond to either bile salts or dehydrocholine. This was so in 3 of 12 cases treated with bile salts and 2 of 12 cases treated with copper sulphate. On the other hand it was found that clotrimazole *administration had no effect on diabetes in 5* cases *in which it was tried,* even though copper and bile salts had previously controlled the disease in these cases.

XVI. The effects of anti-protozoal drugs on cases of migraine

It has been seen that collagen diseases, specially when accompanied by "fibrositis" of the neck or rheumatoid cervical spondylitis, may be accompanied by migraine, often of great frequency and intensity, or by "cluster" headaches. Moreover, migraine may be associated with eczema and asthma, which are often manifestations of collagen and auto-immune disease. Reference has been made to the frequent reports of improvement of migraine by the giving of anti-amoebic drugs. The author tried the effect of chloroquine in a number of cases of classical migraine which had resisted all other types of treatment. Nine such cases · were treated and in 7 the effect was dramatic as the headaches practically ceased immediately treatment was commenced.

Case 95 Female, aged 56 years. At the age of 36 years she began to suffer from occasional left-sided headaches, usually waking her in the early morning and lasting all day. At first these were not accompanied by visual disturbance or vomiting. They gradually increased in frequency over the next few years and began to affect the right side only at times and then to be accompanied by fortification spectra and vomiting. At the end of 3 years they were occurring 3-4 times a week and often lasted 2 days. At the age of 40 years she

had an hysterectomy for fibroids causing menorrhagia without any beneficial effect on the headaches. She found no benefit or effect on the frequency of the headaches from any form of drug and her life became completely dominated by them. She was regarded as a case of depression with paranoia. Examination showed no abnormalities except for marked tenderness on pressure over the cervical structures on both sides. The blood pressure was 130/80 roms. Serum RF and thyroid auto-antibodies were present and X-rays of the cervical spine showed the changes of rheumatoid spondylitis. Treatment with chloroquine 200 mgms. daily was commenced and her symptoms ceased immediately. Within a month she was able to begin work as a typist again after 15 years without working. Treatment was continued for a year without return of symptoms. She was followed for 4 years and remained perfectly fit.

XVII. The effects of anti-amoebic drugs on cases of myasthenia gravis

The effects of anti-amoebic drugs on the collagen-auto-immune disease, myasthenia gravis, was tried in one case as follows:-

Case 96 Male, aged 81 years. Past history nil relevant. He was admitted with a three months history of intermittent diplopia and rapid tiring of the jaws during mastication and also generalized muscular weakness in the evenings. He found his grip tended to tire rapidly. *Examination* showed right-sided ptosis and an intermittent lateral rectus palsy of the right eye. Chewing food showed a rapid weakening of the bite and this tiring was also shown by repeated pumping up· of a sphygmanometer to a fixed pressure. Intravenous injection of Tensilon abolished all these symptoms. A diagnosis of myasthenia gravis was made.

Investigations Chest X-rays and tomography of the mediastinum showed no evidence of a thymic tumour with normal heart and lung shadows. Blood count, Hb 13.2 G per 100 mls. E.S.R. 26 mms. per hour. W.B.C. 8,700 per cu. mm. L.F.T. and plasma proteins normal. P.B.I. 6.3 µG per 100 mls. Rose-Waaler and latex fixation tests negative. ANF negative. Thyroid auto-antibodies, gastric parietal cells and smooth muscle antibodies all positive.

He was treated with prostigmine 15 mgms. t.d.s. with partial relief of symptoms and then 30 mgms. t.d.s. with further relief, but the tiring of his grip was still evident. The drug was then stopped with return of symptoms and he was then given dehydrocholine 750 mgms. t.d.s. This resulted in immediate disappearance of all symptoms, including the tiring of the grip. The tablets were continued for two months and then stopped. After 6 weeks the symptoms began to return, though less severely than before. He was then given clotrimazole 100 mgms. per kilo. with immediate relief of symptoms after taking a single dose of the tablets. They remained completely absent during the six months he took the drug.

Further observations on the effects of antiprotozoal imidazole drugs in cases of rheumatoid disease

The effects of clotrimazole in cases of active rheumatoid disease was reported first by the author to the IX International Congress of Chemotherapy in 1975 and later by others from a multicentre trial to a seminar held in San Francisco in July 1977. The effects closely resemble those obtained with levamisole, another antiprotozoal drug containing an imidazole group. The results confirmed the author's findings. Otterness and Niblack (1976) and Lund-Olesen (1977) have suggested that the effects of clotrimazole on cases of active rheumatoid disease are due to the fact that the drug stimulates the adrenal glands

and the former also that it has an anti-inflammatory action. The author (Wyburn-Mason, 1976), however, pointed out that in both these papers the dosage of the drug was abnormally high and its effect on active rheumatoid disease could be obtained in a dose of 1-2 G daily, that is less than one twentieth of the doses used by the above workers. Such doses produce a concentration in the body so low that according to the figures of Otterness and Niblack there are no anti-inflammatory or adrenal stimulating effects at this level. Furthermore, the drug may be effective when either cortisone preparations or ACTH have failed to relieve the symptoms. In addition such explanations as the above authors suggest cannot explain the occurrence of an Herxheimer reaction which sometimes involves the affected tissues with clotrimazole administration.

It has been shown above that the drug tinidazole, a purely antiprotozoal substance, which consists of an imidazole group with a short side chain containing a sulphone group, can produce a dramatic effect in relieving the active inflammation in rheumatoid disease and this is often proceded by an Herxheimer reaction in which the affected tissues become more inflamed and tissues previously unknown to be involved also become inflamed. This is followed by a diminution in the inflammatory changes and a general improvement or gradual disappearance of the inflammation in the affected tissues.

It was stated above that metronidazole, an imidazole compound closely related to tinidazole and active against various protozoa, was without effect in rheumatoid disease, but repetition of the trials of this substance showed that this initial impression was false. In the original trials a dose of 200 mgms. three times daily was used. This dose had no effect. Later larger doses of the drug were used. The effects were examined in 10 cases of active rheumatoid disease which were not controlled by other drugs. Their previous treatment was continued and the metronidazole added to this. When used in doses of 400 mgms. the drug has an identical effect to that of tinidazole, either causing an exaggeration of the inflammatory changes around the joints and elsewhere followed by a disappearance of the inflammation or by a rapid diminution in the inflammatory changes without an initial increase. When first administered, either drug can cause a general influenza-like condition with shivering, fever, head and neck-ache and sweating, which may begin within a few hours of the first administration of the drug and last up to 24 hours. Because of the increase in the symptoms the administration of the drug may have to be interrupted after 7-10 days, when, after a rest, the inflammatory activity of the disease will be found to have manifestly diminished as compared with before treatment was begun. Several courses of the drug may have to be given before the maximum effect is obtained and all active inflammatory changes disappear. When administered to cases of amoebic dysentery or trichomonas infection neither tinidazole nor metronidazole cause such effects.

Later the drug was given in doses of 800 mgms. eight hourly. With this the exaggeration of the symptoms produced by the smaller dose was avoided and administration is followed by a gradual lessening of the active inflammation in the tissues beginning in about a week and gradually progressing. This dose of the drug does tend to cause nausea and perhaps vomiting after about ten days, when it has to be withdrawn for a while. The course can be repeated in about two weeks and this may require to be done 4-5 times before the full beneficial effect of the drug is obtained and all inflammatory changes disappear and do not return after the treatment is stopped.

Confirmation of these findings has been independently reported to the author by a number of American doctors in the case of metronidazole. Dr. J.M. Blount, of Philadelphia, Missouri, U.S.A., is an excellent example of the beneficial effect of metronidazole in cases of rheumatoid disease. His symptoms began as a systemic illness in his teens with muscle pain, metatarsalgia, lumbago, intercostal pains, iridocyclitis, psoriasis and eventually pains in the joints, generalized arthritis with effusions, carpal tunnel syndrome, paraesthesiae, ulcerative colitis, aseptic necrosis of a femoral head for which a prothesis was inserted, etc. He was reduced to total invalidism and took to alcohol, morphine-containing drugs, barbiturates and was a terminal case. He had had to give up his practice in March 1974 and had taken steroids for more than twenty years. He began treatment with metronidazole 750 mgms. t.d.s. and noticed subjective and objective improvements within a week with relief of soreness, stiffness, swelling and pain. The previous periods of sweating and chills gradually abated and the dysentery and tenesmus decreased day by day. The cyanosis of the feet and the paraesthesias stopped over the next six months. Nasal stuffiness and discharge ceased. His mental functions changed remarkably. The feelings of despair and hopelessness disappeared and over a period of three months he was able to stop the steroids. He now had no colitis symptoms. He took metronidazole in this dosage over four periods of eleven days with a rest between treatments. The course lasted about six months. The period of his recovery lasted eight months. He now scarcely needs to take anything except the occasional aspirin. He is now about to resume his medical practice after 3½ years. He has now treated about thirty rheumatoid arthritis patients on the same lines. The majority of them have experienced similar remarkably favourable results.

Both tinidazole and metronidazole are antiprotozoal drugs with an antiprotozoal spectrum embracing tric'homonas, various species of amoebae, giardia, etc. The occurrence of the Herxheimer reaction around the joints and the general malaise after administration followed by lessening or disappearance of the inflammatory changes affecting the joints or other tissues indicates conclusively the protozoal nature of rheumatoid disease.

Summary of the effects of antiprotozoal drugs on collagen and auto-immune diseases

It, thus, appears that all the various manifestations of active collagen and auto-immune disease, whether presenting as generalized rheumatoid arthritis, systemic lupus erythematosus or dermatomyositis or as involvement of a single organ or tissue, and including diabetes, myasthenia and hyperkeratoses, may in *early* cases *lessen or completely disappear when the patient is treated with* antiprotozoal *drugs, such as imidazole compounds, including tinidazole, metronidazole (pure antiprotozoal compounds), clotrimazole, levamisole and nitro-imidazole derivatives, bile salts , pentamid ine,* copper *salts, 4-aminoquinolines, daraprim, mepacrine* or *dehydroemetine. Many of these* drugs *produce amelioration of the rheumatoid process within 24 hours and clinical cure may be complete within 72 hours.* There may be a mild Herxheimer reaction, recalling the effect of diethylcarbamazine on cases of filariasis. None of the above antiprotozoal drugs are anti-inflammatory agents. This suggests a parasitic infection. RF, ANF and organ specific auto-antibodies may disappear from the blood gradually. These effects it must be emphasized consist of a complete reversal of the disease process in contrast to the effects of anti-inflammatory drugs.Pha nquone (Entobex) , suramin and furamide are ineffective. The swelling of the thyroid gland in Hashimoto's thyroiditis and the accompanying hypothyroidism may be re-lieved in early cases. Idiopathic Addison's disease may be cured. The atrophic changes in the gastric mucosa and diabetic neuropathy of long-standing are not affected by treatment with such anti-protozoal drugs, though early diabetic neuropathy may be cured. In subjects exhibiting no clinical lesions, but RF or auto-antibodies in the blood treatment with these substances often causes the antibodies and RF to disappear gradually. None of these diseases respond to antibiotics, as they would do if caused by bacteria. All the *drugs effective* in the above *conditions are antiprotozoal and in particular anti-amoebic* or *shown* to *be* active *against limax* amoebae. Most significant is the finding that imidazole *drugs, bile salts,* copper *sulphate, pentamidine and dehydro-emetine produce immediate effects and these may be evident within a* **few** *hours, recalling the action* of *an antibiotic in a bacterial disease.*

Conclusions on the nature of collagen and auto-immune diseases (rheumatoid disease)

In the foregoing pages it has been concluded that collagen and auto-immune diseases form, in fact, one disease, comparable to syphilis, in which all the tissues of the body are affected, but the brunt of the disease may fall on one or several organs, such as the thyroid gland, gastric mucosa, etc. RF, ANF and various auto-antibodies may be present in the blood in any form of this condition. It has been pointed out that: –

1) RF, ANF and various tissue antibodies may be present in the blood in many infections, especially leprosy, and in particularly high concentrations, comparable to those found in cases of rheumatoid disease, in cases of infections with protozoa, such as malaria and trypanosomiasis. Successful treatment of these diseases causes the RF, ANF and tissue auto-antibodies to

disappear.

2) Collagen-auto-immune (rheumatoid) diseases appear to be an infection.

3) Free-living (limax) amoebae have been isolated from all cases of these diseases examined.

4) Many substances known to be amoebaestatic or amoebaecidal to limax amoebae may completely and rapidly relieve all the manifestation of local or generalized rheumatoid (collagen-auto-immune) disease and result in the disappearance of all the abnormal antibodies from the blood, including RF and ANF. This effect may be complicated by an Herxheimer reaction indicating an organismal cause for the diseases.

5) Phenomena closely resembling those of rheumatoid disease and including *vasculitis* result from injection of free-living amoebae into lower animals in which the organism can often not be distinguished in the tissues.

Thus, all Koch's postulates as to the *causation of collagen-auto-immune* disease by *strains* or *species of free-living amoebae are satisfied.* These can sometimes be demonstrated by special methods. The various serum factors, such as RF, ANF and organ specific auto-antibodies must be produced in the body by stimulation by the antigens of the organisms and, since all, some or none may occur in any case of collagen-auto-immune disease, it seems that the causative organisms must differ antigenically with strain or species. Different species of amoebae must possess antigens common to certain tissue cells, such as thyroid, gastric parietal cells, striated muscle and adrenal cortical cells. In subjects in whom such factors are present in the serum without obvious lesions it seems the infection is latent. Most significant is the finding that while copper salts, bile salts, pentamidine and imidazole drugs are all rapidly effective in relieving and curing most cases of rheumatoid disease and in preventing recurrence, in a small proportion of cases no beneficial

effect is obtained. Similarly in most cases of diabetes the manifestations of the disease disappear rapidly when treated by copper and bile salts, yet clotrimazole was found to be without such an effect. This suggests that, if an organismal cause for the manifestations exists, then different organisms or different strains or species of the organism are responsible for different manifestations of collagen-auto-immune disease.

Free-living amoebae live on the earth and tend to proliferate in stagnant warm pools, such as bathing pools. Three cases in the author's experience are thus of significance. A fit man of 34 years was walking in a field near Toronto when an insect flew from the ground and lodged in one nostril. He experienced severe irritation and a foul smell and developed a foul smelling discharge lasting 3 weeks. Within a day or two he developed generalized arthropathy and dysentery lasting 11 months and severe sweats, especially at night, with a pyrexia. No cause for the dysentery was found. Within 9 months the serum RF was found to be positive. Two years later scleroderma began and became generalized. A second fit man, aged 44 years ploughed a dusty field in the Middle West of U.S.A. and got much dust in his nostrils. Next morning he woke with generalized rigidity and polyarthropathy a nd high temperature and sweats and later developed RF in the serum. A fit girl aged 15 years, swam in a little used stagnant bathing pool in Puerto Rico. That evening she suffered coryza, pyrexia, sweating and next day generalized polyarthritis eventually proving to be of rheumatoid nature. Such cases suggest that rheumatoid disease arises from infection from the ground or stagnant water.

It *seems highly probable that various* species *of free-living amoebae are the aetiological agents of the above disturbances,* but different species show different tropisms and so affect different organs. While in general collagen-auto-immune diseases l:how every gradation and combination with one another, they are not due to a single organism, but to a number of similar organisms. Such a parasitic infection would explain the urticaria, asthma and eosinophilia observed in many cases of collagen or auto-immune disease as an allergic response to its presence and similar Herxheimer reactions in the patients on treatment with imidazole drugs. It will be recalled that no explanation of the effect of chloroquine, daraprim and mepacrine in cases of rheumatoid arthritis and other collagen diseases was found by Nielson and Lansbury (1961), Hiraki and Kimura (1964) and Sams (1971). The failure *to* find such organisms in ordinary sections of tissues is due to the fact that they appear like macrophages. In experiments in lower animals in which amoebae are injected a similar failure to demonstrate the organisms is found. They may be shown up, however, by immunofluorescent techniques as shown above. Experimentally it has been seen that infection with limax amoebae produces an amoebic pyelitis in animals, while an abacterial *pyelonephritis* has been seen to be common in rheumatoid disease and it must be supposed that in the latter it is produced by the causative amoeba.

Paget's disease appears to be a limax amoebic osteitis produced by a special strain or species of amoeba.

Ulcerative colitis and its arthropathy forms part of the collagen-auto-immune spectrum. In this condition RF is not usually present in the blood. The colitis and the arthropathy respond to drugs which inhibit limax amoebae. The condition would thus appear to be due to a species of free-living limax amoeba different from that causing rheumatoid arthritis. The organism, like E. histolytica, shows a tropism for the large intestine, presumably not affecting the small intestine because the trophozoites are killed by bile salts in this situation.

In cases of *myasthenia gravis* substances active against limax amoebae produce a rapid disappearance of symptoms and if treatment is prolonged a cure of the disease. It seems that in this condition there is a substance derived from the amoebae which affects the neuro-muscular junction. This appears to be the serum blocking factor reported by Ringel et al. (1975) and Pinching et al. (1976).

Many cases of *diabetes* respond immediately to chloroquine, copper and bile salts, but none were found to benefit from clotrimazole administration. It seems, therefore, that while many cases of diabetes are due to limax amoebae infection, the organisms concerned differ from those causing rheumatoid disease.

Ankylosing spondylitis and psoriatic arthropathy are generally regarded as separate conditions from rheumatoid arthritis, though they have many features in common. They could well be due to different strains or species of limax amoebae from that causing rheumatoid arthritis.

Species of limax amoebae are present in the gastrointestinal tracts and faeces of most individuals and animals. They appear to be present in the tissues of almost every adult human individual and grazing animals. In this respect the situation resembles that in endemic areas of malaria, amoebic dysentery or trypanosomiasis, where many subjects are infected with and carry the infecting protozoon without showing signs of disease. In other words rheumatoid disease is latent in everyone. With increase in age so there occurs increasing evidence of infection by the organism, shown by the increasing tendency to collagen and auto-immune diseases with age. It seems probable that different strains of limax amoebae must possess different invasive properties and also that there is a difference in the resistance of different subjects to invasion by the organism. Moreover, recurrent infection by different strains of the organism must occur throughout life and thus, if these are pathogenic, so collagen or auto-immune

—208

diseases may occur at any time in life. Probably infection may occur many years before clinical manifestations of disease appear, possibly as a result of lowered resistance. Infection may occur at any time and may even be congenital (see below).

As indicated previously limax amoebae may be recovered from the tissues of some apparently healthy patients. Their presence is shown by a number of observations made by the author. Metallic copper and copper preparations, tinidazole, metronidazole and levamisole are all effective in killing various protozoa, including amoebae. When administered to a patient with rheumatoid disease, they may, in fact, cause an Herxheimer reaction with exaggeration of the joint inflammation before the inflammatory changes die down. In apparently normal patients the same effects may occur with any of these substances. The author suggested that a healthy female of 45 years exhibiting no evidence of disease should wear a prophylactic specially made wide copper bracelet in order to obtain maximum absorption of copper into the body. Within a few days this produced pain and stiffness of the hands and knees and rheumatoid swelling of the ankles with tenosynovitis around the ankles and intense burning and hotness of the feet, which only gradually died down after taking off the bracelet. This suggests an Herxheimer reaction to the presence in the oody of un:::uspected organisms (amoebae) sensitive to copper in a symptomless patient. Exactly the same result occurred when tinidazole or metronidazole was administered to several apparently healthy patients, the reaction lasting up to two weeks *to* be followed by complete disappearance of any symptoms. Segal et al. (1977) reported transient inflammatory arthropathy when using levamisole in patients not suffering from rheumato:d disease. The collective findings are confirmation of the presence in the "normal" body of a protozoal organism, similar to that causing rheumatoid disease.

It must be stressed that the effects of anti-amoebic agents, such as copper sulphate and dehydrocholine on rheumatoid disease may be only short-lived after cessation of their administration, suggesting • that they do not kill the amoebae, but temporarily inhibit them, that is, they are amoebaestatic not amoebaecidal in the dosages it is possible to use in man. Clotrimazole, however, in high dosage over a long period may abolish all manifestations of rheumatoid disease which do not return when the drug is stopped. It may be it sterilizes the tissues of the amoeba. These considerations raise the possibility of a *cure* of rheumatoid disease, Hashimoto's thyroiditis, Sjtigren's syndrome, ulcerative colitis, diabetes and myasthenia using long courses of anti-amoebic drugs. It will be noted that many of the lesions produced by limax amoebae, such as Hashimoto's thyroiditis, atrophic gastritis, ulcerative colitis and Paget's disease, are premalignant.

In this connection the protozoal disease, African trypanosomiasis, is of interest. The causative organism produces an exoantigen which can change with remission in the infection, thereby favouring the long survival of the organism. In the advanced disease where lesions are maximal, the smallest numbers of trypanosomes are found. It has, therefore, been concluded that the lesions are due to an *exaggerated immune response* in the host, rather than to any direct effect of this relatively non-toxic organism (Ormerod, 1957) . In many animals latent infections with trypanosomes exist without producing any signs or symptoms (Wenyon, 1926). *In other words pathological changes are only produced by the* protozoa *in sensitive individual animals.* The response to such infections is often genetically control!ed (Leading Article, Brit. med. J., 1969, 4, 317). In other cases increase in virulence of the organism may occur and when this happens, the organism becomes pathogenic.

This phenomenon occurring with infections resembles the finding that certain individuals react unusually to drugs and this again may have an immunological or genetic basi (Bearn, 1971). Such conclusions seem to apply to protozoal infections in general. It follows that infection with Iimax amoebae may exist in the body without producing lesions, symptoms or serological evidence of their presence in subjects who are not sensitive to its existence in the body. When subjects are sensitive to the infecting organism, that is it produces a pathological reaction, the latter may be accompanied by an eosinophilia commonly found in collagen and auto-immune disease. In other words, when it produces manifestations of disease, these are cell-hypersensitivity reactions, so that proponents of both infective and immunological theories of the causation of symptoms of collagen and auto-immune diseases are correct. Such sensitivity is manifested by the urticaria and asthma w.hich mav occur as part of the collagen allu auto•1mu\une diseases. In such sensitive subjects there are often found allergies to many other substances, such as drugs, a common finding in cases of intrinsic asthma, Sjtigren's syndrome and rhinitis. In other words sensitivity to limax amoebae is but one manifestatitm of a condition of hypersensitivity to many different agents, a state often genetically determined. In this respect the HL A antigens are of interest. They are a group of histocompatability antigens on the surface membranes of human leucocytes, platelets and fibroblasts and are deterrnined by two closely linked autosomal genes on a pair of chromosomes (6). The many genes in the HL A region are concerned with graft versus host reactions, transplantation antigens and immune responses (Leading Article, Brit. med. J., 1975, 2, 238). HLA-A8 is associated with coeliac disease, derrnatitis herpetiformis and myasthenia gravis. The striking associations of HL A antigens are with the rheumatic diseases, while individuals possessing HLA-A8 and W15 tissue antigens are prone to develop insulin-dependent diabetes (Cudworth et al. (1975) and HLA-B27 antigens are associated with the development of ankylosing spondylitis, ulcerative colitis and iritis. Pachman et al. (1977) point out the increased frequency of HLA-B8 tissue antigens associated with dermatomyositis, dermatitis herpetiformis, coeliac disease, myasthenia gravis, Sjogren's syndrome, idiopathic Addison's disease, chronic active hepatitis, insulin-dependent diabetes mellitus and thyrotoxicosis (literature). They suggest that these disease' may be due to an increased susceptibility to an exciting agent or altered immune response to such an agent.

Entry into and spread of limax amoebae infection in the body

Limax amoebae being *universally* present in human and animal faeces, it appears that the entrance of cysts or trophozoites of Iimax amoebae into the body occurs from the environment in the air and from soil or raw food or milk via the mouth, nose, conjunctivae, pharynx and lungs. On becoming invasive Jimax amoebae may enter the body by way of any of these organs. They appear to spread directly from the mouth .up the ducts of the salivary glands to invade the substance of these glands and result in the development of *Sjogr en-Mikulicz's* syndrome. This may be preceded by recurrent swelling of the salivary glands, so-called *"auto-immune parotitis"*. The tissue invasion may also occur by way of the tonsils and adenoids, which develop chronic reactive hyperplasia and local lymph node swelling. lt seems highly probable that the *hyperplasia of tonsillar and adenoidal tissue which occurs in childhood marks the entrance of the organism into the body and is the first manifestation of infection.* Extension to the nasal mucosa produces *catarrhal* or *atrophic rhinitis, Eustachian salpingitis* ' *anCil dea fness* and to the pharynx, larynx and lungs inflammation followed by atrophy of the mucosa of these organs, often

—210

with asthma *and chronic bronchitis*. Direct spread down the oesophagus to the stomach presumably leads to *oesophagitis and gastritis,* which may later become atrophic in type. It mlty well be that *local* spread from the floor of the mouth may extend to the thyroid and parathyroid glands.

It has been seen above that experimental infections with amoebae occur by gaining access to *blood vessels* from which the amoebae may escape into the perivascular tissues producing an *arteritis and peri-arteritis* as they pass through the vessel wall. Since vasculitis and peri-arteritis are common in collagen and auto-immune diseases, it seems highly probable that limax amoebae spread in a similar manner and *migrate through the vessel walls.* Lymphadenopathy also occurs frequently in collagen and auto-immune disease. It, therefore, appears that *lymphatic spread* also occurs in this condition.

Localization of collagen and auto-immune diseases to certain tissues

Different subjects suffering from rheumatoid arthritis may exhibit different auto-antibodies, RF or ANF in the serum in various concentrations or no antibodies are demonstrable at all. It thus appears that either different strains or species of limax amoebae have different antigenic properties or different individuals show different antibody responses to the same organism. Collagen and auto-immune diseases may have a major effect on one organ, for example gastric mucosa, thyroid or colon, and tend to affect the same organ or tissues in certain families, producing atrophic gastritis, pernicious anaemia, thyroid disease and diabetes. In such cases auto-antibodies against the especially affected organ tend to be present in the serum of the patient and of unaffected relatives. Since organ-specific auto-antibodies in the blood in cases of auto-immune disease appear to play a part in causing the lesions in specific organs, so these lesions could be produced by special strains or species of limax amoebae giving rise to antibodies active against certain organs, and since any given species of the amoebae may be local in its geographical distribution, so families affected by these species might be expected to have the same organ disease.

Addendum: Reference has been made earlier to the fact that infectious organisms introduced into the body tend to localize in areas of trauma or chronic inflammation. This obviously applies to amoebic infection, since not infrequently rheumatoid disease starts in an injured joint.

Chapter VI

The mode of production of certain features of collagen and auto-immune diseases

The effects of lesions of the hypothalamus and the neighbouring reticular formation on bodily and cerebral function

The hypothalamus directly or indirectly controls all functions of the body, including the cerebrum, the discharges of the autonomic nervous system, the subcortical motor centres and the pituitary secretions and also forms certain neurohormones. Lesions of the hypothalamus and third ventricle region, whether from tumours, vascular disturbances, trauma, damage from infections, such as encephalitis lethargica, or from other conditions, may be associated clinically with a great variety of bodily and cerebral disturbances. These are considered by Gagel (1936), Riddoch (1938), Fulton (1943), Wyburn-Mason (1949) and Walsh (1957). They include the following:–

1) Disturbances in *fat metabolism.* There may be gross obesity, which is often in part due to increased ingestion of food (bulimia), but which also occurs in the absence of such excess appetite. On the other hand marked loss of fat with extreme emaciation and anorexia may result from hypothalamic lesions.

2) Disturbances in *carbohydrate metabolism.* There may be diminished sugar tolerance, glycosuria and polyuria accompanied by marked wasting, loss of fat and insulin resistance. Conversely and abnormal sensitivity to insulin an hypoglycaemia may complicate hypothalamic lesions and are often associated with obesity.

3) Disturbances in *protein metabolism* with excess output of urea may complicate diabetes due to hypothalamic lesions.

4) Disturbances of temperature regulation resulting in either hyperthermia or hypothermia.

5) Changes in the *basal metabolic rate* which may be increased or decreased to a marked extent and are independent of changes in thyroid function.

6) Disturbances in *sweat* secretion. This may be excessive or diminished.

7) Disturbances in *water excretion.* These occur when the supra-optic nuclei, the tuber cinereum or the posterior lobe of the pituitary are affected, producing the condition of diabetes insipidus. This is often accompanied by hyperthermia and a rise in the basal metabolic rate. On the contrary hypothalamic lesions may result in oliguria (diabetes tenuifluus).

8) Increased *adrenaline secretion* by the suprarenal may result from lesions of the posterior hypothalamus.

9) Disturbances in *skin pigmentation.*

10) *Hypertrichosis.*

11) Disturbances in *pupillary function.* The pupils may be unequal in size.

12) Disturbances in *lacrimal secretion.* There may be an increased or diminished secretion of tears.

13) Disturbance in *salivary secretion,* which may be diminished or excessive.

14) Disturbances in *bladder function.* The bladder may be overactive quite apart from polyuria.

15) Disturbances in *cardiac and vasomotor function.* Attacks of p9.roxysmal tachycardia or extra-systoles may result from hypothalamic lesions. In some cases marked vasodilatation and oedema may be found in areas of skin. This sometimes

occurs in attacks. In other cases arteriolar vasoconstriction and hypertension are found. Thus, paroxysmal hypertension and glucose intolerance may be associated with cerebral tumours or concussion (Stalder, 1972).

16) Disturbances of *respiratory rhythm.* Various respiratory disturbances, such as Cheyne-Stokes breathing and hiccoughing, may complicate lesions of this region.

17) Disturbances in function in the gastro-intestinal *tract.* These consist of ulceration of the upper alimentary tract, hypermotility and hypertonicity of the gut and hyperchlorhydria. Experimentally it has been shown in dogs that lesions of the hypothalamus produce atrophic states, haemorrhages and gangrenous changes in all tissues of the body, including the bowel.

18) Disturbances in *sleep.* These may consist of hypersomnia, insomnia or attacks of narcolepsy or cataplexy.

19) Changes in the number of circulating *blood cells.* Increase in the red cell count, alterations in the numbers of white cells in the absence of infection or haemorrhages may occur with lesions of the hypothalamus. This may result in polycythaemia or leucocytosis. These may be found in association with other manifestations of hypothalamic disturbance.

20) Disturbances in development and function of the *secondary sex characters,* resulting either in pubertas praecox or failure of development of secondary sex characters and infantilism.

21) Epilepsy. These constitute so-called centro-encephalic epilepsy and may be of various types, both generalized and localized. Attacks emanating from the hypothalamic region may be accompanied by various manifestations of hypothalamic disturbance, such as flushing, slow respiration, lacrimation, sweating, salivation, exophthalmos, hiccoughing and a strong rapid pulse (diencephalic autonomic epilepsy) .

22) Changes in the *electroencephalogram.* The electroencephalogram usually shows widespread abnormalities in all areas of the cortex which may resemble those occurring in deep sleep. In other cases all waves disappear from the electro-encephalogram, indicating that lesions in the hypothalamic region alter function in all areas of the cortex.

23) *Mental and intellectual disturbances.* Lesions of the hypothalamus and third ventricle regions are always associated with mental and intellectual changes. Lesions of the anterior parts of the hypothalamus tend to produce states of excitement, while those of the posterior part cause lethargy, indifference or a tendency towards catatonia. Stimulation of the posterior portion may induce all the signs of sham rage in animals. Lesions of the hypothalamus elicit emotional, intellectual and personality changes and psychoses which may be summarized as follows:-

a) Psychotic manifestations, including Korsakoff's psychosis, confusion, disorientation, hallucinations, manic excitement, depression and a schizophrenic syndrome.

b) Intellectual impairment is constant and may reach a stage of dementia.

c) Personality changes consisting of loss of inhibitions, carelessness in habits, amorousness and indifference to surroundings.

d) Emotional excitement is constant. There may be manic-like reactions, often episodic and lasting only as long as the stimulus. There are often swings of mood, such as alternating depression and excitement, or emotional lability, uncontrolled laughter and crying, feelings of anxiety, apathy and depression and irrascibility. These effects are independent of the previous mental make-up of the patient.

e) A state of akinetic mutism affecting both intellect and emotion producing a state of "arrested consciousness".

The vascular system of the hypothalamus and the pathways of pituitary secretion

The blood vessels of the pituitary and hypothalamus are arranged as a portal system and those of the anterior, intermediate and posterior lobes pass up in the infundibular stalk to be distributed to the various nuclei of the hypothalamus, including the supra-optic (Wislocki and King, 1936). They are surrounded by a sheath. The colloid bodies of the pars intermedia and tuberalis are often present in the portal vessels and their sheaths. Colloid is seen in contact with the unmyelinated fibres in the tuber and infundibulum and has been observed to pass between the ependymal cells of the third ventricle. There is a great body of evidence indicating that the secretions of all portions of the pituitary pass into the third ventricle, in the walls of which they can often be found. The action of such secretions on the cells of the hypothalamus was demonstrated by Cushing, who instilled extracts of the posterior pituitary into the third ventricle and caused a general stimulation of hypothalamic activity. He found that no such effects were produced when the patient was under an anaesthetic or if the hypothalamus was destroyed by disease (Wyburn-Mason, 1949). He concluded that the secretions of the anterior and posterior pituitary produced their effects on target tissues partly by their action on centres in the walls of the third ventricle. Other endocrine secretions, such as insulin, thyroxin and steroid bodies, also have such an effect. The general effects of intoxications and infections, such as anorexia, Joss of weight, fever, rise in B.M.R., tachycardia, changes in the blood corpuscles, changes in blood pressure, disturbances in water metabolism, hyperglycaemia and glycosuria, etc., appear to be produced, at any rate in part, by toxic substances derived from the infection in the blood acting on the hypothalamic centres (Wyburn-Mason, 1949). *The same effects must be expected from infections with limax amoebae.*

The possible aetiology of diabetes mellitus

The nature of diabetes mellitus occurring in man in the absence of obvious disease of the pancreas is unknown. This is especially so because in most early cases of the disease no lesion is found in the pancreas. It seems certain that in long-standing diabetics exhaustion of the ,8-cells of the pancreas occurs. The condition has, therefore, been ascribed to one or more of the following disturbances:-

a) Abnormality of pancreatic ,8-cell function.

b) Secretion of an abnormal form of insulin.

c) Increased demand for the hormone.

d) Imbalance between production and demand for the hormone.

e) The existence of plasma antagonists to insulin seen, for example in insulin-resistant diabetics and in the "synalbumin" of Vallance-Owen (1966).

f) Resistance of peripheral cells to insulin action, for example in obesity.

g) Destruction of insulin at an increased rate.

h) The existence of antibodies which inhibit the action of insulin.

However, diabetes may be due to damage to or dysfunction of the hypothalamus from various causes. Moreover, it is well-known that diabetes may be precipitated, unmasked or aggravated by infections of any sort in which hypothalamic function is altered. Furthermore, in normal subjects transient hyperglycaemia and glycosuria may occur in acute infections. In addition diabetes occurs in association with any manifestation of collagen or auto-immune disease, which appears to be due to infection with limax amoebae. Moreover, it has been shown above that diabetes can often be lessened in severity or abolished slowly by treatment with chloro-quine, or immediately by bile or copper salts, but not by clotrimazole, all of which are anti-amoebic substances. In fact, *dia-*

betes may, thus, *commonly be a manifestation of disturbance of hypothalamic function by chronic infection with limax amoebae other than those causing rheumatoid disease*. This would explain why other infections or emotional upset, which also disturb the hypothalamus, may cause diabetes or may aggravate pre-existing diabetes and why in most diabetics it is unusual to find any lesions in the pancreas. It would seem possible that in cases of chronic infection with limax amoebae there also occurs an interference with the normal function or carriage of insulin by the presence of an abnormal protein or other substance in the blood, perhaps the "synalbumin" of Valiance-Owen. This is perhaps a metabolite derived from limax amoebae circulating in the blood. This is in accord with the recent Nobel Prize-winning work of Dr. Rosalyn Yalow, who showed that in maturity-onset diabetics the blood contains normal or larger than normal quantities of insulin.

The causation of many cases of thyrotoxicosis

The pathogenesis of thyrotoxicosis is unknown. It was at one time thought to be due to increased stimulation of the thyroid gland by TSH hormone from the pituitary, but the evidence is against this. Evidence that thyrotoxicosis is a manifestation of collagen and auto-immune disease has been adduced above, but the exact nature of the condition is still not clear. The theory most favoured until recently is that there exists in the blood a substance known as long-acting thyroid stimulator (LATS), believed to be an antibody, the source of which is unknown. However, this cannot be demonstrated in all cases of thyrotoxicosis. Its role in the causation of thyrotoxicosis is now dismissed (Solomon and Chopra, 1972 Werner, 1972).

Thyrotoxicosis may occur with various changes in the thyroid gland, including Hashimoto's thyroiditis, nodular goitre and diffuse hyperplasia. It may exist, however, in the complete absence of the thyroid gland, as, for example, when complete thyroidectomy was formerly practiced for a recurrence of the condition after partial thyroidectomy (Kocher, 1919-27; Crotti, 1938). In such cases the signs are a mixture of those of myxoedema and thyrotoxicosis. Again, thyrotoxicosis may develop after pituitary ablation for carcinoma of the breast (Baron and Gurling, 1959; Gurling et al., 1959). Hence, it appears that neither the pituitary (Werner, 1972), nor the thyroid gland are essential for the development of thyrotoxicosis.

In cases of thyrotoxicosis there occurs a general stimulation of the autonomic nervous system and not infrequently glycosuria, a rise in the B.M.R., loss of weight, tremor, exophthalmos, lid-lag and retraction and oedema of the eyelids, all of which may result from hypothalamic stimulation. Thyrotoxicosis also occurs in cases of Albright's syndrome or lipodystrophy (lipoatrophic diabetes) when it is thought to arise from hypothalamic overactivity. The case reported by Greene and Oliver (1968) is of interest in relation to the causation of the symptoms of thyrotoxicosis. These authors report the case of a woman of 22 years who developed obstruction of the aqueduct of Sylvius and all the signs of thyrotoxicosis, including exophthalmos unequal on the two sides, lid-lag, an enlarged thyroid gland, nervousness, a feeling of tremulousness, but no excess sweating. Tests showed overactivity of the thyroid gland. All these manifestations rapidly returned to normal when surgical drainage of the third ventricle was carried out, the eye signs, thyroid swelling and abnormal thyroid function tests disappearing. Furthermore, complete disappearance of the manifestations of thyrotoxicosis may result from treatment with the ,8-blocking agent propranolol, thyroid function returning to normal (see McLarty et al., 1973). Such observations suggest that thyrotoxicosis arises from overactivity of the hypo-

Addendum: Muggeo M, ˙r JG, Ham˙ n LC and ˙ w England J. Med. 1979, 300, 477-480- Treatment by

thalamus, the thyroid disturbance being secondary. Emerson and Utiger (1972) and Pittman {1972} also suggest such a possibility. Solomon and Chopra (1972) also consider the role of the nervous system in the aetiology of thyrotoxicosis. The hypothalamic disturbance would appear to be produced in many cases by irritation by secretions from limax amoebae as part of collagen and auto-immune disease. Such a conception is in keeping with the frequent finding that in other cases thyrotoxicosis follows emotional stress which involves hypothalamic stimulation. It would appear that in some cases of thyrotoxicosis hypothalamic function has become autonomous and escaped from normal control. The thyroid overactivity is presumably secondary to this and is a factor in causing the continued hypothalamic overactivity since thyroidectomy may cause a disappearance of the symptoms of thyrotoxicosis. In addition it has been shown that the ocular disturbances of "endocrine exophthalmos" appear to be due at least in part to limax amoebae infiltration of the orbital tissues, since as shown above anti-amoebic drugs may cause their disappearance, while thyroidectomy may not benefit, but exacerbate the condition.

Primary gonadal failure with limax amoebae infection

Sexual precocity or infantilism and failure to menstruate may be features of hypothalamic lesions. Attention has been drawn to the fact that in association with collagen or auto-immune diseases, such as thyroid diseases and diabetes, there may be a late menarche and/or early menopause or failure to menstruate at all when the onset of the collagen or auto-immune disease occurs early in life. Subjects are often obese. In these cases usually no abnormality is found in the ovaries and it is tempting to suppose that the presence of infection with limax amoebae results in

the appearance in the blood of a substance which either inactivates the ovarian secretions or the pituitary gonadotrophic hormone or disturbs hypothalamic control of the gonads in exactly the same way as it does insulin in cases of diabetes.

The mode of production of leukoderma and melanoderma in cases of collagen and auto-immune disease

Disturbances in skin pigmentation and polycythaemia can be produced by hypothalamic lesions. The same disturbances are also manifestations of collagen and auto-immune disease, but their manner of causation has not been elicited. It is tempting to suppose that the above disturbances occurring in cases showing evidence of infection with limax amoebae are the result of the accompanying disturbance of hypothalamic function. Since expansion and contraction of the melanophores in animals and probably in man is under nervous control (Wyburn-Mason, 1949), in the case of *leukoderma and melanoderma* the patchy distribution on the body could perhaps be explained by a patchy disturbance in the innervation of the melanophores of the skin from hypothalamic centres.

The possible aetiology of certain neurological diseases

Paralysis agitans may be accompanied by loss of emotional control, mental disturbances, loss of weight, polyuria, sialorrhoea, vasomotor disturbance, cold extremities, hot flushes, hyperidrosis, oedema and cyanosis of the extremities and excess sebaceous secretions, all manifestations of hypothalamic disturbance. Certain drugs, such as tranquillizers, and toxins, such as metal compounds (Wilson, 1940), may result in the appearance of Parkinsonism without producing pathological changes in the brain and the syndrome usually disappears when the drug is stopped. In early cases of paralysis agitans changes in the brain are often minimal. In 'fact, the eminent neuropathologist, the late Dr. J.G. Greenfield, used to say jokingly that it was an hysterical manifestation! Moreover, the symptoms of Parkinsonism are often relieved temporarily by acute pyrexial illness in which function in the hypothalamus and related centres is altered. Later organic changes are found in the brain. These facts suggest that idiopathic paralysis agitans may be the result in the early stages of dysfunction rather than organic changes in the central nervous system. Since an infection may cause postencephalitic Parkinsonism and syphilis may lead to Parkinsonism, it has recently been suggested that an infection, possibly with a slow virus, might be the cause of idiopathic paralysis agitans. Similarly amyotrophic lateral sclerosis has been suggested to be of infective and slow virus nature. Yoshiro Yase (1972) states that pathologically and clinically the fundamental changes in the central nervous system in amyotrophic sclerosis, paralysis agitans and presenile and senile dementia form part of an ALS and/or Parkinsonian-dementia complex and fade into one another. They are part of the aging process occurring in selected areas of the central nervous system. This raises the question as to whether infection with limax amoebae which increases with age is the cause of these conditions. Behan et al. (1976) suggest an association between HLA A2 and A28 histocompatability_ antigens and motoneurone disease which may indicate a special genetic susceptibility of motor neurones to the secretions of these organisms.

A description of the pathological changes -in the central nervous system and peripheral nerves in cases of collagen and auto-immune diseases has been given. Reference was also made to various neurological, psychoneurotic and psychotic disturbances which may be associated with these changes. Attention was drawn to the frequency with which cases of rheuma-

toid arthritis developed *Parkinsonism* in the series of cases in the geriatric series (10 of 100 cases). This was also found in Case 1 and in one case in this series there was associated *motoneurone disease.* In this respect Wilson (1940) and Bing (1939) both mention rheumatoid disease as preceding paralysis agitans. This again raises the question as to whether paralysis agitans is due to limax amoebae infection. The effect of anti-amoebic substances, bile salts and copper sulphate, on cases of paralysis agitans was, therefore, tried on five cases of paralysis agitans with a varying duration of symptoms. In none of them was there any evidence suggesting a previous encephalitis. Two of them showed rheumatoid changes in the toes, Two of them showed the presence of ANF, one gastric parietal cell and another thyroid auto-antibodies in the serum. Two had achlorhydria. In two of the cases no tremor was present. These two responded best to treatment. The effects of copper sulphate and bile salts were similar in nature and degree in the dosage used. They caused a general lessening of the rigidity and in the paucity of movement. Walking tended to revert to normal. The "demarche a petit pas" disappeared a nd in early cases the patient began to swing his arms and to smile spontaneously again. When present, the tremor tended to lessen and the patient volu nteered he felt very well. After leaving off the treat ment, the condition reverted to what it was previously in about six weeks.

Case 97 Male, aged 59 years. He gave a six month history of uselessness of the right hand. On examination he had typical Parkinsonian facies with paucity of movement of the face (Fig. 52). He did not smile spontaneously. No tremor was present, but he did not swing the right arm in walking. There was increased tone in the right arm. He was treated with dehydrocholine 1 G t.d.s. There was rapid improvement in his mobility. His gait returned to normal and spontaneous smiling

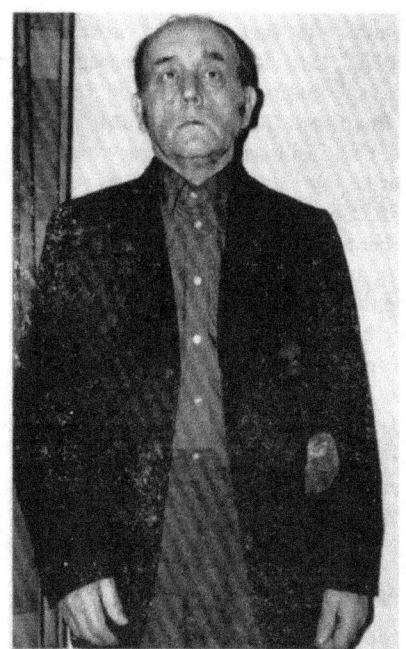

Fig. 52-A

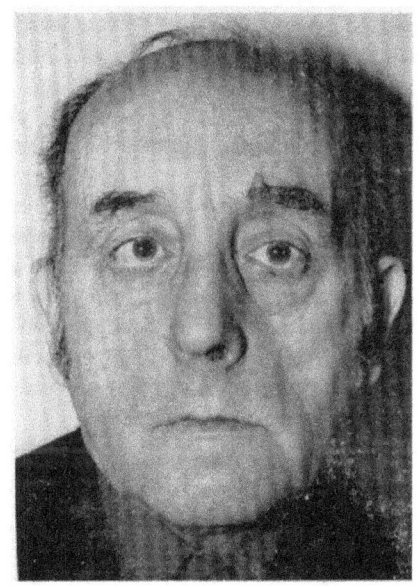

Fig. 52-B

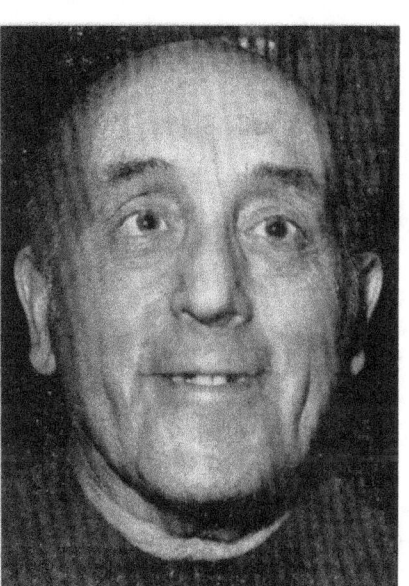

fig. 52-C

Fig. 52 Male, aged 59 years. Parkinsonism of six months
duration showing typical posture and facial appearances at
"A" and "B". Treated with bile salts for 2 weeks which
produced relief of all manifestation of the disease and a return
to spontaneous smiling, "C" (Case 97).

218 —

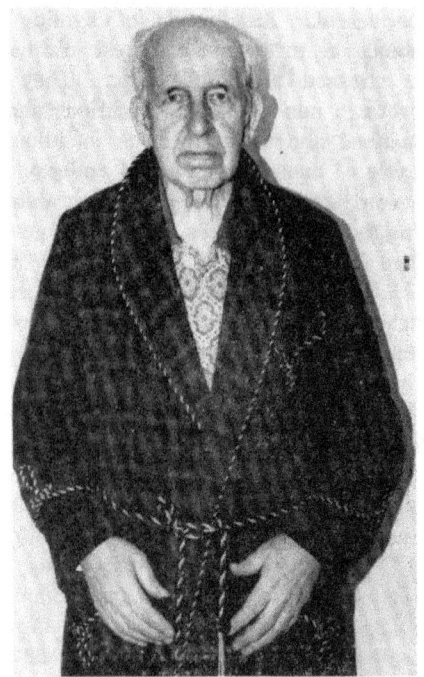

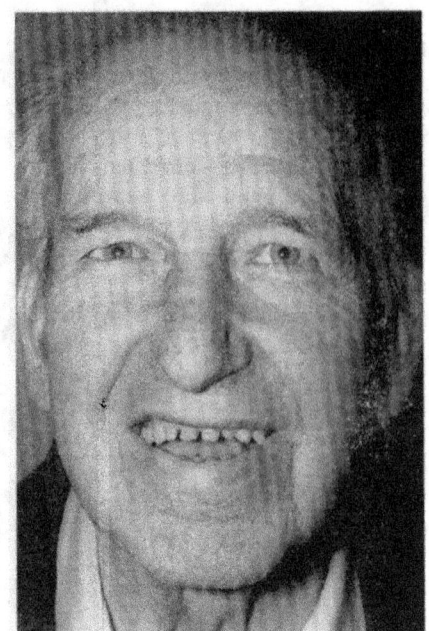

Fig. 53-A   Fig. 53-B

Fig. 53 Male, aged 73 years. Parkinsonism of two years
duration. Typical expressionless face and posture seen at "A".
After 2 weeks treatment with bile salts he was almost symptomless and exhibited normal spontaneous movements of the face'
"B" (Case 98).

reappeared (Fig. 52). Treatment was continued for 5 weeks and then was stopped.
His symptoms had returned after six
weeks.

Case 98 Male, aged 73 years. He had
been under treatment for rheumatoid arthritis for 4 years. He was noticed to exhibit Parkinsonian signs during treatment
and showed no tremor, but loss of spontaneous movement and shuffling gait, increase in muscle tone and a typical posture (Fig. 53). Dehydrocholine vastly
lessened these disturbances (Fig. 53).

It seems, therefore, that in early cases
of paralysis agitans the disturbances are
not due to organic disease, but to alterations in nervous function in the region of
the hypothalamus and corpus striatum
produced by substances liberated from

limax amoebae. In early cases the effect
of these substances can be reversed.
Later organic changes occur and the symptoms cannot be relieved by treatment.

Since some cases of presenile dementia
appear related to and merge with cases
of paralysis agitans, it seems highly probable, therefore, that many examples of
presenile dementia result from limax amoebae infection too.

"Idiopathic" psychoneuroses, affective psychoses and epilepsy

It has been seen that dementia or any
type of affective psychotic disorder or
epilepsy and sleep disturbance may be
produced by hypothalamic lesions. They
may also be produced in a previously nor-

mal subject by intoxications or infections, such as pneumonia, typhoid, influenza or alcoholism, presumably by their effect on the hypothalamus. In all these conditions there may be found changes in laminae III-V of the cortex, Ammon's horn, the hypothalamus, reticular formation of the brain-stem and around the aqueduct of Sylvius. Such changes are well described in Wilson (1940) and Wyburn-Mason (1948). In "idiopathic" cases of schizophrenia and manic-depressive psychoses and cases of idiopathic epilepsy *degenerative changes in the central nervous* system id:mtical *with those found in intoxications and non-specific infections are described.* A summary of these changes has been given by Taft (1916), Josephy (1930), Morgan (1940) and Wyburn-Mason (1948). In acute cases of "idiopathic" schizophrenia, especially those with catatonia and patients dying in status epilepticus, there is a typical "Hirnschwellung" with oedema of the pia. Histologically there is marked swelling of the ganglion cells and amoeboidosis of the glia. Adjacent to the fresh changes are found old ones in the form of sclerosis and "ausfall" of cells. The changes are present in the same areas as in the chronic cases mentioned below, including the deeper layers of the cortex. In the chronic cases there is an "ausfall" of cortical cells occurring in small fleck-l!ke areas, especially in laminae III and V of the cortex. In these the ganglion cells are reduced in number, separated from one another and irregularly placed. There are of ten small oedematous areas in which the nerve cells are affected. The ganglion cells show various degrees of degeneration. There may be perivascular lymphocytic collections (see Torrey and Peterson, 1973). The changes are discontinuous and occur especially around the ca pillaries. They are found in all areas of the cortex, but especially in the premotor areas, superior frontal gyri and in the temporal lobes and cerebellum, Ammon's horn, the globus pallidus and hypothalamus. There is a

perivascular distribution of hyaline substance in these areas. These changes it is stressed are non-specific. They also occur in non-specific intoxications and infections and their presence in idiopathic cases of mental disease and epilepsy is in accord with an infective or toxic aetiology for these disturbances. Again, in generalized intoxications the same changes in the E.E.G. may be found as occur in cases of schizophrenia, manic-depressive psychoses and idiopathic epilepsy, further suggesting that the latter are due to an unknown infection or intoxication.

Transitions or combinations of manic-depressive, depressive or schizophrenic disorders may occur "idiopathically" (Slater and Roth, 1969). It has been seen already that any type of affective psychosis, psychoneuroses or epilepsy may complicate collagen diseases. A relationship between coeliac disease and schizophrenia has been suggested by Dohan (1969). Most diabetics are psychiatrically disturbed, even when the diabetes is controlled (Bondy, 1971). Thyrotoxicosis is frequently associated with psychoneurotic or psychotic disturbances, even when the patient is rendered euthyroid. Psychoneuroses and psychoses are common in patients suffering from ulcerative colitis or intrinsic asthma. Alopecia areata or universalis are commonly associated with psychoneurosis or psychoses and are often seen in mental hospitals. Thus, any psychoneurotic or psychotic disturbance may result from limax amoebae infection. Since this infection is almost universal and often latent, it may be that it is the cause of many cases of "idiopathic" psychoneuroses or affective psychoses, in which evidence of collagen or auto-immune disease would be found if specifically sought for. These would be more obvious with increasing age, but especially around the menopause. These changes include skin lesions, rheumatoid disease, thyroid disease, atrophic gastritis, etc. Manic-depression may be precipitated by the menopause, when rheumatoid arthritis tends to occur, and manic-depression, schizophrenia, paraphrenia and dementia appear more frequently with increasing age (Slater and Roth, 1969). In this connection Burch (1964, a, b, c), by a statistical method comparing manic-depressive psychoses, schizophrenia and involutional psychoses with collagen and auto-immune diseases, concludes that all three major syndromes of affective disorders are "auto-immune" disturbances. It seems reasonable to suppose that many cases of "idiopathic" mental disturbances result from the effect of products of infection with limax amoebae on the hypothalamus carried to it by the circulation. This would readily explain the spontaneous fluctuations in the severity of the symptoms and why some patients recover spontaneously. However, a number of rheumatologists state that rheumatoid arthritis is uncommon in mental hospitals. This suggests that the amoeba concerned is usually different from that causing rheumatoid disease.

a) Manic-depressive psychoses

In manic states the skin is flushed and sweating and there is increased lacrimal and salivary secretion. The growth of hair is luxuriant. The bronchial and tracheal secretions are increased. Idiopathic depression may be accompanied by dryness of the mouth, anorexia, dyspepsia, dryness and wrinkling of the skin. Hair growth is slowed or ceases and the hair becomes dry. In both states these are changes which may result from hypothalamic disturbances as described above and indeed mania and depression may be symptoms of lesions of this region of the brain. Idiopathic mania or depression with similar features to organic reactions may end in stupor and delirium, confusion or coma, like that resulting from infections. This is in accord with the possibility that the conditions result from a chronic latent infection. In manic depressives signs of collagen and auto-immune disease may be found when sought. The hair may fall out, either pat-

chily (alopecia areata) or sometimes completely (alopecia universalis). Menstrual function may cease. There may be hyperglycaemia or glycosuria. As described in Chapter II vitiligo may be found. Scleroderma may also complicate cases of depression (Sack, 1933; Cassirer and Hirschfeld, 1935). This suggests that manic-depression results from infection with limax amoebae and could be influenced by anti-amoebic drugs. This, in fact, occurred in the following case.

Case 99 Male, aged 58 years. Family history nil relevant. Patient had a normal education, and many different jobs. Aged 52 years prostatectomy for benign enlargement. Six months later feelings of depression with periods of agitation began. These were associated with profuse sweating and weight loss. He also suffered from delusions and ideas of reference and persecution. He was several times so ill and retarded as to amount to mutism and stupor. He attempted suicide on two occasions in periods of tenseness. He also complained of periodic dizziness and was subject to recurrent chest infections. He had had five admissions to a mental hospital in 5 years during which he was treated with antidepressant drugs and E.C.T. He was transferred to hospital from a mental hospital because of deep vein thrombosis of the left leg. Examination showed he was confused and retarded; depressed and unable to give an account of himself. He was fully investigated. WR negative. C.S.F. protein 40 mgms. per 100 mls. E.S.R. 31 mm. per hour. Serum albumin and globulin both 3.8 G per cent. Achlorhydria present. RF negative. AU serum auto-antibodies negative. He was taking Nitrazepan 5-10 mgms. nocte and valium 10 mgms. t.d.s. He was treated with copper sulphate 25 mgms. t.d.s. which he has now taken for 9 months. He rapidly returned to normal mentally, lost his depression and ideas of reference and influence and became intellectually normal. He was discharged from hospital 6 weeks later and took a job as a gardener, the first one for 5 years. He has worked satisfactorily at this for 6 months. He is still under observation.

Another case which came under the writer's care was that of a man of 80 years of age, a victim of chronic rheumatoid arthritis for over 40 years. With the onset of the arthritis the patient developed severe mental disturbance which consisted of hyperactivity and a tendency to run away from his home and get lost. *These symptoms varied with the activity of the rheumatoid arthritis* and responded to tranquilizers under which he immediately ceased to function at all, spending more and more time sleeping in an almost hypnotic semiconscious state when his bowels failed to function and he refused food and any fluids. Stopping the tranquilizers caused a return of the hyperkenetic state when he was very alert and completely lucid but lacked the ability to take any responsibility and any immediate decision whatsoever. In a further case a previously extremely healthy woman of 80 years there was a simultaneous onset of acute rheumatoid disease and mental changes consisting of dementia with complete withdrawal symptoms.

Such cases suggest that idiopathic mania and depression are often due to intoxication by limax amoebae infection, which explains the cyclical nature of the condition by variations in the severity of the intoxication.

b) Schizophrenia

In idiopathic cases of schizophrenia the condition may end in delirium and in fatal catatonia there may be high fever and vascular collapse (Torrey and Peterson, 1973) as in cases of severe infections. In evidence summarized in Slater and Roth (1969) there are repeated observations which suggest that in schizophrenics the body fluids contain an unidentified substance, which exerts toxic or lethal effects when injected into animals and produces behaviour changes and impairment of

learning capacity in the rat and catatonia and other schizophrenic symptoms in monkeys and man. Moreover, rheumatoid disease may be complicated by schizophrenia (see Chapter II). Apart from this, in "idopathic" cases of schizophrenia there may occur lesions of various other body tissues. There may be increased salivary secretion, amenorrhoea or menstrual irregularities, and generalized melanoderma or pemphigus (Wiener, 1947), pruritus, urticaria, seborrhoeic eczema and psoriasis, dryness or keratosis of the skin, partial or complete alopecia (see Galewsky, 1932; Wiener, 1947), rheumatoid arthritis and oedemas, and abnormalities in the serum proteins (Torrey and Peterson, 1973). In fact, collagen and auto-immune disease obviously occur just as frequently in cases of schizophrenia as in mentally normal subjects and in any case limax amoebae infection obviously occurs just as often and as early in schizophrenics as in others. Checkley and Birley (1977) describe a man of 52 years who developed schizophrenia at the age of 23 years and rheumatoid arthritis at 47 years following which there was a close parallel between the arthritis and the severity of the mental symptoms. A number of examples of this in the author's experience are as follows: –

A woman, aged 56 years, developed seropositive rheumatoid disease for which she was treated. This was accompanied by delusions of persecution and fixed obsessions that she had cancer or syphilis. The severity of her mental state ran parallel with the severity of her joint condition.

A woman of 41 years had been eccentric for years and had developed systematized delusions of anti-semitic nature in recent years. At the age of 36 years she had a hysterectomy for fibroids and an operation for bilateral benign ovarian cysts at the age of 38 years. Since that time she had developed symptoms of Sjögren's syndrome and swellings in both parotid glands, which proved to be due to benign

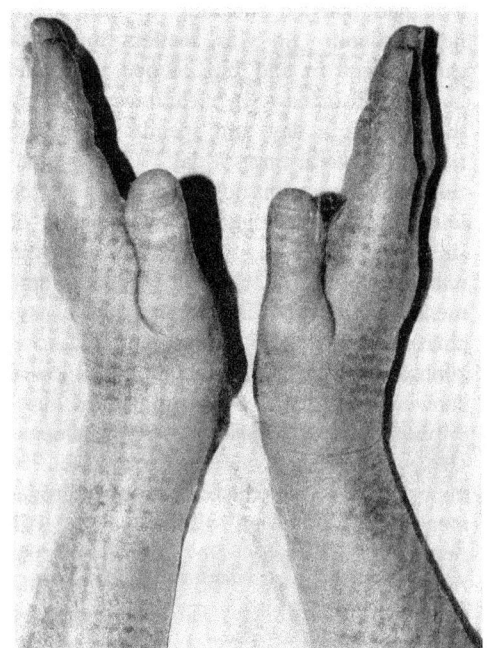

Fig. 54-A

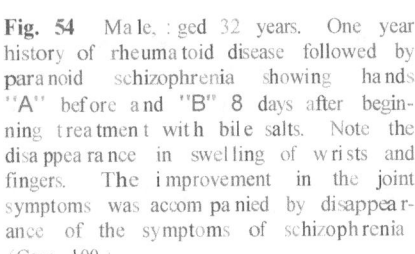

Fig. 54 Male, : ged 32 years. One year history of rheumatoid disease followed by paranoid schizophrenia showing hands "A" before and "B" 8 days after beginning treatment with bile salts. Note the disappearance in swelling of wrists and fingers. The improvement in the joint symptoms was accompanied by disappearance of the symptoms of schizophrenia (Case 100).

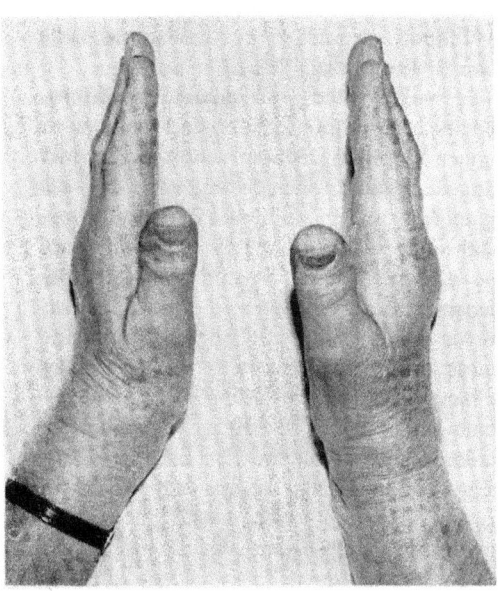

Fig. 54-B

lympho-epithelial lesions. RF was present in the serum. A man, now aged 29 years, whose father was an alcoholic and suffered from eczema, developed severe intrinsic asthma in childhood, which had persisted. At the age of 16 years he developed schizophrenia, which had necessitated frequent hospitalization ever since. It was noted that exacerbations in the asthmatic condition frequently preceded an exacerbation of his mental state. The following case is of considerable importance.

Case 100 Male, aged 30 years. Pakistani from Kenya. Family and past history irrelevant. He first presented with a two months history of pain and swelling of the ankles and both shoulders, especially on waking and tending to pass off in the course of the day. Examination showed swelling, tenderness and restricted movements of the fingers, wrists, elbows, knees and ankles (Fig. 54). Chest X-ray normal. Hb 15 G per 100 mls. W.B.C. 4,900 per cu. mm., 58 per cent polymorphs, 40 per cent lymphocytes. E.S.R. 3 rpms. in 1 hour. No lupus erythematosus cells seen in the blood. RF negative.

He was treated with naxogin and tabs. codeine co. without relief and later with copper sulphate 25 mgms. t.d.s. The last caused a rapid disappearance of all his symptoms within 48 hours. He left hospital and failed to attend for follow up. He presented again 8 months after discharge with a two months history of return of his joint symptoms, especially in the hands and ankles and a 6 weeks history of mental symptoms. His memory had become defective. His relatives stated he walked about all night. He began to read religious books and spent long hours in prayer. He kept a long knife about his person and cut the pulps of all his fingers "to let out the devils". He wrote all over his body with a biro pen religious texts to ensure his safety and to propitiate devils. He kept hearing noises and voices telling him he had sinned and a girl friend

who had married speaking to him about her husband. He was restless and continually got in and out of bed. He had become obsessed with cleanliness, shaving three times a day and spending hours in the bath several times a day. On examination there was marked swelling of the joints of the phalanges and wrists and of the ankles and feet. He was confused and unable to tell the date or to do simple mental arithmetic. He was seen by a psychiatrist and a diagnosis of paranoid schizophrenia was made. Lumbar puncture showed a normal C.S.F. All serum auto-antibody tests were normal. RF was negative. He was given dehydrocholine 750 mgms. t.d.s. This caused a rapid improvement in his condition within 2 days. His restlessness ceased. He stopped cutting his fingers, writing on the skin and praying and gave up bathing. He also ceased to hear voices. The joint sy.mptoms disappeared within 4 days (Fig. 54). He was now given copper sulphate 25 mgms. t.d.s. in addition. In 14 days he was symptomless. He was discharged on this regime and followed over two months without return of symptoms.

Such observations suggest that many cases of idiopathic schizophrenia are due to chronic limax amoebae infection, which is presumably the source of the unidentified substance in the body fluids.

c) Psychoneuroses

It was recorded in Chapter II that many different types of collagen or auto-immune disease may be associated with psychoneuroses, obsessions and psychopathic features. Many skin lesions of collagen and auto-immune type may be associated with hysteria, neurasthenia or other psychoneuroses. These include urticaria, psoriasis, eczema, pruritus, seborrhoea (Nob!, 1928; Torok, 1932; Sack, 1933). Many "psychoneurotic" symptoms with fatigue, headache, etc., may be relieved by antiprotozoal drugs (see Elsdon-Dew, 1972), suggesting they are due to a protozoal infection.

The author observed a dramatic case in

which a severe anxiety state preceded by a number of years the appearance of manifestations of collagen disease. The patient was a woman of 26 years who at the age of 18 years developed an acute anxiety state for no apparent reason. This necessitated several periods in a mental hospital. She then began to gain an enormous mount of weight and three years after the onset of her nervous symptoms was found to be hypothyroid, treatment of which with !-thyroxin had no effect on her weight gain or her anxiety symptoms. This was followed six years after the development of her first anxiety symptoms by a severely painful peripheral arthropathy and by the presence of RF, ANF and lupus erythematosus cells in the blood. A diagnosis of systemic lupus erythematosus was made, but in spite of treatment by various anti-inflammatory drugs, aspirin and steroids, she continued to gain in weight and the peripheral arthropathy progressed rapidly so that her hands, feet, wrists, elbows, ankles and knee joints became markedly swollen and painful making walking ext remely difficult and the hands practically useless. Her anxiety state was extreme. All treatment, except !-thyroxin, was stopped and dehydrocholine 1.5 grams t.d.s. was substituted. Within 10 days she was completely symptomless, both from the mental and physical aspects. She lost 18 pounds in weight within that time without dieting. Her shoes became three inches too long for her. She was discharged home on this regime and remained quite symptomless over the next six months. She was still losing weight. The lupus erythematosus cells disappeared from the blood within three weeks.

Such observations suggest that, in fact, psychoneuroses are frequently a manifestation of limax amoebae infection. Thus, psychiatric and psychoneurotic disturbances appear to be of organic nature. Surely the time has arrived for a scientific approach to mental and psychological disturbances and to forget the fanciful non-

rcnsc and mumbo-jumbo of Freud, Jung, Adler and others.

d) The possible aetiology of many cases of idiopathic epilepsy

Epileptic attacks of various types may result from hypothalamic lesions, from acute infections of various kinds, especially the acute fevers of childhood, and they nny also result from chronic infections, su(:h as syphilis. Furthermore, epilepsy may complicate cases of rheumatoid arthritis or Sjogren's syndrome (see previous section). In cases of idiopathic epilepsy, the attacks may be identical with those of symptomatic epilepsy, but no cause is found. The pathological changes in the brain and the changes in the E.E.G. in suC"h cases are nonspecific and similar to those of chronic generalized infections. Again, in cases of status epilepticus the patient may pass into a state of confusion, delirium, hyperpyrexia and eventually die in coma with marked cerebral oedema, all of which are features of a severe infection. Morecwer, it is well known that in some subjects idiopathic epilepsy may be associated or alternate with intrinsic asthma, which it has been suggested above is frequently caused by Iimax amoebae infection. Eosinophilia, which may be caused by such an infection, may also be a feature of some cases of idiopathic epilepsy, especially about the time of an attack and during status epilepticus (Wyburn-Mason, 1948). All these considerations suggest that, in the absence of any special physical causes or cerebral lesions, many cases of idiopathic epilepsy may be a manifestation of the wide-spread infection with Iimax amoebae.

The presence in the blood of some unknown factor in cases of collagen and auto-immune disease

In considering the various manifestations of collagen and auto-immune disease separately certain conclusions have been reach,-ed both by others and by the author as to the presence in the blood of some agent producing various disturbances. Thus-

1) In cases of Henoch-Schonlein's purpura a number of workers have concluded that some unknown factor in the blood is damaging the capillary walls.

2) In those skin diseases which form part of the spectrum of collagen and auto-immune diseases Kohner's phenomenon is often seen. This indicates the existence in all parts of the skin and deep tissues and presumably in the blood of some generalized abnormal factor which becomes localized at sites of trauma, and results in the skin lesions.

3) In cases of diabetes it has been concluded that some abnormal factor is present in the blood interfering with the activity of the hypothalamus and possibly with the action of insulin.

4) In early cases of paralysis agitans it appears that some substance is present in the blood which interferes with the function of the basal ganglia and reticular formation.

5) In some cases of collagen and auto-immune disease it is possible that an abnormal factor in the blood either disturbs the hypothalamus or intereferes with the action of the female sex hormones leading to disturbance of normal menstruation, late menarche, premature menopause or "primary gonadal failure".

6) In cases of idiopathic affective psychoses and psychoneuroses and some cases of epilepsy the symptoms appear to result from some circulating toxin originating from limax amoebae which acts on the hypothalamic centres.

7) In female cases of myasthenia gravis (an effect of collagen or auto-immune disease) pregnancy may result in the birth of an infant with transient myasthenia (neonatal myasthenia). This indicates the presence in the blood of the mother of a circulating substance which crosses the placenta to affect the foetus. In cases of myasthenia the administration of anti-amoebic drugs immediately relieves the symptoms, suggesting these substances neutralize or abolish the circulating substance.

8) In migraine the onset of symptoms appears to be due to the presence of a humoral agent in the blood (Plum, 1971).

All these arguments point to the presence in the circulation of a substance derived from limax amoebae, which interferes with function in vessel walls to produce purpura, with liberation of acetylcholine at nerve endings and with various serum factors and also acts on various hypothalamic centres. It has been suggested that this circulating substance might interfere with normal functioning of the hypothalamic centres producing obesity.

Collagen and auto-immune disease and aging

The currently favoured theories of aging relate our decline over the years to accumulating errors in the body machinery. Different theories back different types of error in mutation (see Franks, 1972), for instance cross-linking between polymeric molecules, free-radical attacks and Orgel's theory of the deterioration in the synthesase enzymes that carry out protein synthesis leading to "error catastrophe". Hayfli c) has shown that mammalian cells in culture never seem to proliferate indefinitely. They seem to be able to undergo only a fairly constant number of cell divisions before they succumb to rapid deterioration. If cell proliferation is equally circumscribed in vivo, then limits are obviously set on the survival of organs containing rapidly dividing cells, and Burnet (1967) points out the thymic cortex has the most rapid cell turnover of any organ in the body.

Walford (1969) argues that the key process in aging is the accumulation of mutations in immunocytic clones. Aberrant immunocytes are ideally placed to cause havoc. If their antigenic properties are changed, they attack healthy body cells.

generating auto-immune disease, while at the same time they may themselves be attacked by unmutated immunocytes-civil war within the body's defence forces. Burnet (1967) argues that the prime function of the thymus-dependent immune system is "immunological surveillance"-the quality control of cell manufacture, whereby mutant cells are weeded out. Now, if the supply of thymocytes does wane as the thymus approaches its Hayflick limit, then the body will become increasingly susceptible to cellular anomalies like malignancy and auto-immune disease. Its defences against them will crumble.

If the author's present deductions about the nature of so-called collagen and "auto-immune" disease are correct, such theories as Burnet's and Walford's are untenable. The collagen and auto-immune phenomena appear to result from an infection with a protozoon. As life progresses there is an increased incidence of the various manifestations of collagen and auto-immune disease, presumably due to decreased resistance to limax amoebae. These include rheumatoid arthritis, thyroid disease, atrophic gastritis and other atrophic conditions of the mucosae of the body, Sjogren's syndrome, atrophic stomatitis with the falling out of the teeth, atrophic gastritis with achlorhydria, ichthyosis acquisita, alopecia, senile hyperkeratoses, Paget's disease of bone with its complications, osteoporosis, polycythaemia with all its complications, deafness, diabetes, contracted kidney with hypertension and its complications, renal tubular acidosis and its complications, coeliac disease and ulcerative colitis and their complications, heart and lung diseases and their complications,

senile psychoses, paralysis agitans, thromboses and various ocular lesions. Spontaneous amyloidosis (senile amyloidosis), a phenomenon produced by chronic antigenic stimulation and a feature of chronic rheumatoid disease, is a related finding in old subjects. and pathologists commonly encounter "non-specific" infiltrations of lymphocytes in sections of organs of aged individuals and periarteritis (Blumenthal and Berns, 1964). Such infiltrations are typical of collagen and auto-immune diseases. Again, it has been suggested that motoneurone disease may be a manifestation of infection with limax amoeba. McComas et al. (1973) point out that it is, in fact, an accelerated form of the normal aging process. Thus, in the aged there is an accumulation of collagen and auto-immune diseases and often the E.S.R. is persistently raised for no apparent reason. With this there occurs a gradually increasing tendency to malignant disease.

In so far as various collagen and auto-immune disease may shorten life. so infection with the limax amoebae plays a very important part in the aging process. Since limax amoebae infection depresses resistance to infection and, thus, to limax amoebae themselves, so the aging process gains momentum and the aging subject becomes prone to further infections. The conclusions reached by the author as to the role of the protozoon in causing human disease would appear to cast serious doubt on the validity of the auto-immune theory put forward by Burnet, including his ideas on aging. It would seem possible that repeated courses of imidazole drugs would postpone the aging process.

· Chapter VII

The effect of limax amoebae on the embryo and foetus

Congenital malformations, hamarto-mata and tumours (anomalies) in the foetus and placenta

Congenital malformations are generally divided into several principle groups — 1) those due to alterations in differentiation of tissues that have arisen from a single area in the embryonic disc, 2) those due to errors of migration of cells from the neural crest, such as melanoblasts and leading to pigmentary disturbances, or from the somites leading to misplacement or absence of organs, and 3) those due to a duplication of the germinal area, thus giving rise to individuals whose body structures are partially, but not completely duplicated, 4) those due to failure of fusion of the neural folds, 5) those due to failure of two parts of a primordial organ to come together, for example the two parts or portions of the teeth or kidr.ey, 6) those due to failure of organs to reach their normal position in the body, for example the ascent of the kidney or descent of the testis, 7) those due to overdevelopment of local tissues, unexplained on an embryological basis. Among these are congenital tumours, for example teratomata or hamartomata. The malformations of the first group, though apparently limitless in variety, fall into well-defined categories, in which individual members show remarkable similarity despite minor variations. The majority result from a local arrest in the normal process of tissue development, fusion and migration. A few; such as polydactyly, may be attributed to excessive division and some from complete local failure of tissue growth.

The developmental anomalies, hamarto-mata or congenital tumours which may exist in the embryo, including its membranes, may affect:-

a) The *blood vessels* giving rise to benign angiomata and angiomatosis, but no sharp line of distinction exists between angiomas and vascular malformations. While most are congenital, some do not develop until later in life. They may be associated with congenital malformations of the skeleton. Occasionally they become invasive. They may be multiple and may involve the placenta.

b) *Lymph vessels.* These may be associated with blood vessel hamartomata and may be accompanied by foetal hydrops and abortion may occur. The placenta may show hydatiform change. Hamartomata of lymph vessels in the limbs may be associated with multiple enchondromata or cysts of the phalanges.

c) *Skeleton.* These may appear as i) multiple exostoses or ii) multiple enchondromata (Oilier's disease) and are often associated with vascular hamartomata (Mafucci's syndrome).

d) *Adipose tissue*, giving rise to numerous or single congenital lipomata, which may be present at birth and are often accompanied by angiomata and other anomalies. Multiple congenital lipomata with congenital anomalies of the limb skeleton was described by Adair et al. (1932). They may occur in the choroid plexus, base of the brain and spine, or they may be associated with defects of the skull, malformed irises, absence of the kidney, hare-lip and cleft palate (see Baker and Adams, 1938). Such congenital fatty tumours may rarely undergo malignant change to liposarcoma.

e) *Combinations* of *a, b, c, and d* may occur. Thus, in the lumbar region may be found congenital bony defects (spina bifida) associated with abnormal tissues containing blood vessels, lymph vessel:>, fatty tissue, fibrous tissue, etc. This forms a myxolipofibro-angioma.

f) *Congenital benign teratomata*, which may likewise be associated with *congenital anomalies and contain numerous and diverse tissues* and may later become malignant.

Congenital malformations of the central nervous system may be a) major and include neural tube malformations, such as anencephaly, spina bifida, cranium bifidum, prosencephaly, hydrocephalus, microcephaly and agenesis of the corpus callosum found in non-viable foetuses, b) of less severity and due to disorders of migration of neuroblasts from the primitive neural tube to the cortex, leading to localized microgyria, pachygyria and nodular ectopia. The pattern of changes is often irregular and they may be associated with c) reactive changes (gliotic encephalopathy) leading to disturbance of normal growth, liquefaction and scarring resulting in localized ulegyria or granular atrophy. These changes are often inflammatory in nature and b) and c) are the cause of the majority of cases of mental retardation (Crome, 1972), which is thus often a manifestation of congenital developmental anomalies of the brain and are commonly associated with congenital anomalies elsewhere in the body.

The placenta forms an integral part of the foetus and is likewise subject to the development of hamartomata, which include cavernous angiomata, chorionangiomata and angiomyxomata (see Potter, 1953).

The genetic state of the tissues affected by congenital growth anomalies

Heterochromia iridis, congenital hemihyperplasia (hemihypertrophy), or hemihypoplasia (hemiatrophy) or body asymmetry may occur in cases of Von Recklinghausen's or OUier's diseases. These asymmetrical conditions were discussed at length by Wyburn-Mason (1958). There it was pointed out that iris colour is genetically determined. The condition of heterochromia iridis must signify a difference in the genetic material in the chromatophores of the irises of the two eyes. This condition may be associated with unilateral developmental growth anomalies affecting one eye and the tissues surrounding it and sometimes with growth anomalies elsewhere in the body. The localized growth disturbances of one eye and its surroundings include melanosis oculi, trigeminal vascular naevus, unilateral buphthalmos or microphthalmos, neuro-angiolipomata, fibromata and warty excrescences, cranial meningocoele, teratoma of the orbit, deformity of the ear on that side, intracranial lipomata and elsewhere syringomyelia, pigmented or vascular naevi, patches of achromia and metameric depigmentation in the skin and congenital heart disease. Like the differences in iris colour the local growth anomalies and lesions elsewhere might arise from a difference in the genetic make-up of the cellular material which eventually forms the congenital anomalous tissue from that of the rest of the body, that is they are due to somatic mutation in early development of the genes of the cell which eventually gives rise to a clone forming the anomalous tissue.

In cases of congenital hemihyperplasia all the tissues on one side of the body are larger than those on the other, and again, heterochromia iridis may be present (see Wyburn-Mason, 1958). The hair colour and thickness may be different on the two sides. The overgrown side may be associated with a trigeminal naevus or pigmented ⇐ or naevus unius lateralis. The fit"sf may be covered by hyperkeratotic skin or warty growths forming a neuroangiolipofibroma. Buphthalmos, polydactyly, syndactyly, cryptorchidism, an increased number of teeth, cavernous angiomata, phlebectasia, lipomata, angiolipomata and epicanthus may be found on the larger side and congenital heart disease may be present. The chambers of the heart on the overgrown side are larger than on the unaffected side. The whole problem is considered by Wyburn-Mason (1958). Now differences in iris colour, eye size, supernummery teeth and digits (polydactyly), syndactyly and epicanthus occurring on the larger side of the body are characters controlled by genes evidently different from those of the normal side of the individual. Linder (1969) indeed found that the cells of human teratomas, which may occur in association with the other anomalies, exhibited a loss of genes. Such observations suggest that growth anomalies occurring on the *affected side in cases of congenital hyperplasia* or *heterochromia iridis are due to* somatic *genetic mutation of one cell of the two-celled stage of the embryo, which eventually* forms *the affected side of the individual.* Such conditions as differences in the eye size or the size of one half of the body and its component tissues accompanied by the presence of organs not normally present on the transplanted side can, in .fact, be produced experimentally in animals by transplanting tissues from embryos belonging to a different species or genera early in development, so-called heteroplastic and xenoplastic transplantation (see Wyburn-Mason, 1958). Such animals or humans exhibiting congenital asymmetry are, in fact, chimaeras. In man the growth anomalies on the affected side are accompanied by various benign tumours(hamartomata), such as lipomata. angiomata, fibromata and warty excresences, teratoma or malignancies, such as Wilm's tumour, malignant melanoma, astrocytoma (Meyerson, 1967) and sometimes by unilateral cryptorchidism. The *occurrence of these hamartomata and tumours* is *also presumably related to dif-*

ferences in the genetic make-up in the abnormal and normal tissue on the two *sides of the body.* Again in cases of unilateral growth anomalies associated with t,milateral retinoblastoma the evidence suggests a somatic genetic mutation of the affected tissues without germinal cell involvement (Leading Article, Lancet, 1971, 2, 1016). This genetic mosaicism may sometimes be reflected in chromosomal abnormalities. Ellis et al. (1963). Ferrior et al. (1964), Hook and Yunis (1965) and Johnston and Penrose (1966) found chromosomal mosaicism in such cases of congenital hemihypertrophy. *Congenital growth anomalies would thus* seem *to be due to somatic genetic mutation oocurring before birth.* Congenital anomalies may also be found in cases of mongolism and Klinefelter's and Turner's syndromes, where chromosomal anomalies and mosaicism are also found (see below).

The mutual attraction of cells to one another during normal development

During normal development many different cells exhibit attraction to one another, resulting in migrations or a tendency to grow together. (For a discussion see Wyburn-Mason, 1958) . This is seen in the attraction of the growing ends of nerve fibres into relationship with dividing cells and in the migration of neural crest cells and those of the Wolffian body. In the developing kidney the cells of the nephrogenic cord grow into contact with those of the ureteric bud, the outgrowth of the Wolffian duct, to form the secreting and collecting units of the kidney. The twin primitive heart tubes and neural folds also attract one another and grow together. Tyler (1955) demonstrated that the forces responsible for the specific adhesion or non-adhesion of cells and tissues, that is attraction, during development appear *analagous to antigen-antibody reactions,* and through this are *related to genetic action.* Thus, when dissociated cells of different species are mixed in a medium, coalescence is found to occur only between those of the same species. It is also possible that natural auto-antibodies may act directly as inductive agents. *The migration of neural crest cells to their definitive position, the attraction to one another of the different cell elements forming the teeth and kidneys and the growth into a tissue of nerve axons in a developing part* presumably depend on such processes. It follows that, should genetic mutation of a clone of cells occur during development, these mutual forces of attraction and induction between cells will be disturbed and major developmental anomalies may arise, such as errors of neural crest cell migration, innervation of tissues or failure of the two parts of the teeth or kidney primordia to grow together.

T.ransplacental infection with limax amoebae in the foetus and new-born

Many infections cross the placenta. These include syphilis, tuberculosis, malaria and toxoplasmosis (Willis, 1958), leishmaniasis, trypanosomiasis and rubella. It has been shown that all the tissues of most adult healthy and diseased subjects are infected with limax amoebae. This includes the ovary and all layers of the uterus and may lead to ovarian cysts or fibroid formation or ectopic pregnancies. It was also shown that the placenta was similarly infected, whether the birth led to the delivery of a healthy infant or one affected by congenital anomalies (Wyburn-Mason, 1964). This is in accord with the motility of the organism.

The sera of all new-born infants contains fluorescent antibodies to either Aca nthamoeba or Naegleria (Leading Article, Lancet, 1977, 2, 1165) and thus all humans are infected transplacentally with free-living amoebae or their antigens. Again, collagen and auto-immune diseases may be present at birth. Thus, congenital rheumatoid arthritis is describ-

ed (Willis, 1958). The author has observed four such cases. Scott (1976) reviewed 16 cases of neonatal systemic lupus erythematosus. Congenital non-hereditary ichthyosis is well-known and is then often associated with multiple allergies (Lightwood and Brimblecombe, 1963). This is identical with ichthyosis acquisita. Intrinsic asthma may be present almost from birth (Lightwood and Brimblecombe, 1963). Apart from cases of mongolism, Klinefelter's and Turner's syndromes the thyroid frequently exhibits abnormalities at birth. In such cases the gland is infiltrated with lymphocytes as in adult diseases and this may be clinically associated with thyrotoxicosis or hypothyroidism and congenital hamartomata may be found in other parts of the body (Willis, 1958). Congenital acanthosis nigricans, an "auto-immune" manifestatidn, may also be present at birth or soon afterwards associated with various congenital anomalies, such as congenital heart disease (Costello, 1972), dwarfism, cryptorchidism, achondroplasia, genital hypoplasia, mental defects (Johne et al., 1955; Curth et al., 1962) or congenital total lipodystrophy (Brubaker et a!., 1965). In addition, infants may be born with myasthenia gravis (congenital myasthenia) of apparently normal mothers or of mothers with myasthenia (neonatal myasthenia) (Rowlands, 1971). The former indicates that congenital auto-immune disease exists, while the latter shows that a humoral agent from the mother passes the placenta into the foetus. The author had a remarkable case under his care. The patient, a woman of 51 years, was born of a mother suffering with chronic rhinitis and asthma. At birth she showed arthropathy, congenital ichthyosis and eczema and soon after birth developed severe intrinsic asthma from which she had suffered all her life. She showed well-marked rheumatoid changes and suffered from diabetes. The joint and, skin changes and asthma partly responded to steroids. The blood contained RF and ANF. This case shows that such collagen and auto-immune conditions may all be congenital and result from transplacental passage of limax amoebae into the foetus.

There is an increased incidence of Hashimoto's thyroiditis in mongols and also alopecia areata and auto-immunity (Du Vivier and Munro, 1975). Many exhibit chronic rhinitis and bronchial spasm from birth (personal observation). Ortig-New and LeRoy (1969) and Price et al. (1976) describe six patients with Klinefelter's syndrome and systemic lupus erythematosus and Salmon and Ashworth (1970) a case of Klinefelter's syndrome and scleroderma and another, a girl of 11 years of age with an abnormal X chromosome and gonadal dysgenesis with rheumatoid arthritis. Cases of Klinefelter's syndrome are prone to intrinsic asthma (Daly and Rickards, 1964; Bomers-Marres, 1964). In Klinefelter's syndrome goitre is not uncommonly present (Burt et al., 1954 (6 cases of the syndrome); Barr et al., 1960; Davis et al., 1963; Clinico-Pathological Conference, Brit. med. J., 1963, 1, 866). Plunket et al. (1964) studied 27 cases of Klinefelter's syndrome and 17 bowed a low radio-iodine uptake by the thyroid. Boyle and McGirr (1965) and Kibei (1965) described athyroidal cretinism in cases of Klinefelter's syndrome. The cretinism is presumably due to prenatal destruction of the thyroid by collagen-auto-immune disease. In the case of Klinefelter's syndrome reported in the Clinico-Pathological Conference mentioned above, in addition to the goitre, there were also diabetes mellitus, adenoma of the stomach and unexplained bile duct proliferation with infiltration of lymphocytes and polymorphs and fibrosis around the portal tracts in the liver. Williams et al. (1970) found thyroiditis of varying severity in 8 of 25 patients with Turner's syndrome with thyroid auto-antibodies in the blood of 20 cases while Hashimoto's thyroiditis was reported in two cases of Turner's syndrome by Sparkes and Motulsky (1963) and also by Mellon et al. (1963). Chaves-Carballo and Hayes (1966) review Turner's syndrome occurring in males. Of 86 cases 6 exhibited Hashimoto's thyroiditis. Diabetes mellitus is also stated to be common in Turner's syndrome. McHardy-Young et al. (1970) confirm the frequent existence of focal thyroiditis and Hashimoto's thyroiditis in Turner's syndrome. They review the literature on this association. They mention also the occurrence of Turner's syndrome with diabetes, with achlorhydria, with Addison's disease and with both hypothyroidism and diabetes. Thus, there is a high incidence of collagen and auto-immune disease at an early age in subjects exhibiting errors of gametogenesis.

These observations indicate that transplacental transmission of the protozoal infection can occur from mother to foetus and destroy the thyroid and presumably other tissues and produce collagen or auto-immune disease before birth or soon afterwards. This transplacental infection to the foetus is comparable to that which occurs in many other diseases. It is to be observed that not only may the offspring exhibit evidence of congenital auto-immune disease, but also growth anomalies and chromosomal abberations (see below).

Chromosomal abnormalities

Mongolism, Klinefelter's and Turner's syndromes are all conditions in which abnormalities of chromosomes have been identified. In most cases of mongolism 47 chromosomes are present in the body cells as compared with the normal 46 (trisomy 21). This is due to an error of dysjunction of chromosomes in the mother's ovum. In a small proportion of cases of mongolism (4.5 per cent) the normal 46 chromosomes are present, but one is abnormally large due to translocation of parts of 2 chromosomes (Polani et al., 1960). In many cases mosaicism is present, while in other cases of mongolism the normal chromosome content is found. Mongolism

-232-

may affect several siblings or twins. It may be associated with galactosaemia or with retinoblastoma or Klinefelter's syndrome. In mongolism various congenital .anomalies are also present, but many are inconstant.

Klinefelter's syndrome occurs in sterile males, who exhibit hypogonadism (gonadal dysgenesis) and Turner's syndrome in sterile females with hypogonadism. In both conditions an abnormality in the sex chromosomes is present. In Turner's syndrome there are only 45 chromosomes and the sex chromosomes are XO, while in Klinefelter's syndrome there are 47 with the sex chromosomes XXY. In both, however, sex chromosome mosaicism has been described and at least two populations. of cells with different sex chromosome complexes may be found in the same individual. In Klinefelter's syndrome the sex chromosomes may be XXY, XXXY, XXYY or XXXXY or a mosaic of XY/XXY. In Turner's syndrome these mosaicisms may be XO/XY or XO/XYY. Many inconstantly occurring developmental defects may be found in either syndrome, but are not an essential part of it. Mongolism may sometimes be associated with Klinefelter's syndrome. Again, in Bloom's syndrome and Fanconi's anaemia chromosomal abnormalities and congenital anomalies also occur (Shaw, 1971).

All these disturbances particularly occur in the last-born of large families or in children born later in the childbearing life and are particularly found in families in which there may have been previous or later cases of ectopic pregnancies. The inconstant chromosomal findings, the occasional finding of normal chromosomes in these conditions and the association of mongolism with galactosaemia or retinoblastoma, which are genetically determined features, suggest they could be due primarily to genetic rather than merely chromosomal disturbances.

Autosomal anomalies may affect various other chromosome groups producing the so-called group C, D, E and F trisomy syndromes and trisomy 13 and 18 (see Eggen, 1963). Trisomy 22 syndrome was described by Hsu et al. (1971). As in cases of mongolism and Klinefelter's and Turner's syndromes these trisomy syndromes tend to occur with advanced maternal age (Eggen, 1963; Shaw, 1971). The relative rarity of such autosomal trisomies and the severity of the associated defect!> suggest that autosomal disturbances of this magnitude are usually lethal. Penrose and Delhanty (1961) and Kemp (1961) obtained triploid cell cultures from macerated non-viable foetuses. Pergament (1970) states that the incidence of chromosomal abberations in non-viable products of conception exceeds that in a comparable population by twenty times. Thirty per cent of all spontaneous abortions carry a chromosomal defect and at least 5 per cent of all conceptions suffer from chromosomal disorders, most of which are lethal and these changes should be suspected in foetuses with bizarre congenital abnormalities affecting several systems (Thiele, 1967; Shaw, 1971).

Autosomal anomalies have also been reported in many cases of congenital growth anomalies, such as Sturges-Weber syndrome and other disturbances (Evans, 1961; Crawford, 1961; Bain and Gauld, 1963; Eggen, 1963; Gropp et al., 1964; Gordon and Cooke, 1964). Stewart et al. (1969) in 184 unselected live-born children with congenital anomalies found 8 (4.3 per cent) with abnormal karyotypes and 3 of these had abnormal nuclear sex. However, in studying chromosomal details use is made of cells cultured from the skin; buccal mucosa, blood, bone marrow and fascia. It is possible in view of the arguments above that, if cells were taken from the tissues of the developmental growth anomalies themselves, chromosome abnormalities might be found more frequently. Indeed Gropp et al. (1964) in a case of hare-lip and cleft palate found the affected tissues showed abnormal chromosomes not present elsewhere in the body. It may well be that in many cases of congenital anomalies the cells of the congenitally anomalous tissues may exhibit not only genetic, but also chromosomal abnormalities as compared with normal tissues.

The causation of errors of gametogenesis

In mongolism, Klinefelter's and Turner's syndromes there exist 1) errors of gametogenesis, 2) often mosaicism and 3) growth anomalies, the cells of which appear to be genetically different from the tissues of the organism. The last-named are inconstantly present and vary from case to case. All the available evidence favours a maternal origin for the error of gametogenesis, which results in the birth of a mongol child (Leading Article, Lancet, 1971, 1, 1223), or a case of Klinefelter's or Turner's syndrome. In this respect Behrman et al. (1966) recorded the case of a woman who had 3 mongol children all of different fathers, indicating the maternal origin of the condition. Robinson (1973) showed that the error in gametogenesis occurred at the first meiotic division in the mother. Chromosomal mosaicism arises from a further mitotic error in early division after fertilization in a zygote that originally had either a normal or an abnormal chromosome constitution.

Birch et al. (1964), Failkow (1964, 1967), Failkow et al. (1965) and Failkow et al. (1971) draw attention to the increased incidence of thyroid auto-antibodies in the mothers of mongols, in non-mongoloid children of these mothers, in thyroid disease among their relatives and in phenotypically normal relatives of patients with gonadal dysgenesis and the high incidence of mongolism in the children of parents with myxoedema during pregnancy. Vallollen and Forbes (1967) found antibodies to the thyroid, gastric parietal cells or rabbit ovarian cytoplasm or ANF in 31 of 45 patients with gonadal

dysgenesis in 16 out of 23 of their mothers and 9 of 20 of their fathers. The incidence of antibodies was significantly higher in patients than in controls, in patients' mothers than in controls and in patients' fathers than in controls. These findings were confirmed by Dallaire et al. (1969). Morris (1965) describes the case of a woman with ulcerative colitis, who had a mongol child. Dallaire et al. also confirmed Failkow's hypothesis that maternal auto-immune disease is causally related to both the occurrence of aneuploid children (mongols and gonadal dysgenesis) and thyroid disease in them, but that auto-immunity is not necessarily thyroid determined. It is considered that auto-immune disease in the mother is responsible for the development of chromosome abnormalities in the offspring, possibly by damage to ovarian cellular genetic material. Since the incidence of collagen and auto-immune disease increases with age, this would explain why mongolism and Turner's and Klinefelter's syndromes are commoner in the offspring of women towards the end of the child-bearing period.

The known causes of congenital malformations of the foetus, including the placenta

The known causes of congenital malformations are very numerous, but can be ascertained in only about two to less than five per cent of cases. The question is discussed by Willis (1958) and Lowe (1972). Although some of the rarer malformations show straightforward Mendelian ratios in their familial aggregations, most of the common ones do not conform to the pattern of dominant, recessive or sex-linked inheritance. In most malformations no major aetiological factor can be identified. While there is strong evidence that environmental factors are concerned, there is little to show that virus diseases, maternal ingestion of drugs or maternal irradiation make a significant contribution to the

Addendum: Lobo, E. de H., Kahn, M. and Tew, J. Community Study of Hypothyroidism in Down's Syndrome, Brit. med. J., 1980, 280, 1253. Down's syndrome is associated with auto-immune diseases affecting the thyroid, pancreas, gastric mucosa and adrenal glands and patients have an increased tendency to produce antibodies. They may also develop hyperthyroidism or diabetes.

common malformations, though these factors materially increase the frequency of certain *specific* malformations (Beam, 1971). The known causes may be grouped as follows:-

A) Genetic disorders (Mendelian) for example Von Recklinghausen's disease, tuberose sclerosis. The genes concerned may be single, multiple or sex-linked.

B) From extrinsic causes

a) Hypoxia and CO_2 poisoning.

b) Prolonged anaesthesia in pregnancy.

c) Administration of hormones, such as steroids.

'd) Administration of teratogenic drugs and chemicals, such as thalidamide and aminopterin.

C) From intrinsic causes

a) Rhesus incompatibility.

b) Vitamin deficiency in the mother during pregnancy.

c) Endocrine disturbances in the foetus as in association with free-martins.

d) Infections in the mother, including rubella and possible other viruses, toxoplasmosis and syphilis.

There is an increased frequency of congenital abnormalities in siblings and other relatives of patients with congenital abnormalities, but these abnormalities are not necessarily of the same type as in the patient and the incidence does not obey Mendelian laws (Lober, 1972). Carter (1969) has shown that in genetically determined congenital abnormalities that many of the common malformations are caused by combined genetic and environmental factors. Mental retardation may be a manifestation of congenital abnormalities of the brain (Crome, 1972).

The effects of collagen and auto-immune disease in the mother on the foetus and new-born

It has been seen that many maternal infections may cross the placenta and produce disease and congenital anomalies in the foetus and new-born. Limax amoebae occur in the ovary and uterus of the mother, where they may produce disease, and may also be present in the tissues of the foetus. Ovarian infection with the protozoon appears responsible for damage to ovarian cellular genetic material and, thus, chromosomal abnormalities in the ova, resulting in mongolism, Klinefelter's and Turner's syndromes, cases of which exhibit inconstant congenital anomalies. There seems no reason why abnormalities affecting chromosomal pairs other than the 21st. or the sex chromosomes, for example trisomy 13 and 18, etc., should not be similarly produced and result in non-viable foetuses and spontaneous abortions of foetuses showing congenital anomalies. Since limax amoebae infection of the mother may damage ovarian cellular genetic material and the foetus is often infected with the organism, it would be surprising if this foetal infection did not damage genetic material in the developing cells of the embryo and produce somatic mutation in a cell, which after division into a clone, would thus result in congenital anomalies of growth. That this may be so is shown by the following observations:-

1) Congenital anomalies tend to occur in the offspring of mothers suffering from diabetes (see Willis, 1958; Navarrete et al., 1970). Diabetes is generally a manifestation of limax amoebae infection.

2) Congenital anomalies tend to occur in the foetus of ectopic pregnancies and in cases of faulty implantation and malposition of the foetus, including placenta praevia (Willis, 1958). These have been seen above to be often the result of collagen and auto-immune disease in the mother.

3) Congenital anomalies tend to occur in foetuses in uteruses affected with fibraids, which appear to result from limax amoebae infection.

4) Congenital anomalies in the new-born may be associated with the presence of congenital acanthosis nigricans (see above), a manifestation of collagen or

auto-immune disease.

5) Congenital anomalies, inconstant and differing from case to case and accompanied by congenital collagen and auto-immune disease occur in subjects of mongolism and Klinefelter's and Turner's syndromes, which appear to result from limax amoebae infection in the mother.

6) Like mongolism, Klinefelter's and Turner's syndromes, congenital anomalies, such as anencephaly, spina bifida, hydrocephalus and other central nervous system deformities, tend to occur with increasing maternal age, that is with increasing possibility of the presence of the effects of infection with limax amoebae.

7) It was seen above that spontaneous abortions of non-viable macerated foetuses commonly result from errors of gametogenesis. In some families there may be an unusual frequency of off-spring with congenital abnormalities often associated with repeated spontaneous abortions or mongolism, mental deficiency or Klinefelter's or Turner's syndromes in other siblings (see Lowe, 1972). One apparently healthy mother under the author's care, aged 28 years at her last pregnancy, had four spontaneous abortions, then a normal child, three further abortions and then a child born with hydrocephalus and spinal meningomyelocoele. The mother's blood contained ANF and thyroid auto-antibodies. Another apparently healthy mother, aged 24 years, had three miscarriages followed by a normal child and then a child with hydrocephalus and spinal meningo-myelo-coele born after threatened abortion. The blood contained ANF and RF. A third woman, aged 26 years, had a normal child, then two abortions and then a mentally retarded child, who exhibited vascular and pigmented naevi and polydactyly in the right hand. Her blood contained thyroid and gastric parietal cell auto-antibodies. Another patient, a woman with ulcerative colitis and intrinsic asthma had 4 pregnancies, one resulting in a spontaneous abortion, the second in a child with severe rhinitis and asthma from an early age, the third in hydrocephalus and meningomyelocoele and the fourth in a mongol with congenital anomalies and myxoedema with severe rhinitis from birth. Another woman, aged 40 years, developed thyrotoxicosis ten years previously and was treated by thyroidectomy. She afterwards had repeated abortions and then developed atrophic gastritis and iron deficiency anaemia. The blood contained thyroid and gastric parietal cell antibodies. In one remarkable case the mother, aged 51 years, had 7 pregnancies, 6 children were normal, the last being born when the mother was 39 years of age. At the age of 43 years rheumatoid arthritis began. The last child was born when the mother was 44 years of age and was autistic and had congenital ichthyosis. The mother's blood contained RF and thyroid auto-antibodies. Another woman had 5 spontaneous abortions between the age of 30 and 38 years, then a healthy child at the age of 39 years and a mongol exhibiting various congenital anomalies at the age of 41 years. At the age of 46 years she had an hysterectomy for fibroids and an enormous benign left ovarian cyst was also removed. At the age of 51 years she developed thyrotoxicosis and the blood contained ANF and thyroid auto-antibodies. In a remarkable family studied by the writer who live in Perth, Australia, the wife's father had severe <;eropositive rheumatoid arthritis, the wife herself had mild symptoms of rheumatoid disease with a positive RF in the blood from the age of 20 years. Her husband was healthy. The chromosomes were normal in both. They had 5 children. The first died a few hours after birth with multiple congenital anomalies, the second a boy was born with enormously hypertrophied tonsils and adenoids which required removal at the age of 9 months. The third, a girl, was found to have ::celiac disease at the age of one year, the fourth was born with congenital aortic valve atresia and other cardiac anomalies and

the fifth with cleft palate, flat feet, kypho-scoliosis, congenital deafness and seroposi-tive rheumatoid arthritis, but she was nor-mal mentally.

8) Abrahams et al. (1972) report two patients who had recurrent abortions and who showed thrombocytopenia and ANF but no lupus erythematosus cells in the blood. One had systemic lupus erythema-tosus and the other possibly did so.

Such considerations suggest a common cause for fibroids, many spontaneous abor-tions due to lethal chromosomal disorders, Klinefelter's and Turner's syndromes and ongolism and for many congenital ano-malies. To conclude, it appears that *col-lagen and auto-immune* disease *in* the *mother may lead to* similar disease *and congenital* anomalies, errors *of gametogene-sis and collagen disease in the off-spring* and frequently results in non-viable foe-tuses and *recurrent spontaneous abortions* and in many cases in mental deficiency. Limax amoebae infections could be the factor responsible for many of the 98 per cent of non-genetically dependent congeni-tal abnormalities, the cause of which is unknown. *It must be that* in so *far* as *limax amoebae may cause genetic changer* in *thovum that* it is *a factor in controll ing the direction of human and perhaps animal evolution* and moreover, it will be responsible for the sudden appearance in a family of genetically controlled disease not previously known in ancestors, for ex-ample achondroplasia Von Recklinghau-sen's disease. Thus, contrary to the con-clusion of Jacques Monad (1972) the di-rection of evolution is not a totally chance occurrence, but could be related to limax amoebae infection.

Part III
The relationship of "collagen" and "auto-immune" disease to human tumour formation

Your Notes

Chapter VIII

Some factors in the causation of human tumours

The relationship of lymphomata and myelomata to one another

Before considering the various collagen and auto-immune diseases and their possible relationship to malignant disease certain facts must be borne in mind.

1) The first histological diagnosis made on lymph nodes in many cases of malignant lymphoma is commonly that of reactive hyperplasia or chronic inflammation (Ackerman and del Regato, 1954). Such an histological picture is that produced by an infection and is in favour of such a causation of malignant lymphomata.

2) In any case of lymphoma, including Hodgkin's disease, histologically there may be found in the affected lymph nodes every gradation from one type of lymphoma to another, either in different parts of the same lymph node, in different lymph nodes of a group removed at the same time, in different lymph nodes from different parts of the body or in lymph nodes taken at different times in the disease (for literature see Wyburn-Mason, 1964; Cooper, 1970, Wisniewski and Taker, 1973), and these changes show every transition to the changes of mere reactive hyperplasia.

3) In cases of myelomatosis with lymph node involvement the lymph nodes may show every histological transition from plasmocytoma to or combination with lymphosarcoma and reticulosarcoma in different parts of the same node or in nodes from different parts of the body (Snapper et al., 1953; Eder, 1953; Marchal et al., 1954; Wagner and Neun, 1955; Da Silva et al., 1958; Schmaman and Isaacson, 1960; Wisketich and Siegmund, 1961; Padovani, 1962; Larsson, 1962; Hellard *et* al.,

1965; Kutschera and Faldini, 1965; Durant et al., 1966; River and Schorr, 1966; Cooper, 1970). The author had under his care a woman aged 56 years suffering from multiple myelomatosis whose son developed malignant lymphoma at the age of 33 years, which also points to a relationship between the two. Such observations suggest that *all forms of lymphoma and myeloma are closely related aetiologically and these again to chronic inflammatory changes.*

Taylor (1974) investigated intracellular immunoglobulin components identified in plasma cell neoplasms (myelomas), in Reed-Sternberg cells and within the cells of some cases of reticulum cell sarcoma and of follicular lymphomas. His findings *strongly* suggest *a* close *relationship between all these conditions* and that at least some so-called "malignant reticulum cells" are, in fact, neoplastic derivatives of the transformed lymphocyte or of the immediate precursors or progeny thereof. Immunoglobulin production is thought to be confined to members of the B lymphocyte series. Thus, immunoglobulin-containing neoplastic cells are related to the B lymphocytic series. Diffuse lymphocytic lymphoma cells do not contain immunoglobulins usually, *The various malignant lymphomas develop after a prolonged plasma cell hyperplasia and maturation arrest related to a period of sustained lymphocytic transformation.*

Multiple cancers in one patient

Multiple cancers may occur in the same patient. These include:-

a) multiple cancers developing in one

Addendum: Cossman, J., Sdhnitzer, B., and Deegan, M.J., Amer. J. Clin. Pathol., 1978, 70, 409-415, report the case of a man of 4.1 years, who suffered from two distinct lymphomas in separate sites. One was a nodular poorly differentiated lymphocytic lymphoma and the other a diffuse histiocytic lymphoma. This is in accord with a common causation for all forms of lymphoma.

organ from different foci, such as in the large intestine, stomach, breast, meninges, etc. (multifocal cancers).

b) multiple cancers of different structures, including lymphoma and leukaemia or myelomatosis, developing in different organs, or

c) multiple cancers of different structure in the same organ, such as simultaneous Hodgkin's disease or lymphoma associated with a carcinoma, for example of the stomach.

The subject of multiple primary tumours affecting different tissues in man has been much studied in recent years. They have been considered by Warren and Gates (1932), Moertel et at. (1959), Canev (1960), Carnes (1960), Moertel et al. (1961), Werhamer et al. (1961), Tees (1961), Collins (1962), Thoma (1964), Fisher and Ketchum (1966), Baldwin and Wisner (1966), Bachulis and Williams (1966), Bordet (1966), Slomska (1967) and Veiga Fernandes et al. (1969). Slomska described a case in which there occurred six primary tumours in different organs and there are many cases of quadruple malignancies reported. Wilson et al. (1965) describe a case of dermatomyositis with three primary cancers (rectum, breast and transverse colon), Schapira and Oppenheimer (1963) report a patient with adenocarcinoma of the stomach, carcinoma of the anus and prostate and basal cell carcinoma of the skin, and list 9 other reported cases of the simultaneous occurrence of 4 primary cancers. Johansson and Holingvist (1963) recorded a case of a woman of 44 years with right mammary cancer, cervical cancer, gastric cancer and comedo cancer of the left breast, Aliev (1964) one with cancer of the uterine body, stomach and caecum. Noxan (1972) described the case of a man, who in the last 17 years of his life developed an osteosarcoma, alveolar cell carcinoma of the lung, an adenocarcinoma of the colon and two skin cancers. Coley et al. (1971) report the case of a man with Klinefelter's syndrome, who over 17 years developed six primary tumours, a sacral chordoma, four large benign lipomata, a spongioblastoma of the brain, a carcinoma of the right breast, a papillary carcinoma of the thyroid and a separate carcinoma of the left breast. Bakker and Tjon (1971) describe a case of multiple sebaceous gland tumours, kerato-acanthomata of the skin and, who over 21 years, developed carcinoma of the colon twice and carcinoma of the stomach. They mention two other similar cases in the literature. Filippova (1973) describes a case of concomitant chronic lymphatic leukaemia, meningioma, adenoma of one kidney and hypernephroma of the other. Cabrera et at. (1966) draw attention to the development of lower genital carcinoma in female patients with anal cancer (5 of 64 cases), indicating the existence of a local carcinogenic agent.

Of special significance is the association of lymphoma or leukaemia with other primary tumours in the same patient. These have been reported by Warren and Gates (1932) Moertel and Hagedorn (1957), Wallace (1957), Fried (1958), Razis et a!. (1959), Corner et al. (1961), Faber and Borum (1962), Tabakova (1966), Berg (1967), Whitelaw (1968) and Coeur (1969). Fried (1958) found lymphoblastoma and leukaemia associated with bronchial adenocarcinoma. Moertel et al. (1958) also found 4 cases of leukaemia or lymphoma associated with bronchial carcinoma. Whitelaw (1968) described the case of a patient who developed Hodgkin's disease at the age of 29 years and in the next 27 years suffered from 11 primary cancers of four distinct histological types. Wallace (1957) in 71 patients with multiple primaries found 5 cases in which *lymphoma* was accompanied by a second primary tumour affecting breast, mucosa of the mouth, bladder, stomach or corpus uteri. Comes et al. (1961) and Cuilleret et aL (1973) also report second cancers in patients suffering from *leukaemia, lymphoma or plasma cell* disorders. Tabakova

(1966) described two cases, one a patient with both acute leukaemia and renal carcinoma and another with chronic lymphatic leukaemia and carcinoma of the oesophagus. Softie (1964) reported the case of a patient, a woman of 54 years, with acute myeloblastic leukaemia, cancer of the breast and mixed parotid tumour and Gilbert et al. (1971) Hodgkin's disease, Kaposi's sarcoma and malignant melanoma in the same patient. Coeur (1969) found malignant tumours in 27 out of 365 cases of *chronic lymphatic leukaemia*. Warren and Gates (1932) collected 1259 cases of multiple cancers from the literature in which the following lesions were observed: -

One case of both lymphosarcoma and adenocarcinoma occurring in the liver, 2 of lymphosarcoma and carcinoma of the stomach, 1 of lymphosarcoma and carcinoma of the caecum, 1 of lymphosarcoma of the stomach and adenocarcinoma of the liver, 1 of lymphosarcoma of the kidney and carcinoma of the bile duct, 1 of lymphosarcoma of the base of the tongue and carcinoma of the larynx, 1 of generalized lymphosarcoma and carcinoma of the ovary, 1 of lymphosarcoma of the mediastinum and carcinoma of the labia, one case each of lymphosarcoma and carcinoma of the prostate, bronchus and rectum and 1 *oi* lymphatic leukaemia and basal cell carcinoma of the skin. The authors suggested the action of some generalized common factor was responsible for the m:.tk·tip!e malignancies.

Moertel and Hagedorn (1957) report on 62 of 2,134 patients with leukaemia who had additional primary cancers. In 27 the diagnosis was made simultaneously, in 18 the I.: ukaemias preceded and in 16 followed the primary tumour. Of 2,340 patients with *malignant lymphoma* 68 had second primaries, 25 being diagnosed simultaneously, while in 23 the other lesion preceded the diagnosis of lymphoma and in 17 was made afterwards. They reviewed the literature of leukaemia or malignant lymphoma

occurring with second primaries. Of 104 cases of *chronic lymphatic leukaemia* 36 exhibited cancer of the skin or lips (29 single, 7 multiple), 12 of the stomach, **8** of the bronchus, 6 of Kaposi's sarcoma, 6 of breast, 4 of larynx, 4 with malignant melanoma, 3 each of colon, cervix or prostate, 2 each of kidney, bladder, tongue and carcinoid and 1 each of oesophagus, appendix, liver, bile ducts, ovary, pleura, lung, kidney and leiomyosarcoma, prostate and fibrosarcoma. Of 17 cases of *chronic myeloid leukaemia* there were 3 cases each associated with cancer of the stomach or bronchus, 2 with carcinoma of the cervix and 1 each with carcinoma of the skin, jejunum, colon, breast, ovary, kidney, adenosarcoma of liver, cerebral astrocytoma and Kaposi's sarcoma. Of 9 cases of *acute leukaemia* 2 were associated with cancer of the colon, rectum or thyroid and 1 each with cancer of the bronchus, breast, cervix, malignant teratoma of the ovary and sarcoma of the kidney. Of 62 cases of *malignant lymphoma* 13 were associated with Kaposi's sarcoma, 15 with skin cancer, 10 with cancer of the stomach, 4 of bronchus, 4 of colon or rectum, 2 of prostate, 2 with malignant melanoma and 1 with 3 adenocarcinomata of the ileum, 2 each with cancer of the ovary and vulva simultaneously, 1 with cancer of the lip and skin, 1 with cancer of the oesophagus and liver, skin and uterus, skin and cervix, skin and testis, colon and kidney, uterus and breast and multiple myeloma. Stavraky et al. (1970), Djaidane et al. (1972) and Russell and Cochran (1973) also describe chronic lymphatic leukaemia with later development of cancer of various organs. In Moertel and Hagedorn's 52 cases of leukaemia the association of *chronic lymphatic leukaemia* with cancer of the skin, hreast, bronchus, stomach, colon or rectum, kidney, bladder and prostate was recorded. In one case leukaemia was associated with cancer of the larynx, mandible and prostate in the same patient and another with

Addendum: Rubins J., Sischy B, Lee T C K. Am. J. Clin. Pathol. 1980, 74/5 696·700. Non-Hodgkin's lymphoma following treatment for Hodgkin's Disease. Case report and review of the literature. Authors report non-Hodgkin's lymphoma appearing following treatment for HD.

Addendum: Leinkram C, Chou S T, Iser J, Sali A. Med. J. Aust 1980, 1/7, 309·11 Multiple primary cancers arising from different organs and tissues. Report a case of lymphoma and adenocarcinoma of the stomach in the same patient and a metastatic squamous carcinoma in the axillary nodes from an unknown primary.

cancer of the prostate and skin. In 11 cases of *chronic myeloid leukaemia* the blood disease was associated with cancer of the skin or lips, breast and in 2 cases with cancer of the colon or rectum and the skin and in another with cancer of the pharynx, bronchus, bladder and prostate. In 8 cases of *acute leukaemia* 3 were associated with carcinoma of the colon or rectum, 1 with carcinoma of the stomach and 1 with carcinoma of the colon or rectum, prostate and seminoma of the testis at the same time. In 68 cases of *malignant lymphoma* 16 were associated with cancer of the skin or lips or both, 7 with cancer of the colon or rectum, 1 with cancer of the colon and rectum and of the skin, 1 with cancer of the colon or rectum and the vulva and there were also cases with an association with cancer of the breast, prostate, thyroid, stomach and bladder, penis, ovary, uterine body, cervix, mouth, pharynx, parotid, oesophagus, malignant teratoma of the testis, melanoma of the choroid, skin melanoma and Kaposi's sarcoma. In one case malignant lymphoma was associated with Kaposi's sarcoma and carcinoma of the breast and in another with seminoma of the testis and cancer of the skin and mouth. Bachulis and Williams (1966) report 220 patients with multiple malignancies. In many one tumour was a reticulosis.

Malignant lymphomata, including reticulosarcoma and Hodgkin's disease, may develop into or co-exist with chronic lymphatic or myeloid or acute leukaemia. Reference to such cases are given by Razis et al. (1959), Joseph et al. (1966), Johnson et al. (1966), Wilson and Vanslyck (1966), Hollard et al. (1967), Lazlo and Grove (1967) and Velez Garcia et al. (1969). Again, acute leukaemia may develop in cases of myelomatosis (Leading Article, Brit. med. J., 1971, 1, 568), though whether this is due to treatment or nautral progress of the disease is uncertain. Rosenberg et al. (1961) reviewed 1,269 cases of lymphosarcoma. They found co-existent

malignancies in 50 cases compnsmg 56 cancers. Of these there were 21 involving the skin, 4 bronchogenic carcinomata, 4 each of the breast, colon and prostate, 3 of the cervix, 2 each of the larynx, rectum, stomach, kidney and malignant carcinoid and one each of the tongue, bladder, chondrosarcoma of the pelvis, malignant melanoma, Kaposi's sarcoma and pituitary ependymoma. Friedmann and MUller (1967) describe the development of reticulosarcoma four years after removal of a medulloblastoma. Fodor and Krutsay (1964) record the simultaneous occurrence of reticulosarcoma and adenoma of the salivary glands of the pharynx, and Parolari (1963) reticulosarcoma of the tonsil with squamous carcinoma of the larynx; reticulosarcoma of tonsil and jaw and basal cell carcinoma of the lip; and multiple myeloma and basal cell carcinoma of the skin of the nose. There is an increased incidence of skin cancers associated with both lymphoma (Green, 1972), chronic lymphatic leukaemia (Stavraky et al., 1970) or visceral cancer (Gilbertson, 1972). More *significant are* cases *where lymphoma and cancer of different types are associated in a single organ.* Warren and Gates (1932) describe lymphosarcoma and adenocarcinoma of the liver, 3 cases of lymphosarcoma and carcinoma of the stomach and lymphosarcoma and carcinoma of the caecum, lymphosarcoma, reticulosarcoma or Hodgkin's disease associated with carcinoma of the stomach (Jernstrom and Murray, 1960; Mainzer et al., 1968; Coppola et al., 1969; Popov and Kurilovich, 1973) or primary lymphosarcoma and carcinoma of the bladder (Stitt and Colapinto, 1966). The case of Coppola et al. (1969) was also associated with macroglobulinaemia. Primary lymphosarcoma and carcinoma of the thyroid has also been described (see later). Tsuzi et al. (1970) recorded glomus tumours and leiomyoma of the stomach occurring together, Leopold and Mogg (1964) both carcinoma and leiomyosarcoma affecting a single adult kidney,

Komorn et al. (1973) simultaneous squamous carcinoma and adenocarcinoma of the larynx and Larrauri et al. (1974) gastrointestinal tract adenocarcinoma with carcinoid tumour areas.

Again, when multiple cancers affect a single organ, the histological structure of the different tumours may be different. Merrick et al. (1972) recorded 15 cases of multiple carcinoma of the lungs in which this was so. Kaye et al. (1971) and Brief et al. (1972) described similar findings in cases of multiple carcinoma of the breasts.

In the large series of cases of malignant disease seen in succession by the author and fully investigated and which are reported later, the following cases of multiple tumours were found:-
Chronic lymphatic leukaemia with reticulasarcomatosis; chronic lymphatic leukaemia with lymphosarcomatosis, 2 cases; reticulasarcomatosis and malignant melanoma of the choroid of one eye; multiple rodent ulcers of the face and chest with lymphosarcoma of the stomach; lymphosarcomatosis and transitional cell carcinoma of the left renal pelvis and transitional cell papillomata and carcinoma of the bladder, benign lympho-epithelial tumour of the parotid and Hodgkin's disease; mixed parotid tumour and Hodgkin's disease; dermoid cyst of the left ovary and Hodgkin's disease; carcinoma of the bronchus and carcinoma of the stomach; carcinoma of the thyroid and Hodgkin's disease; carcinoma of the prostate, malignant lymphoma, carcinoma of the male breast and separate carcinoma of the bronchi in the two lungs; malignant lymphoma and malignant melanoma; eosinophilic pituitary adenoma and myelomatosis; monocytic leukaemia and malignant hepatoma; sarcoma of the shoulder and acute myeloid leukaemia; chronic lymphatic leukaemia and carcinoma of the bronchus; chronic lymphatic leukaemia and carcinoma of the larynx; chronic lymphatic leukaemia and cortical adrenal adenoma; rodent ulcer of the face and carcinoma of the stomach; rodent ulcer of an eyelid and adenocarcinoma of the thyroid gland; separate carcinomata of both breasts and pancreas; carcinoma of the right breast and myelomatosis; carcinoma of the thyroid and myelomatosis; rodent ulcer of the neck and malignant melanoma of the left nostril; malignant melanoma of the umbilicus and carcinoma of the breast; carcinoma of the breast and fibrosarcoma of the right upper arm; rodent ulcer of the face and carcinoma of the bronchus; carcinoma of the larynx and mixed parotid tumour; simultaneous carcinoma of the thyroid and bronchus; carcinoma and neurofibroma of the stomach; carcinoma of the stomach and carcinoma of the colon; carcinoma of the cervix and carcinoma of the stomach; carcinoma of the colon and carcinoma of the bronchus; carcinoma of the stomach, two carcinomata of the colon, carcinoma of the pancreas and of both ovaries; cortical adrenal adenoma and malignant insulinoma; rodent ulcer of the eyelid and carcinoma of the bladder; multiple rodent ulcers of forehead and neck carcinoma of the anal canal and carcinoma of the bladder; multiple rodent ulcers and carcinoma of the bladder; carcinoma of the breast and chromophobe pituitary adenoma; cerebral meningioma and fibrosarcoma of the mesentery; right .frontal cerebral glioma with overlying rodent ulcer; carcinoma of the breast and carcinoma of the cervix; neurofibroma of the forearm. malignant lymphoma of one breast and carcinoma of the other; carcinoma of the transverse colon followed by carcinoma of the rect m and bronchus together; carcinoma of the body of the uterus with carcinoma of both ovaries (3 tumours); carcinoma of the vagina and carcinoma of the body of the uterus; .eosinophil adenoma of the pituitary and carcinoma of the bronchus; carcinoma of breast, colon and bladder; carcinoma of the ovary and of the colon; carcinoma of the breast and carcinoma of the colon; multiple mY-elomatosis and acute lymphoblastic leukaemia; and carcinoma of the breast and

Addendum: Prat, J. and Scully, R.E., Cancer (Philadelphia) 1979, 44, 1327-1331. Sarcomas in ovarian mucinous tumours. A report of two cases. The authors report two cases of ovarian cysts. One a cyst adenocarcinoma in which the walls contained solitary nodules of sarcoma. It shows a common aetiology of sarcoma, adenoma and adenocarcinoma.
Addendum: Peyhonen, L, Heikkinen, J and Vehkalaht, S. Two different primary tumours of the brain in a patient with breast cancer. Eur. J. Nucl. Med., 1979 4/6 483-484. The authors report a case who had primary breast cancer and later meningioma and a glioblastoma multiforme were found at autopsy.

carcinoma of the body of the uterus. In a large number of other cases in this series a malignant tumour was associated with fibroids or benign ovarian cysts (see below).

Thus, these observations suggest that–

1) *Every kind of benign or malignant tumour, myelomatosis or lymphoma and any type of leukaemia may occur in the same patient or in the same organ.*

2) *In cases of multiple malignant tumours, whatever their histological structure, and* of *malignant tumours associated with benign tumours occurring in Europe and U.S.A. a single factor generalized throughout the body often appears to be causally responsible for the tumourous change occurring in the various organs.* In these cases Gilbert et al. (1971) also raised the possibility of a general mesenchyme susceptibility to tumour induction. Dellon et al. (1975) likewise conclude that multiple neoplasms arise from a single cause.

3) *The same factor which induces the development of malignant lymphoma, myeloma or leukaemia, is also responsible for the development of the cancers or benign tumours affecting any organ or tissue, which may be found associated with the myelomatosis, lymphoma or leukaemia, either acute or chronic, in any particular case of multiple malignancy.* It has been suggested above that in the case of such benign tumours as uterine fibroids or ovarian cysts this factor is that causing collagen and auto-immune disease. As Savic et al. (1966) point out, such cases prove that can er in Western Countries at least, is usually a *generalized rather than a local disease* caused by unknown biological factors. Again, multiple malignancies affecting a single organ or system, such as the urinary tract from kidney to bladder or the bowel and mouth and respiratory tract, suggest a field of precancerous change. Jimmerson and Merrill (1970) call attention to multiple malignancy in the cervix, vagina, vulva and peri-anal skin, indicating a localized tumour-producing agent for all the tumours. A similar explanation can be reached for the case described by Bochenek et al. (1973) in which three different neoplasms affected neighbouring tissues, namely carcinosarcoma of the larynx, carotid body tumour and a mixed type thyroid carcinoma with local metastases.

Known factors in the genesis of human cancer

A number of factors are known to be concerned in the genesis of human cancer:-

A. Hormonal factors

Cancer of certain organs, notably the breast before the menopause, of the prostate and possibly of the uterus and ovary and of the thyroid in a proportion of cases have been thought to be due to hormonal causes and non-environmental in aetiology.

B. Genetic factors

In man malignant disease is known to develop sometimes in the abnormal tissues in certain heredo-familial, that, is genetically controlled diseases, such as Von Recklinghausen's, Von Hippel-Lindau's or Gartin's syndromes and in xeroderma pigmentosa, though it is thought that some environmental factor is necessary to precipitate the malignant change in such cases. Genetic factors are also important in the development of multiple endocrine adenomatomas (see Evans, 1966; Johnson et al., 1967). Fanconi's anaemia is also a genetically controlled disease. Swift (1971) found that in cases of Fanconi's anaemia heterozygotes the risk of death from neoplasm is three times as great as normal. Again genetic factors are known to play a highly significant part in the development of malignant change or resistance to malignant change in experimental animals in certain organs, as in the breast cancer of certain breeds of mice. Horn and Horn (1971) describe fou r patients with clear cell carcinoma of the kidney in a family.

Tht gGnetic factors are important in man in predisposing to cancer generally is now well established (Oettle, 1967; Bottomley and Condit, 1968; Lynch, 1969). Bryant and Rush (1967) reported multiple primary neoplasms in identical twins. A family in which numerous cancers occurred (Family "G") was first described by Warthin in 1913 (Warthin, 1913). This has be-:m brought up to date by Lynch and Crush (1971). The progenitor died of cancer of the stomach or intestine. Six of his 10 children developed cancer. Of the ten branches of the family two have never had a case of cancer, but the eight other branches now contain 82 patients who have developed single primary malignant tumours and 13 with multiple tumours. The 650 blood relations have now been afflicted with 113 verified tumours. Fifty-two were in the colon, 18 endometrial and the rest include leukaemia, lymphoma and even sarcoma. Buehler et al. (1975) report a large inbred family in Newfoundland in which 7 cases of Hodgkin's disease, 3 of lymphosarcoma, 2 of thymoma, 2 of common variable immunodeficiency and single cases of retinoblastoma, neuroblastoma and rhabdomyosarcoma occurred, strongly suggesting a genetic basis for the above conditions and that immunological defects are of importance. Creagan and Fraumeni (1973) describe carcinoma of the stomach in 12 members of an inbred kindred over four generations. In 16 members of the family a high frequency of auto-antibodies to gastric parietal cells and cell-mediated immune defects were found, suggesting that a uto-immunity is involved in the familial susceptibility to stomach cancer. Potolski et al. (1971) report a sibship of 10 adults of which 5 died of lymphoreticular malignancy. In 4 surviving siblings there were immunological abnormalities of humoral and cellular type, suggesting a genetic relationship between immunological abnormalities and susceptibility to neoplasia of lymphoid tissue. Fraumeni et al. (1969) reported a similar family. Cohen

et al. (1958) record the case of a woman aged 29 years, who developed a number of maligancies over 3¥2 years. These included Hodgkin's disease, carcinoma of the breast and Paget's disease, pleomorphic sarcoma in the mastectomy scar, superficial malignant melanoma of the skin, leukaemia and atypical glandular proliferation of the endometrium. One month after her death her father developed Hodgkin's disease and her son a cerebral tumour. A man, aged 63 years, under the author's care died of carcinoma of the bronchus. His only sibling, a male, also died of carcinoma of the bronchus at the age of 50 years. Both their parents died of cancer, the father of the stomach, the mother of the breast. The patient's wife died at the age of 50 years of cancer of the breast and his only child, a woman, died at the age of 43 years of cancer of the breast.

In a family investigated by the author, the patient, a woman of 58 years, died from carcinomatosis of the breast, her mother died of cancer of the large bowel, her brother of cancer of the stomach and her grandmother of cancer of an unknown primary. She had no other brothers or sisters. In Case VII, 3, a man of 19 years, developed a malignant lymphoma and gave a marked family history of cancer. His paternal grandfather died of carcinoma of the bladder and his paternal grandmother of carcinoma of the ovary and had been treated also for carcinoma of the breast. His maternal grandfather died of carcinoma of the stomach and suffered from numerous lipomata. His maternal grandmother died from carcinoma of the bronchus. His only maternal aunt had a mixed parotid tumour. His parents were so far not affected, but his mother suffered from, rheumatoid arthritis.

Apart from the susceptibility to cancer of various organs illustrated by the above, families may also exhibit a special tendency to specific cancers. Familial lymphatic leukaemia and its relation to Waldenstrom's disease was discussed by Gordon

(1963) and Dreyfus et al. (1966), familial Hodgkin's disease by Vettori and Erie (1967, familial lymphoma by Hambleton (1969) and Zachau-Christiansen and Christensen (1966), familial multiple myeloma by Robbins (1967), familial leukaemia and lymphoma by Rigby et al. (1966) and familial acute leukaemia by Heath and Moloney (1965), Gunz et al. (1966) and Lundmark et al. (1967). Heath and Moloney reported 5 cases of acute leukaemia in three generations, three being of one generation, with two cases of breast cancer and probable pernicious anaemia and in another generation there was a case of mongolism. The familial tendency to breast cancer is well-known. Lynch et al. (1974) describe the familial occurrence of cancer of the breast and ovary. In all recent reviews of the genetic factors in human cancer (Gettle, 1967; Willis, 1967; Lynch, 1969; Anderson, 1970) it is concluded that in every case of cancer a *combination of genetic and non-genetic (exogenous or environmental) factors is of importance*, but vary in their relative importance in different cases.

C. Congenital anomalies

It is well known that the cells of many congenital anomalous tissues, which as seen above may often differ genetically from normal cells, are especially liable *to* malignant change. It is thought, however, that some environmental factor is also necessary for this change.

D. Chromosomal abnormalities predisposing to malignant change

In a number of conditions associated with chromosomal abnormalities in the body cells there occurs a predisposition to malignant change (Hamden, 1976). These include mongolism, Klinefelter's and Turner's syndromes, Bloom's syndrome and Fanconi's anaemia. These will be considered below.

E. Radiation

In any form X-irradiation is known to cause any type of human cancer.

F. Conjugal cancers

Occasionally conjugal cancers have been reported (Walach and Horn, 1973). These include conjugal Hodgkin's disease (see Hoster and Dratman, 1948) and acute leukaemia of the same type and at the same time in husband and wife recorded by Amos et al. (1967), who review reported cases. Such cases point to an environmental or infective causation.

G. Clusters of leukaemia cases are described. The author had experience of four cases of leukaemia occurring in one house in unrelated subjects more or less contemporaneously. Orchard (1961) described the occurrence of two cases of malignant lymphoma and one of acute lymphatic leukaemia occurring together in workers in an East African meat packing house where they were exposed to raw meat (in which limax amoebae are found). Such cases would again appear to be envir m-mental or infective in causation. Smithers (1967) pointed out the occurrence of Hodgkin's disease and leukaemic lymphoma in siblings and in adjoining houses, supporting an infective rather than an inherited origin. Schimpff et al. (1975), in studying leukaemia and lymphoma patients interlinked by prior social contact, suggested the possibility that apparently different diseases of the lymphoid system may be caused by the same agent and may be transferred from person to person. These include different leukaemias, Hodgkin's disease, lymphoma, lymphosarcoma and reticulum cell sarcoma.

H. Environmental factors

Geographically cancer patterns in different countries show wide variations. Migrant populations to an area tend to take on the pattern of the indigent population, for example negroes have the same incidence of cancer of different organs as whites in U.S.A. This indicates that an environmental factor rather than race plays an essential role in causing tumours in Western industrialized states. This might be chemical, physical or infective in nature. Such environmental factors operate even in the case of congenital anomalies and genetically predisposed individuals. A few such environmental factors are known, such as exposure to radiation, chemicals as in the case of carcinoma of the bladder in dye workers, aromatic amines, asbestos, haematite ores, nickel and chromium compounds, smoking in the case of carcinoma of the bronchus, trachea, larynx and pharynx and possibly of the bladder, exposure to arsenic, exposure to the sun in cases of skin cancers and melanomata, exposure to burns as in Kangri cancer, the chewing of Betel nut in mouth cancer in India, chemical carcinogens in chimney sweeps, mule-spinners cancers and those of tar workers, cancer of the naso-pharynx in wood and boot and shoe workers in this country, trauma in the case of skin cancers and other tumours, such as meningiomas (Leading Article, Brit. med. J., 1969, 3, 369-370) and low standards of sexual hygiene in uterine cervical cancer. In Africa the role of aflotoxins and nitrosamines in the production of cancer appears to be important. Occasionally metazoan parasites, such as flukes or schistosomes, play a part in the production of human and ani al cancer. Boyland (1969) suggests that not more than 10 per cent of huma n tumours are caused by radiation or viruses, leaving about 90 per cent attributable to exogenous or endogenous chemicals. In the large majority of human cancers no cause is evident. It must be stressed that in all parts of the world free-living limax amoebae exist in the environment and infect man.

Fields of origin of epithelial tumours

The strict unicentric view of the origin of tumours is untenable. Tumours arise from small or large fields of tissue from a multifocal origin in an epithelium and not only by cellular proliferation, but also by progressive neoplastic conversion of tissue within those fields. In many cases the extent of the potentially neoplastic field is much greater than the small size of the initially appearing tumour would suggest. Tumours of the skin, for example, display evidence of a progressive hyperplastic-neoplastic change still taking place in a centrifugal direction over fields of epidermis. The actual size of the potentially cancerous field round a tumour of the skin is much greater than the tumour, since there are wide zones of epidermal hyperplasia around the growth. The frequently multicentric or diffuse mode of origin of basal cell growths of the skin is well-known and there is often evidence of multifocal origin from groups of sweat glands and ducts or from several hair follicles and sheaths or from both. A similar origin of cutaneous melanomas by a progressive neoplastic change from considerable fields of epidermal cells is demonstrable. Similar findings are associated with epithelial tumours of mucous membranes, such as the mouth, oesophagus, stomach, large intestine and bladder, of glandular organs such as the breast, prostate, liver, pancreas, kidney, salivary glands and testis, and fields of origin of non-epithelial mesodermal tumours, such as leiomyomas of the uterus (fibroids), lipomas, meningiomas and gliomas. The whole question of the origin of tumours from fields of potentially neoplastic material is considered by Willis (1967).

Willis (1967) states "Neoplastic change does not take place suddenly, but in a gradual and cumulative manner, long-standing hyperplasia often passing insensibly into neoplasia or an early benign or non-invasive tumour by progressive stages into a malignant invasive one without any sudden change in. cellular characters, the degree of differentiation or rate of growth. This neoplastic change takes place either simultaneously or successively in vast numbers of cells over more or less extensive fields of tissue. Benign and malignant tumours are not sharply distinct. In many tumour classes every possible gradat.:on of structure and behaviour is to be found, from the most malignant to the ;:: ost benign".

"If, then, there exists any single common factor underlying neoplastic change, it must *apply* to *benign* as *well as* to *malignant tumours.* To suppose that all the variant members in a particular histogenic class of tumours are due to "mutations" would be to suppose there are almost as many different "mutations" as individual "tumours".

Now the subepithelial tissues control the metabolism of overlying epithelia and access to the cells of the latter, including carcinogenic agents, is controlled by the subepithelial tissues. An extensive precancerous field in an epithelium may mean a *large* epithelial *area containing a carcinogenic factor* in the subepithelial tissues. It will be recalled that large areas of epithelia may be affected in cases of collagen and auto-immune disease, that is there is a disturbance extending over a large field in many subjects, while the benign tumours, called benign ovarian cysts and fibroids, appear to be causally related to collagen and auto-immune diseases.

Congenital or primary acquired agammaglobulinaemia or hypogammaglobulinaemia and tumour formation

These conditions may be divided into 1) congenital, 2) acquired primary cases evidently occurring as the first manifestation and precursor of other evidence of collagen and auto-immune disease, and 3) cases associated with the presence of malignant lymphomata. In the first two groups of these conditions it has been pointed out that there is a special liability to the development of collagen and auto-immune disease. This occurs in at least one-third of the cases. This tendency is also accompanied by a predisposition to the development of lymphomas or cancers. Doll and Kinlen (1970) remark on the close association between the immunological disorders and tumour formation, especially of the reticulo-endothelial system.

In primary (congenital) immunodeficiency states the frequency of malignancy is roughly 10,000 times that in the general matched population (Penn, 1974) Classical congenital agammaglobulinaemia of the Bruton type predisposes to leukaemialymphoma (Page et al., 1963; Gabrielson et al., 1969), that of the Aldrich syndrome to reticulum cell sarcoma or reticuloendotheliosis (Gabrielson et al., 1969) and of ataxia-telangiectasis to lymphoma (Peterson et al., 1964; Hetch et al., 1966). Von Bermuth et al. (1970) describe a child of 5 months of age with thymic alymphoplasia, severe anaemia and a low IgG level which developed rashes and frequent intercurrent infections, including Pneumocystis carinii (a protozoal) infection, and Hodgkin's disease in lymph nodes, liver and lungs. In a Clinico-Pathological Conference at Charing Cross Hospital the case of a 14 year old boy with agammaglobulinaemia who developed rheumatoid arthritis and four years later lymphoma was described.

In some cases of primary acquired disease there occurs an hyperplasia of the germinal centres in lymph nodes and spleen with splenomegaly and often with hypersplenism. The changes in the lymph nodes approach those of follicular lymphoblastomas and occur in perhaps 10-15 per cent of cases of the acquired type (Green et al., 1966; Janeway, 1967; Gabrielson et al., 1969). Pancytopenic changes of hypersplenism may be found in the blood. The condition may go on to generalized lymphoma. This has been frequently observed and in these cases the antibody deficiency syndrome has antedated the development of lymphoma by as much as 26 years. In some cases of hypogammaglobulinaemia with steatorrhoea a nodular hyperplasia of the small intestine is

Addendum: Voelcker, H.E. and Naumann, G.O.H., Br. J. Ophthalmol., 1978, 62, 408-413, report a case of two separate malignant melanomas of the choroid in one eye, which contained two additional uvea I naevi. They found seven further cases in the literature and eleven of bilateral multicentric malignant melanomas of the uvea. Such cases illustrate the occurrence of malignancies in a "field."

Addendum: Louis, S. and Schwartz, R.S., Semin. Haematol., 1978, 15, 117-138, emphasizes the frequent association between immunodeficiency and the development of malignant lymphoproliferative diseases, suggesting an infective cause for the latter.

found. Three of 9 patients with this developed malignancy of the gastro-intestinal tract (2 stomach, 1 rectum) (Janeway, 1967; Gabrielson et al., 1969). The working party on hypogammaglobulinaemias in the United Kingdom Report (1969, Lancet, i, 163) describes 8 malignancies as occurring in this condition, 6 being lymphomas. Migueres et al. (1969) report a case of hypogammaglobulinaemia with RF, lupus erythematosus cells, antiglobulin antibodies in the blood and malignant lymphoma. Potolski et al. (1971) report a sibship of 10 adults of which 5 died of lymphoreticular malignancy. In 4 surviving siblings there were immunological abnormalities of humoral-cellular type suggesting a genetic relationship between immunological abnormalities and susceptibility to neoplast!a of lymphoid tissue. Fraumeni et al. (1969) reported a similar family. Wolf (1962) described a case of primary acquired hypogammaglobulinaemia with a high incidence of haematologic abnormalities in the family. These included systemic lupus erythematosus, idiopathic thrombocytopenic purpura, leukaemia, reticuloendotheliosis and Hodgkin's disease. Furthermore, patients with primary acquired hypogammaglobulinaemia may develop thymoma (Gehrmann and Engstfeld, 1965) in association with pancytopenia or myasthenia (Velve et al., 1966; Mallinson. 1971). This is in contrast to the general atrophy of lymphoid tissue.

The fact that in cases of *congenital* hypogammaglobulinaemia *there* is *no special liability* to *virus* diseases, but lymphoma and cancer are especially common, is strongly against a viral causation for the latter. It also suggests that various kinds of tumour have the same causation in many cases. Moreover, the special liability to both collagen and auto-immune diseases and to malignancy found in both congenital and primary acquired cases of hypo- or a-gammaglobulinaemia suggests that such cases are especially liable to show signs of limax amoebae infection and that this may perhaps be related to tumour formation of various kinds.

Viruses and cancer in man

In the last few years the virus causation of many animal cancers and leukaemias has been demonstrated and by analogy such an aetiology for human cancer has naturally been suggested. The author (Wyburn-Mason, 1952 a and b), in fact, reported the development of cancer in the human skin directly out of the lesions or scars of herpes simplex or zoster. Kwasnicka (1965) confirmed this in the case of herpes simplex of the lips. Recent work has raised the possibility of an herpes virus playing a role in the development of cancer of the cervix (Rawls et al., 1970). The earlier work of Moore and Sarker (1972) appeared to favour the view that human cancer may be due *to* a virus. Now, however, these workers (Moore and Sarker, 1972) have reported that further work shows no evidence to substantiate such an idea. McAllister et al. (1972) studied human adenoviruses. These may induce tumours in laboratory animals and transform rodent cells in vitro. They conclude, however, that adenoviruses are not likely to be an important cause of human cancers. Burkitt (1969) has suggested the role of a virus in causing African lymphoma or nasopharyngeal growths in subjects of chronic malaria, a protozoal disease. However, tumours identical with African lymphoma have been reported from many parts of the world where malaria is unknown in subjects who have never left the area and even in cats in the Bristol area. It has also been suggested that nasopharyngeal carcinoma and African lymphoma may be caused by Epstein-Barr virus. Banatzala et al. (1972) found Epstein-Barr virus specific IgM present in the serum of cases of infective mononucleosis for 7-10 days, but absent in cases of nasopharyngeal carcinoma, Hodgkin's disease and African lymphoma. Burkitt

-251-

Addendum: Sauer, O. and Spelger, G. (Monatschr Kinderheilkd., 1977, 125, 885) describe Duo:'itz's syndroe in 2 sisters, one had hypogammaglobulinaemia and neuroblastome, the other complete IgA deficiency and malignant lymphoma.

(1970) mentions that the tumour rejection phenomena observed in African lymphoma appear to be related to a high degree of antigenicity, which is characteristic of virus-induced animal tumours. Such a degree of antigenicity is not found in the majority of human cancers (Klein, 1970). Again, as was seen above in cases of congenital or primary acquired a- or hypo-gammaglobulinaemia there is no special liability to virus diseases, though lymphoma and/or carcinomata tend to occur with an increased frequency. In general, however, even after intensive work in all parts of the world all modern reviews conclude that no human cancers have been shown to be viral in aetiology. In reviewing all the evidence available up to 1967 on the relationship of viruses to human tumour formation Willis (1967) concludes that "There is no evidence that viruses are the .... cause of any kind of human neoplasm, except possibly acute leukaemia". Indeed, this author throws considerable doubt on the claim that virus-induced "tumours" and "leukaemias" in rodents are tumours in the sense of human cancer. In viral cancers in animals the malignancies show no association with collagen or auto-immune disease as they will be seen to do in man, and virus infections do not cause the precancerous field ,changes described above. Human cancer would seem to differ from animal virus-induced cancer in its aetiology. It seems that the time has arrived to discard the virus theory and look elsewhere for the causation of many human cancers. If ever the causes of malignant disease in man are to be determined, then the cause of those lesions which are known to be premalignant in man must be found. This is not to be discovered from experiments on cancers in rats and mice, but by clinical observation in man, that is "The proper study of mankind is man". (Alexander Pope, An Essay on Man). Many premalignant lesions will be seen below to be those of collagen-auto-immune disease, for

example atrophic gastritis, cystic mastitis, Paget's disease of bone and Hashimoto's thyroiditis. Thus, collagen-auto-immune disease may be one of the primary causes of human cancer.

Prolonged antigenic stimulation and malignancy

Virchow concluded that the cause of cancer was chronic irritation. This idea must be modified. However, there is a great deal of evidence that prolonged cellular multi-antigenic stimulation may give rise to malignancy in genetically predisposed individuals.

a) Experimental lymphoma formation in animals

Schwartz and Beldotti (1965) injected ⊢ week old F1 hybrid mice with parental living spleen cells. They were given an immuno-suppressive drug to reduce mortality from the graft-host reaction. Long term survivors of the reaction developed neoplasms resembling Hodgkin's disease and lymphosarcoma, the tumours containing giant cells and eosinophils. The tumours were transplantable to isogenic recipients, indicating fkat they were of host rather than donor-origin. These mice were chimaerae, but the parental cells present within their spleens had specific immunological tolerance towards the host antibodies. The tumours did not involve the thymus. Certain immunological theories of neoplasia are of interest in this respect. One of these theories (Dameshek and Schwarz, 1959) has as its basis the cellular proliferation that characterizes the response of lymphoid tissue to antigen. It proposes that a continuous or repetitive exposure to an antigen could result in a sustained proliferation response, which culminates in neoplasia. The concept is supported by Metcalf's (Metcalf, 1965) experiments, in which an increased incidence of reticulum cell sarcoma and plasma cell tumours was found in mice which had been given repeated injections of bovine serum albumin or salmonella Adelaide vaccine.

b) Organ transplants leading to tumour formation

Reference will be made later to the greatly increased liability to the development of both lymphoma and carcinomata in cases of organ transplants. Myking (1971) suggests this is due to the chronic antigenic stimulation by the graft cells.

c) Chronic antigenic stimulation and myelomatosis

The plasma cells and lymphocytes produce antibodies to antigens. In cases of myelomatosis or plasmocytoma there is a proliferation of plasma cells and a resultant paraproteinaemia and cryoglobulinaemia. This suggests a prolonged antigenic stimulation as preceding their proliferation, but again the nature of the prolonged antigenic stimulation is not known.

d) Chronic antigenic stimulation by infections or allergens and reticuloses and leukaemias

Scheuer-Karpin and d'Heureuse-Gerhardt (1965) point out that reticuloses and leukaemias may be the result of chronic antigenic stimulation ·by various infections, such as chronic acti tuberculosis, malaria, osteomyelitis, owfs media and urinary infections. Imahori.'and Moore (1972) report two cases of plasma cell dyscrasia developing after prolonged hyposensitization therapy.

Tan et a!. (1974) studied 19 patients with mycosis fungoides, a condition closely related to malignant lymphoma. They found auto-antibodies in 13 of the cases. Their findings support the hypothesis that mycosis fungoides is a chronic granulomatous response to persistent unidentified antigen (s) , upon which immune imbalance can develop, resulting in auto-immune phenomena and in a few cases various lymphoreticular neoplasms.

Thus, it appears that both experimentally and clinically in many cases of myelomatosis and lymphomata there *must be a chronic and persistent cellular and multi-*

antigenic stimulation in the body, and, since many human cancers, myelomata and lymphomata can often be attributable to one cause, this may apply to many carcinomata also. Such a chronic antigenic stimulation occurs in chronic collagen and auto-immune diseases and it is also a feature of other chronic infections, such as malaria and leprosy. Burch (1963), Innis (1966, 1969) and Barclay (1969) suggest that auto-immune reactions may be the cause of malignant lesions by removal, inhibition or alteration of the differentiating factor within the cell. Their proposal that all cancer originates in the reticulo-endothelial system explains the vagaries of the circulating "cancer" cell and the reason why some metastases regress and others do not. It relates the malignant process to inflammatory and degenerative processes. It is, therefore, possible that the cause of collagen and auto-immune disease is the source of the chronic antigenic stimulation in many cases of human can:::er, but other chronic infections may play a part.

e) Metazoon parasites in the pathogenesis of cancer in man and animals

Infestation with a number of metazoan parasites is known to lead to malignant change in some animals and man. The subject up *to* 1931 was reviewed by Strong (1931). These parasites include:-

1) Trematodes

Schistosomiasis is generally regarded as responsible for malignant change in the bladder in some subjects, though it does not appear to be so in the liver, intestine or lung where the parasites may also be found. The part played by secondary bacterial infection is not yet determined. In animals and man, infestations of the liver and bile ducts with *Opisthorchis felinis* may lead to cirrhosis and carcinomatous change in the liver or bile passages, and in man this is also true of infestation of the liver with the fluke, *Clonorchis sinensis.*

2) Nematodes

Addendum: *Protozoal infection and cancer.* Infection with protozoa may predispose to malignant change. Thus heavy malarial infection is an important factor in the development of African lymphoma, both in Africa and New Guinea, while cancer of the oesophagus, uterine cervix and urinary system appears to be more common in sufferers from Chaga's disease than in non-Chaga's subjects. Association of Chaga's disease and cancer. De Lustig ES, Puricedi L, BalE and LanzettiJC. Medicina (B. Aires) 1980, 40, 43-96. Furthermore trichomonas vaginalis infect on of the vagina may cause atypical cell alterations of the cervix. Trichomonas vaginalis and cytological findings. Hotho H. Arch, Geschwulstforsch. 1977, 471, 455-461.

In rats the nematode, *Capillaria hepatica,* which is a common parasite of this animal, may induce gastric carcinoma and another nematode, *Trichosomoides crassicauda,* which inhabits the urinary bladder, ureter and renal pelvis may produce papillomata and malignant growths. In some pheasants the nematode, *Heterakis isolanche,* which is confined to the caecum, may lead to local spindle-cell sarcomatous change. Bourne and Sandground (1939) described the development of gastric epithelial tumours bordering on malignancy as a result of the presence of the nematode, *Nochtia nochti,* in monkeys in Batavia, and they produced similar tumours experimentally in these animals. Doerr and Menzi (1934) and Schmidt-Lange (1935) found experimental feeding of trichinella larvae to rats and mice produced spindle cell sarcoma of the diaphragm or liver, the tumours developing in relation to the encysted larvae. As will be seen later infestation with filaria may produce lymphadenopathy closely resembling that of Hodgkin's disease (see Galliard and Mallarme, 1955).

3) Cestodes

In both dog and man *Taenia multilocularis* cysts of the liver, but of no other organ, have been found associated with primary carcinoma or sarcoma of the liver. Cysticercus fasciolaris is the cystic form of the tape worm of the cat, *Taenia crassicolis,* and, by feeding rats with the eggs of the worm, Bullock and Curtis (1925) obtained single or multiple tumours of the liver. The sarcomas developed from the connective tissue around the cysts. They were mostly spindle-cell or polymorphous celled, but there were some fibrosarcomas, and one liposarcoma and cartilaginous tissue was present in several tumours and in one case in the metastases. Only rarely did carcinoma develop. Dunning and Curtis (1946, 1953) further investigated and confirmed the findings of Bullock and Curtis that sarcoma is an almost inevitable result of infestation of the liver or subcutaneous tissues of rats with the

cysticercus. Sarcomas of the peritoneum could be produced in 90 per cent of cases by intraperitoneal injection of freshly ground up larvae and the active principle was associated with the calcium carbonate fraction of the parasite. It is not present and active in filtrates of the sarcoma. The responsible agent is present in suspension!:: of washed freshly ground taenia larvae from *rats* of *the same* strain bearing a cysticercus sarcoma. Berkfeld filtrates of the suspension were inactive. The liability to malignant change is thus *dependent* on *genetic make-up.* The larvae seem to develop the carcinogenic agent after about 12 months of age. The tumours develop on an average 89 days after inoculation. The neoplastic change is produced by a carcinogen liberated from the worm and not as a result of chronic irritation.

Thus, it appears that metazoan tissue parasites may lead to locally induced malignant change in some animals and man after a latent period and that this may be *genetically dependent.* Parasites within the lumen of the hollow viscera may also do so locally. Thus, *local fo-reign cells may induce malignant change in some animals.*

Cancer and the aging process

Cancer is predominantly a disease of the elderly (see Willis, 1967) and about four-fifths of all fatal carcinomas occur in the oldest one-third of the community and about two-thirds occur at ages ovr 60 year::;. Cancer is mainly a d;sease of the elderly, not because senile tissues are "predisposed" to cancer, but cancer is indeed part of the aging process, be::ause of the usually long latent period elapsing between the application of carcinogenic stimuli and the development of tumours. Such a long-standing antigenic stimulus exists in the form of the cause of long-standing collagen or auto-immune disease. The causation of many cancers seems to lie in the causation of the aging process, of which collagen and auto-immune disease forms an important element.

The significance of the rarity of primary cancer of the duodenum and small intestine

Bile acids exist in the bile in a conjugated state in which cholic acid (a sterol) is combined with glycocoll (glycine) or with taurine, which is related to cystine. Percy-Robb and Collee (1972) point out that these are deconjugated by many intestinal bacteria and that this unconjugated bile acid may have bacteriocidal and bacteriostatic properties, which are pH dependent. Bile salts are secreted into the duodenum and are present unconjugated throughout the small intestine down to the ileo-caecal junction, being reabsorbed into the circulation during their transit. Reference has already been made to the finding that unconjugated bile salts in the concentration existing in the small intestine destroy trophozoites of many amoebae. This may be the explanation of why E. histolytica lesions are not found in the small intestine where the amoebae would be killed by unconjugated bile salts, but occur in the liver and other organs where bile salts are conjugated or absent. The rarity of primary cancer of the small intestine, including the duodenum, in man is well-known, but no real explanation of this fact has been put forward. Furthermore, while malignant change is common in gastric ulcers, it practically never occurs in duodenal ulcers, while primary cancer of the liver, bile ducts and gall bladder is not uncommon. This could be explained if chronic limax amoebae infection were responsible for many cases of malignant disease, but the unconjugated bile salts present in and being absorbed through the duodenum and small intestine destroyed it, whereas the conjugated bile salts in the bile passages would have no such effect.

Chapter IX

The effects of anti-amoebic substances on cases
of human malignant disease

Human and many animal malignant tumours contain large numbers of limax amoebae, which must be presumed to exert a harmful effect on the host. Moreover, Culbertson et al. (1972) in experimental infections of guinea pigs with the free-living amoeba, N. aerobia, found that the organism produced in these animals a condition which closely resembles the effects of malignant disease. It appeared important to try to determine the part played by the amoebic infection in the manifestations of human malignant disease.

The effects of various anti-amoebic substances on different types of malignant disease have been studied and the results described below under the following headings:-

I. Reticuloses
   a)   The effects of 4-aminoquinolines.
   b)   The effects of dehydro-emetine.
   c)   The effects of indo-methacin.
   d)   The effects of copper sulphate.
   e)   The effects of bile acid.
   f)   The effects of clotrimazole.
   g)   The effects of levamisole.

II. Leukaemias
   a)   The effects of 4-aminoquinolines.
   b)   The effects of dehydro-emetine.
   c)   The effects of copper sulphate.
   d)   The effects of bile acid.
   e)   The effects of clotrimazole.
   f)   The effects of metronidazole.

III. Gliomata
   a)   The effects of 4-aminoquinolines.
   b)   The effects of copper sulphate.
   c)   The effects of clotrimazole.

IV. Carcinomatosis
   a)   The effects of 4-aminoquinolines.
   b)   The effects of dehydro-emetine.
   c)   The effects of copper sulphate.
   d)   The effects of bile acid.
   e)   The effects of streptomycin.
   f)   The effects of clotrimazole.
   g)   The effects of other imidazole-containing anti-amoebic drugs.

V. Myelomatosis

I. a)   Effects of chloroquine in cases of reticuloses

Hiraki and Kimura (1962) treated a case of advanced generalized lymphosarcoma with chloroquine and obtained marked regression in size of lymph nodes and spleen, disappearance of ascites and pleural effusions and a return to normal appearance in the lymph nodes. In two cases of giant follicular lymphoma a similar regression occurred and the lymph node histology returned to that of chronic inflammation. In one case of reticulasarcoma and another of Hodgkin's disease no improvement occurred. Rossberg (1963) treated a case of plasmocellular reticulosis of the skin with chloroquine diphosphate, 250 mgms. daily for 47 days with regression of the lesions. Kennedy et al. (1963) and Damron et al. (1965) also obtained similar results. Tanneberger and Bacigalupo (1967) found that chloroquine in cases of lymphoma had a corticosteroid-like action and was anti-pruriginous and fever-lowering, but it was not cytostatic.

The author (Wyburn-Mason, 1964) studied the effects of chloroquine on 25 cases of malignant lymphoma, including Hodgkin's disease. Only four, which were all in the last stages of the disease and who had previously had various types of treatment, failed to respond in any way to treatment. Two of these were cases of Hodgkin's sarcoma. Response may occur whether the patient has had previous X-ray or antimitotic drug treatment or not. Complete disappearance of symptoms and signs of disease occurred in 10 cases. In Cases 3, 4 and 5 of this series the results ere dramatic. The sweating, pruritus, pyrexia, skin lesions, lymph node enlargement, serous effusions, anaemia, raised E.S.R. and signs of neuropathy vanished. This usually occurred in early cases who had no previous treatment. In the follow up, which varied from four months to over five years, in five of these cases there was no sign of disease up to over five years after cessation of treatment. In the other five cases, after a period varying from two months to two years, symptoms and signs of disease returned. A further course of chloroquine treatment may or may not have a beneficial effect. In eleven cases improvement was not so marked and complete disappearance of symptoms and signs of disease did not occur. In these cases the lymph node enlargement regressed, but did not disappear, sweating, pruritus and pyrexia ceased and the E.S.R. fell. Two further cases treated in the same way are now described : —

Case VII, 3 Male, aged 19 years. Student. Family history-His paternal grandfather had died of carcinoma of the bladder. His paternal grandmother died of carcinoma of the ovary and had been treated for carcinoma of the breast. His maternal grandfather died of carcinoma of the stomach and suffered from multiple lipomata. His maternal grandmother died of carcinoma of the bronchus. His only maternal aunt suffered from a mixed parotid tumour. His pJ.rents were free

of cancer, but his mother suffered from rheumatoid arthritis. Two weeks before hospital attendance he noticed a painless lump in the anterior wall of the right axilla rapidly increasing in size. There was no disturbance of his general health. Examination showed a generalized enlargement of the lymph nodes of the neck, axillae and groins and one larger node about 3 ems. in diameter at the lower border of the right pectoral muscle in the anterior axillary wall. The nodes elsewhere varied from 1 to 3 ems. in diameter. The spleen and liver were not enlarged clinically. There was no pyrexia. A chest X-ray was normal. A blood count showed Hb 100 per cent, W.B.C. 6,000 per cu. mm., polymorphs 70 per cent, lymphocytes 20 per cent, monocytes 5 per cent, eosinophils 5 per cent, E.S.R. 35 mms. per hour, plasma proteins-albumin 4.3 gms. per cent, globulin 1.7 gms. per cent. Biopsy of the largest lymph node was carried out. Cross section showed a homogeneous grey tissue. Microscopically the structure of the lymph node was completely obliterated. Numerous reticulum cells were scattered in the lymphatic tissue, sometimes forming small aggregations. In other parts there were collections of lymphocytes and plasma cells with local areas of eosinophils. A few multinucleated giant cells were present. The structure was that of early Hodgkin's disease. He was treated with amodiaquine 200 mgms. twice daily for 2 months and then 200 mgms. daily. Within two weeks all the lymph node enlargement had disappeared and an E.S.R. at the end of three weeks was 3 mms. in 1 hour. The blood count remained normal, the eosinophilia falling to one per cent of 7,600 W.B.C. per cu. mm. A year later he suffered from herpes zoster in the left D10 segment accompanied by painful enlargement of the lymph nodes in the left axilla and groin. The latter subsided after two weeks. He has remained completely well over the last ten years with a normal blood count

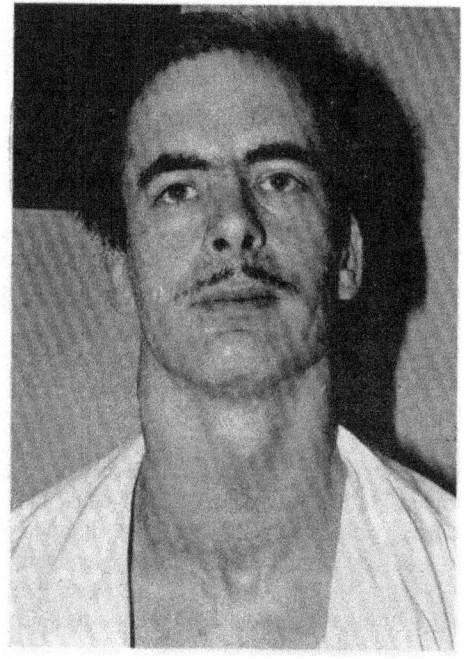 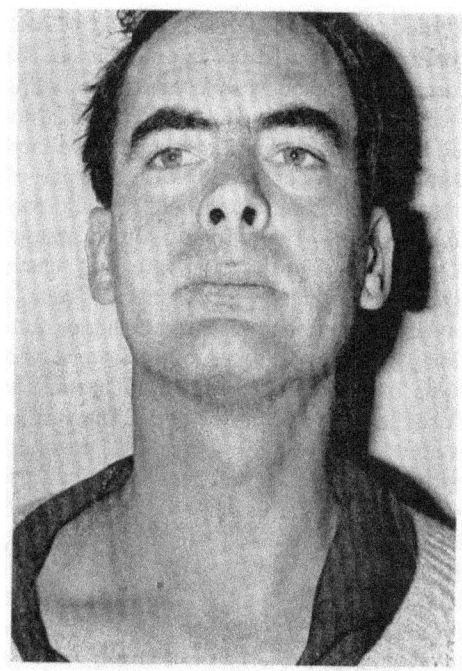

Fig. 55-A   Fig. 55-B

Fig. 55 Male, aged 32 years. Hodgkin's disease of right
cervical lymph nodes. "A" before and "B" one momh after
treatment with amodiaquine (Case VIII, 28).

and E.S.R. Treatment was stopped after two years.

tJase VIII. 28 Male, aged 32 years. He suffered from asthma until the age of 14 years and since the age of 17 years had been subject to the development of itching wheals on the back occurring irregularly, but especially after physical exertion. Ten months before being first seen he developed slight fever and sweating followed by the appearance of a large persistent painless swelling of the lymph nodes on the right side of the neck. Examination showed a hard non-tender mass of enlarged lymph nodes beneath the upper part of the right sternomastoid muscle (Fig. 55). Less enlarged nodes were present In the posterior triangle of the left side of the neck and in the right axilla. The liver and spleen were not palpable.

He was running a fever of 99_0- $99.8°$ F. A blood count showed Hb 90 per cent, W.B.C. 7800 per cu. mm., polymorphs 73 per cent, monocytes 9 per cent, lymphocytes 8 per cent, eosinophils 10 per cent, E.S.R. 36 mms. in 1 hour. Chest X-ray was normal. Biopsy of one of the enlarged cervical lymph nodes was carried out and the histological report was as follows—The normal structure of the node is completely destroyed. In some areas lymphocytes form diffuse sheets mingled with proliferating reticulum cells, plasma cells and eosinophils. Scattered among these are multinucleated giant cells. The picture is typical of Hodgkin's granuloma.

He was treated with amodiaquine 200 mgms. twice daily for two months. The temperature fell to normal the next day.

Within three days the mass on the right side of the neck began to subside. At the end of 5 weeks the lymphadenopathy had completely disappeared (Fig. 55). A blood count now showed Hb 97 per cent, W.B.C. 5600 per cu. mm., polymorphs 56 per cent, lymphocytes 39 per cent, eosinophils 5 per cent. The E.S.R. was now 1 mm. per hour. He was followed for 20 months during which time there was no recurrence of symptoms, but then after developing a sore throat there was a short-lived painful swelling of the left cervical lymph nodes lasting about a week. This subsided spontaneously. The wheal formation ceased to occur after the beginning of treatment. After another six months the swelling of the cervical lymph no:Jes recurred and there was only a partial regression of the swelling after recommencing treatment with amodiaquine. Eventually he was treated with prednisolone and chlorambucil, but in spite of this the disease progressed and X-ray therapy was commenced with improvement in his condition.

I, b) Effects of dehydro-emetine (DUE) in cases of reticuloses

Abd-Rabbo (1967, 1969) in Egypt reported favourable responses in cases of Hodgkin's disease and ·lymphosarcoma to the administration of dehydro-emetine in doses of 500 mgms. orally daily or on alternate days. In cases of Hodgkin's disease it caused the lymph nodes to swell and a pyrexia and this was followed by regression of the lymph node enlargement as may occur in the treatment of filariasis with diethylcarbamazine (Herxheimer reaction).

I, c) The effects of indomethacin on cases of Hodgkin's disease

The anti-rheumatoid drug, indomethacin, has been used in the treatment of Hodgkin's disease by Silberman et al. (1965)

and Paver() and della Pietra (1966). They found that the drug reduced the fever, but had no effect on the course of the disease.

I, d) The effects of copper sulphate on cases of malignant lymphoma

The effect of administration of copper sulphate was observed on one case of malignant lymphoma with myelofibrosis and chronic myeloid leukaemia.

case VII, 40 Female, aged 89 years. Fifteen years before admission she was operated on for an enormous uterine fibroid weighing 15 lbs. and at that time the spleen was found to be grossly enlarged. She made few complaints until shortly before admission, when she began to lose weight. Examination at that time showed marked rheumatoid changes in the hands and feet and in addition a spleen reaching down to the left iliac fossa. There were widespread pigmented keratoses of the skin. An enlarged lymph node was present above the left clavicle. fhe urine contained 2 per cent of sugar. She was markedly deaf and also incontinent. A random blood sugar showed a level of 250 mgms. per 100 mls. X-rays of the chest showed a very large heart and marked bilateral hilar lymph node enlargement and fluid at the right base (Fig.56). X-rays of the abdomen showed a markedly enlarged spleen with a calcified splenic artery low in the left iliac fossa. A blood count showed Hb 7.4 grams per 100 ml. (51 per cent), W.B.C. 7700 per cu. mm., 90 per cent neutrophils, 2 per cent myeloblasts, 5 {:er cent lymphocytes, 3 per cent monocytes, serum albumin 2.4 G, globulin 3.7 G per 100 mls. E.S.R. was 60 mms. per hour. Serum iron, folate and vitamin B12 concentrations normal. Serum bilirubin less than 1 mg. per cent. The sternal marrow showed increased cellularity with preponderance of premyelocytes and myeloblasts. Leucopoiesis and megakaryocytes normal. The changes were suggessive of early myeloid leukaemia.

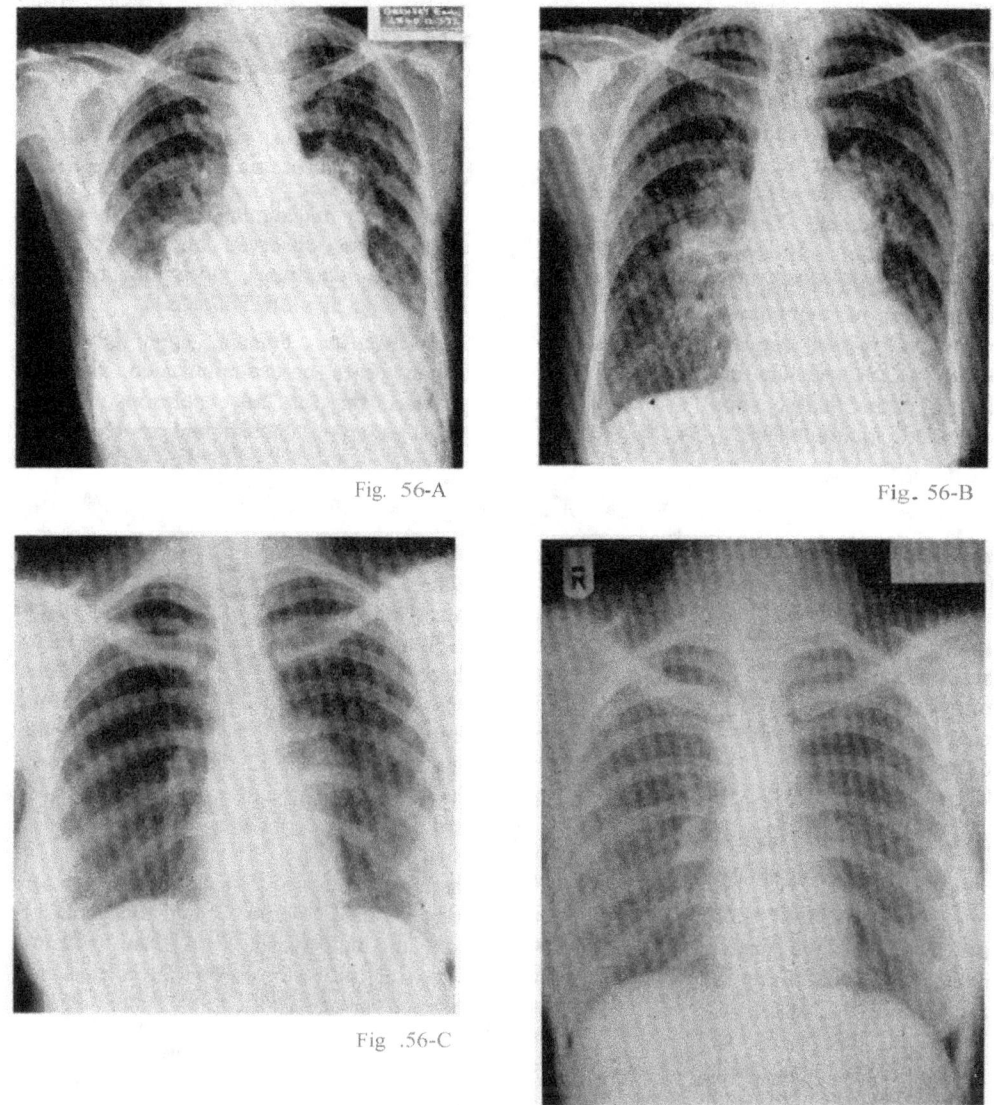

Fig. 56-A

Fig. 56-B

Fig .56-C

Fig. 56-D

Fig. 56   Female, aged 89 years.   Myclofibrosi with malignant lymphoma and myeloid leukaemic cha nges.   "A" X-ray
of chest before treatment showing pleural effusions and hilar
lymphadenopathy and "B" after treatment "'ith copper sul-
pha te showing disappearance of effusions and diminution of
hilar shadows (Case VII, 40).

Female, aged 28 year.   Hodgkin' di case.   X-rays of chest
showing left hilar lrmphadenopath y "C" before and "D" 3
weeks after begi nning trea tment with copper sulphate. showing
disappearance of lymph node enlargement.

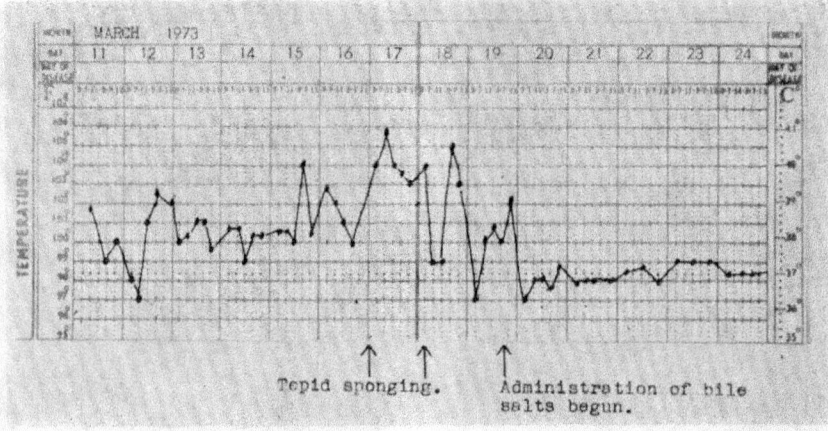

MARCH 1973

Tepid sponging.

Administration of bile salts begun.

Fig. 57

Fig. 57 Case of a woman, aged 28 years, suffering from Hodgkin's disease, showing the effect of administration of bile acid on the temperature.

Biopsy of a lymph node showed the changes of lymphosarcoma. X-rays of the long bones showed evidence of myelofibrosis. Lupus erythematosus cells absent. Serum RF negative. Thyroid and gastric parietal cell auto-antibodies negative. Free HCL present in gastric secretion. Electrophoresis showed diffuse increase in $\alpha 1$ and $\alpha 2$ globulins. No Bence-Jones protein present in urine. A diagnosis of myelofibrosis, malignant lymphoma and chronic myeloid leukaemia with diabetes mellitus and long-standing rheumatoid arthritis was made. She was given a transfusion of 4 pints of packed red cells with general improvement in her condition. The leukaemic changes and hilar lymph node enlargement persisted. She was, therefore, treated with copper sulphate 25 mgms. t.d.s. and there was a rapid general marked improvement in her condition. The E.S.R. fell to 26 mms. per hour. Within 3 weeks the total white cell count fell to 3.300 per cu. mm. Neutrophils 70 per cent. The white cell precursors had vanished from the peripheral blood at that time. The hilar lymph node enlargement lessened (Fig. 56) and the glycosuria disappeared. She was kept on this regime for 6 weeks and discharged home, but was lost to follow-up.

I, e)   The effects of bile acid on reticuloses

This was tried in 3 cases, all suffering from Hodgkin's disease. It was found that bile acid produced a slight diminution in the size of the lymph nodes, a fall in temperature and E.S.R., improvement of appetite, some gain in weight and disappearance of "toxic" effects as demonstrated in the accompanying figures (Figs. 57–60).

I, f)   The effects of clotrimazole on reticuloses

This was tried on two cases of Hodgkin's disease with the following results:—

Case 101 Female, aged 65 years. Past history nil relevant. She presented with a string of several lumps below the left breast. Examination showed three hard discrete mobile masses about one inch in diameter running transversely below the

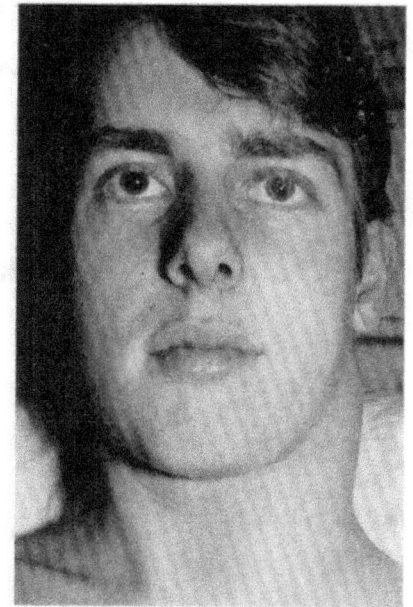

Fig. 58·A

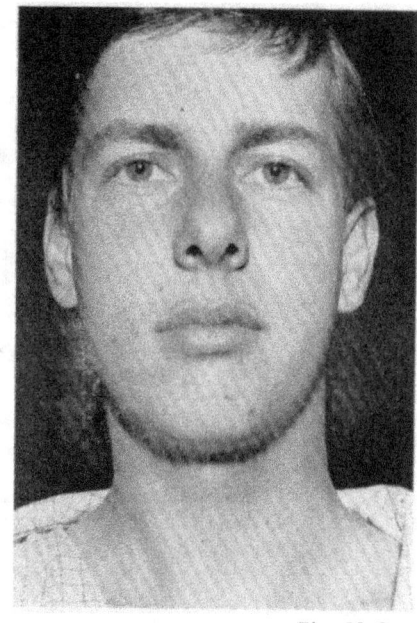

Fig. 58·C

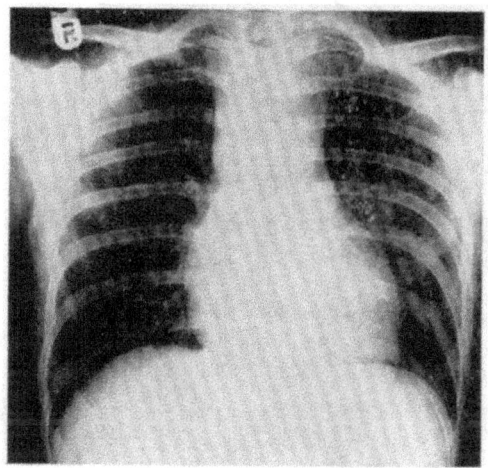

Fig. ss.n

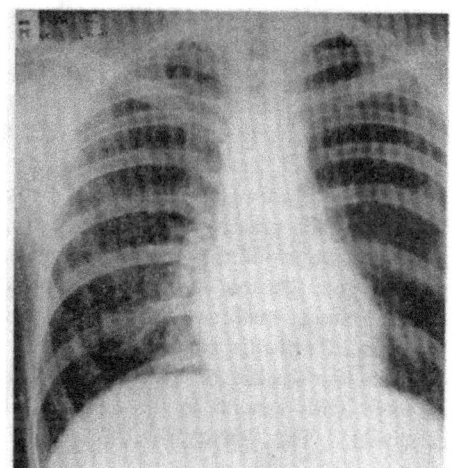

Fig. 58·O

Fig. 58   fale, aged 18 year.   Hodgkin's disea(' of lrft
cervica l and superior media tina! lymph nodes.   "A" and "B"
before and   "C" and "D" af ter trcatm<'nr with bil(' acid for
one month.

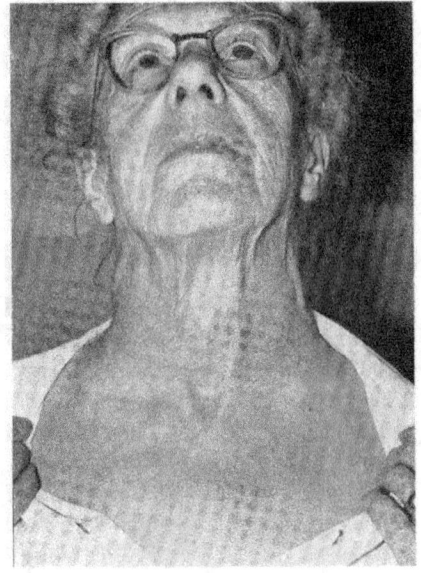 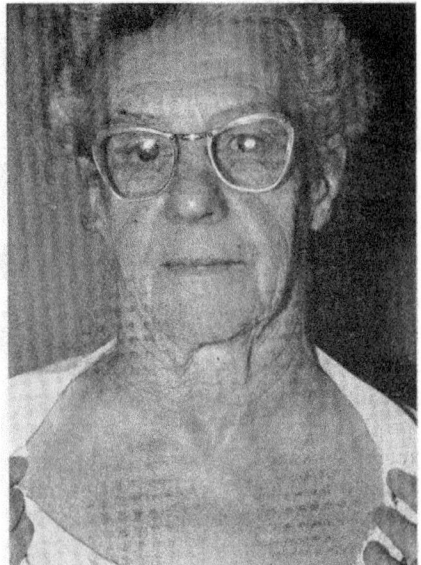

|Fig. 59-A|Fig. 59-B|

Fig. 59 Female, aged 70 years. Hodgkin's disease of cervical lymph nodes. "A" before and "B" 2 months after continuous treatment with bile acid showing disapp<'arance of swellings.

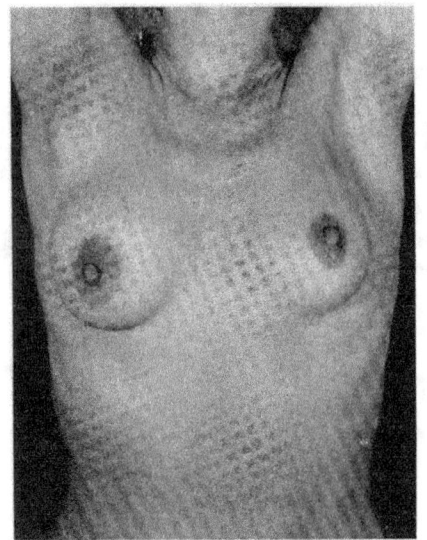 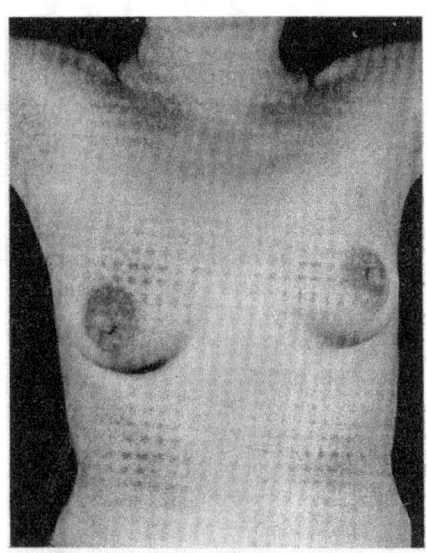

|Fig. 60-A|Fig. 60-B|

Fig. 60 Female, aged 29 years. Hodgkin's disease of 3 years duration showing mass of lymph nodes beneath the right pectoral muscle "A" and disappearance of mass after treatment with bile acid "B".

left breast, but nothing else was found abnormal elsewhere in the body. Temperature was normal. *Investigations.* Blood count, Hb 15.1 G per 100 mls., W.B.C. 8,500 per cu. mm., leucocytes 81 per cent, E.S.R. 129 mm. per hour. Achlorhydria present. RF, ANF and all auto-antibodies absent from the serum. Liver function tests normal. Plasma proteins, albumin 3.2 G per 100 mls., globulin 2.8 G per 100 mls. A chest X-ray normal. Excision of the three masses showed the changes of Hodgkin's disease. After recovery she was treated firstly with bile acid and later with copper sulphate without any change in the E.S.R. She was then given clotrimazole 2 G t.d.s. Within two days there was a rise in temperature to 99.8° F with general malaise and sweating and then a markedly enlarged tender node appeared above the left clavicle. This persisted for 3 weeks and then spontaneously subsided. The E.S.R. a week after beginning clotrimazole rose to 152 mm. per hour and later fell to 85 mm. per hour. The treatment was continued. She remained unchanged over the next six months.

Case 102 Male, aged 22 years. Nothing of significance in the past or family history. For two years he had been subject to irregular bouts of influenzal-like symptoms. Three weeks prior to admission he developed an attack in which the temperature ranged from 99-102°F. for 3-4 days and this was followed by the development of lymph node swelling in the left side of the neck. *Examination.* He was markedly thin, pale and sweating with a temperature of 102.2°F. and there was lymphadenopathy of varying degree ranging from the size of a pea to that of a gooseberry in the posterior triangle of the left side of the neck. There were also slightly enlarged tender nodes in the left axilla and left inguinal regions. The liver and spleen were not palpable. Nothing abnormal was found in the abdomen or the rest of the body. *Investigations.* Chest X-ray was normal. There was no enlargement of the mediastinal lymph nodes. Biopsy of a cervical lymph node showed loss of normal follicular pattern and proliferation of reticulum cells among numerous lymphocytes and occasional binucleate cells were seen. The appearances were those of Hodgkin's disease. Liver function tests were normal (alkaline phosphatase 9 KA units per 100 mls.). Plasma proteins, albumin 2.9 G per 100 mls., globulin 4.1 G per 100 mls. Blood count, R.B.C. 4.46 mil. per cu. mm. Hb 11.8 G per 100 mls. W.B.C. 9,200 per cu. mm., neutrophils 76 per cent. lymphocytes 24 per cent. E.S.R. 127 mms. per hour. Electrophoresis showed diffuse increase in alpha 2 globulin fraction.

He was treated with clotrimazole 100 mgms. per kilogram daily. This produced a dramatic effect. Within 48 hours there was a massive tender swelling of all the lymph nodes on the left side of the neck and a tender mass appeared in the epigastrium. After 48 hours the temperature rose to 104°F. There was profuse sweating and rigors and these symptoms persisted for 3 days after which time the temperature began to settle and the swelling of the lymph nodes rapidly subsided. Within 5 days of beginning treatment his temperature became normal and after a week to ten days the enlarged cervical lymph nodes were hardly palpable. The patient felt well and he began to eat. The E.S.R. fell to 83 mm. per hour and he gained 5 pounds in weight in 2 weeks. He was discharged still taking clotrimazole and two weeks later, whilst feeling well he attended a wedding and took some champagne. Within one hour he developed epigastric aching. The temperature rose rapidly and he began to sweat profusely again. He was readmitted to hospital, but in spite of continuing clotrimazole, he continued to run a temperature and to lose weight. He was then treated by quadruple chemotherapy.

I, g) The effects of levamisole on reticuloses

Levamisole is an antiprotozoal drug containing an imidazole group like clotrimazole and tinidazole. Phillips et al. (1977) report on two cases of advanced Hodgkin's disease with pronounced sweating and fever unaffected by other anti-mitotic drugs, but these symptoms were abolished by levamisole, though it had no other effect on the course of the disease.

In conclusion drugs acting on limax amoebae may cause regression of the lesions in cases of lymphoma and disappearance of the toxic symptoms of the disease. Most significant is that *these may cause a rapid exacerbation* of *the disease manifestations and a painful swelling* of *the affected nodes like an Herxheimer reaction* similar to that produced in syphilis and filariasis by drugs active against the causative organism. This confirms the presence in the lymph nodes of an organism sensitive to clotrimazole, such as limax amoebae as already demonstrated.

II, a) The effect of 4-aminoquinolines on cases of leukaemia

Hiraki and **Kimura** (1962) treated two cases of acute and two of chronic lymphatic leukaemia with chloroquine. In both cases of the latter the lymphadenopathy regressed. No improvement in the blood count occurred. Allan and Watson-Williams (1964) and Watson-Williams and Allan (1968) describe the beneficial effect of antiprotozoal drugs on cases of chronic lymphatic leukaemia in Nigeria, where the condition appears to be related to tropical splenomegaly. Wyburn-Mason (1964) reported an improvement in cases of leukaemia treated with chloroquine. Of the six cases of acute leukaemia treated all were in young children and all but one had previously received treatment with corticosteroids and/or 6-mercaptopurine at other hospitals and were rapidly deteriorating in spite of this. This treatment was continued and in addition 4-aminoquinoline was given by mouth as chloroquine 50

mgms. t.d.s. Three of the cases, one of which was a mongol, died within 7-20 days of beginning treatment. Of the other three all showed a response to chloroquine. The corticosteroids and 6-mercaptopurine in the two cases receiving them were discontinued. In all of them the blood count returned completely to normal within ten weeks and all symptoms disappeared. In two the bone marrow appearances also became normal. These two cases were followed for a year without evidence of recurrence. One of them died later of leukaemia. In the other case the marrow appearances, though not returning to normal, approached it more nearly so than before. This patient died of acute leukaemia a year after beginning the treatment.

The five cases of chronic leukaemia were all myeloid in type. Three of these had received treatment with corticosteroids and myeleran and were in the last stages of the disease with marked splenomegaly, hepatomegaly, ascites, serous effusions and bleeding from the mucosae and into the skin. The blood count in all cases showed severe anaemia, deficient platelets and white cell counts ranging from 260,000 to 400,000 per cu. mm. with many myeloid precursors. In the other two only hepatomegaly and splenomegaly were present and the white cell count was 98,000 and 111,000 W.B.C. per cu. mm respectively with myeloid precursors in the film. Neither had received any other treatment. In all cases the sternal bone marrow showed the typical picture of chronic myeloid leukaemia. All five cases were given daily intravenous injections of 300 mgms. of antrycide (a 4-aminoquinoline). Two of the advanced cases died within 14 days of beginning treatment. The other advanced case and two early cases showed a good response to treatment, which was continued for two months. The advanced case then deteriorated and died three months after beginning treatment, but the other two continued to improve. The total W.B.C. count progressively fell and the precursor cells disappeared from the peripheral blood. The anaemia, hepatomegaly and splenomegaly gradually disappeared. The blood counts reached normal in 6-8 weeks. These two cases were followed for 12-18 months and remained symptomless and their blood counts normal. In one case a repeated sternal puncture showed a normal appearance. Both of these patients later died of leukaemia in spite of continuing treatment.

Since the author's original account ar.- other case of chronic myeloid leukaemia and three cases of chronic lymphatic leukaemia have been treated with 4-aminoquinolines.

Case 103 Male, aged 56 years, developed fainting attacks. There were no abnormal physical signs. A blood count showed Hb 14.0 G per 100 mls. W.B.C. 38,600 per cu. rom. 80 per cent being polymorphs, 12 per cent lymphocytes and 4 per cent eosinophils. Occasional myeloid precursors were present. The bone marrow showed the typical changes of *chronic myeloid leukaemia*. He was maintained on chloroquine 200 mgms. daily for 6 years remaining symptomless throughout this time, the W.B.C. remaining at about 36,000 per cu. mm. At the end of this time he suddenly developed purpura and it was then found that the platelet count had fallen to 40,000 per cu. rom. and myeloid precursor cells rose to 20 per cent of the total of 37,000 W.B.C. In spite of treatment with busulphan, prednisolone and copper sulphate he ra pidly went downhill and died from gastrointestinal bleeding. The spleen was not palpable at any time during the course of his illness.

Case 104 Male, aged 49 years. He developed tiredness and had lost 10 lbs. of weight over the previous 3 months. Examination showed a liver enlarged 4 fingers breadth below the costal margin with a smooth edge and the spleen was also markedly enlarged. A blood count showed Hb 13.8 grams per cent., W.B.C. 20,000 per cu. rom., neutrophils 22 per cent, eo-

sinophils 2 per cent, lymphocytes 63 per cent, monocytes 30 per cent. The excess lymphocytes were chiefly small and mature. The E.S.R. was 4 rom. in 1 hour. A sternal bone marrow showed fairly active erythropoiesis, normoblastic in type. Leucopoiesis showed marked lymphoid infiltration amounting to 60 per cent of all the nucleated cells. The lymphocytes were chiefly small with little cytoplasm, but occasionally large lymphocytes and lymphoblasts were noted . Thrombopoiesis was normal. The diagnosis was that of *chronic lymphatic leukaemia*. He refused treatment at first, but he continued to lose weight rapidly and this amounted to 30 lbs. over five months. Six months after the onset of symptoms the liver had increased enormously in size and the spleen was enlarged to 5 fingers breadth below the costal margin. The blood Hb by this time had fallen to 11.5 grams per cent and the E.S.R. to 35 mm. in 1 hour. Treatment with plaquenil 200 mgms. a day was then commenced. From that time he made steady improvement. He began to gain weight. Gradually all his symptoms disappeared and the liver and splenic enlargement lessened. After one year he had gained 11 lbs. in weight. The liver remained smooth and was now only 2 fingers enlarged and the spleen was only just palpable. By that time he had returned to all his normal activities, both business and sport, the latter including off-shore sailing. A blood count at this time showed Hb 15.0 grams per cent, W.B.C. 8,000 per cu. rom., neutrophils 25 per cent, lymphocytes 34 per cent, eosinophils 2 per cent, monocytes 12 per cent. Occasional large lymphocytes were present in the blood, but no lym phoblasts. In view of this blood picture the haematologist felt a further bone marrow biopsy was unjustified. He has remained well over four years.

case X, 24 Female, aged 66 years. She was treated by radiation for carcinoma of the left vocar' cord 18 months previously:

She had recently developed enlarged lymph nodes in the right groin and right side of the neck. A blood count showed Hb 106 per cent, W.B.C. 18,700 per cu. mm., neutrophils 20 per cent, lymphocytes 79 per cent, E.S.R. 9 mm. per hour, platelets 800,000 per cu. mm. Sternal bone marrow showed that the predominant cell was a small lymphocyte compatible with the diagnosis of chronic lymphatic leukaemia. Biopsy of a lymph node showed generalized infiltration with lymphocytes compatible with the diagnosis of chronic lymphatic leukaemia. She was treated with chloroquine 200 mgms. daily over the next 12 years, during which time her total white cell count never rose above 21,400 per cu. mm. and mostly remained at 12-13,000 per cu. mm. and the neutrophils formed 43-48 per cent of the total white cell count. At the end of this time she moved from the district, having remained perfectly well during the period of treatment.

Case 105 Male, aged 63 years. Presented as a case of chronic bronchitis and emphysema discovered. A blood count at that time showed Hb 10.2 G per 100 mls. (70 per cent). W.B.C. 115,600 per cu. mm., 100 per cent being lymphocytes. Platelets were within normal limits. Sternal bone marrow revealed changes compatible with chronic lymphatic leukaemia. E.S.R. 20 mms. per hour. Biopsy of an axillary lymph node showed a Joss of the normal follicular architecture with proliferation of immature lymphocytes throughout the tissue compatible with chronic lymphatic leukaemia. He was treated with chloroquine 100 mgms. t.d.s. and within one week the W.B.C. had fallen to 53,000 per cu. mm. The dose of chloroquine was then reduced to 200 mgms. daily. He was kept on this regime for the next 5 years, the W.B.C. averaging 50,000 per cu. mm. of which about 3 per cent were polymorphs and the rest lymphocytes. At the end of this period the W.B.C. suddenly rose to 340,000 per cu. mm. He died in congestive heart failure.

II, b) The effect of dehydro-emetine and emetine on cases of leukaemia

Abd-Rabbo (1967, 1969) reported favourable responses to the administration of dehydro-emetine in cases of chronic myeloid leukaemia and Wyburn-Mason (1966) likewise described marked improvement in some cases of leukaemia with the same drug.

II, c) The effect of copper sulphate on cases of leukaemia

This treatment was used in a number of cases of leukaemia. In one case (Case X, 23 or VI, 31 or 15 (page 304) with chronic lymphatic leukaemia and Sjogren's syndrome already described (page 77), the manifestations of Sjogren's syndrome disappeared and the white blood count approached more nearly to normal. In Case VII, 40 already mentioned copper sulphate administration caused the disappearance of chronic myeloid leukaemic changes in the blood. Two other cases of leukaemia were similarly treated.

II, d) T.he effect of bile acid on cases of leukaemia

This was tried in three cases of chronic lymphatic leukaemia and one with the changes of chronic lymphatic and monocytic leukaemia.

Case X, 21 Female, aged 67 years, Indian from Kenya. Onset with Raynaud's phenomena and blisters in the mouth, pains in the right side of the face and neck and both knees and numbness of the left heel. On examination no abnormal physical signs were made out. Pyrexia of 99-100.20F. X-rays of chest showed a slight pleural reaction at the right base. A blood count showed Hb 120 per cent, W.B.C. 3,000 per cu. mm., neutrophils 34 per cent, lymphocytes 63 per cent. Free hydrochloric acid present in gastric secretion.

Occult blood in stools negative. Lupus erythematosus cells present in blood. Serum iron, folate and B12 content normal. P.B.I. 6.2 $p.G$ per 100 mls. RF negative. ANF positive. Thyroid and gastric parietal cell auto-antibodies negative. Sternal marrow showed increased cellularity and excessive activity in all cell systems. Neutrophils showed shift to the left with signs of primitive forms. Later her blood count showed Hb 11.7 G per 100 mls. (80 per cent), W.B.C. 3,300 per cu. mm. Neutrophils 1 per cent, lymphocytes 96 per cent, monocytes 3 per cent. E.S.R. 31 mms. per hour. A diagnosis of systemic lupus erythematosus and chronic lymphatic leukaemia was made. She was treated with prednisolone 10 mgms. t.d.s. without improvement in her symptoms. She was then given dehydrocholine 750 mgms. t.d.s. over 6 weeks. At the end of this time W.B.C. was 2,600 per cu. mm., 37 per cent neutrophils, 53 per cent lymphocytes, 5 per cent monocytes. She was now symptomless. She remained on this regime for the next year. At the end of this time the W.B.C. was 5,000 per cu. mm., 50 per cent polymorphs, 43 per cent lymphocytes.

Case 10G (X, 20) Female, aged 61 years. Admitted with a three months history of tiredness, mild memory failure and occasional ankle swelling. Examination showed some oedema of the eyelids, hoarseness, one inch (2.5 ems.) swelling of the liver below the costal margin. No splenomegaly. Blood pressure 190/110 mms. Pulse rate 60 per minute, regular. Investigations: Chest X-ray, considerable enlargement of the left ventricle, P.B.I. 0.4 $p.G$ per 100 ml. Albumin 5.2, globulin 3.5 G per 100 ml. L.F.T. bilirubin less than 1 mgm. per cent. Alkaline phosphatase 12.7 K.A. units per 100 ml. Thymol turbidity 10 units. E.S.R. 6 mms. per hour. Hb 11.4 G per 100 ml. (78 per cent), W.B.C. 38,300 per cu. mm., neutrophils 2 per cent, lymphocytes 98 per cent. A repeat W.B.C. 40,600 per cu. mm., 3 per cent neutrophils, 97 per cent lymphocytes.

Some abnormal lymphocytes present in the film. Sternal biopsy confirmed the diagnosis of chronic lymphatic leukaemia. Liver biopsy showed the changes of chronic active hepatitis. RF negative, ANF positive, gastric parietal cell antibodies and all thyroid antibodies strongly positive. A diagnosis of chronic lymphatic leukaemia, chronic active hepatitis and myxoedema was made. She was treated with L-thyroxin 0.1 mgms. twice daily. At the end of a month the serum P.B.L had returned to within normal limits, but the liver function tests and blood count remained unchanged. She was then given copper sulphate 50 mgms. t.d.s. over a period of 7 weeks without any change in the blood count. She was then treated with dehydrocholine 750 mgms. daily and 7 months later the Hb had risen to 14 G per cent, W.B.C. 5,600 per cu. mm., 70 per cent neutrophils, 30 per cent lymphocytes. The liver function tests were normal. The E.S.R. had fallen to 4 mms. per hour. She was symptomless and has remained so over the last 2 years.

Case 107 Female, aged 62 years. Eight years history of sero-positive rheumatoid arthritis, now moderately severe. Four years previously she was discovered to have chronic lymphatic leukaemia. Examination showed typical moderately severe rheumatoid changes in hands, wrists, feet and ankles. Hb 12.5 G per 100 mls. (86 per cent). E.S.R. 35 mms. per hour. W.B.C. 16,700 per cu. mm. Polymorphs 27 per cent, lymphocytes 72 per cent. Film showed excess of small lymphocytes. Rose-Waaler test positive 1 in 128. Rheumatoid arthritis latex test positive greater than 1 in 20. Sternal marrow showed marked infiltration with lymphocytes. Treated with dehydrocholine 750 mgms. t.d.s. One month later the blood count had returned to normal. Hb 13 G per 100 mls. W.B.C. 7,000 per cu. mm. Polymorphs 66 per cent. Lymphocytes 30 per cent, and remained so over the next six months at the end of which time treatment was stopped. Six months later the changes of lymphatic leukaemia were again observed in the blood.

Case 108   Male, aged 75 years. Six years history of increasing dyspnoea and Raynaud's phenomena. Examination showed no abnormality apart from mucosal pallor. Blood count showed Hb 7.8 G per 100 mls. (56 per cent). W.B.C. 1,100 per cu. mm., neutrophils 8 per cent, lymphocytes 18 per cent, monocytes 74 per cent. Platelets 225,000 per cu. mm. E.S.R. 42 mm. per hour. Erythrophagocytosis, hypochromia, anisocytosis and abnormal monocytes present in the blood film. A bone marrow biopsy showed diminished haemopoiesis and leucopoiesis and infiltration of the marrow with monocytes. Lupus erythematosus cells absent from the blood. Cold agglutinins present 1 in 128. RF, ANF, thyroid and gastric parietal cell auto-antibodies absent from serum. He was treated with dehydrocholine 1 G t.d.s. After .6 weeks the blood count showed Hb 63 per cent, W.B.C. 1,500 per cu. mm., neutrophils 37 per cent, lymphocytes 40 per cent, monocytes 23 per cent. E.S.R. 16 mm. per hour. The Raynaud's phenomena disappeared and the patient was now otherwise symptomless. He is still under observation.

Case X, 27   Male, aged 68 years. Nine years history of diabetes, reasonably well controlled on diet alone. Six months previous to admission he developed purpura and was found to have hepatosplenomegaly and slight lymphadenopathy and the blood showed a thrombocytopenia. A preleukaemic phase of chronic lymphatic leukaemia was diagnosed at the London Hospital. Three months before admission he developed a chest infection and was pyrexial and became disorientated. Chest X-rays showed a right basal pneumonia. He was treated with antibiotics and slowly recovered. It was noted that during this illness there was no leucocytosis, his platelet count varying between 40,000 and 121,000 per cu. mm. He was discharged

on a diabetic diet and glibenclamide 5 mgms. each morning, showing glycosuria intermittently during the day.

On first attendance he complained of vague abdominal discomfort, but no abnormal physical signs were made out, except for rheumatoid changes in the feet and hands. There was well-marked arteriosclerosis present. The urine contained 2 per cent of sugar. A blood count showed Hb 11.1 gms. per 100 ml., (77 per cent.) W.B.C., 4,100 per cu. mm., neutrophils 42 per cent, lymphocytes 53 per cent. Platelets 48,000 per cu. mm. E.S.R. = 50 mms. per hour. A random blood sugar 3¥2 hours after a light breakfast showed 162 mgms. per 100 mls. Bilirubin 1.3 mgms. per 100 mls, alkaline phosphatase 26 K.A. units per 100 mls. Thymol turbidity 9 units. Liver biopsy showed the changes of active chronic hepatitis. Plasma proteins, albumin 2.6 G per 100 mls, globulin 6.2 G per 100 mls. Total 8.8 G per 100 mls. Electrophoresis showed raised a• and an M band in the gamma region. Immunophoresis showed IgG 4,800 mgms. per' 100 mls. Skeletal X-rays normal. No Bence-Jones protein was found. Bone-marrow biopsy showed excess of lymphocytes and depression of megakaryocytes. A diagnosis of paraproteinaemia, diabetes, chronic active hepatitis, chronic lymphatic leukaemia and thrombocytopenia was made.

He was treated with dehydrocholine, 750 mgms. t.d.s. Within 36 hours the glycosuria disappeared and after this the glibenclamide had to be stopped owing to hypoglycaemic attacks. His abdominal pains and the spontaneous bruising ceased. He stated that he felt better than for years. Treatment was continued for two months. During this time there had been no sugar in the urine. At the end of this time a random blood sugar was 108 mgms. per cent. The liver function tests showed bilirubin < 1 unit per 100 mls., alkaline phosphatase 12 K.A. units per 100 mls. Thymol turbidity 2 units. Blood count

Hb 14.2 G per 100 mls., W.B.C. 6,600 per cu. mm., neutrophils 56 per cent, lymphocytes 38 per cent. Plasma proteins, albumin 3.6 gms. per 100 mls., globulin 5.8 gms. per 100 mls. IgG 3,000 mgms. per cent.

II, e) The effects of clotrimazole on cases of leukaemia

This was tried on two cas.3s of acute leukaemia with pyrexia and toxic symptoms and one case of chronic lymphatic leukaemia associated with a peri-anal undifferentiated carcinoma (Case 111). In the two former cases, while the drug was being administered, it caused a rapid fall in the temperature and sweating and improved the appetite, but it had no effect on the blood count and fatal course of the disease. In the third case, which was apyrexial, the peri-anal mass disappeared and the total white count fell, but not to normal levels (Case 111).

II, f) The effects of metronidazole in chronic lymphatic leukaemia

This was tried in one case. Female, aged 60 years. Under treatment for mild late onset diabetes for 10 years with diet and tolbutamide, which satisfactorily controlled the disease. After a "cold" she developed a severe herpes simplex affecting the whole of both lips and surrounding areas and extending to the nares and cheeks accompanied by severe ulceration of the inside of the cheeks, gums and fauces with pyrexia of 105°F, sweating, severe dysphagia and general malaise. The submaxillary and cervical lymph nodes were enlarged and tender. No abnormal physical signs elsewhere. A full blood count showed haemoglobin 14.0 G per cent with a total W.B.C. of 30,000 per cu. mm., 100 per cent lymphocytes. The urine contained a trace of sugar and the sternal bone marrow was heavily infiltrated with fully formed lymphocytes consistent with

the diagnosis o(chronic lymphatic leukaemia. Swabs from the stomal ulcers revealed a mixed growth of organisms, including staphylococci and spirillae, sensitive to numerous antibiotics, including tetracycline, ampicillin, etc. She was treated by a course of tetracycline and later by ampicillin, neither of which had any effect on the patient's condition and the urine began to contain more than 2 per cent sugar, while the random blood glucose level rose to 400 mgms. per cent. Treatment was then changed to metronidazole 800 mgms. t.d.s. This was followed within 24 hours by the most dramatic improvement in her condition. At the end of this time the temperature had settled to normal. The general malaise had disappeared and within 5 days the skin lesions and the ulcers within the mouth and pharynx were crusted and healing. At the same time the glucose in the urine disappeared and a random blood glucose estimation fell to 100 mgms. per cent. A repeat blood count showed W.B.C. had now fallen to 15,000 W.B.C. per cu. mm., 70 per cent lymphocytes. Three weeks after beginning treatment with metronidazole she was symptomless and evidence of diabetes had disappeared. She was discharged to a convalescent home still taking the drug and later observed for 6 months when she suddenly died for no obvious reason and an autopsy showed that all tissues were mildly infiltrated with fully formed lymphocytes.

In this case an anti-amoebic drug had completely abolished the toxic manifestations associated with chronic lymphatic leukaemia as well as the signs of diabetes.

In conclusion as to the effects of anti-amoebic substances on cases of leukaemia, it seems that in cases of acute or chronic myeloid leukaemias these substances may have little or no effect on the blood count, but they may temporarily abolish the symptomatology of the disease, such as the pyrexia, sweating, etc. In some cases of chronic lymphatic and some cases of chronic monocytic leukaemia they may cause not only disappearance of symptoms and signs of disease, but also the blood count may return to normal or nearly so and remain so over many years.

III, a) The effects of 4-aminoquinolines on cerebral gliomata

Three cases of cerebral gliomata treated with the 4-aminoquinoline, antrycide, were reported by Wyburn-Mason (1964). All were in a comatose state when treatment began. One showed no response to treatment. In the other two the most surprizing improvement in the condition of the patient was observed. The coma and papilloedema disappeared and the physical signs in the central nervous system decreased. After a while the symptoms returned, however, and the patients died in spite of recommencing the injections.

III, h) The effect of copper salts on cases of cerebral glioma

This treatment can produce the most astonishing improvement. It was tried in one case, a man of 60 years, who was admitted for terminal care from the Atkinson Morley's Hospital, where craniotomy and biopsy revealed a Grade III astrocytoma of the left parietal lobe. On admission he was in extremis, only just rousable and able to swallow. He was doubly incontinent and showed bilateral papilloedema and complete inability to move all four limbs. A bed-sore was present over the sacrum. He was given copper sulphate 25 mgms. t.d.s. Within 48 hours he began to respond to stimuli and within a week was able to sit up in bed. In two weeks he could use his left limbs and he began to talk. He could now feed himself. The dose of copper sulphate was increased to 25 mgms. six times daily. This was well tolerated. He was then able to sit in a chair. Within three weeks the bed-sore had healed. After 6 weeks move-

ment returned to his right arm and leg and with physiotherapy and exercises he learnt to walk again. The papilloedema receded. He was able to go home after 2 months on the same medication. He is still being followed up.

III, c) The effects of clotrimazole on cases of cerebral glioma

This was tried in 3 cases, all of which showed a dramatic response to treatment. All three had had craniotomy and confirmation of the tumours by biopsy. An example of this was the following:-

Case 109 Male, aged 55 years. Previous history not relevant. One year previously he began to complain of morning headaches, memory impairment and for the last 3 months of Jacksonian epileptic attacks affecting the right upper limb, which later developed considerable weakness. After investigations craniotomy revealed a Grade II astrocytoma of the right frontal lobe extending into the motor area. After the operation he remained stuporose and was doubly incontinent. A complete right hemiplegia was present and there was considerable papilloedema. He was fed through a nasal stomach tube.

He was treated with clotrimazole 100 mgms. per kilogram introduced through the stomach tube. Within 3 days his stuporose state had improved and he began to answer questions. Within the next fortnight improvement was so advanced that his incontinence had disappeared. He was able to sit up in a chair. He was no longer confused. He had a dense right hemiplegia. Within a month he was able to watch television and read the newspaper. The papilloedema had now subsided. His response to questions was now normal. He remained under treatment for 6 months, during which his condition was unchanged.

Thus, drugs active against limax amoebae may have a dramatically beneficial effect on cases of glioma.

IV, a) The effect of 4-aminoquiolines on human carcinomata

Fukuhara et al. (1963) report that, when chloroquine is instilled into the serous cavity, it may inhibit hydrothorax formation in cases of carcinoma of the bronchus. Hiraki et al. (1963) treated 40 cases of human carcinomatosis with once or twice weekly intravenous injections of 250 mgms. of chloroquine. The treatment failed to produce improvement in 11 cases. In one an "obscure result" was obtained. The drug had no effect in the last stages of the disease. In 28 cases (70 per cent) the drug was effective in causing subjective and general improvement, relief of pain, regression in size of tumours in some cases, decrease in serum lactic acid dehydrogenase and a tendency for necrosis of tumours. When injections were continued for two months to up to one and a half years "they never resulted in therapeutic failure". The effects were most pronounced in lung and bladder cancer and less so in gastric cancer. The authors claimed that treatment was more effective in tumou rs rich in connective tissue. They stressed that the drug is not an antimitotic agent, but acts in some other way which they consider is on the connective tissue stroma of the growths. The author (Wyburn-Mason, 1964) reported on the effect of the drug on 45 cases of human carcinomatosis in an advanced stage of the disease, often with enormous masses of malignant tissue in chest or abdomen, ascites, pleural effusions or jaundice. Some of the cases of carcinoma of the breast had had mastectomy and postoperative radiation, but all but one of the other cases had had only diagnostic procedures carried out. Of the twenty cases with very large masses of tumour tissue only three showed an obvious response to treatment. Two of these were cases of carcinoma of the ovary and another a primary carcinoma of the liver without jaundice. None of the cases with jaundice due to liver secondaries showed any improvement as a result of treatment; of the other 25 cases with smaller masses of tumour tissue, 18 showed a response to treatment. This was evidenced by absorption of serous effusions, decrease in size of tumour masses, fading or decrease in size of skin metastases, fall in E.S.R. and temperature, decrease in anaemia or by a temporary cessation of tumour growth. In two cases of scirrhous carcinoma of the breast attached to the deep tissues, the tumours became mobile. Thus a total of 21 of the 45 cases benefitted from the administration of plaquenil or other 4-aminoquinolines, which were continued until improvement ceased to occur. It appeared that the smaller the mass of malignant tissue and the better the patient's general condition the more likely was benefit obtained from the treatment. Improvement is only temporary, however, and some time after cessation of treatment varying from two months upwards, the disease continues its course. Two cases of scirrhous carcinoma of the breast, however, remained immobilized for two years.

IV, b) Effects of dehydro-emetine in in cases of cancer

Wyburn-Mason (1966) described complete regression of a rectal carcinoma after administration of DHE. Abd-Rabbo (1967, 1969) reported favourable responses to DHE in cases of tongue and bladder cancer. Street (1972) reported marked improvement in cases of carcinoma of the lung after administration of cyclophosphamide and emetine.

IV, c) The effects of copper sulphate on cases of carcinomatosis

This treatment was tried in a number of cases, of which the following are examples:-

Case XV, 37 Male, aged 69 years. Known diabetic for 5 years. This was

272

controlled with diet and insulin. Two months before admission the control of his diabetes became impossible and a month later he complained of aching, weakness and ataxia of his legs. If he forced himself to walk, he would collapse and lose consciousness. He fell down 2-3 times a day. He also complained of tingling in the feet. Examination showed severe dementia, bilateral grasp reflexes, slurring dysarthria, inability to stand unaided, gross ataxia in the finger-nose and heel-knee tests and all tendon reflexes were absent. There was gross weakness and wasting of the proximal limb girdle muscles. The urine contained more than 2 per cent of sugar all the time. A chest X-ray showed a large shadow at the left hilum typical of carcinoma of the bronchus. Free hydrochloric acid was present in the gastric contents. The blood E.S.R. was 71 mms. per hour. Thyroid auto-antibodies were present in the serum. The white cell count was normal. The question arose as to whether the neurological disturbance was due to carcinomatosis of the bronchus or to his diabetes and it was found impossible to control the latter. His condition was rapidly deteriorating and his speech became impossible to understand. He could only be roused from a semicomatose state with difficulty. He was then put on copper sulphate 50 mgms. t.d.s. with the most dramatic effect, for within 48 hours he became completely rational, his dysart hria had disappeared and in 4 days he was able to stand and walk unaided and the attacks of unconsciousness ceased. By the fifth day the tendon reflexes had returned. Within 48 hours the glycosuria had ceased and he now developed hypoglycaemic attacks necessitating stopping the insulin injections and for a month remained free of evidence of diabetes or of neurological disease. The chest X-ray appearances were unchanged. The copper sulphate administration was now stopped after a month of normal life and

he died within 16 hours in coma. Autopsy showed the presence of an oat-cell carcinoma at the hilum of the left lung with metastases in the mediastinal lymph nodes. No involvement of the brain or peripheral nerves by carcinoma was present.

Case XV, 21 Male, aged 67 years. Admitted with a 6 weeks history of generalized headaches and slight unsteadiness on his feet. There was a slight and variable memory loss for recent events and a 6 months history of dryness of the skin. Examination showed a somewhat euphoric individual with well-marked rheumatoid changes in the hands and feet and severe ichthyosis acquisita. A bursitis was present over the left olecranon process. There was euphoria, moderate dementia, slight ataxia of gait, right-sided foot drop, all tendon reflexes were absent and a bilateral grasp reflex was present. A chest X-ray showed slight fluid in the costaphrenic angles. An E.C.G. was normal. Blood E.S.R. was 53 mms. in 1 hour. Blood urea and electrolytes normal. Blood count Hb 106 per cent, W.B.C. normal, lupus erythematosus cells absent, free hydrochloric acid present in the gastric contents. Liver function tests and plasma proteins normal. C.S.F. under normal pressure. Protein content 120 mgms. per cent, WR negative in blood and C.S.F. RF and all auto-antibodies negative in serum. E.E.G. showed minor diffuse disturbances. During his hospitalization he ran an occasional pyrexia of 99.4°F. He was investigated neuro-surgically with carotid arteriography and radio-active scanning, but no cerebral lesion could be located. Repeated X-rays of the chest eventually showed a shadow in the left lower lobe suggestive of a carcinoma. He was given copper sulphate 50 mgms. t.d.s. with a rapid and dramatic improvement in his condition. Within 36 hours his mental state had returned to normal. Within 5 days the tendon reflexes had reappeared, the foot drop had disappeared and ataxia could not be demonstrated. The ichthyosis cleared within a

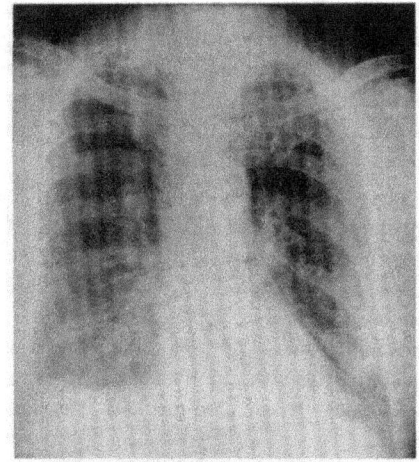 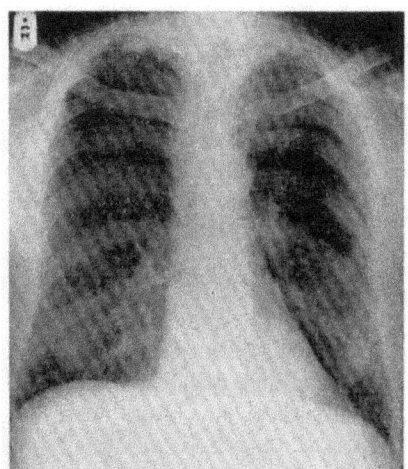

Fig. 61-A   Fig. 61-B

Fig. 61   Male, aged 67 years.   Oat cell carcinoma of the left
lower lobe bronchus with paraneoplastic neuropathy and encephalopathy.   Chest X-ray before "A" and "B" a week after
beginning treatment with copper sulphate, showing dramatic
changes in appearances, which were accompanied by the di-
appearance of the encephalopathy and neuropathy (Case
XV, 21).

week. The bursitis cleared in 5 days and the pleural effusions in two weeks. The temperature fell to normal. He remained completely symptomless in spite of the presence of the shadow in the left lower lobe (Case 60) (Fig. 61). After one month the copper sulphate administration was stopped. He died within 36 hours of this, rapidly passing into coma. At autopsy a primary oat cell carcinoma of the left lower lobe of the lung was present. No metastases could be found.

IV, d)   The effects of bile acid on cases of carcinoma

This simple treatment was tried in a number of cases of advanced cancer in doses of 1 G-1.5 G t.d.s. combined with kaolin and proved to be the most effective of the anti-amoebic substances used, sometimes producing the most dramatic, rapid and unexpected improvement in the pa-

tients condition, continued over a long period. Among the cases treated were the following:–

Case 110 Male, aged 73 years. Moderate smoker. Fourteen months previously he suffered a coronary thrombosis and was found to be a mild diabetic. The latter was controlled by diet alone. He recovered from the coronary thrombosis, but had recently developed shortness of breath, swelling of the feet and ankles and cough and had lost 40 pounds in weight over the last three months. On examination there was a mild glycosuria. The liver was enlarged three fingers breadths. Chest X-rays showed a large right pleural effusion. Liver function tests showed bilirubin 2.0 mgms. per cent. Alkaline phosphatase 23.5 K.A. units per 100 mls. Plasma proteins, albumin 3.2 G, globulin 3.7 G per 100 mls. The pleural effusion was aspirated. It contained malignant cells. Tomograms done immediately after aspiration revealed

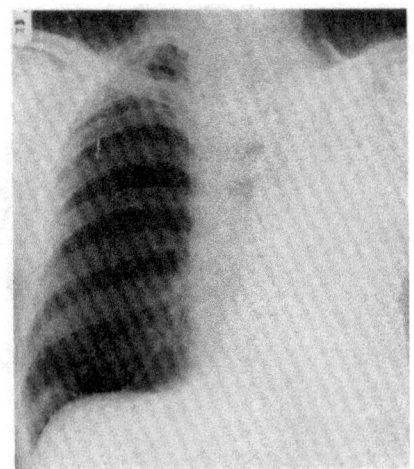
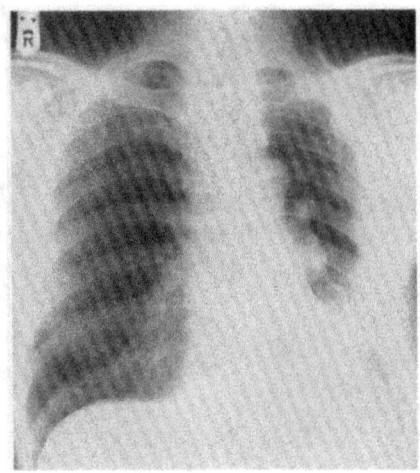

Fig. 62-A   Fig. 62-B

Fig. 62 Male, aged 73 years. Adeno-carcinoma of left lower lobe bronchus. Chest X-ray showing blacking out of the left lung with partial collapse and deviation of trachea to the left with pleural effusion. "A" before and "B" after 3 weeks treatment with copper sulphate. Note the absorption of the pleural effusion and the reaeration of the lung.

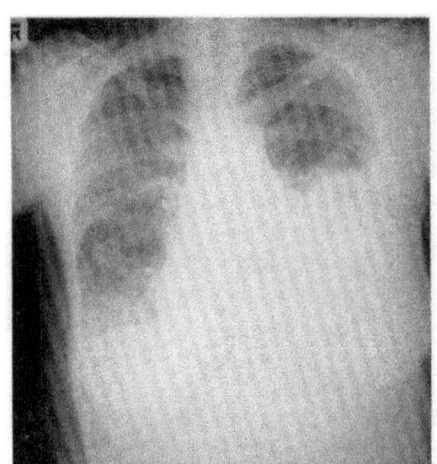
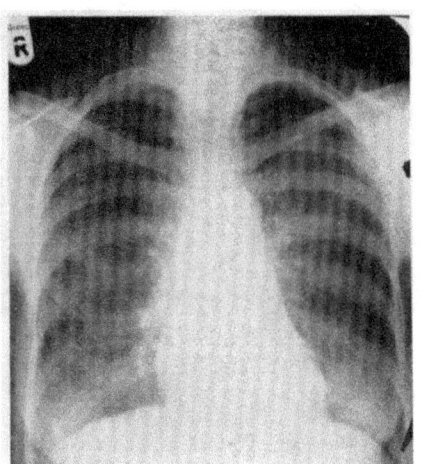

Fig. 63·A   Fig. 63-B

Fig. 63 Female, aged 60 years. Carcinomatosis of the pancreas. "A" shows X-ray appearance of chest before and "B" 6 weeks after beginning treatment with copper sulphate.

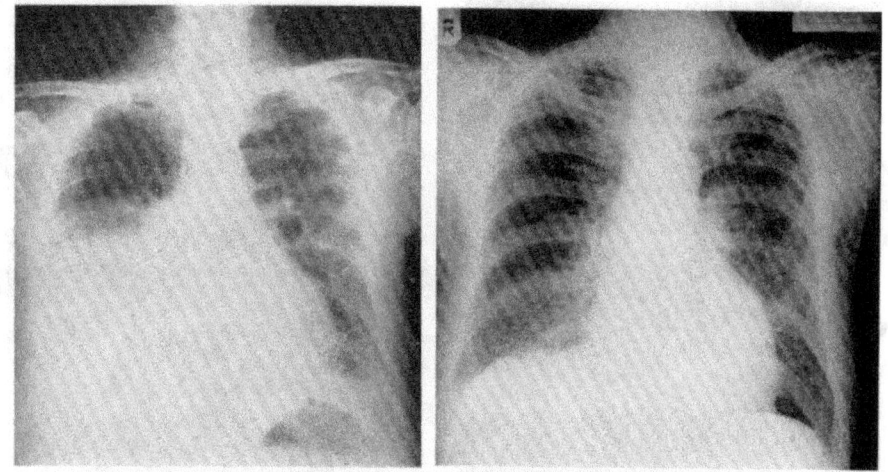

Fig. 64-A   Fig. 64-B

Fig. 64 Male, aged 73 years. Oat cell carcinoma of right
lower lobe bronchus with collapse of right lower lobe and
right plrural effusion at "A". After 3 wrrks treatment with
bile acid patient was symptomless and chest X-ray was as
"B" (Case 95).

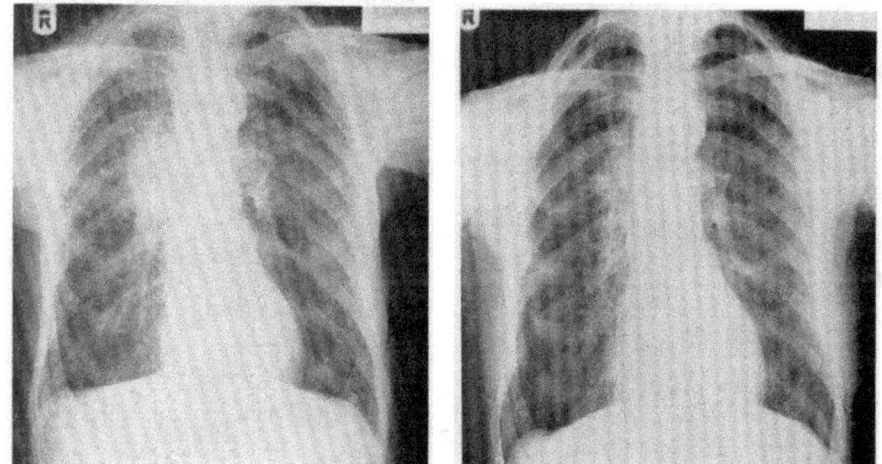

Fig. 65-A   Fig. 65-B

Fig. 65 Male, aged 70 years. Squamous cell carcinoma of
the right bronchus with continuous haemoptysis and severe loss
of wright. Apprarances of chest X-ray before, "A" and after
6 weeks treatment with bile acid,
"B".

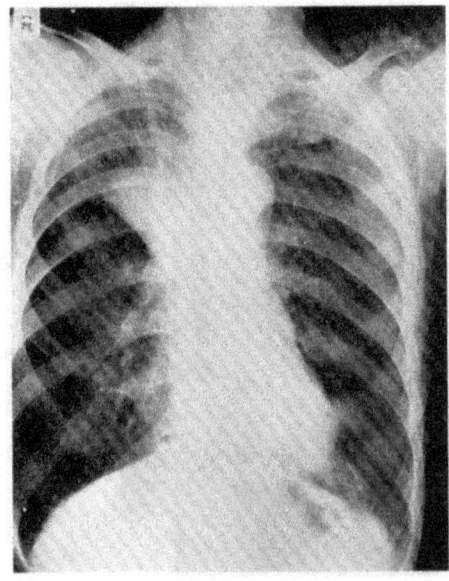 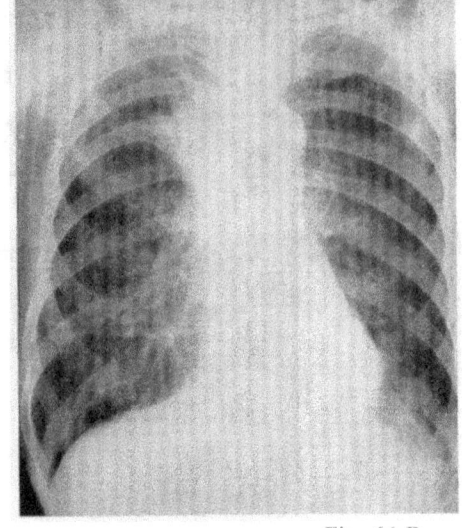

Fig. 66-A   Fig. 66-B

Fig. 66   Male, aged 72 years.   Squamous cell carcinoma of
the right upper lobe bronchus.   Chest X-ray before "A" and
after 3 weeks treatment with bile salt, showing partial clearing of hilar shadows "B".

a mass in the lower lobe of the right lung. An enlarged lymph node appeared above the right clavicle. This was biopsied and showed metastases of an adenocarcinoma. The pleural effusion reappeared. He was treated with dehydrocholine 1 G t.d.s. The effect was dramatic. His appetite became enormous. He gained 10 lbs. in weight in 10 days. The dyspnoea lessened and the pleural effusion disappeared (Fig. 62). The diabetes was no longer present. The liver function tests returned to normal. He has been maintained feeling well and with no laboratory evidence of disease over six months.

IV, e)   The effects of streptomycin on cases of carcinomatosis

Streptomycin may inhibit the growth of amoebae (Hawkins, 1973). On several occasions in the author's experience in investigating patients with abdominal symp-

toms, pyrexia and sweating the differential diagnosis lay between tuberculosis and malignancy. Therapeutic tests for abdominal tuberculosis by antituberculous treatment with streptomycin injections were tried. They were found to result in some cases in a rapid fall in temperature to normal, a cessation of the sweating and improvement in the patients condition. They had no effect on the ultimate outcome of the disease in spite of continued treatment though the temperature remained normal. All proved to have abdominal malignancies at autopsy, but no evidence of tuberculosis.

IV, f)   The effects of clotrimazole on cases of carcinomatosis

This was tried in 6 cases, in two of which the tumours were subcutaneous and could be directly observed.

Case 111   Male, aged 45 years. He was

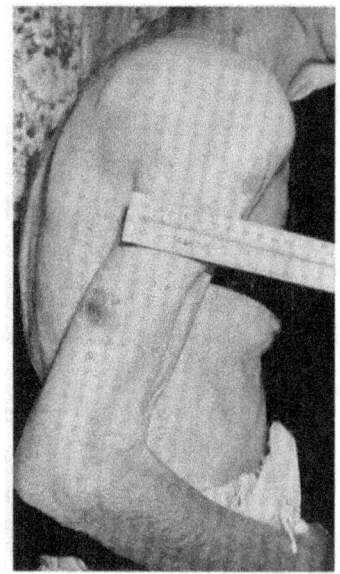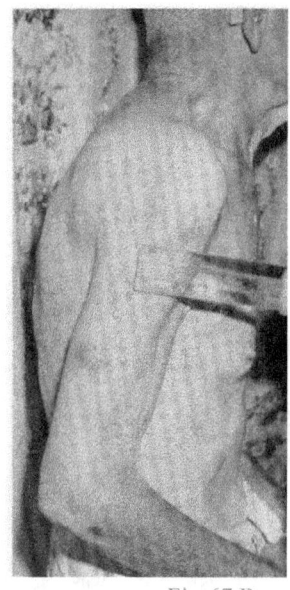

Fig. 67·A   Fig.67·B

Fig. 67 Case 112. Male, aged 79 years, with multiple subcutaneous metastase of an unknown primary carcinoma showing A, the appearan\cs of two subcutaneous masses in the
right upper arm with marked redness, tenderness and inflammatory change around and B. the same one week after treatment with clotrimazole. Note the decrease in th size and
the inflammatory redn SS. This was accompanied by disappearance of the tendern SS.

admitted complaining of a hard lump beside the anus. This was biopsied and
showed the presence of an anaplastic carcinoma. A barium enema was normal. A
blood count at this time showed W.B.C.
55,000 per cu. mm., 7 per cent neutrophils,
70 per cent lymphocytes, 20 per cent smear
cells. Hb 13.4 G per 100 mls. E.S.R. 22
mms. per hour. Sternal marrow biopsy
showed widespread diffuse increase of
small lymphocytes compatible with chronic
lymphatic leukaemia. He was treated with
clotrimazole 100 mgms. per kilogram daily
without untoward effects for 2 months.
During this time the peri-anal mass disappeared and the W.B.C. fell to 31,000 per
cu. mm. of which 13 per cent were neutrophils and 87 per cent lymphocytes. The
patient remained symptomless over the

next six months and the white blood count
varied between 30,000 and 39,000 per cu.
mm. with about 10 per cent neutrophils
and the rest lymphocytes.

Case 112 Male, aged 79 years. He presented with multiple painful subcutaneous
lumps on both upper arms, left side of the
trunk, the front of the chest and over the
left scapula and right mandible, which had
been present for the last month. There
was anorexia and weight loss. *Examination.* The lumps were hard, tender and
firm and some were fixed to the deeper
tissues. They were surrounded by markedly reddened areas of inflammatory
reaction. They varied in size from $1\frac{1}{2}$
ins. (3.75 ems) to $\frac{1}{2}$ in. (1.25 ems) in diameter (Fig. 67). His temperature varied
between 99°F. – 102°F.

Investigations. Biopsy of one of the nodules showed them to consist of a metastatic poorly differentiated carcinoma (?adenocarcinoma), but no useful indication of the primary site could be given. Chest X-ray and barium meal were normal. Liver function tests were normal. Thyroid and gastric parietal cell antibodies were negative. ANF and RF were negative. Alkaline phosphatase 15.5 K.A. units per 100 ml. Plasma proteins, albumin 2.4 G per 100 mls., globulin 3.6 G per 100 mls. Blood count, R.B.C. 3.79 mils. per cu. mm., Hb 10.4 G per 100 mls. W.B.C. 15,600 per cu. mm., neutrophils 89 per cent. Hypochromia and anisocytosis were present. E.S.R. 130 mms. per hour.

He was treated with clotrimazole 1 gram t.d.s. and after three days there was an obvious change in the secondary cancers. The redness, inflammatory reaction and the tenderness had disappeared (Fig. 67). His temperature fell to normal. Treatment was continued over two months during which time the serum alkaline phosphatase fell to 11 K.A. units per 100 mls. Plasma proteins changed to albumin 2.6 G per 100 mls., globulin 3.5 G per 100 mls. but the E.S.R. remained unchanged. During the whole of this time there was no increase in size of the secondary deposits which remained painless, non-tender and no longer inflamed. The patient, however, gradually lost weight.

IV, g) The effects of other imidazole-containing anti-amoebic drugs on cases of carcinomatosis

Miconazole and levamisole both contain imidazole groups and are anti-amoebic drugs. Scheff et al. (1974) treated seven cases of carcinomatosis, which were pyrexial, with miconazole, a drug closely related to clotrimazole in both structure and action. Five became subfebrile, while in the other two no effect was obtained. Ward (1976) treated a series of patients with disseminated cancers with levamisole and this often caused temporary regression or disappearance of nodules.

Thus, drugs active against limax amoebae may have a *dramatically beneficial effect on the "toxic" and especially the neurological paraneoplastic disturbances of carcinomatosis.* The temperature may fall to normal. They may cause regression or immobilization of the tumour and diminish the inflammatory response associated with the tumour.

V. Myelomatosis

The effects of chloroquine, copper salts, bile salts and clotrimazole were tried on 6 cases of myelomatosis. None had any demonstrable effect.

Summary of the effects of anti-amoebic substances in cases of malignant lymphoma, leukaemia and carcinomatosis

It has been shown in the foregoing pages that many of the toxic manifestations of malignant disease, including pyrexia, sweating, effusions, arthropathy and neurological and psychotic disturbances may disappear or improve very rapidly for a while at least on administration of various substances active against limax amoebae. In cases of chronic lymphatic or monocytic leukaemia the blood abnormalities may disappear completely. This effect may be long-lasting or the manifestations return sooner or later after discontinuance of treatment. The lymphadenopathy in cases of lymphoma may disappear or become less marked, or in other cases there results a rapid painful temporary increase in size and inflammatory changes in the nodes when treated with large doses of clotrimazole, indicating an Herxheimer reaction and proving conclusively that an organism reacting to this drug is present in the lesions. In cases of carcinomatosis there is usually only limited regression of the growth itself, but inflammatory changes around the tumour may disappear. Reference has been made to the finding of limax amoebae in the tumours and in all the tissues of the body in all cases of human carcinoma, lymphoma and leukaemia and especially in carcinomatous tumours. These can someti?les be demonstrated by special methods. ,.Culbertson et al. (1972) in experimentally induced disease from Naegleria aerobia remarked that this produced a state apparently identical with that of advanced malignant disease.

It will be seen later that the appearance of a malignancy of any sort may be immediately preceded or accompanied by the development of any of the various manifestations of limax amoebae infection in the shape of rheumatoid arthritis (so-called carcinomatous arthropathy), of systemic lupus erythematosus, dermatomyositis, scleroderma, polyarteritis, thyrotoxicosis, diabetes, acanthosis nigricans, peripheral neuropathy, cerebellar disturbance, dementia, psychotic states, etc., as so-called paraneoplastic conditions again showing the close association of cancer with limax amoebae infection. Many cases of leukaemia, lymphoma or myelomatosis present as cases of pyrexia of unknown origin, suggesting the existence of limax amoebic infection as an essential feature of these conditions. In the acute or late stage of human leukaemia and the toxic and especially the late manifestations of any type of lymphoma and in some late cases of carcinomatosis the same disturbances are found. These include pyrexia, sweating, which is often severe and occurs during sleep, rigors, anorexia, weight loss, a raised E.S.R., hypergammaglobulinaemia, splenomegaly, peripheral neuropathy, mental (manic-depression, schizophrenia and confusional states), intellectual and cerebellar disturbances, oedemas and effusions into the serous cavities, a disturbance in previous diabetic control or the first appearance of diabetes and finally delirium and coma. *All these* symptoms *and* signs *are typical of a severe infection, which appears to be the same in the late* or *acutely toxic stages of* most *forms of human cancer, lymphoma and leukaemia and* to *be the ultimate cause of death in many cases.* The symptoms involve disturbance of hypothalamic function. These disturbances, moreover, are identical with those of disseminated eosinophilic collagen disease and acute rheumatoid disease. Such observations appear to show that in *patients with malignant disease death often occurs from a state identical with acute collagen disease as a result of proliferation of limax amoebae, especially in solid tumours.* **It** follows that the *paraneoplastic neurological disturbances, peripheral and central, are manifestations of collagen and auto-immune* disease and probably due to limax amoebae infection.

-280-

Chapter X

The possibility that "collagen" and "auto-immune" disease may be related to malignant disease in many cases

In the various types of collagen and auto-immune disease the tissues contain limax amoebae which appear to be the causative agent. Likewise limax amoebae are present in all the tissues of human malignant disease, especially in the solid tumours. It has been shown above that many of the general manifestations of carcinomatosis and all those of chronic lymphatic and monocytic leukaemia and malignant lymphoma may disappear on administration of drugs active against these amoebae. The amoebae might thus appear to be the causative agent of many cases of chronic lymphatic leukaemia and lymphomas. Could they also be the cause of the solid tumours and other leukaemias? In cases of disseminated eosinophilic collagen disease the condition may be complicated by the development of chronic myeloid leukaemia with eosinophilia, eosinophilic leukaemia, chloromata, myeloblastomiita or lymphomata, while in subjects of rheumatoid arthritis and systemic lupus erythematosus changes closely resembling, if not true malignant lymphoma may occur in lymph nodes and spleen. Moreover, collagen and auto-immune disease in the mother appears to induce errors in gametogenesis and somatic mutations in the embryo and foetus. Furthermore, it may result in the development of paraproteinaemia and Waldenstrom's macroglobulinaemia, which is considered to be a form of lymphosarcoma. It has been shown that collagen and auto-immune disease may result in excessive stimulation of the haemopoietic elements in the bone marrow resuiting in the development of polycythaemia vera, often with accompanying fe"ucocytosis and thrombocytosis. In collagen and auto-immune disease there may also be a proliferation of the plasma cells in the bone marrow. Fields of change in epithelium occur in such diseases. Furthermore, in the mucosa affected by atrophic gastritis metaplasia of the epithelium is frequently seen and similar changes occur in cases of atrophic rhinitis. Again, in thyroid glands affected by Hashimoto's thyroiditis squamous metaplasia of the epithelium of the acini is frequently found (Dube and Joyce, 1971). These changes often precede malignancy. In cases of chronic cholecystitis there occurs a stimulation of epithelial growth to form Rokitansky-Aschoff sinuses (see above). In cases of Paget's disease of bone there is again an excessive stimulation of bone forming cells. Both conditions are premalignant.

In cases of coeliac disease there is an interference with the normal process of "enteropoiesis" (Booth, 1970) in the cells of the jejunal mucosa, presumably brought about by the causative infection. There is, thus, a maturation defect which has been compared with the interference in haemopoiesis which occurs in leukaemia. Again, the special liability of cases of congenital a- or hypo-gammaglobulinaemia to both collagen or auto-immune diseases and to lymphoma or cancer may point to a relationship between the two sets of conditions. Such considerations as these point to the possibility that collagen and auto-immune disease may be concerned in inducing malignancies.

A familial association of collagen and auto-immune disease and lymphoma

Holman (1963) concluded that in certain families rheumatic diseases, such as rheumatoid arthritis, systemic lupus erythematosus, hypogammaglobulinaemia and lymphoma of one type or another, including multiple myeloma, occur especially frequently. Creagan and Fraumeni (1972) refer to studies of familial Hodgkin's disease and describe a family in which 3 cases of Hodgkin's disease occurred and also various collagen and auto-immune diseases. The proband had Hodgkin's disease, liver failure and anto-immune haemolytic anaemia. A sister developed idiopathic thrombocytopenic purpura (ITP), then systemic lupus erythematosus and Hodgkin's disease. Her son had ITP alone. A maternal aunt developed Hodgkin's disease. A maternal cousin once removed died of acute monocytic leukaemia. A son of the proband suffered from Crohn's disease. One of his children had multiple congenital anomalies and necrotizing encephalitis. The mother of the proband had operations for duct carcinoma of one breast and colloid carcinoma of the other. Wolf (1962) described a case of primary acquired hypogammaglobulinaemia with a high incidence of haematological abnormalities in the family. These included systemic lupus erythematosus, idiopathic thrombocytopenic purpura, leukaemia, reticuloses and Hodgkin's disease. Potalski et al. (1971) report a sibship of 10 adults of which 5 died of lymphoreticular malignancy. In 4 surviving siblings there were immunological abnormalities of humoral and cellular type, suggesting a relationship between immunological abnormalities and susceptibility to lymphoid neoplasms and familial tendency to these. Fraumeni et al. (1969) reported a similar family. Such observations suggest a close relationship between collagen diseases and lymphoma.

Statistical evidence on the relationship of rheumatoid arthritis to malignancy

Statistically contradictory reports as to the frequency of malignant lymphoma in cases of rheumatoid arthritis are forthcoming. This is discussed by Druet et al. (1969) and others. Abbott and Lea (1956) found a statistical relationship between "rheumatoid diseases" and leukaemia. Lea (1964) reported a statistical correlation between the "rheumatic diseases", the nature of which are not specified, and the reticuloses. The figures of Etcheverry et al. (1959) do not favour the predisposition of cases of rheumatoid arthritis to develop lymphoma. Neither Miller (1967) nor Oleinick (1967) could find statistical evidence in favour of such a predisposition. Cobb et al. (1953) found no case of lymphoma in 191 cases of rheumatoid arthritis. Dubois (1966) found one instance of malignant lymphoma in 58 autopsies of cases of systemic lupus erythematosus. As regards the relationship between rheumatoid arthritis and non-lymphomatous malignant disease Ragan and Snyder (1955), Duthie et al. (1964), Cobb (1967) and Owen et al. (1967) found no increased incidence of cancer in subjects of rheumatoid arthritis. Again, these statements depend on the criteria for diagnosing rheumatoid arthritis, which must vary from person to person and whether the source of the cases was a rheumatism clinic or a surgical clinic where rheumatoid arthritis is likely to pass unnoticed. As already mentioned above many cases of rheumatoid arthritis never attend hospital for this. In contrast to these reports in 16 cases of rheumatoid arthritis Sinclair and Cruikshank (1956) found one case of lymphoma and one with carcinoma and chronic lymphatic leukaemia. Siurala et al. (1965) in 71 cases of collagen diseases of various kinds found one case of carcinoma of the large bowel. Strandberg and Jarløv (1961) followed 53 cases of classical rheumatoid arthritis over a number of years and of these no less than 26 (50 per cent) developed malignant lymphoma, leukaemia, myelomatosis, carcinoma, melanoma or osteosarcoma. Gardner (1969) in 142 cases of rheumatoid arthritis found 25 (18 per cent) developed tumours of various organs. Gardner irt a personal communication described the tumours found. There were two benign, one haemangioma of the liver and one lymphangioma of the jejunum. The malignant tumours recorded were as follows-cancer of the bronchus, 7 cases; cancer of the colon and rectum, 4 cases; uterus, 2 cases, ileal carcinoid 2 cases. The rest were one each of carcinoma of the ovary, breast, stomach, gall-bladder and oesophagus and malignant hepatoma, sarcoma and mesothelioma of the pleura. In the geriatric series of 100 cases of rheumatoid arthritis, reported previously, I6 died of cancer of various organs. These were cancer of the bronchus in non-smokers 4 cases, stomach 5 cases, colon and rectum 3 cases and one each of the senile breast, pa ncreas, body of uterus and kidney. Moesmann (1969) encountered malignant disease in 14 per cent and 43 per cent of series of 85 and 28 rheumatoid patients respectively, figures which he says are 2.0-2.2 times those expected to occur in a random matched population. There was 'no correlation between malignancy and sex, disease class, RF titres, X-ray changes, serum a2-globulin or serum alkaline phosphatase levels. The malignancies were cancer of the pancreas (I), stomach (1), bronchus (4), breast (5), ovary (1), bladder (I), pleura (I), caecum (I), skin (1), uterus (2), unknown primary (1), malignant melanoma of skin (I), Hodgkin's disease (I), plasmocytoma (1) and multiple myelomatosis (1). Cecil and Kammerer (1951) report cancer as present in 5 of 14 (36 per cent) of cases of subacute rheumatoid arthritis in old age and Mackenzie and Scherbel (1963) describe 77 cases of connective tissue syndromes with cancer (but included hypertrophic osteoarthropathy) .

Thus, rheumatoid arthritis has been reported as associated with lymphoma, Hodgkin's disease, leukaemias, myelomatosis, melanoma, plasmocytoma, osteosarcoma, sarcoma, mesothelioma of pleura and carcinoma of various organs, including skin, carcinoid and benign haemangioma or lymphangioma.

The figures of the later-quoted authors are striking and in marked contrast to those quoted earlier. The former have compared the incidence of cancer in cases of rheumatoid arthritis with those of subjects who do not exhibit severe manifestations of this condition. Such comparisons are of no significance since as shown above 1) many patients with rheumatoid arthritis never attend hospital, 2) many apparently normal subjects are infected with the causative organism of rheumatoid arthritis without showing any arthritic manifestations, 3) they do not take into account the fact that any of the controls could be suffering from a manifestation of limax amoebae infection as shown by the presence of Hashimoto's thyroiditis, Sjogren's syndrome, atrophic gastritis, pernicious anaemia, etc., without evidence of rheumatoid arthritis. In fact, it is at present impossible to conceive of a controlled series of subjects in which infection with the organism does not exist. *This, therefore, renders such comparisons of the incidence of malignant disease in cases of rheumatoid arthritis or indeed of any collagen or auto-immune disease with controls as quite meaningless.*

The occurrence of collagen or auto-immune disease in cases of malignant disease recorded at the South West Metropolitan Cancer Registry in the years 1961-6

Through the courtesy of the Director of the South West Metropolitan Cancer Registry, Mr. P.W. Payne, the author was allowed to examine the records of the Registry for the years 1961 inclusive of those cancer cases in which the presence of other diseases was mentioned. Those in which collagen or auto-immune diseases were recorded were noted. The recording of various complications of cancer cases on the forms of the Registry usually depends on junior doctors or even records officers at the hospitals concerned, some of whom only do so from the case notes and only very obvious complications can be expected to be recorded. Only severe rheumatoid arthritis may be noted. Minor degrees of arthritis, atrophic gastritis or euthyroid goitre due to Hashimoto's thyroiditis and various other signs or the occurrence of auto-immune disease are not sought for in cases of cancer in most hospitals, so that the figures given are quite unreliable as indications of the frequency of collagen or auto-immune disease in cases of malignant disease. In many cases the duration of the symptoms of the collagen or auto-immune disease before the onset of malignancy was not stated on the forms. The findings are, however, recorded. They represent the conditions preceding or associated with the development of malignancy in a proportion of cases, but they must be a considerable underestimate of the frequency of collagen and auto-immune disease in cancer cases. They occurred in a total of 202,791 cases of malignant disease.

1) *Rheumatoid arthritis preceding malignant disease*

Carcinoma of skin- 3 cases, aged 65-81 years, of unexposed areas.

Malignant melanoma- 3 cases, 2 of unexposed areas, 1 of eye, aged 67–78 years.

Carcinoma of tongue – 1 case (with psoriasis) male, aged 76 years.

Carcinoma of pharynx- 1 case, female, aged 79 years.

Carcinoma of post-cricoid region – 1 case, female, aged 71 years.

Carcinoma of oesophagus – 6 cases, 4 female, 2 male, aged 70-93 years.

Carcinoma of stomach – 16 cases, 8 males, 8 females, aged 50-85 years, all but 2 over 60 years: one case had a history of rheumatoid arthritis extending over 38 years.

Carcinoma of the colon and rectum – 22 cases, *18 females*, 4 males, 1 with longstanding psoriasis, aged 58-83 years.

Primary cancer of the liver – 1 case, a female, aged 63 years.

Carcinoma of the gall-bladder – 1 case, a female, aged 77 years.

Carcinoma of the pancreas – 7 cases, 3 female, 4 male, aged 58-96 years.

Lymphoma and leukaemia –

Reticulosarcoma – 5 cases, aged 55-78 years.

Malignant lymphoma – 1 case, female, aged 60 years.

Hodgkin's disease- 3 cases, aged 43-73 years.

Chronic lymphatic leukaemia – 3 cases, aged 65-78 years.

Chronic myeloid leukaemia- 1 case, aged 57 years.

Acute lymphoblastic leukaemia – 2 cases, aged 6 and 72 years.

Acute monocytic leukaemia – 1 case, aged 71 years.

Erythromyeloblastic leukaemia – 1 case, aged 52 years.

One of the cases of acute lymphoblastic leukaemia was noteworthy. It occurred *in* a 6 year-old boy, who one year before had developed juvenile rheumatoid arthritis.

Myelomatosis- 3 cases. All occurred after long-standing rheumatoid arthritis, aged 56-81 years.

Carcinoma of bronchus – 63 cases, of which 14 were female. The male cases varied in age from 50-90 years and the females from 48-80 years; only one case below 50 and 15 cases below 60 years.

Pleural endotheliorria – 1 case, aged 74 years.

Carcinoma of kidney – 1 case, female aged 68 years.

Carcinoma of bladder – 3 cases, 1 male, aged years.

Carcinoma of prostate - 11 cases aged 61-77 years.

Carcinoma of breast - 38 cases, 1 male, 1 bilateral, 1 with long-standing psoriasis, aged 36-89 years; 27 cases were over 60 years of age.

Carcinoma of cervix - 13 cases, aged 37-75 years with up to 10 years preceding history of rheumatoid arthritis; 5 cases were below 50 years of age.

Carcinoma of body of uterus – 7 cases, aged 55-74 years.

Carcinoma of ovary – 3 cases, 1 bilateral, aged 36-75 years.

Carcinoma of vulva - 2 cases, aged 68-71 years

Haemangioblastoma of cerebellum - 1 case, aged 48 years.

Ependymoma of cauda equina – 1 case, aged 31 years.

Fibrosarcoma of muscle – 1 case, aged 67 years

Unknown primary cancer - 1 case, aged 80 years

2) *Systemic lupus erythematosus preceding malignant disease* - 4 cases, all in females aged 37-76 years. They consisted of carcinoma of cervix, kidney and bronchus and acute monocytic leukaemia at intervals of 4 years to 9 months after onset of systemic lupus erythematosus.

3) *Rheumatoid* arthritis *and Hashimoto's thyroiditis preceding malignancy* – 2 cases a) female, aged 64 years, developed malignant lymphoma, b) male, aged 46 years, developed carcinoma of the thyroid.

4) *Rheumatoid arthritis and thyrotoxicosis preceding malignancy* - 2 cases a) female, aged 73 years, developed reticulosarcoma, b) female, aged 66 years, developed multiple basal cell carcinoma.

5) *Rheumatoid arthritis and myxoedema preceding malignancy* – 1 case, female aged 65 years, developed myelomatosis.

6) *Rheumatoid arthritis and long-standing diabetes preceding malignancy* – 14 cases, *all but one in females,* aged 40-83 years. The male case was one of carcinoma of the prostate. There were six cases of malignant lymphoma and four cases of carcinoma of the senile breast.

7) *Rheumatoid arthritis, long-standing diabetes and pernicious anaemia preceding malignancy* – 2 cases, both in females, one developed malignant lymphoma, aged 46 years, the other carcinoma of the stomach aged 76 years.

8) *Dermatomyositis preceding malignant disease* – 3 cases, all males, aged 53 1 years, 2 cancer of the bronchus, 1 of male breast. They occurred 14 to 3 years after onset of skin rash.

9) *Sclera-dermatomyositis preceding malignancy* – 1 case, female, aged 36 years, with 8 years history of skin disease preceding cancer of the bronchus.

10) *Scleroderma preceding malignancy* - 3 cases of long-standing scleroderma, all in females, aged 39-79 years, one with a 9 years history of skin disease. The growths originated in the pancreas, bron-;, chus and senile breast.

11) *Sjogren's syndrome preceding malignancy* – 2 cases a) male, aged 46 years, developed malignant lymphoma, b) male, aged 56 years, developed cancer of the breast.

I2) *Hashimoto's thyroiditis preceding malignancy* - 14 cases, *2 male, 21 female,* aged 39-81 years. One developed carcinoma of the thyroid, two carcinoma of the bronchus in females and four carcinomata in senile female breasts.

13) *Myxoedema preceding malignancy* - 29 cases, *7 males and 22 females,* aged 38-82 years. Two were cases of chronic lymphatic leukaemia and one of Hodgkin's disease; II cases affected the senile breast and three the bronchus in women.

14) *Thyrotoxicosis preceding or coinciding with malignancy* - 77 cases, *16 in males and 61 in females,* aged 32-81 years. There were 20 cases of carcinoma of the bronchus (11 females), 19 cancer of the female breast, 2 of thyroid carcinoma, 7 of colon or rectum, 4 of stomach, 2 of pancreas, 2 of body of uterus, 1 of both ovaries, 1 of a single ovary, 2 cases of Hodg-

kin's disease (female, aged 43 years, female, aged 32 years) and one case of reticulosarcoma in a female, aged 58 years. There was one case of acute monocytic leukaemia (female, aged 34 years).

15) *Thyrotoxicosis and diabetes preceding malignancy* – 1 case of cancer of the female breast, aged 68 years.

16) *Myxoedema and diabetes preceding malignancy* – 3 cases, all in females, aged 68-81 years, affecting breast, uterine body and haemangio-endothelioma of the skin of the face.

17) *Pernicious anaemia preceding malignancy* – 4 cases aged 60-82 years. One case of malignant lymphoma and one each of cancer of prostate, bronchus and skin.

18) *.Pernicious anaemia and diabetes preceding malignancy* – 8 cases, 4 male and 4 female, aged 60-82 years. One case of chronic lymphatic leukaemia, 2 of malignant lymphoma, 1 of myelomatosis and 1 each of carcinoma of the pancreas, bronchus and colon and one case of malignant melanoma.

19) *Diabetes mellitus* – 1,979 cases of which 60 immediately preceded the development of carcinoma of the pancreas and were symptomatic, and 58 were of long-standing diabetes and developed cancer of the pancreas. Of the rest 81 were cases of long-standing diabetes developing malignant lymphoma, including Hodgkin's disease or leukaemia of various types. The rest comprised malignant disease of practically every organ.

20) "Idiopathic" *Addi son's disease preceding malignancy* – Addison's disease was present for up *to* 15 years prior to the ap - pearance of malignancy. Ten cases, 8 in females aged 33-81 years, 3 were malignant lymphoma, 2 were carcinoma of the bronchus in females.

21) *Coeliac disease preceding malignancy* – 6 cases, 2 males and 4 females, aged 38-71 years; 3 cases of malignant lymphoma, one after having coeliac disease for 15 years, 1 case had co-existing asthma, another dermatitis.

22) *Fibrosing alveolitis* – 1 case, male aged 64 years, developed generalized lymphosarcoma after 15 months.

23) *Ulcerative colitis preceding malignancy* – 2 cases, 1 affecting the stomach, the other the female breast. In 4 other cases diabetes was also present, all affecting men, aged 38-71 years, and comprised carcinoma of the pancreas, bronchus and bladder. One case developed chronic lymphatic leukaemia.

24) *Idiopathic hypoparathyroidism preceding malignancy* – 1 case, male, aged 57 years, of carcinoma of the pancreas.

25) *Non-alcoholic cirrhosis of the liver* or *active chronic hepatitis developing malignancy* – 42 cases, 21 female, 21 male, aged 38-78 years. Four cases of primary carcinoma of the liver, 6 cases of malignant lymphoma. Two also suffered from long-standing diabetes. Three cases of carcinoma of the oesophagus, seven of cancer of the stomach, six of carcinoma of the *bronchus* (4 *in females)*, two of cancer of the larynx, five of colon or rectum and three of carcinoma of the pancreas with preceding diabetes.

26) *Chronic relapsing pancreatitis preceding malignancy* – 3 cases, one of carcinoma of the pancreas preceded by long· standing diabetes and two of carcinoma of the bronchus.

27) *Paget's disease of bone* – 37 cases, aged 43-89 years, 29 in males, 4 of bone sarcoma, 2 of reticulosarcoma, 1 of Hodgkin's disease, 1 of acute lymphoblastic leukaemia, 1 of multiple myelomatosis, 4 of carcinoma of the bronchus, 2 of cafcinoma of the oesophagus, 2 of the stomach, 1 of the gall-bladder, 2 of the pancreas, 4 of the large intestine, 1 of the kidney, 5 of the prostate, 2 of the bladder, 3 of the female breast, 1 of the nostril.

28) *Klinefelter's syndrome* – 1 case, male, aged 48 years, with cancer of the rectum.

Thus, of these 2,475 cases of cancer recorded as developing in pre-existing cases of collagen or "auto-immune" disease there were 144 cases in which malignant lymphoma, including Hodgkin's disease, acute or chronic leukaemia or myelomatosis appeared. The other primary cancers involved almost any organ. They were found in a total of 202,791 cases, that is 1.2 per cent. While this estimate of the frequency of the occurrence of cancer in cases of collagen and auto-immune disease is obviously far too low, certain facts emerge from the figures.

1) As with collagen and "auto-immune" disease, so the age of the patients tended to be over 50 years.

2) There was often a long-standing history of systemic lupus erythematosus, rheumatoid arthritis, dermatomyositis, scleroderma or auto-immune disease preceding the onset of malignancy. This extended up to 38 years.

3) The case of the boy who developed juvenile rheumatoid arthritis at the age of 5 years and a year later acute lymphoblastic leukaemia would seem significant.

Systemic investigation of successive cases of malignant disease for the presence of collagen and auto-immune disease

It seemed necessary to investigate fully a series of *consecutive* cases of cancer encountered over a long period in a general hospital for the presence of collagen and "auto-immune" disease preceding, accompanying or following the appearance of the cancer. The investigations included:-

1) Questioning the subject on the existence or previous history of collagen or auto-immune disease, such as rheumatoid arthritis, pernicious anaemia, goitre, thyrotoxicosis, myxoedema, chronic cholecystitis, diabetes, asthma, fibroids, ovarian cysts, etc.

2) Examining the patient for signs of rheumatoid arthritis in any degree, thyrotoxicosis, myxoedema, thyroid enlargement or operation scars for cholecystectomy, hysterectomy, ovariectomy, etc. Careful note of the condition of the feet and cervical spine was made. No attempt at strict classification of rheumatoid arthritis according to the American Rheumatism Association System was attempted, but the clinical diagnosis of rheumatoid arthritis was only made in the presence of the typical deformities of hands and/or feet, often combined with typical rheumatoid disease of the cervical spine with or without the presence of RF in the serum and with typical radiological changes. Degenerative arthrosis of the hands was carefully excluded.

3) Questioning of the patient on a family history of collagen or auto-immune disease.

4) X-raying the cervical spine, hands and feet for evidence of rheumatoid disease.

5) Examining the blood for evidence of diabetes, signs of anaemia, pernicious anaemia, lupus erythematosus cells, etc.

6) Estimating the blood calcium for idiopathic hypoparathyroidism.

7) Carrying out a histamine fractional test meal for evidence of achlorhydria, probably always indicative of the presence of atrophic gastritis.

8) Estimating blood electrolytes and prednisol content indicative of adrenal function.

9) Estimating protein bound iodine for signs of hypo- or hyper-thyroidism (myxoedema and Hashimoto's thyroiditis).

10) Carrying out serum tests for RF, ANF, thyroid auto-antibodies (thyroid cytoplasmic fluorescent antibody, thyroid tanned red blood corpuscles agglutination titre and thyroid complement fixation tests), gastric parietal cell fluorescent antibody, adrenal cortical cell antibody, auto-immune bodies against red blood corpuscles and cryoglobulins. In the case histories recorded below the presence or absence of any kind of thyroid auto-antibody is simply recorded without reference to the type.

11) At autopsy or operation examinmg the thyroid, gastric mucosa, adrenal glands and liver for signs of auto-immune disease.

In many cases not examined at post mortem "auto-immune" lesions may exist, but give no evidence of their presence in life, for example atrophic gastritis or infiltration of the thyroid with lymphocytes. Hashimoto's thyroiditis may be found at autopsy in patients without clinical signs of thyroid disease (Furszyter et al., 1970). It is *important* to emphasize that antibodies may not be found in the serum in typical cases of collagen and auto-immune disease, especially in cases of burnt-out rheumatoid arthritis. *The diagnosis of the presence of these diseases is made on clinical and histological grounds and not by serological tests.*

It will be recalled that, when a lymphoma, myelomatosis or leukaemia develops, RF, ANF and auto-antibodies tend to disappear from the serum and then serological evidence of preexisting collagen and auto-immune disease may not be found in such cases.

Table VII. Malignant Lymphoma

Case	Sex	Age	History	Presence of achlorhydria	Serum auto-antibodies
VII, 1	M	40	Indian from Bombay. Resident in this country many years. Ten years previous, ly acute inflammatory swelling of left *spermatic cord* and testis. Biopsy showed generalized *lymphocytic in filtration*. At same time some transient generalized lymphadenopathy. *Diabetes* for 6 years. **Recent onset** of left inguinal lymphadenopathy. Biopsy showed reticulosarcoma, *paraneoplastic peripheral neuropathy* present.	+	Thyroid + ANF +
VII, 2	F	72	Long history of *arthropathy* of hands, wrists, knees and feet with at one time a left frozen shoulder. Treated with prednisolone. Aged 60 years onset of generalized lymphadenopathy and the blood showed changes of *chronic lymphatic leukaemia*. Biopsy of lymph node=*reticulosarcoma*. P.B.I. showed marked *hypothyroidism*.	+	
VII, 3	M	24	Marked family history on both sides of cancer of various organs. One year previously onset of generalized lymphadenopathy and later of herpes zoster. Biopsy=malignant lymphoma. Treated with chloroquine with **regression**.		Thyroid + **present 5 years** after onset and in total remission
VII, 4	M	51	Nine years history of *rheumatic* pains and swelling of *shoulders, hips, feet and ankles*. Followed by digestive symptoms. Operation showed malignant lymphoma of stomach with *atrophic gastritis*.	+	Thyroid + Gastric parietal cell +
VII, 5	M	49	Long history of hypertension and proteinuria with transient *Bence-Jones proteinuria* and *paraproteinaemia*. Later lymphadenopathy + **malignant** lymphoma, *paraneoplastic peripheral neuropathy*.		Thyroid + Gastric parietal cell +
VII, 6	M	55	Left eye removed for malignant melanoma of choroid 8 years before. Now **goitre**, *rheumatoid arthritis* of hands. **Post mortem** malignant melanomatosis of liver. *Hashimoto's thyroiditis. Paget's disease* of **bone**, reticulosarcoma of thyroid and lung. (Two malignancies).	+	Thyroid tt ANF +
VII, 7	F	79	Aged 49 years removal of area of *cystic mastitis* of left breast. Aged 69 years onset of *severe rheumatoid arthritis*. Under continuous treatment since. Now lymphosarcoma of left orbit.	+	RF + ANF + Gastric parietal cell +
VII, 8	M	70	Primary lymphosarcoma of stomach with gastrectomy and recurrence **in gastric** stump. Showed severe *rheumatoid arthritis* of hands and multiple rodent ulcers of nose, forehead and front of chest. (Multiple tumours).	+	ANF tt Thyroid +
VII, 9	F	88	One years history of a **mass in the left** breast, enlarged lymph nodes in left axilla. Biopsy of both showed presence of malignant lymphoma. Advanced *rheumatoid arthritis* of hands, wrists, elbows, feet **and ankles** present.	+	ANF - Thyroid +

Table VII (continued)

Case	Sex	Age	Clinical details		Serology
VII, 10	M	48	Six years previously sudden-;Onset of seropositive s.evere *rheumatoid arthritis*. Under continuous treatment and now bedbound. Two -mnths history of a rapidly enlarging mass **in the** right axilla =reticulosarcoma rapidly becoming generalized.		RF + ANF **tt**
VII, 11	F	54	*Raynaud's phenomena* for several years. Sixteen months history of *recurrent swelling of the salivary glands* accompanied by *polyarthritis* and *polyneuropathy* followed by lymphadenopathy. Autopsy 8 years later showed reticulosarcomatosis and widespread *arteritis* with reticulosarcoma developing in the enlarged parotid salivary gland (Sjogren-Mikulicz).		ANF **tt** speckled variety. Lupus erythematosus cells ++ in blood
VII, 12	F	72	Marked *rheumatoid arthritis* of hands.' Retro-peritoneal sarcoma.		Thyroid + RF +. ANF +
VII, 13	M	58	Severe *rheumatoid arthritis* for 10 years. Now chair bound. Recent onset of generalized lymphadenopathy =malignant lymphoma.	+	
VII, 14	M	58	*Alopecia universalis* for 10 years. *Chronic active hepatitis* 2 years. Malignant lymphoma 1 year.		Thyroid +++ becoming negative.
VII, 15	F	56	Severe *rheumatoid arthritis* for 10 years. *Myxoedema* for 4 years. Reticulosarcoma _of right humerus.		RF =+. NF + **Thyroid**+
VII, 16	M	66	*Diabetes* of unknown duration. Now lymphosarcoma.	+	ANF + Thyroid +
VII, 17	F	69	Menarche aged 17 years. Periods always scanty. Menopause aged 43 years. Aged 53 years hysterectomy for *fibroids* and lumps in periphery of both breasts **due to cystic mastitis** accompanied by mild *peripheral arthropathy*. Aged 60 years *diabetes* found. Aged 69 years lymphadenopathy in right groin. Biopsy=reticulosarcoma. Examination showed *mild rheumatoid arthritic* changes of fingers, wrists, ankles and feet.	+	ANF + Thyroid + Gastric parietal cell ++ C.F.T. platelet **antibodies**.
VII, 18	M	74	Under treatment for *rheumatoid arthritis* for several years. Now generalized lymphadenopathy and splenomegaly=lymphosarcoma.	+	ANF **tt** RF **tt** Thyroid tf-
VII, 19	F	72	Benign mass in left breast *(cystic mastitis)* aged 46 years. Now malignant lymphoma of cervical nodes.	+	Thyroid +++
VII, 20	F	46	*Vittiigo and melanoderma* 3 years. Eosinophilia in **blood**. Now malignant lymphoma of atdominal nodes.		ANF + Thyroid + Gastric parietal cell ++ prior to onset of lymphoma

Table VII (continued)

VII, 21	F	57	White. Lived in Central Africa in youth until 4 years prior to being seen. Aged 19-37 years recurrent attacks of *malaria*. Aged 24 years and 26 years two attacks of sleeping sickness (*African trypanosomiasis*) treated with Bayer 205. Aged 37 years attack of jaundice due to hepatitis of unknown causation. Now lymphosarcoma.		RF +
VII, 22	M	80	Anglo-Indian. Elephant shooter. Many years in India and Burma. **Frequent** malaria. Well-marked chronic *rheumatoid arthritic* changes and now giant follicular lymphoma in left inguinal nodes.	+	RF + Gastric parietal cell +
VII, 23	M	63	Left *epididymo-orchitis* 3 years ago. Now reticulosarcoma.	+	Thyroid +
VII, 24	F	74	Mild *rheumatoid arthritis* of hands and wrists over an indefinite period. Now malignant lymppoma of mediastinum.	+	RF + ANF + Thyroid ++
VII, 25	F	65	Ten years, 5 years and 6 months previously developed *recurrent* painless left *parotid salivary gland swelling*. On last occasion this left an enlarged mass below the left ear. During this 10 year period she developed dryness of the mouth and eyes=*Sjogren's syndrome*, and also of the nasopharynx and nose leading to nasal and nasopharyngeal crusting. During this period also subject to **intermittent** *joint pains* with morning stiffness of the joints, *swelling of the right knee* and left wrist and a *butterfly rash*. Examination showed well marked *rheumatoid changes* in the hands and feet and enlargement of the liver with a rash suggestive of *systemic lupus erythematopsus*. The mass below the left ear was fixed. Biopsy showed a nodular area of *lymphocytic* and *plasma cell infiltration* with a few islands of lymphoid tissue. The changes were a mixture of *malignant lymphoma* merging into *medullary plasmocytoma*. The bone **marrow** showed excess of lymphocytes. X-rays showed narrowing of the disc spaces in the cervical spine and typical *rheumatoid arthritic* changes **in** the hands and feet. No Bence-Janes protein was present in the **urine and** no bony lesions of myelomatosis. Electrophoresis showed no M band, but a diffuse increase **in** globulins and immunodiffusion showed IgA=440 mg. per 100 ml. IgG 5,200mg. per 100 **ml.** IgM 170 mg. per 100 ml. E.S.R. 75 mm. per hour. Blood count, Hb 128 G per cent. Later enlargement of the para-aortic, pelvic and left cervical lymph nodes appeared.	+	ANF ff+RF ff+Thyroid and gastric parietal cell and anti-bodies negative. Coombs test also negative.
					RF +
VII, 26	F	46	*Juvenile rheumatoid arthritis* aged 10-15 years. *Fibroids* aged 31 years. Myomectomy. Now lymphosarcoma and huge *fibroids*. Sister died of reticulosis.		Thyroid +
VII, 27	M	45	*Hypothyroidism* for 4 years. Now lymphosarcoma in cervical lymph nodes.		
VII, 28	M	49	Sudden onset of ascites and oedema of feet. Laparotomy showed liver cirrhosis and lymphosarcoma of spleen. Liver biopsy showed *chronic active hepatitis*.	+	RF +, ANF + Thyroid + Smooth muscle liver cell auto-antibodies **1 in** 80

Table VII (continued)

	Sex	Age			
VII, 29	M	40	**Father died of carcinoma of pancreas. Five years previously removal of almost painless right parotid *swelling*=*auto-immune parotitis*. Followed by cervical lymphadenopathy=malignant lymphoma.**	+	ANF +
VII, 30	M	28	Life-long *chronic rhinitis* and *drug sensitivity*. Now Hodgkin's disease with high pyrexia and spinal compression. Eosinophilia in blood.	+	ANF +
VII, 31,	M	54	*Atrophic rhinitis* with *crusting* and deafness due to *adhesive otitis*. Now malignant lymphoma of cervical nodes.	+	
VII, 32	F	72	Non-smoker. Fifteen years well marked *rheumatoid arthritis*. Now *myxoedema*. *Hashimoto's thyroiditis*. *Fibrosing alveolitis*, mediastinal lymphoma and *diabetes*.	+	RF + Thyroid tilt Gastric parietal cell +
VII, 33	M	64	Painless swelling of right parotid gland. *Biopsy*=*Mikulicz's disease* with dense lymphocytic infiltration. Three years **later malignant lymphoma beginning in cervical nodes.**	+	RF +
VII, 34	F	74	One brother died of cerebral glioma and one sister died of C.Irainoma of the breast. Patient had uterine polyp 20 years ago. Now lymphosarcoma.	+	
VII, 35	F	82	*Paget's disease* of right tibia. *Myxoedema*, *Sjogren's syndrome*. *Rheumatoid arthritic* changes. Now widespread reticulosarcomatosis.	+	ANF + Thyroid +
VII, 36	F	65	Aged 52 years transitional carcinoma of left renal pelvis. One year later several transitional cell papillomata and later carcinoma of bladder. Now generalized lymphosarcoma. Mild generalized *rheumatoid arthritic* changes. (4 tumours).	+	ANF +
VII, 37	F	64	One brother died of cerebral tumour. One niece has diabetes. One cousin has diabetes. Aged 38 years operation for *bilateral benign ovarian cysts and fibroids*. Aged 52 years *diabetes*, severe hypertension. Aged 61 years *auto-immune haemolytic anaemia*. Aged 63 years Kaposi's sarcoma. Mild *rheumatoid arthritic* changes.	+	ANF +
VII, 38	F	68	Hysterectomy for *fibroids* aged 48 years. *Thyrotoxicosis* operation aged 57 years. Now retroperitoneal sarcoma.	+	
VII, 39	F	75	*Fibroids* operation aged 45 years. Severe *rheumatoid arthritis* for 10 years. Now retroperitoneal sarcoma.	+	ANF +
VII, 40	F	89	Aged 74 years operation for removal of uterus containing a 15lb. *fibroid*. Severe splenomegaly found at this time. Now has *diabetes*, *ichthyosis acquisita*, severe *rheumatoid arthritic* changes in feet, *myelosclerosis*, malignant lymphoma and chronic myeloid leukaemia. (2 cancers).	+	ANF +

292

Table VII (continued)

VII, 41	F	73	Mother suffered from severe rheumatoid arthritis. Patient under treatment for 4 years for seropositive *rheumatoid arthritis*. Now developed lymphadenopathy. Biopsy=lymphosarcoma and blood showed chronic lymphatic leukaemia. (2 tumours).	+	RF + Thyroid + becoming negative with onset of lymphoma.
VII, 42	F	50	Acute onset of pyrexia, oedema, sweating and generalized lymphadenopathy, acute lymphoma. *Paraneoplastic peripheral neuropathy.*	+	Thyroid + Auto-immune haemolytic anaemia.
VII, 43 (Case 5)	F	53	Nine years previously aged **44** years hysterectomy for flooding. Specimen showed numerous *fibroids* of various sizes. Operation followed by onset of acute *dermatomyositis*. Treated by **prednisolone** resulting **in** the development of a peptic ulcer, for which partial gastrectomy performed. Immediately post-operatively the dermatomyositis resolved spontaneously. Remained well for 8 years when onset of malignant lymphoma.	+	ANF + Thyroid + Nine years previously. All tests now negative.
VII, 44	M	48	Five years previously onset of *pernicious anaemia* with *atrophic gastritis* and blood showed ANF and **gastric parietal and intrinsic factor** auto-antibodies positive. Later developed rashes and *lymphadenopathy=reticulosarcoma.*	+	Tests negative with onset of lymphoma.
VII, 45	M	48	Acute onset of stem-cell lymphoma of retroperitoneal tissues.	+	ANF + RF +
VII, 46	M	67	Generalized lymphosarcoma. *Paraneoplastic peripheral neuropathy.*	+	Thyroid +
VII, 47	M	76	Mild *rheumatoid arthritis* of hands and feet. Now follicular lymphoma of right groin.	+	RF +
VII, 48	M	51	Onset of *pernicious anaemia* and *coeliac disease* many years before followed by development of abdominal lymphoma.	+	
VII, 49	F	59	Ten years previously enlargement of right lobe of **thyroid**. Partial thyroidectomy showed *focal lymphocytic infiltration*. Thyroid auto-antibodies in blood. Now pathological fracture of head of right femur and D10 vertebal collapse. Biopsy=lymphocytic lymphoma.	+	Thyroid auto-antibodies now negative.
VII, 50	M	29	Sudden haematemesis without previous symptoms. Operation showed primary lymphoma of stomach.		
VII, 51	M	40	Ten years ago onset of *dermatomyositis*. Two years ago right orchidectomy for tumour=malignant lymphoma. Now generalized enlarged lymph nodes= lymphoma.		ANF + Thyroid + Gastric parietal cell +

Table VII (continued)

	Sex	Age			
VII, 52	M	75	For 20 years generalized *rheumatoid arthritis*, including cervical spine. Ten years ago bilateral *choroiditis*. Four years ago *alopecia mucinosus*. **One year later mycosis fungoides** of scalp, abdomen and legs.		RF +, ANF + Thyroid + disappearing with development of mycosis.
VII, 53	F	63	Developed pain **in hip** joints, which showed bony involvement of **the** heads of both femora. Examination showed signs of mild *generalized rheumatoid arthritis*. Biopsy of femoral heads showed reticulosarcoma. Later developed multiple lymphadenopathy=reticulosarcoma.	+	RF + ANF + Thyroid
VII, 54	M	71	Generalized lymphadenopathy. *Rheumatoid arthritis* of feet. Biopsy=reticulosarcoma.	+	ANF +.
VII, 55	F	33	Malignant lymphoma confined to duodenum and local lymph nodes.		
VII, 56	F	79	One of four siblings. One brother and one sister both died of "cancer". **Patient** suffered from *intrinsic asthma* since her teens and developed *chronic bronchitis*. Since aged 40 years suffered from widespread *dermatitis*. **Now has a** retroperitoneal sarcoma.	+	RF +
VII, 57	M	46	**Patient and three brothers** suffered from gou t. **Father and** one brother both died of leukaemia (type **unknown)**. Two sisters are alive and well. Patient had a lump in the groin and biopsy showed a follicular histiocytic lymphoma.	+	ANF +
VII, 58	M	51	Under treatment for *rheumatoid arthritis* for 3 years. Simultaneous onset of malignant melanoma of **the** dorsum of the right hand and lymphosarcoma of the tonsils.		Thyroid +
VII, 59	F	28	Aged 18 years operation for chronic *follicular appendicitis*. *Cystic right ovary and fibroids* discovered. Aged 26 years *fulminant pyorrhoea* **with loss of all her teeth** and onset of *Sjogren's syndrome* and *atrophic rhinitis*. Now *chronic active hepatitis*. Cervical lymphadenopathy due to lymphosarcoma also affecting nasopharyn x and chronic lymphatic leukaemia.		RF -+ ANF + Thyroid +
VII, 66	M	70	Under treatment for *rheumatoid arthritis* for several years. Onset of adenocarcinoma of the **prostate**. Opera tion 1 year later showed lymphosarcoma of inguinal lymph nodes. Two years later retroperitoneal sarcoma and at same time carcinoma of right breast (male). Three years later carcinoma of right upper lobe of bronchus and a year later separate and different histological cancer of left lung. (Multiple malignancies).	+	RF
VII, 61	F	30	Painless right pre-auricular lymph node enl argement followed by mass in **right** parotid salivary gland and right cervical lymphadenopathy. AU showed follicular lymphadenopathy.		ANF + Thyroid +
VII, 62	M	47	Ly phosarcomatosis with multiple rodent ulcers(multiple malignancies).	+	ANF +

294

Table VIII. Hodgkin's Disease

Case	Sex	Age	History	Presence of achlorhydria	Serum auto-antibodies
VIII, 1	F	78	Well-marked *rheumatoid changes* in hands, feet, wrists and elbows for 10 years. Thyroid adenoma present. Developed abdominal mass =Hodgkin's disease. Post mortem-thyroid adenoma with focal *thyroiditis, atrophic gastritis,* Hodgkin's disease of abdominal nodes.	+	Thyroid +
VIII, 2	M	78	*Alopecia universalis* for 12 years. Now generalized Hodgkin's disease.	+	Thyroid +
VIII, 3	F	77	Severe generalized *rheumatoid arthritis* for many year>. Now Hodgkin's sarcoma of left cervical lymph nbdes.	+	ANF + Gastric parietal cell +
VIII, 4	M	23	*Acute rheumatism* aged, 16 years. Now Hodgkin's disease.		ANF +
VIII, 5	M	22	Hodgkin's disease. *Rheumatoid granulomatous myocarditis* at autopsy.		
VIII, 6	F	69	Sister died aged 29 years of pernicious anaemia. Patient had *rheumatoid arthritis* for 9 years. Under treatment ever since. Now Hodgkin's disease.		RF + ANF +
VIII, 7	M	38	*Diabetes.* Now Hodgkin's disease.		ANF +
VIII, 8	M	33	*Diabetes* 6 years ago. Now Hodgkin'S disease.		Gastric parietal cell +
VIII, 9	M	64	Four years *myxoedema.* Now Hodgkin's disease.		Thyroid +
VIII, 10	M	28	Indian from Calcutta. Aged 22 years cervical lymphadenopathy subsiding spontaneously. Aged 23 years fever and axillary lymphadenopathy with 27 per cent eosinophils in white blood cells. Biopsy=Hodgkin's paragranuloma. Spontaneous regression. One year later severe *alopecia.* Five years later again lymphadenopathy, which subsided, but soon followed by xecurrent high fever up to 106°F., rigors, sweating, lymphadenopathy, splenomegaly, pleural effusions and oedema of right leg. High eosinophilia in blood throughout.		Thyroid + ANF +
VIII, 11	F	28	Mother has rheumatoid **arthritis.** Brother has pernicious anaemia. Patient has Hodgkin's disease of axillary and inguinal lymph nodes.		Lupus erythe-matosus cells + ANF +
VIII, 12	M	49	*Intrinsic asthma* for 15 years. Allergic to penicillin, etc. Now Hodgkin's paragranuloma of right axillary nodes.		ANF + Thyroid +

Table VIII (continued)

VIII, 13	M	33	Six months "rheumatic" pains and now simultaneous onset of thyrotoxicosis and Hodgkin's disease.		ANF + RF Thyroid + all becoming negative during course of illness. *
VIII, 14	F	64	Premature menopause aged 38 years. Aged 48 years onset of dryness of mouth and eyes with recurrent Painless swelling of both parotid glands. Schirmer's test positive for Sjögren's syndrome. Aged 53 years developed benign lympho-epithelial tumour. Operative removal showed benign lympho-epithelial tumour. Aged 53 years onset of dysparaunia due to atrophic vulvitis and vaginitis. Aged 64 years cervical lymph-adenopathy and swelling of both submaxillary glands. Lymph node biopsy= Hodgkin's disease. (2 tumours)	+	ANF +. RF + Gastric parietal cell + at onset of Sjogren's syndrome becoming negative with onset of Hodg-kin's disease.
VIII, 15 (Case 18)	M	44	Aged 28 years onset of severe rheumatoid arthritis for which under continuous treatment till time of death. Aged 41 years onset of symptoms of coeliac disease and Sjögren's syndrome. Schirmer's test positive. Achlorhydria present. RF strongly positive. Treated with gluten-free diet with some improvement in diarrhoea, but later developed pernicious anaemia. Three years later onset of Hodgkin's disease and died 5 years after this. Autopsy— severe rheumatoid arthritis, atrophic gastritis, atrophy of small intestinal mucosa, wide-spread Hodgkin's disease.	+	RF, ANF and gastric parietal cell becoming negative at onset of Hodgkin's disease.
VIII, 16	M	39	Indian employed at Embassy. Frequent malarial attacks in past. Two years previously in Saigon onset of acute painful swelling of left ankle followed by severe rheumatoid swelling of small joints, hands and feet, fever and night sweats. Six months after onset blood showed a marked eosinophilia. Eighteen months later lymphadenopathy in left axilla and left side of neck. Biopsy showed Hodgkin's sarcoma and the eosinophilia persisted.		RF and ANF + 6 months after onset. Both be-came negative with appearance of lymphadeno-pathy.
VIII, 17	F	22	Aged 15 years thyrotoxicosis; treated for 3 years. Since then vague rashes. Now Hodgkin's disease of cervical nodes.		
VIII, 18	F	63	Seven years mild diabetes. Now Hodgkin's disease.		Thyroid +
VIII, 19	F	48	Thyroidectomy for thyrotoxicosis aged 24 years. Aged 26 years herpes zoster of right side of abdomen. Aged 34 years removal of multilocular cyst from the canal of Nuck. Aged 44 years onset of arthropathy of peripheral joints for which under continuous treatment. Now night sweats, pruritus and lymphadenopathy in left side of neck and right axilla. Biopsy=Hodgkin's disease.	+	RF + Thyriod + at onset of rheuma-toid arthritis. Now negative.
VIII, 20	M	31	Onset 18 months previously with "influenza!" symptoms (fever, night sweats, malaise, tiredness), joint swellings and muscular cramps, followed by generaliz-ed alopecia. After 18 months lymphadenopathy in neck, groin and mediastinum. Biopsy=Hodgkin's disease.		RF + Thyroid+ after one year

Table VIII (continued)

VIII, 21	M	40	Over 5 years recurrent painless enlargement of left submaxillary gland. *Biopsy=diffuse lymphocytic infiltration with plasma cells.* Now Hodgkin's disease of cervical nodes.		RF +
VIII, 22	M	32	Mother died of cancer when patient aged 7 years. *Intrinsic asthma* as long as remembers. Onset of Hodgkin's disease 2 years previously.		**Thyroid** +
VIII, 23	F	17	Aged 13 years onset of Hodgkin's disease. Not yet menstruated. Puberty not reached. Cytogenetically a mosaic.		
VIII, 24	F	38	One year ago onset of Hodgkin's disease. Now carcinoma of the thyroid in gland showing changes of *Hashimoto's thyroiditis.* (2 tumours).	+	Thyroid +t
VIII, 25	F	61	One sister died of diabetes. One sister died of leukaemia. Aged 36 years erythema nodosum, *peripheral jollt swelling* and later lymphadenopathy. Diagnosed sarcoidosis. Aged 56 years recurrence with positive Coombs *test=auto-immune haemolytic anaemia.* Now Hodgkin's disease in left axilla and neck.		
VIII, 26	M	30	Aged 2d years recurrent almost painless swelling of submaxillary glands. Biopsy, lymphocytic infiltration. *Sjogren-Mikulicz's syndrome.* Twelve months la ter pain and swelling in the right inguinal region=Hodgkin's disease.		ANF +
VIII, 27	F	26	Onset of widespread *vitiligo* 3 years previously. Now generalized Hodgkin's disease.		ANF + / Thyroid ttt
VIII, 28	M	32	Since age of 17 years frequent *urticarial wheals,* especially after exercise. Onset of Hodgkin's disease aged 32 years.		RF + / **Thyroid** + becoming negative
VIII, 29	M	40	*Eczema, hay-fever and intrinsic asthma* from early age. In one attack of asthma aged 21 years enlarged node in right axilla. Eczema cleared aged 31 yea rs. Aged 40 years after an attack of severe *asthma* axillary node increased in size and others enlarged. Biopsy=Hodgkin's disease.		Eosinophilia, ANF tit. RF + **Gastric** parietal cell +
VIII, 30	F	26	Two years *atrophic vaginitis* accompanied by mild *arthropathy.* Then lymphadenopathy in groins and axillae. Biopsy=Hodgkin's disease.		ANF +. RF + **at onset of** Hodgkin's disease.
VIII, 31	F	50	Onset of *myxoedema* 5 years previously, followed by generalized Hodgkin's disease.	+	
VIII, 32	F	42	Aged 38 years onset of *joint pains and swelling* and flooding. Hysterectomy for *fibroids.* Aged 42 years partial gastrectomy for primary Hodgkin's disease of stomach and surrounding lymph nodes on lesser curvature.	+	RF + **Thyroid** +

297

Table VIII (continued)

	Sex	Age			
VIII, 33	M	26	Four years crusting and dryness of the nasal mucosa=atrophic rhinitis, followed by epistaxis and blocking of right side of nose and cervical lymphadenopathy. Biopsy=Hodgkin's disease.		ANF +
VIII, 34	F	27	One year previously removal of dermoid cyst of left ovary. Now Hodgkin's disease in cervical lymph nodes. (2 tumours).		ANF + Thyroid + Gastric parietal cell +
VIII, 35	F	42	Fifteen years previously partial thyroidectomy for thyrotoxicosis. Now lymphadenopathy of left axillary nodes Hodgkin's disease,		Thyroid +.
VIII, 36	M	47	Severe rheumatoid arthritis since aged 27 years with several surgical operations on hands and knees. Now generalized nodular-sclerotic Hodgkin's disease.		ANF tf., RF tf. Thyroid +
VIII, 37	M	47	Generalized lymphadenopathy=Hodgkin's disease. Paraneoplastic peripheral neuropathy.		Thyroid +
VIII, 38	M	52	Generalized lymphadenopathy. No arthropathy or other diseases. Biopsy=Hodgkin's disease.	+	
VIII, 39	F	50	Onset of bilateral reticulosarcoma of tonsils treated by D.X.T. 4 years. Later abdominal lymphadenopathy=Hodgkin's disease. Eight years later onset of myxoedema. Died aged 67 years of carcinomatosis of skin of the irradiated area of neck.	+	
VIII, 40	F	60	Generalized lymphadenopathy.	+	ANF + Thyroid +
VIII, 41	M	46	Onset 15 years before in India with painless swelling of left salivary parotid gland, which subsided slowly. Two years later 2 attacks of painless swelling of the left cervical nodes in which the left parotid again enlarged and remained so. A mixed parotid tumour was removed. After another 5 years the tumour recurred and the cervical nodes again enlarged. Biopsy=Hodgkin's disease. (2 tumours).	+	RF +
VIII, 42	M	47	One year previously onset of acute seronegative polyarthritis affecting aU peripheral joints. Two months previously he suffered from anorexia and obstructive jaundice. White blood count=12,000 (12 per cent being eosinophils). Chest X-ray, three opacities in the right lung. Laparotomy, lymphadenopathy in the porta hepatis and the jejunal mesentery. Biopsy showed Hodgkin's disease with numerous eosinophil, plasma and reticulum cells.	+	Thyroid +
VIII, 43	M	25	Severe Raynaud's disease since aged 15 years. Now Hodgkin's disease.		ANF + Lupus erythematosus cells tf.

Table VIII (continued)

VIII, 44	M	47	Mother died of Parkinsonism. All his three brothers died of "leukaemia". Patient has Hodgkin's disease.	—	ANF **+**, Lupus erythematosus cells **+**
VIII, 45	M	47	*Psychotic* (manic depressive) for 5 years. Now Hodgkin's disease.		RF **+**, ANF +
VIII, 46	F	64	*Benign lympho-epitheliomatous lesion of parotid* with Hodgkin's disease.	+	
VIII, 47	M	35	Doctor. Left dental sepsis followed by left cervical lymphadenopathy= Hodgkin's disease.		Thyroid **+**
VIII, 48	F	34	*Thyrotoxic.* Bilateral cervical lympha<denopathy and mass present in **right** side of thyroid gland. Lymph node biopsy showed Hodgkin's disease. Removal of thyroid, mass revealed Hodgkin's disease developing in *Hashimoto's thyroiditis.*		Thyroid +
VIII, 49	M	44	Under treatment for severe *rheumatoid arthritis* for 20 years. Now Hodgkin's disease of right axillary nodes.	+	RF + Thyroid +
VIII, 50	F	74	Aged 50 years *myxoedema.* Now Hodgkin's disease and *rheumatoid arthritis* of feet.	+	Thyroid **+**
VIII, 51	M	52	Under treatment for *rheumatoid arthritis* for 10 years. Now Hodgkin's disease.	+	RF **+**
VIII, 52	F	68	Hodgkin's disease.	+	
VIII, 53	M	60	*Rheumatoid arthritis* for 9 years. Given various treatments including gold injections. Hodgkin's disease for one year. Now rodent ulcer. (Twin malignancies).	+	RF **+**

299

Table IX. Myelomatosis

case	Sex	Age	History	Presence of achlorhydria	Serum auto-antibodies
IX, 1	F	56	Grandfather died of myelomatosis. Three attacks of herpes zoster over 20 years. Intermittent *painful arthropathies of hand*. One year symptoms of myelomatosis. Died under treatment with melphelan with acute lymphoblastic leukaemia. (Twin malignancies).	+	
IX, 2	F	70	Long history of *recurrent asthma* and chronic bronchitis, now mild *peripheral arthropathy* and *rheumatoid arthritic* changes in hands and feet. *Thyroid* diffusely enlarged. Now myelomatosis.	+	
IX, 3	F	60	Onset with spontaneous compression of a dorsal vertebra. Mild *rheumatoid arthritic* changes in hands. Thyroid moderately and diffusely enlarged.	+	Thyroid +
IX, 4	M	45	Onset with lymphadenopathy and later vertebral collapse.	+	
IX, 5	F	64	Aged 43 years *cystic mastitis* upper outer quadrant of left breast. Aged 45 years carcinoma of outer part of right breast. Mastectomy followed by elephantiasis of *right arm* 15 years later. Aged 45 years menopause with generalized *arthropathy* lasting 2-3 years settling after prolonged treatment. Aged 54 years E.S.R. markedly raised and remained so over the next 10 years when onset of myelomatosis. (Two tumours)	+	ANF + Thyroid + becoming negative
IX, 6	F	62	Operation for *fibroids* aged 40 years. Now myelomatosis.	+	
IX, 7	M	57	Onset with cord compression followed by laminectomy. L. F. T. and liver biopsy showed *active chronic* hepatitis.	+	
IX, 8	M	63	Onset with *generalized urticaria* and microcytic hypochromic anaemia. Mild *rheumatoid arthritis*. Acromegaly due to eosinophilic pituitary adenoma. Now myelomatosis. (2 tumours).	+	
IX, 9	F	60	Myelomatosis with associated thyrotoxicosis and mild signs of *rheumatoid arthritis*.	+	Thyroid +
IX, 10	F	71	*Myxoedema* aged 46 years. *Rheumatoid arthritis* aged 70 years. Three months previously massive gastrointestinal haemorrhage. Laparotomy and gastrectomy showed *atrophic gastritis* with metaplasia of mucosa. Albumin 3.1 G/100 ml. Globulin 8.2 G/100 ml. E. S. R.=87 mm. per hour. Electrophoresis=M band in gammaglobulins. Skeletal survey showed myelomatosis. Platelets=60, 000.	+	

300

Table IX (continued)

IX, 11	F	70	One sister died of carcinoma of stomach. One sister has diabetes. Five brothers and one sister alive and well. Mild *rheumatoid arthritis* of hands and feet for years. Now myelomatosis with nasal **plasmacytoma.** Bence Jones **protein in** urine. Normocytic anaemia. Hypergammaglobulinaemia of monoclonal type. Immunophoresis, IgG 10 mgs. per 100 mls., IgA less **than** 28 mgms per 100 mls., IgM nil.	+	RF +
IX, 12	F	72	History of *asthma* since her twenties. Now bronchitis and myelomatosis.	+	ANF +
IX, 13	M	58	Mother died two years previously of myelomatosis. Patient has myelomatosis.	+	
IX, 14	M	41	Jamaican negro. Severe and recurrent *malaria* in childhood. Now myelomatosis. Electrophoresis 2 M bands in immunoglobulins. E.S.R. 137 mm/hr. Anaemia. Bence-Jones proteinuria. IgG 5,500 mgms. per cent, IgA 150 mgms. per cent, IgM 40 mgms. per cent.	+	RF +
IX, 15	M	61	Aged 50 years peptic ulcer. *Ichthyosis acquisita* for 5 years. Now Bence.Jones proteinuria and myelomatosis.	+	
IX, 16	M	60	Mother died with severe rheumatoid arthritis. Patient has myelomatosis.	+	
IX, 17	M	47	Chronic rhinitis and intrinsic asthma since childhood. Onset of severe *rheumatoid arthritis* aged 27 years. Aged 42 years papillary carcinoma of thyroid. Treated by excision. Now myelomatosis. (2 malignancies).	+	ANF + RF lft
IX, 18	F	60	Hysterectomy for *fibroids* aged 47 years. Nine years history of joint pains and swelling. Now myelomatosis with Bence-Jones prote.nuria.	+	
IX, 19	F	78	*Cholecystitis* without stones. Calcified *fibroids.* Asymptomatic myelomatosis.	+	RF +

Table X. Leukaemias

Case	Sex	Age	History	Presence of achlorhydria	Serum auto-antibodies
I. Acute leukaemia					
X, 1	F	72	Mother died of diabetes. Fifteen years previously operations for cervical polyp and removal of *ovarian cyst*. For several years painful peripheral *arthropathy* treated with prednisolone and aspirin. Now acute lymphoblastic leukaemia with mouth ulceration.	+	RF +
X, 2	F	44	Aged 40 years onset of severe sero-positive *rheumatoid arthritis* resulting in severe deformities. Now acute leukaemia of stem cell type with extensive mouth ulceration.		RF +
X, 3	M	5	Brother has intrinsic asthma and **rhinitis** and father intrinsic asthma and a family history of asthma and diabetes. Patient aged 3 years migrating *arthropathy* with severe stomatitis and tonsillitis continuing. Aged 4+ years acute lymphoblastic leukaemia.		RF +
X, 4	M	12	Acute onset of *thyrotoxicosis*. Blood showed acute stem cell leukaemia.		
X, 5	M	9	Acute onset of *thyrotoxicosis* with severe stomatitis. Blood showed acute stem cell leukaemia.		
X, 6	F	66	Aged 50 years hysterectomy for *fibroids*. Sudden onset with abdominal pain and swelling of the feet and abdomen. Liver markedly enlarged. Blood showed changes of acute monocytic leukaemia. Liver function tests and liver biopsy showed *chronic active hepatitis*. Bone marrow confirmed monocytic leukaemia. Autopsy showed chronic active hepatitis and malignant hepatoma. (Twin malignancies.)	+	ANF + RF ++ Thyroid +
X, 7	F	69	Aged 36 years a period of acute *painful arthropathy* under treatment for 2 years. Aged 50 years hysterectomy for *fibroids*. Now acute myeloblastic leukaemia with swollen tender gums.	+	Thyroid + RF +
X, 8	F	38	Onset with *thyrotoxicosis*. Heart failure. Acute stem cell leukaemia with severe ulceration of mouth.	+	Thyroid +
X, 9	F	56	Grandfather died of myelomatosis. Three attacks of herpes zoster over 20 years. **Intermittent** *painful arthropathy* of hands. One year symptoms of myelomatosis. Died with acute lymphoblastic leukaemia. (Twin malignancies).	+	
X, 10	M	54	Acute monocytic leukaemia. Found to be *myxoedematous*. Teeth carious and falling out.	+	Thyroid ++

Table X (continued)

X,11	M	16	Very severe painful ulceration of gums, buccal mucosa and pharynx, *joint pains* and *swelling*. Swelling over left shoulder blade which on biopsy showed sarcoma. Blood count–acute myeloblastic leukaemia.		RF +
X,12	F	20	Two years previously onset of *myxoedema* and recurrent sore throats. Now suffers from acute lymphatic leukaemia.		
X,13	M	64	Acute myeloid leukaemia. Found to be *thyrotoxic*.	+	Thyroid + Gastric parietal cell +

II. Chronic lymphatic leukaemia

X,14	M	70	Onset with lymphadenopathy. Long-standing history of severe *rheumatoid arthritis* with deformity of limbs. For 5 years lymphadenopathy and chronic lymphatic leukaemia.	+	
X,15	M	55	*Atrophic gastritis* for 9 years followed by development of chronic lymphatic leukaemia.	+	
X,16	F	65	Aged 43 years hysterectomy for *fibroids and bilateral ovarian cysts.* Long history of rheumatic pains. Marked *rheumatoid deformity* of hands. Now chronic lymphatic leukaemia.	+	Thyroid +
X,17	F	67	Operation for bilateral benign *ovarian cysts* aged 60 years. Marked *rheumatoid arthritic deformity*, of hands wrists and knees. Now chronic lymphatic leukaemia.	+	
X,18	M	60	*Fibrosing alveolitis* for 2 years developing into chronic lymphatic leukaemia.	+	Thyroid +
X,19	M	65	*Pernicious anaemia* for 6 years followed by development of chronic lymphatic leukaemia and then carcinoma of bronchus. Non-smoker (2 tumours).	+	Thyroid + Gastric parietal cell ++ becoming negative with development of leukaemia
X,20	F	61	Onset with *myxoedema, rheumatoid deformities* of hands. *Active chronic hepatitis* and chronic lymphatic leukaemia.	+	ANF + Gastric parietal cell ++

Table X (continued)

X, 21	F	67	Indian from Kenya; in this country for 10 years. *Raynaud's disease for 12 months.* Blisters in the mouth of recent onset with *pains and swelling in knees, right shoulder* and *temporo-mandibular* joints and *pleuritic* pain at right base. Blood showed pancytopenia, *lupus erythematosus cells* +. X-rays of cervical spine showed narrowing of disc spaces. Diagnosed *systemic lupus erythematosus.* In next 3 months changes of chronic lymphatic leukaemia appeared.		ANF :llt
X, 22	F	78	Sister and mother both died of pernicious anaemia. Two years previously patient developed left D 10 herpes zoster and *later ichthyosis acquisita* appeared. Examination showed well-marked *rheumatoid deformities* of hands and feet. Blood showed changes of *pernicious anaemia* and chronic lymphatic leukaemia.	+	Gastric parietal cell + RF +
X, 23	F	44	Mother and her **mother's sister suffered from severe rheumatoid arthritis.** Developed *acanthosis nigricans* 10 years prior to first being seen. Aged 42 years hysterectomy for *fibroids.* Over the **last** 18 months this subject to recurrent bouts of pyrexia, soreness of the throat, swelling of the cervical lymph nodes and night sweats lasting for 4–6 weeks and followed by soreness and dryness of the mouth and sudden *falling out of all the teeth.* The eyes became dry. Examination showed xerophthalmia and enlargement of submaxillary, parotid and sublingual salivary glands, atrophic pharyngitis, stomatitis and angular stomatitis and enlarged cervical lymph nodes (*Sjogren-Mikulicz's syndrome*). Operation for *chronic cholecystitis.* While under investigation developed *chronic active hepatitis* and **arterial** thrombosis in several digits. Investigation showed *chronic active hepatitis* and **arterial** thrombosis in several digits. Biopsy of cervical lymph node=lymphosarcoma. Blood showed monoclonal paraproteinaemia. Developed peripheral neuropathy.		RF :llt Cold agglutinins +
X, 24	F	60	Long-standing *arthropathy,* especially of elbows and knees. Recent radiotherapy for carcinoma of larynx. Six months later developed lymphadenopathy and found to have chronic lymphatic leukaemia. (Twin malignancies).	+	
X, 25	F	64	Known severe hypertensive since aged **48** years. Aged 56 years *thyrotoxicosis* associated with *arthralgias.* Aged 58 years onset of *diabetes.* Now chronic lymphatic leukaemia with mild *rheumatoid changes* in hands and feet. Autopsy showed heavy *lymphocytic change in thyroid gland,* right cortical adrenal adenoma and left cortical adrenal hyperplasia. (Twin malignancies).	+	Thyroid +
X, 26	F	62	Aged 37 years hysterectomy for *fibroids.* Aged 54 years onset of *rheumatoid arthritis.* Aged 59 years chronic lymphatic leukaemia and severe rheumatoid arthritis present.	+	RF :llt
X, 26 a.	M	68	*Diabetes* 9 years. Now *rheumatoid arthritis* of feet, *chronic active hepatitis,* IgG paraproteinaemia and chronic lymphatic leukaemia.	+	RF + Gastric parietal cell+
X, 26 b.	F	63	*Benign ovarian cyst* removed aged 32 years. *Thyrotoxicosis* aged 63 years, treated mediUUy. Two years later chronic lymphatic leukaemia.	+	Thyroid +

Table X (continued)

X. 26 c.	M	37	Carcinoma of the rectum. Chronic lymphatic leukaemia. (Twin malignancies).		Thyroid + Gastric parietal cell +

III. Chronic myeloid leukaemia

X. 27	F	50	Mother suffered from pernicious anaemia ending in carcinoma of the lltomach. Patient gave 2 years hitory of *painful swelling of hands and wrists with morning stiffness* followed by development of a frozen shoulder and diffuse en/ari(emetl *of the thyroid gland.* Developed *myxoedema.* Blood showed thrombocytaemla and later chronic myeloid leukaemia. Biopsy of thyroid Hashimoto's thyroiditis.		Thyroid ++ RF +
			Onset with dyspnoea. Blood count showed chronic myeloid leukaemia.	+	Thyroid +
			Rheumatoid arthritis of hands, *thyroid swelling.* Blood showed chronic myeloid leukaemia.		ANF tt Thyroid ++
			Onset with dyspnoea. No evidence of coHagen or auto-immune disease.		
			Aged 30 years oophorectomy for *bilateral benign ovarian cysts.* Chronic myeloid leukaemia found aged 73 years.		RF + ANF +

Table XI.: Basal and squamous cell carcinoma of skin

Case	Sex	Age	History	Presence of achlorhydria	Serum auto-antibodies
XI, 1	F	83	Sister died 8 years previously of leukaemia. Multiple basal cell carcinoma on back and face. *Chronic rheumatoid arthritic* changes in hands and feet.	+	ANF + Gastric parietal cell +
XI, 2	F	65	Aged 46 years operation for *chronic cholecystitis* and gall-stones. *Severe Paget's disease* of bone. *Mild rheumatoid arthritic* changes in hands. Multiple basal cell carcinoma of **trunk.**	+	
XI, 3	F	55	*Ulcerative colitis.* Basal cell carcinoma of back and face.		ANF + RF + Thyroid
XI, 4	F	86	*Severe rheumatoid arthritis* of hands, etc. Multiple basal cell carcinoma of **trunk.**	+	ANF + Thyroid + Gastric parietal cell +
XI, 5	M	45	Lived in sunny climate for years. Rodent ulcer of side of neck.		ANF +
XI, 6	F	65	Aged 52 years cholecystectomy for *chronic cholecystitis* and gall-stones. Crippled with *rheumatoid arthritis.* Extensive squamous cell carcinoma of scalp.		
XI, 7	F	67	Aged 57 years onset of severe *rheumatoid arthritis* for which under treatment ever since. Aged 61 years operation for *chronic cholecystitis* and gall-stones. Aged 65 years *myxoedema and diabetes.* Aged 67 years multiple squamous cell carcinoma of face and **trunk.**	+	RF + Thyroid tt
XI, 8	M	62	**Heavy drinker in past.** *Rheumatoid arthritis* of fingers. Spider naevl. Rodent ulcer of **tip** of nose.		RF + Smooth muscle antibodies +
XI, 9	F	78	*Severe rheumatoid arthritis* since aged 60 years. Rodent ulcer of forehead.	+	RF +
XI, 10	F	70	*Diabetes* aged 60 years. Large rodent ulcer of nose removel. Now *Paget's disease.*		
XI, 11	M	56	Five years ago rashes on face and neck. *Polycythaemia* one year. Hypochlorhydria. Now heart failure, *rheumatoid arthritis* of hands, nd rodent ulcer and hyper-keratosis of left cheek.	+	ANF +
XI, 12	F	60	All her life skin very sensitive to sun, which caused blisters. For 6 years *thyrotoxicosis* developing in to *myxoedema* with persistent diarrhoea. At same time she developed delirium and was in a mental Hospital off and on. Well-marked *rheumatoid arthritis* of feet. *Raynaud's disease* for years. *Ichthyosis acquisita.* Two years recurrent multiple squamous carcinoma of skin of face and keratoses of skin of lower legs.	+	RF + Thyroid tt

Table XI (continued)

XI, 13	M	84	Aged 65 years cholecystectomy for chronic cholecystitis and gall-stones. Aged 80 years rodent ulcer of nose. Now *Ichthyosis acquisita*. Well-marked *rheumatoid arthritis* of feet and carcinoma of stomach. (Twin tumours).		ANF **+** Gastric parietal cell **+**
XI, 14	F	62	Hysterectomy for fibroids aged 36 years. Rodent ulcer of nose aged 40 years. *Thyrotoxicosis* aged 54 years. Onset of *rheumatoid arthritis* aged 55 years. Aged 56 years onset of *Sjögren-Mikulicz's* syndrome, *atrophic rhinitis* and *adhesive otitis*.	+	Thyroid ++ Gastric parietal cell ++
XI, 15	M	80	Non-smoker. *Rheumatoid arthritis* of hands. Rodent ulcer of scalp. Carcinomatosis of bronchus. *Paraneoplastic peripheral neuropathy*.		ANF **+** Thyroid ++
XI, 16	F	61	Non-smoker. *Pernicious anaemia* for 8 years. Simultaneous carcinoma of the bronchus, carcinoma of the stomach and *paraneoplastic peripheral neuropathy*. (Twin malignancies). Rodent ulcer of back 3 years previously.	+	ANF **+** Gastric parietal cell **+**
XI, 17	F	79	Five years ago intra-epidermal carcinoma of anal canal. One year ago rodent ulcers of forehead and neck. Now carcinoma of bladder. Well-marked *rheumatoid arthritis*. (Multiple malignancies).	+	ANF **+** Thyroid **+**
XI, 18	F	75	Aged 61 years rodent ulcer of right temple. Aged 65 years rodent ulcer in front of **right** ear. Aged 73 years purpura. Aged 75 years transitional cell carcinoma of bladder. (Multiple malignancies).	+	Thyroid ++ Gastric parietal cell+
XI, 19	F	76	Eighteen years ago **rodent ulcer of left lower** eyelid. Now carcinoma of bladder with marked chronic *rheumatoid arthritic* changes. (Multiple malignancies).	+	Thyroid **+** Gastric parietal cell +
XI, 20	M	67	Aged **57** years rodent ulcer of left side of neck. Treated by excision. Now malignant melanoma of left nostril. Severe *rheumatoid arthritic* changes of hands and feet. *Myxoedema*. *Paraneoplastic dementia*. (Multiple tumours).		Thyroid **+** Free *acid*.
XI, 21	F	75	*Rheumatoid arthritis* for 15 years. **Under treatment** the whole time. **Now** squamous cell carcinoma of right temple.		ANF **+** RF **+**
XI, 22	F	75	Severe *rheumatoid arthritis*, hiatus hernia, Bowen's disease of **right** temple.		RF **+** Thyroid **+**
XI, 23	F	93	*Diabetes* 15 years with retinopathy. Widespread *Paget's disease*. Severe *rheumatoid arthritis*. Three years previously rodent ulcer removed from bridge of nose. Now *myxoedema*.	+	ANF **+** Thyroid **+** Gastric parietal cell **+**
XI, 24	F	74	Large rodent ulcer of back aged 60 years. Now very severe *rheumatoid arthritis*.	+	

308

Table XII. Malignant melanoma

Case	Sex	Age	History	Presence of achlorhydria	Serum auto-antibodies
I. Choroid of eye					
XII,1	F	57	Recurrent left episcleritis followed by development of malignant melanoma of choroid with diffuse goitre and *thyrotoxicosis.*	+	ANF + RF +
XII,2	M	60	*Diabetes* for 4 years. Melanoma of right eye with secondaries in liver.	+	RF +
XII,3	F	74	*Diabetes* for 20 years. Melanoma of choroid of **left eye.**	+	RF +
XII,4	M	60	Left eye removed for malignant melanoma 8 years previously. Followed 2 years later by development of a goitre due to *Hashimoto's thyroiditis. Rheumatoid arthritis* of hands noted at this time. Developed *paraneoplastic peripheral neuropathy.* X-rays showed *Paget's disease* of various bones. At autopsy reticulosarcoma of thyroid and lungs present. (Twin malignancies).		ANF + Thyroid +++
XII,5	M	63	Severe bilateral *iridocyclitis* for 27 years with recurrent attacks leaving severe visual impairment followed now by malignant melanoma of left choroid. *Thyroid* diffusely *enlarged.*	+	ANF + RF + Thyroid +++
II. Elsewhere					
XII,6	F	55	*Diabetes* for 3 years. Malignant melanoma of skin of neck.		ANF + RF +
XII,7	F	75	Aged 40 years hysterectomy for *fibroids.* Left benign *ovarian cyst* found. Aged 46 years operation for *chronic cholecystitis* and gall-stones. Carcinoma of right breast aged 65 years. Acute onset of *rheumatoid arthritis* followed by malignant melanomatosis and peripheral neuropathy. Primary unknown. (Twin malignancies).	+	Thyroid +
XII,8	M	70	'Veil-marked *rheumatoid arthritic* changes of fingers and toes. Malignant melanoma of nail bed of left big toe.	+	ANF +
XII,9	F	64	Five years ago malignant melanoma of umbilicus. Two years ago carcinoma of left **breast.** Now melanomatosis. Catarrhal *deafness. Myxoedema. Rheumatoid arthritis* of moderate degree and slow onset. (Twin malignancies).		RF +
XII,10	M	67	Aged 57 years rodent ulcer of left side of neck. Treated by excision. Now malignant melanoma of left nostril. Severe *rheumatoid arthritis* of hands and feet. *Myxoedema. Paraneoplastic dementia.* (Twin malignancies).	+	Gastric parietal cell +

308

Table XII (continued)

			ANF	Thyroid	
XII, 11	M	51	+	+	Under treatment for *rheumatoid arthritis* for 3 years. Simultaneouonset of malignant melanoma of the dorsum of the right hand and lympto arcoma of the tonsils.
XII, 12	F	60			Subungual melanoma right index finger. *Rheumatoid arthritis* of feet.

309

Table XIII. Connective tissue tumours (fibrosarcoma, osteosarcoma, malignant synovioma, etc.)

Case	Sex	Age	History	Presence of achlorhydria	Serum auto-antibodies
XIII, 1	M	60	Slight *rheumatoid arthritic* symptoms for several years with *rheumatoid nodules* and slight arthropathy of fingers. Fibrosarcoma of right upper arm.	+	RF + ANF + Thyroid +
XIII, 2	F	65	Simultaneously fibrosarcoma of right upper arm and carcinoma of right breast. Hands show *rheumatoid changes.* (Twin malignancies).		RF + ANF +
XIII, 3	M	12	*Eczema and intrinsic asthma* since birth. Now Ewing's tumour of bone with secondaries.		ANF +t
XIII, 4	M	7	Aged six months severe *alopecia areata.* Now embryonal sarcoma of liver.		ANF + RF +
XIII, 5	M	20	Indian, native of Malaya. Osteogenic sarcoma of left femur.		Thyroid +t
XIII, 6	F	48	riffuse *goitre.* Three years morning stiffness. Signs of *rhezlmatoid arthritis* of fingers and toes. Malignant synovioma of great toe joint with metastases.		ANF + Thyroid +
XIII, 7	F	70	Between the ages of 25-35 years developed a number of lipomata, one below the left breast metamerically and several on the right forearm and left thigh. Aged 49 years onset of *rheumatoid arthritis* for which she had been treated for many years. Recently she developed onset of *diabetes.*	+	ANF + Thyroid +
XIII, 8	F	80	Severe *rheumatoid arthritis* of feet. Ten years previously development of huge lipoma of left buttock. Now *thyrotoxicosis.*	+	ANF + Thyroid +
XIII, 9	M	62	Aged 33 years onset of *diabetes.* Now fibrosarcoma of vas and testis.	+	RF +

Table XIV. Nasopharynx, nose, middle ear and Larynx

Case	Sex	Age	History	Presence of achlorhydria	Serum auto-antibodies
XIV. 1	F	60	Fifteen years previously carcinoma of the nasopharynx treated by radiotherapy. Now well.	+	ANF +
XIV, 2	F	78	Twenty years previously operation for *thyrotoxicosis*. Now lympho-epithelioma of palate.	+	ANF + Thyroid + Gastric parietal cell +
XIV, 3	M	72	Lived in a menage with male aged 65 years who died of myelomatosis and female aged 69 **with rheumatoid arthritis** and carcinoma of the breast. Cat died of "cancer" during this period. Patient had gout for years. Now sialoma of middle turbinate. Paget's disease.		RF +
Antrum					
XIV, 4	M	53	Five years ago operation and radiotherapy for carcinoma of antrum. Ten months ago onset of myopathy of limb girdles. Now recurrence in right lower lobe of lung. Peripheries of limbs show mild *rheumatoid arthritic* changes.		RF ll+ Thyroid +
XIV, 5	F	69	Under treatment for *rheumatoid arthritis* and *Sjögren's syndrome* for 20 years. Now carcinoma of right **antrum**.	+	Gastric parietal cell +
Middle ear					
XIV, 6	F	60	Chronic *adhesive otitis* for 10 years. Mild *rheumatoid arthritis* for 10 years. Now carcinoma of middle ear. Death from meningitis.		RF + ANF +t
XIV, 7	F	**66**	*Diabetes*. Squamous carcinoma of middle ear.	+	L.E. cells + ANF +
Larynx					
XIV, 8	M	60	Thirty years previously acute onset of *rheumatoid arthritis*, now severe. Now carcinoma of larynx.		ANF +
XIV, 9	M	74	Advanced carcinomatosis of larynx. No evidence of rheumatoid **arthritis**.	+	
XIV, 10	M	60	*Diabetes* for 10 years. Now carcinoma of larynx.		
XIV, 11	M	60	Under treatment for *rheumatoid arthritis* for 10 years. Now carcinoma of larynx.		RF +t ANF +
XIV, 12	F	60	Carcinoma of larynx treated by irradiation, followed by chronic lymphatic leukaemia. Peripheral *arthropathy*. (Twin malignancies).	+	Thyroid +

311

Table XV. Carcinoma of the bronchus

Case	Sex	Age	History	Presence of achlorhydria	Serum auto-antibodies
XV. 1	F	63	Heavy smoker. Under treatment for *rheumatoid arthritis* for 10 years. Now carcinoma of the bronchu.		ANF + RF +
XV. 2	M	i0	Non-smoker. Carcinoma of the bronchu> and *paraneoplastic peripheral neuropathy*.		
-XV. 3	F	76	Mother died of cancer? primary. Non-smoker. Hysterectomy fo r *fibroids* aged 55 years. Onset of *pernicious anaemia* aged 58 years. Now carcinoma of bronchus.	+	RF + Thyroid + Gastric parietal cell +
XV. 4	F	i3	Non-smoker. Ten years previously operation for *nodular goitre. Atrophic vaginitis* discovered. Eight years previou>ly onset of *rheumatoid arthritis*. Under continuou> treatment since. Now carcinoma of bronchus.		ANF + Thyroid †tt
XV. 5	M	53	Heavy smoker. Now carcinoma of bronchus and *paraneoplastic peripheral neuropathy*.		Thyroid +
XV. 6	F	63	["non-smoker. Carcinomat03i> of bronchus. *Paraneoplastic peripheral neuropathy*.		Gastric parietal cell +
XV. 7	F	69	Non-smoker. Carcinomatosis of bronchus.	+	
'XV. 8	F	G3	Non-smoker. Twenty years previou>ly *thyrotoxicosis*. Generalized *rheumatoid arthritis* for last 10 years. Carcinoma of bronchus.		ANF + Thyroid ††
XV. 9	M	63	Non-smoker. Severe *rheumatoid arthritis*. Now carcinoma of bronchus.		ANF' †+ RF †+
XV. 10	M	68	Non-smoker. Onset of severe *rheumatoid arthritis* aged 55 year;:. Now carcinoma of bronchus.	÷	RF 1tt
XV. 11	F	71	Non-smoker. Onset of *rheumatoid arthritis* aged 49 years. Now crippled. Carcinoma of bronchus.		RF 1tt
-XV. 12	M	64	Anglo.Indian. Non-smoker. In England for 15 years. Soon after arrival onset of severe crippling *rheumatoid arthritis, Sjogren's syndrome, crusting of nasa/ mucosa. Atrophy* and dryness of th e skin and desquamation (Ichthyosis acquhita). *Atrophy of oesophageal and gastric mucosa, fibrosing alveolitis, rheumatoid granulomatous myocarditis*, carcinoma of the bronchum.	+	ANF + RF +t. Ga tr|c parietal cell +
XV. 13	M	l°0	Non-smoker. Carcinoma of bronchus with cerebral metastases.	+	

Table XV (continued)

XV, 14	M	72	Smoker. *Diabetes* for 20 years. Now carcinoma of bronchus.		ANF +
XV, 15	F	69	Non-smoker. Now carcinoma of bronchus.		RF + Gastric parietal cell +
XV, 16	M	66	Moderate *rheumatoid arthritis* for 10 years. Severe *Paget's disease.* Now benign adenoma of left lung.		ANF +
XV, 17	M	64	Carcinoma of bronchus and *paraneoplastic peripheral neuropathy.*	+	
XV, 18	M	67	Smoker. Ten years previously right lobectomy for cancer of bronchus. Six years later *paraneoplastic peripheral neuropathy.* Now **intra**thoracic recurrence. *Rheumatoid arthritis* in hands and feet.	+	R.B.C. agglutinins in blood 1 in 6,400
XV, 19	F	67	Since twenties *cervical spondylitis.* Cholecystectomy for chronic *cholecystitis* aged 41 years. *Rheumatoid arthritis* in shoulders, arms, hands for 8 years. Agtd 59 years severe *Raynaud's disease.* Now carcinoma of bronchus.		ANF + RF +
XV, 20	M	51	Three years treatment for *rheumatoid arthritis.* Acute right *epididymo-orchitis* one year before onset of carcinoma of bronchus.		RF + Gastric parietal cell +
XV, 21	**M**	65	*Rheumatoid arthritis* for several years. Recent *ichthyosis acquisita* and left olecranon bursitis. Not smoked for 10 years. Now **bronchial carcinoma with *paraneoplastic peripheral neuropathy, cerebellar and mental disturbance.*		ANF +
XV, 22	M	69	Non-smoker. Severe *rheumatoid arthritis. Fibrosing alveolitis.* Now carcinoma of bronchus.		RF +t Thyroid +
'XV, 23	M	57	Non-smoker. Severe *rheumatoid arthritis.* Carcinoma of bronchus.		
XV, 24	M	Sg	Heavy smoker. Now carcinoma of bronchus and *paraneoplastic peripheral neuropathy.*		
XV, 25	F	**68**	Non-smoker. Now carcinoma of bronchus.	+	ANF -l
XV, 26	F	80	Non-smoker. Severe *rheumatoid arthritis* for 14 years. *Vitiligo* and *myxoedema* for 14 years. *Ulcerative colitis* for 4 years. Now carcinoma of bronchus.	+	
XV, 27	M	65	Non-smoker. Cerebral secondaries from carcinoma of bronchus.		ANF +
XV, 28	**M**	74	Moderate smoker. Now carcinoma of bronchus.		ANF +
XV, 29	M	80	Non-smoker. *Rheumatoid arthritis* of hands. Rodent ulcer of scalp. Carcinomatosis of bronchus. (Two malignancies).	+	ANF + Thyroid +

313

Table XV (continued)

	Sex	Age			
XV, 30	F	57	Non-smoker. *Rheumatoid arthritis* for 10 years. *Hashimoto's thyroiditis.* Simultaneous carcinoma of thyroid and bronchus. (Twin malignancie>).		RF + Thyroid +
XV, 31	F	87	Non-smoker. Severe *rheumatoid arthritis*. Now carcinoma of **bronchus**.	+	
XV, 32	M	69	Moderate smoker for **many years**. Old case of *thyrotoxicosis*; now carcinoma of bronchu>. *Paraneoplastic peripheral neuropathy.*		ANF +
XV, 33	M	83	Occasional smoker. Severe *Raynaud's phenomena* for many years. Severe *rheumatoid arthritis* for 10 years. Now carcinoma of **bronchus**.		ANF **+** Gastric parietal cell **+**
VX, 34	F	55	Non-smoker. Known *polycythaemic* for **8 years**. Now carcinoma of bronchus.	+	ANF **+** Thyroid +
XV, 35	M	72	Non-smoker. Thirty years ago *benign lympho-epithelial lesion* of right parotid. Nine years *diabetes.* Now carcinoma of bronchus and gall-stones.		ANF +
XV, 36	M	42	Non-smoker. Aged 32 years sudden onset of *rhinitis* and *intrinsic asthma.* Now carcinoma of bronchus.		ANF **+** RF **+**t Eosinophilia **in** blood.
XV, 37	M	70	*Diabetes*> for **8 years**. Non-smoker. Mild *rheumatoid* arthritic changes. Now carcinoma of bronchus.		ANF **+** Thyroid +
XV, 38	F	60	Non-smoker. Aged 50 years onset of acute *rheumatoid* arthritic symptoms persisting. Aged 52 years thyroidectomy for *thyrotoxicosis.* Now carcinoma of bronchus.	+	RF **+** ANF **+** Thyroid
XV, 39	F	79	Moderate smoker 20 years. Under active treatment for *rheumatoid arthritis* for 10 years. *Thyrotoxicosis* for 5 years. *Diabetes* for 2 years. Now carcinoma of bronchus.	+	ANF **+** Thyroid + Gastric parietal cell **+**
XV, 40	M	70	Non-smoker. Now carcinoma of bronchus. No history or signs of *rheumatoid arthritis.*	+	ANF **+**t
XV, 41	M	57	Moderately severe smoker. Squamous carcinoma of bronchus. Post-mortem showed *thyroid heavily infiltrated with lymphocytes.*		ANF **+**
XV, 42	M	69	Moderate smoker. Carcinomatosis of bronchus.		Thyroid +
XV, 43	M	78	Thirty years history of severe *rheumatoid arthritis.* **Subpleural anaplastic** carcinoma of bronchus.		RF **+**t ANF **+**

Table XV (continued)

XV, 44	M	78	Twelve years under treatment for severe *rheumatoid arthritis* and now carcinoma of bronchus.	+	ANF + Gastric parietal cell+
XV, 45	M	70	Heavy smoker. Advanced carcinoma of bronchus. No history or signs of rheumatoid **arthritis.**	+	
XV, 46	M	62	Heavy smoker. Now carcinoma of bronchus.	+	Gastric parietal cell +
XV, 47	M	72	Moderate smoker. Now carcinoma of bronchus. *Paraneoplastic peripheral neuropathy.*	+	
XV, 48	M	67	Non-smoker. Wide3pread *Paget's disease.* Carcinoma of bronchus.	+	
XV, 49	M	60	Non-smoker. *Still's disease* aged 10 years. Treated for years. Aged 30 years severe recurrence of *rheumatoid arthritis* of knee3 and hands. Now carcinoma of bronchus.	+	ANF + RF +t
XV, 50	F	58	One brother died of cerebral glioma aged 47 years. One brother died carcinoma of bronchu3 aged 65 years. Patient moderate smoker over many vea ra. Aged 31 years hy3terectomy for *fibroids.* Aged 33 year3 oophorectomy for *benign cyst* of left ovary. Aged 42 years cholecystectomy for *chronic cholecystitis.* Aged 56 years right *cystic mastitis.* Operation. Now carcinoma of bronchus. On examination severe *rheumatoid arthritis* of feet.	+	RF +
XV, 51	M	65	Non-smoker. *Pernicious anaemia* for 6 years followed by development of chronic lymphatic leukaemia and then carcinoma of bronchus. (Twin malignancie3).	+	Thyroid + Gastric parietal cell + teecomlng negative
XV, 52	F	63	Non-smoker. *Pernicious anaemia* for 6 years. Now carcinoma of bronchus and carcinoma of stomach. (Twin malignancie3).	+	Gastric parietal cell + ANF +
XV, 53	M	60	Non-smoker. Resection of carcinoma of transverse colon aged 50 years. Now simultaneous carcinoma of rectum and bronchu3. *Paraneoplastic peripheral neuropathy.* (Twin malignancies).	+	ANF +t
XV, 54	M	76	Sudden appearance of severe *ichthyosis acquisita.* Some *rheumatoid arthritis* of feet. Now carcinoma of bronchus.	+	RF +
XV, 55	M	66	Smoker for years. Now *Paget's disease* of bone, carcinoma of bronchus and *paraneoplastic peripheral neuropathy.*	+	ANF +

Table XV (continued)

XV, 56	M	53	14 years history of *diabetes*. Now oatcell carcinoma of the left upper lobe bronchus with loss of diabetic control.		Thyroid +
XV, 57	F	52	Under treatment for severe *rheumatoid arthritis* since aged 35 years. Non-smoker. Oat-cell carcinoma of bronchus.		ANF +
XV, 58	F	52	Since aged 35 years under treatment for severe *rheumatoid arthritis* requiring calipers. Non-smoker. Now oat cell carcinoma of lung with metastases.		RF +
XV, 5J	M	58	Heavy smoker. Under treatment for *rheumatoid arthritis* off and on for 9 years. Now carcinoma right lower lobe bronchus.		RF +t Thyroid +
XV, 60	M	70	IY-oderate *rheumatoid arthritis*. Carcinoma of bronchus.	+	Thyroid +t
XV, 61	M	60	*Parkinsonism.* Carcinoma of bronchus.	+	Thyroid +
XV, 62	M	80	Non-smoker. *Psoriasis* and *vitiligo* for years. Six years *iron deficiency anaemia* and achlorhydria. Now *pernicious anaemia, rheumatoid arthritis* of hands and feet. Carcinoma of bronchus. Fodent ulcer of forehead (t:ouble malignancy).		
XV, 63	M		Carcinoma of bronchus. Non-smoker. Peripheral neuropathy.	+	RF +
XV, 64	M		Ten years ago *alopecia areata*. Five years ago onset of acromegaly due to eosinophil adenoma of pituitary. Now *rheumatoid deformities, ichthyosis acquisita, diabetes* and carcinomatosh of the tronchus. (t:ouble tumours).		RF + Thyroid +

Table XVI. Gastro-intestinal tract

Case	Sex	Age	History	Presence of achlorhydria	Serum auto-antibodies
I. Tongue					
XVI, 1	F	55	Leukoplakia and cancer of the tongue. No evidence of rheumatoid arthritis. After treatment developed *paraneoplastic peripheral neuropathy* with recurrence.		Thyroid ++
XVI, 2	M	72	Moderately severe *rheumatoid arthritis* for 15 years. Leukoplakia of the tongue with underlying haemangioma.	+	ANF + Thyroid +
II. Palate					
XVI, 3	M	35	*Ulcerative colitis* for 4 years. Now cancer of the hard palate.		
III. Parotid					
XVI, 4	M	70	Generalized *rheumatic pains* for 20 years. Fifteen years *bilateral lympho-epithelial tumours* of both parotids. *Myxoedema.*		RF + ANF +
XVI, 5	M	65	Unilateral adenolymphoma (benign lympho epithelial lesion) of parotid.	+	
XVI, 6	M	55	*Raynaud's disease* for 23 years. Mixed parotid tumour removed 3 years ago. Spastic paraplegia=multiple sclerosis.		RF +
XVI, 7	M	66	Aged 22 years onset of *ankylosing spondylitis* and *rheumatoid arthritis.* Now *Paget's disease* and carcinomatosis of parotid gland.	+	RF +
XVI, 8	M	46	Fifteen years before in India onset with painless swelling of *left parotid salivary gland,* which subsided slowly. Two years later two attacks of painless swelling of the left cervical lymph nodes in which *left parotid again enlarged* and remained so. Biopsy= Mikulicz's syndrome. After another 5 years the tumour increased *in size* and a mixed parotid tumour found. The cervical nodes again enlarged. Biopsy=Hodgkin's disease. (Twin tumours).	+	RF + ANF + Gastric parietal cell + at time of parotid swelling. Disappeared with onset of Hodgkin's disease.
XVI, 9	F	55	One son was born with two toes absent from left foot. Patient has parotid cyst (=mixed parotid tumour).		ANF + Thyroid +
XVI, 10	M	64	Operation for mixed parotid tumour aged 60 years. Now carcinoma of larynx. *Rheumatoid arthritis* of hands and feet.	+	RF +

317

Table XVI (continued)

IV. Oesophagus

XVI, 11	F	51	Marked family history of rheumatoid arthritis. Hysterectomy for *fibroids* aged 38 years. Severe *rheumatoid arthritis* at menopause aged 48 years leaving moderate joint changes. Now carcinoma of oesophagus.	+	ANF + RF + Gastric parietal cell +
XVI, 12	F	38	*Pernicious anæmia* 12 years. Now carcinoma of oesophagus.	+	Gastric parietal cell + Thyroid +
XVI, 13	M	64	Carcinoma of oesophagus. No history or signs of rheumatoid **arthritis**.	+	RF +
XVI, 14	F	60	Aged 42 years removal of bilateral *benign ovarian cysts*. Well-marked *rheumatoid* arthritic changes in fingers and *ichthyosis acquisita*. Leio-myo-sarcoma of oesophagus.		RF + Thyroid +
XVI, 15	M	62	Operation for *toxic goitre* 18 years previously: *Hashimoto's thyroiditis*. Recent morning *swelling of hands* and *"fibrositis"* of shoulders. Now carcinoma of oesophagus.		RF + Thyroid + Gastric parietal cell +
XVI, 16	F	56	Carcinoma of oesophagus.		Gastric parietal cell +
XVI, 17	F	63	Cholecystectomy for *chronic cholecystitis* aged 46 years. Now carcinoma of oesophagus.	+	Thyroid +
XVI, 18	M	80	Old carcinoma of colon 12 years ago. Now carcinoma of oesophagus. (Double malignancy).	+	RF +

V. Stomach

XVI, 19	M	60	Carcinoma of stomach	+	
XVI, 20	M	72	Life-long history of *polycythaemia vera*. Now carcinoma of stomach.	+	Thyroid + Gastric parietal cell +
XVI, 21	F	78	Carcinoma of stomach	+	
XVI, 22	F	56	*Pernicious anæmia* for 7 years. *Thyroid adenoma* for 2 years. Now carcinoma of stomach.	+	ANF + Thyroid + Gastric parietal cell +

318

Table XVI (continued)

XVI, 23	F	80	Severe *rheumatoid arthritis* since age of 46 years. *Hashimoto's thyroiditis* aged 52 years. Now carcinoma of stomach.	+	ANF +
XVI, 24	F	59	Aged 40 years onset of progressively severe *rheumatoid arthritis*. Two years later goitre due to *Hashimoto's thyroiditis* and now *Sjogren's syndrome* found. *Paget's disease* of bone. Five **primary** carcinomata found at autopsy (stomach, colon (2), pancreas and both ovaries). (Four malignancies).	+	ANF +, RF +t, Thyroid ++
XVI, 25	M	84	Aged 65 years cholecystectomy for *chronic cholecystitis* and gall-stones. Rodent ulcer of nose removed 3 years ago. Now carcinoma of stomach with metastases, *ichthyosis acquisita*, well-marked *rheumatoid arthritis* of feet. (Twin malignancies).	+	ANF +, Thyroid +
XVI, 26	F	58	Moderately severe *rheumatoid arthritis*. *Acanthosis nigricans* for 4 years. Now carcinoma of stomach.	+	RF +
XVI, 27	M	74	*Scleroderma* of face and hands. Now carcinoma of stomach.	+	ANF +
XVI, 28	M	57	Carcinoma of stomach. No rheumatoid arthritis observed.	+	
XVI, 29	M	65	No rheumatoid **arthritis** observed. **Old gastric ulcer.** Scirrhous carcinoma (leather tattle) stomach with neurofibroma in stomach wall (Twin tumours).	+	
XVI, 30	F	85	*Rheumatoid arthritis* for 15 years. *Pernicious anaemia* for 6 years. Now carcinoma of stomach.	+	ANF +, RF +, Gastric parietal cell +
XVI, 31	M	46	Carcinoma of stomach. No evidence of **rheumatoid** arthritis.	+	ANF +
XVI, 32	M	72	Well-marked *rheumatoid arthritis*. Now carcinoma of stomach.	+	ANF +
XVI, 33	F	82	Old partial gastrectomy for duodenal ulcer aged 50 years. Severe *rheumatoid arthritis* 50-65 years. Middle ear *deafness* progressive due to *adhesive otitis* since 68 years of age. Now gastric carcinoma.	+	ANF +, Thyroid +, Gastric parietal cell +
XVI, 34	M	46	Marked family history of rheumatoid arthritis and cancer. Onset of severe *rheumatoid arthritis* aged 40 years. Now carcinoma of stomach.	+	RF 1tt, Gastric parietal cell +
XVI, 35	F	81	Terminal carcinoma of stomach. No **evidence** of rheumatoid **arthritis**.	+	ANF +
XVI, 36	F	80	Severe *rheumatoid arthritis. Acanthosis nigricans.* Now carcinoma of stomach.	+	

Table XVI (continued)

XVI, 37	M	90	Well-marked *rheumatoid arthritis* of hands and feet. *Atrophic gastritis.* Now carcinoma of stomach.	+	ANF + RF + Thyroid + Gastric parietal cell +
XVI, 38	F	60	*Auto-immune haemolytic anaemia* for 5 years. *Atrophic gastritis.* Now carcinoma of stomach.	+	ANF + Thyroid + Gastric parietal cell +
XVI, 39	F	75	Coombs positive *auto-immune haemolytic anaemia* for 12 years. *AtroPhic gastritis.* Severe *rheumatoid arthritis* for 4 years. Now carcinoma of stomach. *Paraneo Plastic peripheral neuropathy.*	+	RF + Thyroid +++ Cold agglutinins pre,en t.
XVI, 40	M	52	Carcinoma of stomach and oesophagus. No history or signs of rheumatoid arthritis.	+	Gastric parietal cell +
XVI, 41	F	70	Well-marked *rheumatoid arthritis* of hands. Carcinoma of stomach followed by moto-neurone disease and then carcinoma of bronchu>. Non-smoker. (Twin malignancy).	+	
XVI, 42	F	70	*Mild rheumatoid arthritis* for many years. *Atrophic gastritis.* Five years previously carcinoma of stomach with recurrence and later carcinoma of colon. (Twin malignancies).	+	RF + Gastric parietal cell +
XVI, 43	F	86	(Sister to Case XVI, 41). Daughter has rheumatoid arthritis. Fifteen years previously carcinoma of cervix treated by radium. Well-marked signs of *rheumatoid arthritis and ichthyosis acquisita* and *myxoedema.* Now has carcinoma of stomach and oesophagus. (Twin malignancie,:,).	+	RF +
XVI, 44	M	80	Aged 40 years cholecystectomy for *chronic cholecystitis* and gall-stone>. Severe *rheumatoid arthritis. atrophic gastritis.* Now carcinoma of stomach.	+	ANF +
XVI, 45	F	86	Severely crippled with *rheumatoid arthritis. Myxoedema* for 12 year;:. Now *atrophic gastritis* and carcinoma of stomach.		ANF + Thyroid + Gastric parietal cell +
XVI, 46	F	69	Aged 38 years hysterectomy for *fibroids.* Well-marked *rheumatoid arthritis* for 10 years. Now *atrophic gastritis* and carcinoma of stomach.	+	ANF + Gastric parietal cell +
XVI, 47	M	55	*Paget's disease* of Jore. Now carcinoma of stomach.	+	ANF + RF +

Table XVI (continued)

XVI, 48	F	75	Aged 52 years cholecystectomy for chronic *cholecystitis* and gallstone. Hysterectomy for *fibroids*. Long history of *rheumatoid arthritis*. *Atrophic gastritis*. Now carcinoma of stomach.	+	Thyroid +
XVI, 49	F	72	*Intrinsic asthma* from childhood. *Pernicious anaemia* for 3 years. Now carcinoma of stomach.	+	ANF + Thyroid + Gastric parietal cell +
XVI, 50	F	69	Aged 33 years onset of *rheumatoid arthritis*. Aged 37 years *adenoma of right side of thyroid* removed. Aged 37 years hysterectomy for *fibroids*. Aged 42 years two separate operations on right breast, upper outer and lower inner quadrant, for *cystic mastitis*. Aged 44 years dyspareunia due to *atrophic vaginitis*. Now carcinoma of stomach.	+	RF + ANF t+
XVI, 51	F	52	Carcinoma of stomach.		ANF +
XVI, 52	M	63	Non-smoker. *Pernicious anaemia* for 6 years. Now carcinoma of bronchus and carcinoma of stomach. (Twin malignancies)	+	ANF + Gastric parietal cell +
XVI, 53	M	66	Carcinoma of l1tomach and *atrophic gastritis*.	+	RF +
XVI, 54	F	59	Cholecystetomy for *chronic cholecystitis* aged 49 years. *Atrophic gastritis*. Now carcinoma of stomach.	+	ANF ttt
XVI, 55	M	75	Carcinoma of stomach. *Rheumatoid arthritis* of feet.	+	ANF +
XVI, 56	M	75	Well-marked *rheumatoid arthritis* of hands, wrists and shoulders. Now carcinoma of stomach.	+	RF +
XVI, 57	F	81	Carcinoma of stomach.	+	ANF +
XVI, 58	M	59	Carcinoma of stomach.	+	RF + Thyroid +
XVI, 59	F	60	*Pernicious anaemia* for 6 yea rs. *Fibrositg atveoitis*. Carcinoma of bronchus and carcinoma of stomach (leather bottle). *Peripheral neuropathy*. (Twin malignancies).	+	Thyroid +
XVI, 60	M	70	Mild *arthritic symptoms*. Now carcinoma of stomach.	+	ANF + RF +
XVI, 61	M	68	Advanced carcinoma of stomach.	+	ANF +
XVI, 62	M	50	Carcinoma of stomach.	+	

Table XVI (continued)

XVI. 63	F	77	Carcinomatosis of stomach. Osteo.arthritis of hips. Mild *rheumatoid arthritic* signs.	+	ANF tt / Gastric parietal cell + / **Thyroid** +
XVI. 64	F	49	She had an hysterectomy for *fibroids* aged 38 years. Aged 42 years an operation for *cystic mastitis*. Now has carcinoma of the pyloric end of the stomach. Marked *rheumatoid arthritis* of feet and *ichthyosis acquisita*.	+	RF + / Gastric parietal cell +
XVI. 65	F	74	Gross *obesity* since childhood. Aged 15 years developed *severe rheumatoid arthritis*. Now has *diabetes* and carcinomatosis of the stomach.	+	RF +
XVI. (65 a.	F	72	Systemic lupus erythematosus. Carcinoma of the stomach.	+	L.E cells ++ / ANF -tt / Thyroid + / Gastric parietal cell +
XVI. 65 b.	**M**	66	Twenty years severe *rheumatoid disease*. Ten years *atrophic gastritis*. Now carcinoma of stomach.	+	Thyroid +

VI. Leio-myosarcoma of gut

XVI. 66	M	55	Recurrent malaria over 10 years. No evidence of rheumatoid arthritis. Operation showed leio-myosarcoma lying outside gut between jejunal flexure and splenic flexure.	+	

VII. Pancreas

XVI. 67	M	61	Carcinoma of pancreas. Well-marked *rheumatoid arthritic* change In hands.	+	
XVI. 68	M	65	Under treatment for *rheumatoid arthritis* for 6 years. Now carcinoma of the pancreas.	t	RF +
XVI. 69	M	66	Mild *rheumatoid arthritic* change in hands and feet. Now carcinoma of **body** of pancreas.	+	ANF -tt / RF + / Gastric parietal cell +
XVI. 70	F	84	Gross *rheumatoid arthritis* for 14 years. *Diabetes* for 8 years. Now carcinoma of pancreas.	+	Thyroid +
XVI. 71	M	65	evere *rheumatoid arthritis* for 5 years. Adenocarcinoma of pancreas with metasta e; 2 years.		RF -tt / ANF +
XVI. 72	F	50	*Rheumatoid arthritis* for 5 years. Now carcinoma of pancreas.		RF tt. ANF +

Table XVI (continued)

XVI, 73	F	41	Carcinoma of pancreas.		Thyroid +†
XVI, 74	M	80	Twenty years previously thyroidectomy for *thyrotoxicosis*. Four years ago onset of *pernicious anaemia*. Now carcinoma of pancreas.	+	
XVI, 75	F	67	*Melanoderma* present for 6 years. Now carcinomatosis of pancreas.	+	Thyroid ++
XVI, 76	F	85	Pre3ented with congestive cardiac failure and carcinoma of head of pancreas. An old-standing case of *rheumatoid arthritis* with *Paget's disease* of pelvis and lumbar spine.	+	Thyroid **tt**
XVI, 77	F	42	Carcinoma of pancreas.		
XVI, 78	M	56	Carcinomatosis of head of pancreas.		
XVI, 79	M	50	Large areas of *pigmentation* of skin. Eosinophilia in blood. Now carcinoma of pancreas.		Thyroid +
XVI, 80	F	65	under treatment for *rheumatoid arthritis* for 15 years. *Ulcerative colitis* for 6 years. Now *myxoedema* and carcinoma of head of pancreas.		ANF +, RF + Thyroid +
XVI, 81	M	50	Carcinoma of pancreas.		ANF **+**
XVI, 82	M	38	Carcinoma of pancreas.		Gastric parietal cell+
XVI, 83	F	57	Carcinoma of pancreas. No rr.eumatoid **arthritis**.	+	ANF **+**
XVI, 84	M	55	Carcinoma of pancreas.	+	
XVI, 5	F	67	Slight *rheumatoid arthritis* of feet. *Ichthyosis acquisita.* Calcified *fibroids.* Carcinoma of l.ead of pancreas.	+	Gastric parietal cell **+**

VIII, Gall-bladder and bile passages

XVI, 86	M	62	Chronic bronchitis and *Paget's disease* of tone. Now carcinoma of gall-bladder.		ANF ·t†
XVI, 87	M	60	Well-marked *rheumatoid arthritis* of feet. *Now* carcinoma of bile duct.	+	
XVI, 88	F	44	Life long *psoriasis* and recent moderately severe *arthropathy.* Aged 29 years myomectomy for *fibroids.* Aged 36 years *hysterectomy* for fibroids. Mild *rheumatoid arthritis* of feet. Now carcinoma of gall-bladder.		RF **+**
XVI, 89	F	82	.-ery obese patient. Six years ago left-sided D 10 zoster. Has had *rheumatoid arthritis* for 15 years in tands, knees and feet. Ten years ago developed *ichthyosis acquisita.* Severe chronic *cholecystitis.* Now has carcinoma of common bile duct.	+	ANF **tt** RF ·t†

Table XVI (continued)

IX. Large bowel

Case	Sex	Age	Description		Antibodies
XVI, 90	M	55	No symptoms or signs of rheumatoid arthritis. Now has carcinoma of rectum.	+	ANF +
XVI, 91	F	43	Iron deficiency anaemia for 10 years. Amenorrhoea for 4 years. No signs of rheumatoid arthritis. Now carcinoma of colon.	+	**Thyroid**+ Gastric parietal cell **+**
XVI, 92	M	68	Operation for carcinoma of colon two years before. No history or signs of **rheumatoid arthritis**.		ANF + Gastric parietal cell **+**
XVI, 93	M	27	Carcinoma of rectum. Immediately post-operatively generalized *arthropathy*.	+	ANF + . RF ⧸
XVI, 94	M	77	Carcinoma of rectum.		RF +
XVI, 95	F	64	Acute *rheumatoid arthritis* aged 39 years, which gradually cleared. Now carcinoma of colon.		Gastric parietal cell ⧸⧸
XVI, 96	F	61	Carcinoma of colon. No evidence of **rheumatoid arthritis**.		
XVI, 97	M	61	Slight *rheumatoid arthritic* changes in hands and feet. Now carcinoma of rectum.	+	
XVI, 98	M	45	Carcinoma of rectum. Ho history of rheumatoid **arthritis**.		
XVI, 99	M	72	Carcinoma of caecum. Ho history or signs of rheumatoid **arthritis**.	+	
XVI, 100	F	70	Mild *rheumatoid arthritis* for years. *Atrophic gastritis* 5 years previously. Now carcinoma of stomach and later carcinoma of colon. (Twin malignancies).	+	RF + Gastric parietal cell **+**
XVI, 101	F	60	Husband suffers from diabete> and Paget's **disease of tone** with thyroid auto-antibodies +. His bro ther suffered from myxoedema, diabete, and Paget's diseas e of tone with thyroid auto-antibodies **tt**. For 10 years patient suffered from sero-negative *rheumatoid arthritis*. Has *Paget's disease* of **tone** and now carcinoma of caecum.	+	ANF +
XVI, 102	F	62	Carcinoma of colon.	+	ANF +
XVI, 103	F	61	Carcinomatosh of colon.		ANF +
XVI, 104	M	53	*Psoriasis* for many years. *Polycythaemia*. Now carcinoma of transverse colon.		
XVI, 105	F	76	Eevere *rheumatoid arthritis* for many yea rs. Now carcinoma of sigmod.	+	ANF+, Thyroid+ Gastric parietal cell **tt**

324

Table XVI (continued)

XVI, 106	M	77	*Rheumatoid arthritis* of hands. Now carcinoma of colon.		ANF + RF +
XVI, 107	F	fi2	Carcinomatosis of colon.		RF + Thyroid +
XVI, 108	F	61	Carcinomatosis of colon.	+	
XVI, 109	M	60	Non-smoker. Carcinoma of colon 10 years previously treated by colostomy. *Diabetes* for 2 years. Mild *rheumatoid arthritic* changes in fingers. Now carcinoma of bronchus. (Twin malignancies).	+	ANF +
XVI, 110	F	73	*Acanthosis nigricans* for 9 years. Well-marked *rheumatoid arthritic* changes. Now carcinoma of colon.	+	Thyroid +
XVI, 111	F	49	Hysterectomy for *fibroids* aged 40 years. Carcinoma of the rectum aged 42 years. Now carcinomatosis.	+	
XVI, 112	M	60	History of *arthritis*. Now carcinoma of rectum.	+	ANF +
XVI, 113	M	90	Advanced cancer of anal canal.	+	
XVI, 114	M	63	Carcinoma of rectum.		ANF + RF +
XVI, 115	M	82	*Rheumatoid arthritis* began aged 22 years and present with varying severity ever since. Well-marked rheumatoid arthritic changes. Now carcinoma of colon.	+	ANF +
XVI, 116	F	72	Six months ago sudden onset of typical *rheumatoid arthritis* in hands. Now carcinoma of transverse colon.		RF +
XVI, 117	M	81	Carcinoma of colon successfully removed 3 years previously. No history or signs of rheumatoid arthritis.	+	ANF +† RF +† Thyroid +†
XVI, 118	F	5S	Rheumatic mitral disease and ten years history of *rheumatoid arthritis*. Now carcinoma of rectum.		RF + Thyroid +
XVI, 119	M	69	Long history of "indigestion". Mild signs of *rheumatoid arthritis* of hands and knees with deformities. Now carcinoma of colon.	+	ANF + Gastric parietal cell +
XVI, 120	F	70	Carcinoma of colon. No evidence of rheumatoid arthritis.	+	Gastric parietal cell +
XVI, 121	F	63	Well-marked *rheumatoid arthritis* of hands and feet. Now carcinoma of colon.	+	

Table XVI (continued)

XVI, 122	F	72	Husband died of myelomatosis. Sister had diabetes and rheumatoid **arthritis**. Patient has rheumatoid a.rthritis of hands. Now carcinoma of colon.		ANF +
XVI, 123	M	52	Carcinoma of sigmoid.		
XVI, 124	M	66	Carcinoma of sigmoid.		
XVI, 125	M	65	Much "rheumatic" pain over many years. Now carcinoma of colon.		
XVI, 126	F	77	Moderate rheumatoid arthritis of hands and feet. Now carcinoma of colon.	+	
XVI, 127	F	72	Carcinoma of rectum.	+	Thyroid +
XVI, 128	M	73	Carcinoma of colon removed 7 years previously.	+	RF + Thyroid +
XVI, 129	M	66	Five years history of joint pains in lower limbs. Now carcinoma of rectum.		
XVI, 130	F	83	Rheumatoid arthritis of hands. Now carcinoma of rectum.	+	ANF + Thyroid+
XVI.131	M	81	Aged 6years cholecystestomy for chronic cholecystitis. Now carcinoma of sigmoid.	+	
XVI, 132	F	78	Severe rheumatoid arthr tis. Now carcinoma of colon.	+	RF +
XVI, 133	F	75	Paget's disease of bone. Now carcinoma of descending colon.	+	ANF + RF +
XVI, 134	M	68	Diabetes followed after 10 years by carcinoma of colon.		Thyroid + Gastric parietal cell +
XVI, 135	M	52	Carcinoma of transverse colon followed one year later by ulcerative colitis.		ANF + Thyroid -
XVI, 136	M	56	Carcinoma of colon 9 years previously.		Thyroid +
XVI, 137	M	40	Onset of thyrotoxicosis and diarrhoea aged 24 years. Diarrhoea persisted in spite of treatment for thyrotoxicosis. After 4 years ulcerative colitis diagnosed. Now carcinoma of colon.		ANF + Thyroid +
XVI.138	F	76	Very severe rheumatoid arthritis and ulcerative colitis. Now carcinoma of colon.		RF +
XVI, 139	F	62	Severe rheumatoid arthritis of hands and feet. Large intestinal obstruction due to carcinoma.	+	Thyroid +

Table XVI (continued)

XVI, 140	F	85	Severe *rheumatoid deformities.* Carcinoma of the descending colon.	+	Thyroid +
XVI, 141	F	84	Under-treatment for severe *rheumatoid arthritis* for years. Now carcinoma of transverse colon.	+	RF + Gastric parietal cell +
XVI, 142	M	59	Indian. In England 8 years. Carcinoma of ascending colon.	+	RF +
XVI, 143	F	60	*Rheumatoid arthritis* of feet. Carcinoma of colon.	+	
XVI, 144	F	55	Severe *rheumatoid arthritis.* Now simultaneous carcinoma of colon and bladder. (Twin malignancies).	+	RF + Thyroid +

Table XVII. The urinary tract

Case	Sex	Age	History	Presence of achlorhydria	Serum auto-antibodies
I. Kidney					
XVII, 1	M	63	Carcinoma of kidney removed 6 years previously. Now *rheumatic pains* in shoulders and wrists, which are swollen.	+	ANF +
XVII, 2	F	77	Long-standing *rheumatoid arthritis*. Now carcinoma of kidney. *Paraneoplastic peripheral neuropathy.*	+	ANF +t Thyroid ++ Gastric parietal cell +
XVII, 3	M	58	Developed *diabetes* and later hypernephroma.		Thyroid + Gastric parietal cell +
XVII, 4	F	63	*Rheumatoid arthritis.* Calcified *fibroids.* Now carcinoma of left kidney.		RF +
XVII, 5	M	72	Twenty years ago removal of *lympho-epithelial lesion of parotid.* Eight years a *diabetic.* Now carcinoma of kidney.		ANF + RF +
XVII, 6	F	69	Twenty years history of *polycythaema* with present transition to *myelosclerosis.* Carcinoma of upper part of left kidney. Basal cell papillomata of the skin of the legs. Removal of growth had no effect on polycythaemia. (Multiple malignancies).	+	Gastric parietal cell +
XVII, 7	F	76	Daughter has diabetes. Patient has had *diabetes* for 20 years. Now clear cell carcinoma of left kidney.		Thyroid +
II. Bladder					
XVII, 8	M	61	*Diabetes* for 12 years. *Myxoedema* for 8 years. Now carcinoma of bladder.	+	ANF + Thyroid ++ Gastric parietal cell +
XVII, 9	F	70	Well-marked *rheumatoid arthritic* changm in hands and feet. Now carcinoma of bladder.		ANF + Thyroid ++t
XVII, 10	M	58	*Fibrosing alveolitis.* Early changes of *rheumatoid arthritis.* Now carcinoma of bladder.		RF +
XVII, 11	F	76	Well-marked *rheumatoid arthritis* of hands and feet. Now carcinoma of bladder with secondarie3 on labia.		ANF +

328

Table XVII (continued)

XVII, 12	M	73	Ankylosing spondylitis. Atrophic gastritis. Subcutaneous fibroma. Now papilloma of bladder.	+	Thyroid + Gastric parietal cell +
XVII, 13	F	79	Five years ago intra-epidermal carcinoma of anal canal. One year ago rodent ulcers of forehead and left side of neck. Well marked rheumatoid arthritis. Now carcinoma of bladder. (Three malignancies).	+	ANF + Thyroid +
XVII, 14	M	86	Well-marked rheumatoid arthritis for many years. Now carcinoma of bladder.	+	Lupus erythematosus cell **tt** ANF +t **Thyroid** +
XVII, 15	M	75	Diabetes for 10 years. Now carcinoma of bladder.	+	Thyroid tt
XVII, 16	M	56	Carcinoma of bladder.		
XVII, 17	F	86	Family history of malignant disease. Mild rheumatoid arthritis for 6 years. Non-smoker. Transitional cell carcinoma of bladder. Paraneoplastic peripheral neuropathy.		ANF **+** RF **+**
XVII, 18	M	76	Severe rheumatoid arthritis for 18 years. Now carcinoma of bladder.	+	ANF +t
XVII, 19	M	54	Fibrosing alveolitis. Now carcinoma of bladder.		RF **+** Thyroid +
XVII, 20	F	69	Periods scanty and irregular from age of 35 years, ceasing aged 42 years. Onset of rheumatoid arthritis aged 52 years. Aged 55-61 years recurrent papillomata of bladder. Aged 67 years onset of diabetes and myxoedema. Aged 69 years Sjögren's syndrome. Paget's disease of bone, calcified fibroids and iron deficiency anaemia.	+	ANF **+** Thyroid + Gastric parietal cell **+**
XVII, 21	F	75	Aged 61 years basal cell carcinoma of right temple. Aged 65 years basal cell carcinoma in front of right ear. Aged 73 years purpura. Aged 75 years **transitional cell carcinoma of bladder**. (Twin malignancies).		Thyroid + Gastric parietal cell +t
XVII, 22	M	60	Rheumatoid arthritis for one year. Acute left-sided epididymo-orchitis six months ago. Now carcinoma of bladder.		RF **+**
XVII, 23	F	76	Eighteen years ago rodent ulcer of left lower eyelid. Well-marked chronic rheumatoid arthritic changes. Now carcinoma of bladder. (Twin malignancies).	+	Thyroid + Gastric parietal cell **+**
XVII, 24	F	51	Myxoedema discovered at age of 41 years. Now has transitional cell carcinoma of the bladder.		

Table XVII (continued)

XVII, 25	F	61	Onset of *idiopathic* Addison's disease aged 56 years. Now has carcinoma of the bladder.		Thyroid + Adrenal cortical +
XVII, 26	F	58	Operation for *fibroids* aged 41 years. Thyrotoxicosis aged 43 years. Idiopathic Addison's disease aged 53 years. Now carcinoma of the bladder.	+	ANF + Thyroid + Gastric parietal cell +
XVII, 27	M	85	Fourteen years history of *rheumatoid arthritis* and *diabetes*. Ten years **recurrent** papillomata of bladder.	+	Thyroid + Gastric parietal cell +
XVII, 28	F	80	*Parkinsonism*. *Rheumatoid arthritis*. Carcinoma of bladder.	+	RF +
XVII, 29	F	78	Ten years previously right mastectomy for carcinoma. Now well-marked *rheumatoid deformities* and simultaneous carcinoma of bladder and descending colon. (Multiple malignancies).	+	Gastric parietal cell + Thyroid +

330

Table XVIII. Endocrine glands

Case	Sex	Age	History	Presence of achlorhydria	Serum auto-antibodies
I. Adrenal cortex					
XVIII, 1	M	73	Chronic bronchitis. Cor pulmonale. Conn's syndrome. Large adrenal cortical adenocarcinoma.		ANF +, RF +, Gastric parietal cell +
XVIII, 2	F	65	Fibroids operation aged 53 years. Now right adrenal cortical carcinoma.		ANF +, Thyroid +, Gastric parietal cell +
XVIII, 3	F	64	Hypertension since aged 48 years. Aged 56 years thyrotoxicosis treated medically followed by slight arthropathy. Aged 58 years onset of diabetes. Now chronic lymphatic leukaemia and mild rheumatoid arthritic changes in hands. Autopsy showed right cortical adrenal adenoma and left adrenal cortical hyperplasia (Twin tumours)	+	Thyroid +
XVIII, 4	F	71	Psoriasis and arthropathy since her twenties. Autopsy revealed uterine fibroids, malignant insulinoma and adrenal cortical adenoma. (Twin malignancies).	+	
XVIII, 5	F	33	Asthma and eczema of hands aged 7 years to present. Cushing's syndrome onset aged 16 years. Cortical adrenal adenomata bilateral.		RF +, Gastric parietal cell +
XVIII, 6	F	33	Cushing's syndrome with diabetes.		Gastric parietal cell +
XVIII, ea	M	62	Aged 22 years onset of recurrent iridocyclitis leading to blindness. Aged 33 years onset of severe obsessional psychoses requiring leucotomy. Now hyperaldosteronism due to adrenal cortical adenoma. Rheumatoid arthritis of feet.	+	Thyroid +, Gastric parietal cell +
II. Thyroid					
XVIII, 7	F	81	Seven years ulcerative colitis. Well-marked rheumatoid arthritic changes. Now carcinoma of thyroid.	+	
XVIII, 8	M	47	Chronic rhinitis and intrinsic asthma since childhood. Onset of severe rheumatoid arthritis aged 27 years with severe se uelae. Fifteen years later papillary carcinoma of thyroid. No w myelomatosis. (Two malignancies).	+	ANF +, RF †††

Table XVIII (continued)

XVIII, 9	F	45	Indian from Calcutta. Lived in England for 5 years. In India operation for benign *ovarian cyst* aged 33 years. For 15 months suffered **from** *thyrotoxicosis*. Then developed nodule in left thyroid. Left hemithyroidectomy showed *gland heavily infiltrated with lymphocytes* and an area of papillary carcinoma. Now *rheumatoid arthritis* of knees and ankles.		RF +
XVIII, fa M		70	Goitre due to *Hashimoto's thyroiditis* for 5 years. Now adenocarcinoma of thyroid.	+	Thyroid +++
III. Phaeochromocytoma					
XVIII, 10	F	56	*Psoriasis* for 30 years. Mild *rheumatoid arthritis* for 10 years. Now malignant phaeochromocytoma.		ANF +
IV. Islet cells					
XVIII, 11	F	71	*Psoriasis with arthropathy* since twenties. Five years ago hypoglycaemic attacks and now obstructive jaundice. Autopsy showed uterine *fibroids*, malignant insulinoma and cortical adrenal adenoma. (Twin malignancies).	+	Gastric parietal cell +
XVIII, 12	F	27	West Indian Negress. Previous history of repeated *malaria*. Now non-secreting malignant beta-cell tumour of pancreas.		Thyroid +
XVIII, 13	M	55	Father died of cancer of bowel. Mother died of cancer of breast. Patient had asthma aged 7-14 years. Now benign insulinoma of 8 years duration.	+	Thyroid +
XVIII, 14	F	52	*Psoriasis* and *psoriatic eczema* for 12 years. *Psychoneurosis*. Severe *rheumatoid changes* in cervical spine. *Rheumatoid arthritis* of feet. Benign insulinoma of pancreas.		ANF +
XVIII, 15	M	55	Benign insulinoma. Psychoneurosis.	+	ANF +
V. Pituitary					
XVIII, 16	F	79	*Rheumatoid arthritis* for 10 years. Now *acromegaly* and *Paget's disease* of bone.	+	RF + ANF +
XVIIU, 17	F	60	Carcinoma of **breast** aged 42 years. Three years moderately severe symptoms of *rheumatoid arthritis*. Now chromophobe pituitary tumour (Twin malignancies).	+	
XVIII, 18	M	51	Under treatment for *rheumatoid arthritis* for 4 years prior to onset of **pituitary** chromophobe adenoma.		ANF + RF tt Thyroid +
XVIII, 19	F	55	Under treatment for *rheumatoid arthritis* for 14 years. Developed *thyrotoxicosis* 7 years after onset followed by partial thyroidectomy. Now *Paget's disease* of bone and acromegaly due to eosinophil adenoma of pituitary.		ANF + Thyroid +

Table XVIII (continued)

XVIII, 20	N1	54	Mild *rheumatoid arthritic* deformities. Chromopr.ote pituitary tumour.			Thyroid +
XVIII, 21	F	E5	Well-marked *rheumatoid arthritis*. Acromegaly due to eosinophil pituitary adenoma.			ANF + / Gastric parietal cell +
XVIII, 22	F	64	Aged 49 years bilateral carpal tunnel syndrome. Diagnosed *myxoedema* and under treatment s nee. evere *rheumatoid arthritis* for 10 years. T\\O years ago *bilateral ovarian cysts* removed a t operation. Now acromegaly due to pituitary eo3inophil adenoma, *Paget's disease* of bone and hypertension.	+		Thyroid + / ANF +
XVIII, 23	F	70	*Intrinsic asthma* for last 9 years. *Thyrotoxicosis* 6 years ago. Chromophobe pituitary adenoma pre>ent for 4 years. *Ulcerative colitis* for 1 year. Died from *Addison's disease*. No evidence of rt.eumatoid **arthriti**.		+	RF + / ANF +
XVIII, 24	F	47	Aged 10 years "*rheumatic*" swelling of feet lasting a year. Aged 18 years onset of symptoms of Cushing's syndrome due to basophil pituitary adenoma.			RF + / Thyroid ++
XVIII, 25	F	62	*Myxoedema* for 7 year;;. Now eosinophil pituitary adenoma.			RF +
XVIII, 26 (XV, 64)	M	53	Ten year;;; ago *alopecia areata*. Five years ago onset of acromegaly due to eosinophil adenoma of pituitary. Now *rheumatoid deformities, ichthyosis acquisita, diabetes* and carcinomatosis of the bronchus. (rouble tumours).			RF + / Thyroid +

333

333

Table XIX. Cerebral and spinal gliomata

1. Glioma

Case	Sex	Age	History	Presence of achlorhydria	Serum auto-antibodies
XIX, 1	F	64	Hysterectomy for *fibroids* aged 34 years. Thyroidectomy for *thyrotoxicosis* aged 50 years. Now grade 3 cerebral astrocytoma.	+	ANF + Thyroid +
XIX, 2	F	58	Aged 29 years thyroidectomy for *thyrotoxicosis*. Now right parietal astrocytoma grade 3.		RF + Thyroid +
XIX, 3	F	42	Acute *rheumatoid arthritis* aged 18 years. Bilateral *cystic mastitis* aged 40 years. Now oligodendroglioma of right temporal lobe. Moderately severe *rheumatoid arthritis* of fingers.	+	
XIX, 4	F	29	Cerebellar haemangioblastoma.		
XIX, 5	F	30	Frontal Jote astrocytoma grade 1.		
XIX, 6	M	68	Severe *rheumatoid arthritis* for 8 years. Now astrocytoma grade 4.		RF + Thyroid +
XIX, 7	F	52	Glioma of right cerebral hemisphere. *Hypothyroidism* discovered.		ANF + Thyroid +
XIX, 8	F	60	Aged 39 years enormous neurofibroma of right trigeminal nerve removed. Aged 54 years *Hashimoto's thyroiditis*. Now well-marked evidence of *rheumatoid deformities* In hands and feet.		ANF +
XIX, 9	M	59	*Psoriasis* since aged 29 years. *Pernicious anaemia, lupoid hepatitis* since aged 56 years. Now cerebral glioma.		ANF + Thyroid + Gastric parietal cell +
XIX, 10	F	63	Moderate *rheumatoid arthritis* of hands. Now cerebral astrocytoma grade 3.	+	ANF + RF + Thyroid Gastric parietal cell +
XIX, 11	M	63	Severe *rheumatoid arthritis* and cerebral glioma.		
XIX, 12	F	56	Glioma of right frontal region. Rodent ulcer of right frontal region. (Twin tumours. Rodent ulcer overlying glioma).		Thyroid +

Table XIX (continued)

XIX, 13	F	65	evere *rheumatoid arthritis* over 15 years. *Myxoedema* 5 years. *Parkinsonism* 2 years. Frontal lote grade 4 astrocytoma.	+	Thyroid + Gastric parietal cell +
XIX, 14	M	64	*Rheumatoid arthritis* of mild degree in hands and feet. Grade 4 astrocytoma of left cerebral hemisphere.		Nil
XIX, 15	M	10	Intrinsic *asthma* aged 2-7 years. Orchidectomy aged 10 years. Now 4th. ventricle medulloblastoma.		ANF +
XIX, 16	F	56	Family history of 3 brothers, who had severe rheumatoid arthritis. Patient has grade 3 cerebral astrocytoma and moderate *rheumatoid arthritic* changes.	+	RF +
XIX, 17	F	69	Under treatment for *rheumatoid arthritis* for 5 years. Now posterior fossa tumour (8th. nerve neurofibroma).		Thyroid +
XIX, 18	M	51	Simultaneous onset of cerebral glioma in the patient, his wife and their dog.	+	ANF +
XIX, 19	F	49	Aged 31 years myomectomy for *fibroids*. Aged 33 years onet of acute *rheumatoid arthritis*. Aged 42 years hysterectomy for further *fibroids*. Now ependymoma of cervical cord.		RF +
XIX, 20	F	35	Cholecystectomy for *chronic cholecystitis* aged 30 years. Aged 31 years onset of epilepsy. Now hydrocephalus due to temporal lote **grade 3 astrocytoma**.		Thyroid + Gastric parietal cell +
II. Meningioma					
XIX, 21	F	56	Menarche aged *16 years*. *Thyrotoxicosis* 4 years ago. Now meningioma.	+	Gastric parietal cell +
XIX, 22	F	64	Aged 54 years removal of cerebral meningioma. Aged 62 years fibrosarcoma of terminal ileo.entery. Mild *rheumatoid arthritic* deformity of hands. (Twin tumours).		RF + Thyroid + Gastric parietal cell +
XIX, 23	F	53	*Rheumatoid arthritis* of mild degree. *Myxoedema*. Now frontal meningioma.	+	Thyroid +
XIX, 24	M	60	*Paget's disease* of skull and spire. Now right-sided cerebral meningioma underlying Paget's change>.		RF + Thyroid +
XIX, 25	M	52	Simultaneous onset of *thyrotoxicosis*, *Hashimoto's thyroiditis* and spinal meningioma.		Thyroid + Gastric parietal cell +
XIX, 26	M	C4	*Acute rheumatism* aged 16 years. Fractured skull aged 44 years. Now angioblastic meningioma.		R F +

Table XIX (continued)

XIX, 27   M   43   Meningioma. Obvious *rheumatoid arthritic* deformitie; of hands.

RF +
ANF +

Table XX. Breast

Case	Sex	Age	History	Presence of achlorhydria	Serum auto-antibodies
XX, 1	F	72	Onset of acute *rheumatoid arthritis* aged 48 years. Aged 52 years carcinoma of breast.	+	RF tt
XX, 2	F	60	Carcinoma of breast.		ANF tt
XX, 3	F	64	*Rheumatoid arthritis* since menopause aged 52 years. Now *nodular goitre* and *thyrotoxicosis* with polygonal carcinoma of breast. Operation showed *lymphocytic infiltration of thyroid gland.*		RF + Thyroid +
XX, 4	F	72	*Rheumatoid arthritis* for 4 years. Now *thyrotoxicosis* and carcinoma of breast.	+	RF tt Thyroid +
XX, 5	F	74	Aged 46 years *cystic mastitis* in left breast. Now carcinoma in same breast.		ANF +
XX, 6	F	50	Carcinoma in right breast aged 24 years. Now disseminated.		L.E. cells + RF +
XX, 7	F	70	Cholecystectomy for *chronic cholecystitis* and gallstones aged 47 years. Now carcinoma of breast.		Thyroid +
XX, 8	F	86	Severe *rheumatoid arthritis* for years. Fungating cancer of left breast.	+	ANF +
XX, 9	F	86	Acute *rheumatoid arthritis* aged 46 years gradually subsiding. Now papillary adenoma of duct of left breast with well-marked old **rheumatoid arthritic** changes.	+	RF + Thyroid +
XX, 10	F	76	Aged 53 years carcinoma of right breast treated by mastectomy. Eight years later severe *rheumatoid arthritis.*	+	
XX, 11	F	64	Aged 45 years cholecystectomy for *chronic cholecystitis.* Now carcinoma of left breast.		
XX, 12	F	79	Well-marked *rheumatoid arthritis* of hands, knees, shoulders and ankles. Now carcinoma of left breast.		
XX, 13	F	51	*Diabetes* for 10 years. Now carcinoma of breast.		ANF + Thyroid +
XX, 14	F	71	Cholecystectomy for *gall-stones* aged 51 years. Right radical mastectomy for cancer aged 69 years. Now carcinomatosis. *Paraneoplastic peripheral neuropathy.*	+	Gastric parietal cell +

337

Table XX (continued)

Case	Sex	Age	Description		Serology
XX, 15	F	70	Aged 50 years onset of *rheumatoid arthritis*. Under continuous treatment s'nce. Aged 51 years developed an area of *cystic mastitis* in right breast. Aged 60 years bilateral carpal tunnel syndrome and *myxoedema*. Aged 55 years intraduct carcinoma of right breast in an area of cystic mastitis.		ANF +
XX, 16	F	55	Aged 47 years removal of **left** side of thyroid for adenoma. *Histology-Hashimoto's thyroiditis*. Moderately severe *rheumatoid arthritis* since age of 43 years. Operation for removal of *cystadenoma* of left ovary aged 51 years. Recurrent lumps in breast over 6 years showing changes of *cystic mastiti s*. Now duct carcinoma.		ANF + Thyroid + Gastric parietal cell +
XX, 17	F	51	Aged 45 years onset of *rheumatoid arthritis* with cervical spir.e involvement. Aged 50 years carcinoma of left breast and *cystic mastitis* of right breast. Aged 51 years carcinoma of cervix. Periods still **present**. (Twin malignancies).		RF + Gastric parietal cell +
XX, 18	F	59	*Rheumatoid arthritis* of feet. t:cirrhous carcinoma of breast.		ANF +
XX, 19	F	62	Fifteen years mild *rheumatoid arthritis* of hands. Kow carcinoma of breast.	+	Thyroid +
XX, 20	F	39	Carcinoma of breast.		
XX, 21	F	55	Severe *rheumatoid arthritis* for 10 years. Now scirrhous carcinoma of breast of 7 years duration.	+	ANF +
XX, 22	F	78	Severe *rheumatoid arthritis* for 15 years. Now chair bound. *Myxoedema* for 10 years. Now carcinoma of breast.	+	ANF +
XX, 23	F	62	Well-marked *rheumatoid arthritic* changes in hands and feet. Now carcinoma of breast.		RF + Thyroid +
XX, 24	F	63	Successful operation for carcinoma of breast 9 years previously. No signs of rheumatoid **arthritis**.		Thyroid +
XX, 25	F	55	Carcinoma of breast. No **history** or **signs** of rheumatoid arthritis. *Paraneoplastic peripheral neuropathy*.		ANF +
XX, 26	F	64	Carcinoma of breast. No evidence of rheumatoid arthritis.	.+	
XX, 27	F	39	**Father** died of carcinoma of prostate. Marked family history of rheumatoid arthritis. Fatient no w has carcinoma of **left** breast.		ANF +++
XX, 28	F	56	Aged 50 years cholecystectomy for chronic *cholecystitis*. Long hisory of *rheumatic pains* in shoulders. Now carcinoma of left breast.	+	

338

Table XX (continued)

Case	Sex	Age	Clinical details		Pre operation
XX, 29	F	58	Aged 31 years thyroidectomy for *thyrotoxicosis*. Aged 34 years removal of area of *cystic mastitis* in upper outer quadrant of right breast. Now lumps *in* both breasts. No history of joint swelling pre-operation. Bilateral mastectomy performed sl.owing *cystic mastitis* of left breast and carcinoma of right breast developing from cystic **mastitis**. **Operation followed within a week by** *acute polyarthropathy of severe degree.*		lupus erythematosus cell +t / ANF +t, RF +t / Thyroid +
XX, 30	F	58	Long-standing *rheumatoid arthritis*. Now carcinoma of breast.		RF +
XX, 31	F	54	*Intrinsic asthma* for many years. Now carcinoma of breast_		Thyroid + / Gastric parietal cell +
XX, 32	F	69	Many years history of *pain and swelling in knees, ankles and feet.* Now carcinoma of breast_	+	ANF +
XX, 33	F	83	Carcinoma of breast.	+	RF + / ANF +
XX, 34	F	40	Advanced carcinomatosis of breast. *Paraneoplastic periPheral neuropathy.*	+	
XX, 35	F	65	Four years severe *rheumatoid arthritis*. Now carcinoma of breast.		RF +t
XX, 36	F	63	Operation 18 years previously for carcinoma of **breast**. Two years later acute *rheumatoid arthritis* involving neck.		ANF + / Thyroid +
XX, 37	F	77	*Intrinsic asthma* since aged 30 years. *Rheumatoid arthritis* for 10 years. *Myxoedemc* for 3 years. Now carcinoma of right breast.		ANF +
XX, 38	M	70	*Diabetes*. Advanced *rheumatoid arthritis*. Now carcinoma of right breast.	+	RF + / Thyroid +
XX, 39	F	62	Moderately severe *rheumatoid arthritic* changes. Now advanced carcinomatosi of breast.	+	Thyroid +
XX, 40	F	30	Congenital spastic paraplegia. Now carcinoma of breast.		
XX, 41	F	30	Rapidly growing carcinoma of breast. *Paraneoplastic peripheral neuropathy.*		
XX, 42	F	50	*Diabetes* for 10 years. Now carcinoma of breast.		Thyroid + / Gastric parietal cell +
XX, 43	F	70	*Rheumatoid arthritis* for 10 years. Now carcinoma of left breast.	+	RF +t
XX, 44	F	62	Carcinoma of breast.		RF +

Table XX (continued)

XX, 45	F	72	Carcinoma of breast.		RF +
XX, 46	F	75	Two years previously carcinoma of breast. Operation for mastectomy. No recurrence. Now mild *rheumatoid arthritis* of hands, wrists and f t.	+	
XX, 47	F	73	Generalized *rheumatoid arthritis* of hands, elbows, shoulders and feet. Now carcinoma of breast.	+	Thyroid + Gastric parietal cell+
XX, 48	F	60	Carcinoma of left breast aged 50 years. Now well-marked *rheumatoid arthritis*.	+	
XX, 49	F	63	Husband qied of carcinoma of prostate and sarcoma of upper arm. One brother is a diabetic. Patient had bilateral *cystic mastitis* aged 24 years. Breasts nodular since. Aged 40 years *hysterectomy* for *fibroids* and one ovary removed for *benign cyst. Diabetic* for two years. Now carcinoma of left breast and colon. (Twin malignancies).	+	Thyroid + Gastric parietal cell +
XX, 50	F	65	*Diabetic* for 12 years. Now carcinoma of breast.		ANF + Thyroid +
XX, 51	F	56	*Thyrotoxicosis* for 12 months. Now carcinoma of **breast for 2** months.	+	
XX, 52	F	55	Menarche aged 12 years. Menopause aged 18 years. Aged 48 years carcinoma of *body* of uterus. Now carcinoma of breast. Mild *rheumatoid arthritic* changes in hands. Hallux valguS ++ and overlapping toes. (Twin malignancie3).	+	Thyroid ++ ANF +
XX, 53	F	73	Daughter has carcinoma of breast. One brother had carcinoma of bladder. Ten years treatment for *rheumatoid arthritis* of lower limbs. Now *cystic mastitis* of right breast and carcinoma of left breast.		RF +
XX, 53	F	73	Generalized *rheumatoid arthritis*. Now carcinoma of breast.		RF +
XX, 55	F	80	*Rheumatoid arthritis* of hands and feet. Now carcinoma of left breast.		ANF +
XX, 56	F	86	One sister died of carcinoma of breast. Mother died of carcinoma of rectum. Patient had very severe *rheumatoid arthritis* for 30 years. Now carcinoma of right breast.	+	Thyroid +
XX, 57	F	70	Carcinoma of breast 10 years ago. Now mild *rheumatoid arthritis*.		Gastric parietal cell ++
XX, 58	F	64	*Perceptive deafness* from unknown cause for several years. Five years ago malignant melanoma of umbilicus. Two years ago developed lump in left breast=polygonal cell carcinoma. Now *metastase3* and *rheumatoid arthritis* of r.ands and feet and melanomatosi3. (Twin malignancie3).	+	ANF + RF +

Table XX (continued)

XX. 59	F	44	Family history of neurofibromatosis. Patient has neurofibroma of forearm. Simultaneous onset of lumps in both breasts. Excision showed one was a malignant lymphoma and the other a primary carcinoma. (Three malignancies).		RF + ANF +
XX. 60	F	69	Under treatment for *rheumatoid arthritis* for 27 years. Carcinoma of t he right breast aged 60 years and now thrombophlebitis migrans.		ANF + RF +
XX. 61	F	72	Long history of *intrinsic asthma* since her thirties. Under treatment for *rheumatoid arthritis* for 20 years. For 3 years she had suffered from *myxoedema*. Now has carcinoma of the right breast.		RF + Thyroid +
XX. 62	F	51	*Chronic rhinitis* since her twenties and *allergic to many different drugs.* Now simultaneous onset of carcinoma of right ovary and right breast.		ANF +
XX. 63	F	66	Father died of carcinoma of the large intestine. One sister died of carcinoma of the body of the uterus aged 66 years. Her son suffered from Hodgkin's disease. At 50 years the patient developed carcinoma of the left breast which was removed and at the same time hysterectomY for *fibroids* was carried out. Aged 61 years she developed carcinoma of the right breast.	+	Thyroid +
XX. 64	F	50	Doctor's wife, ex-nurse. Aged 36 years cholecystectomy for *chronic cholecystitis.* Aged **38** years operation for *follicular appendicitis.* Aged **40** years onset of severe seropositive *rheumatoid arthritis* for which under treatment ever since. Aged **41** years operation for *bilateral benign ovarian cysts* and myomectomy for *fibroids.* Aged 50 years carcinoma of the left breast of round cell type. Aged 51 years *thyrotoxicosis.*	+	RF -itt Gastric parietal cell +†
XX. 65	F	51	Mother died of carcinoma of breast. Rheumatic fever aged **5 years.** Aged 27 years appendectomy and ruptured *benign left ovarian cyst.* Aged **28** years operation for right renal calculus. Aged 51 years carcinoma of right breast.		RF + Thyroid +
XX. 66	F	50	Under treatment for *rheumatoid arthritis* f or 10 years. Now rapidly spreading carcinoma of left breast.		RF +
XX. 67 (XVI 29)	F	78	Ten years previously right mastectomy for carcinoma. Now well-marked *rheumatoid deformities* and simultaneous carcinoma of bladder and descending colon. (Multiple malignancies).	+	Gastric parietal cell + Thyroid +

Table XXI. Female genitalia

Case	Sex	Age	History	Presence of achlorhydria	Serum auto-antibodies
1. Body of uterus					
XXI, 1	F	58	Acute menopausal *rheumatoid arthritis*. Aged 56 years adenocarcinoma of uterine body and 2 years later papillary carcinoma of both ovaries. (Three malignancies).		Thyroid + ANF +
XXI, 2	F	74	Under treatment for *rheumatoid arthritis* for 8 years. Now carcinoma of body of uterus.	+	RF 1ft
XXI, 3	F	88	Mild stiffness of hands over several years with evidence of *rheumatoid arthritis*. Now carcinoma of body of uterus.	+	ANF +
XXI, 4	F	55	Onset of *thyrotoxicosis* and vaginal bleeding due to carcinoma of body of uterus.	+	Thyroid +
XXI, 5	F	55	Para three. Menopause 2 years previously. Now *atrophic vaginitis*. *Fibroids* ++. Adenocarcinoma of body of uterus with inflammatory reaction of mucosa.		ANF + Thyroid +
XXI, 6	F	60	Severe *rheumatoid arthritis* for 10 years. Now carcinoma of body of uterus.		ANF + RF +
XXI, 7	F	55	Menarche aged 12 years. Menopause aged 18 years. Aged 48 years carcinoma of body of uterus. Now carcinoma of breast. (Twin malignancies).	+	Thyroid ++ ANF +
XXI, 8	F	23	Crippled in chair with *rheumatoid arthritis* for 5 years. Now carcinoma of body of uterus.		ANF + RF + Thyroid +
XXI, 9	F	57	Marked family history of diabetes. Patient aged 53 years discovered to have *diabetes* and *myxoedema*. Now carcinoma of body of uterus.		ANF + RF + Thyroid
XXI, 10	F	70	"Rheumatic fever" in childhood. Onset of *rheumatoid arthritis* aged 27 years. Now well-marked burnt out rheumatoid arthritic changes Carcinoma of vagina aged 55 years and carcinoma of body of uterus aged 65 years. (Twin malignancies).	+	ANF +
XXI, 11	F	59	Aged 49 years carcinoma of body of uterus. Now carcinomatosis and *rheumatoid arthritis* of hands and feet.		ANF + FR 1ft
XXI, 12	F	63	Mild *rheumatoid arthritis* for 7 years. *Diabetes* for 7 years. Now adenocarcinoma of polyp of uterine body.	+	ANF +
XXI, 13	F	70	Severe *rheumatoid arthritis* for 8 years. Now carcinoma of body of uterus.	+	ANF +

Table XXI (continued)

XXI, 14	F	55	Severe *rheumatoid arthritis* for 10 years. Now carcinoma of body of uterus.		ANF + RF + Thyroid +
XXI, 15	F	55	Mild *rheumatoid arthritis*. Fibroids and now carcinoma of corpus uteri. *Paraneoplastic peripheral neuropathy*.		RF + Thyroid +
XXI, 6	F		*Myxoedema*. Three years ago cervical polyp and *atrophic vaginitis*. Now carcinoma of body of uterus.	+	ANF +
XXI, 17	F	65	Under treatment for *rheumatoid arthritis* for 13 years. Now has *thyrotoxicosis* and developed carcinoma of the body of the uterus.		RF + Thyroid +
II. Cervix					
XXI, 18	F	52	*Thyrotoxicosis* with carcinoma of cervix.		Thyroid +
XXI, 19	F	62	Menopause aged 33 years. Aged 42 years *right lobe of thyroid* found enlarged. Onset of severe *rheumatoid arthritis* aged 46 years. Aged 60 years bilateral mammary duct ectasia. Aged 62 years **subtotal** thyroidectomy for *thyrotoxicosis*. Now carcinoma of cervix.		RF + Thyroid + Gastric parietal cell +
XXI, 20	F	64	Multipara. Ten years treatment for *rheumatoid arthritis*. Now carcinoma of the cervix.	+	RF +
XXI, 21	F	65	Multipara. *No evidence* or history of rheumatoid arthritis. Now carcinoma of cervix.	+	
XXI, 22	E	76	Multipara, *diabetes* for 10 years, now carcinoma of cervix.	+	Thyroid +
XXI, 23	F	50	Carcinomatosis of cervix.		Gastric parietal cell +
XXI, 24	F	45	Para 1. Onset of *rheumatoid arthritis* aged 39 years. Now carcinoma of the cervix.	+	ANF + RF +
III. Vagina					
XXI, 25	F	75	*Intrinsic asthma* since age of 44 years. *Rheumatoid arthritis* of hands and feet. Carcinoma in situ of vagina.	+	RF ++
XXI, 26	F	55	*Thyrotoxicosis* and carcinoma of vagina.	+	ANF +
IV. Ovarian tumour					
XXI, 27	F	56	*Rheumatoid arthritis* of feet and ankles. Now carcinoma of ovary.	+	

343

Table XXI (continued)

XXI, 28	F	56	Carcinoma of ovary. Found to have *thyrotoxicosis*.		RF + Thyroid +
XXI, 29	F	59	Aged 54 years oophorectomy for adenocarcinoma of left ovary. Six months later found to have carcinoma of colon. (Two malignancies).	+	ANF + Gastric parietal cell +
XXI, 30	F	56	Marked family history of rheumatoid arthritis and carcinoma of the stomach. Onset of severe *rheumatoid arthritis* aged 49 years with menorrhagia. Hysterectomy for *fibroids*. Now carcinoma of both ovaries.		RF ++
XXI, 31	F	65	Son had diabetes. Patient had *rheumatoid arthritis* of peripheries. Now carcinoma of ovary.		ANF +
XXI, 32	F	60	Menopause aged 53 years. Aged 50 years *atrophic vaginitis*. One year ago *eczema* of hands and *pernicious anaemia* and *thyrotoxicosis* discovered. Now carcinoma of ovary. *Cranial arteritis* aged 50 and 55 years.	+	ANF + Thyroid ++ Gastric parietal cell +
XXI, 33	F	56	Acute menopausal *rheumatoid arthritis* aged 48 years. Aged 56 years adenocarcinoma of body of **uterus**. One **year** later carcinoma of left ovary. (Twin malignancies).		RF ++ Gastric parietal cell +
XXI, 34	F	68	Onset of *rheumatoid arthritis* 20 years previously, now affecting hands, feet, knees and elbows with severe bambooing of spine. Now bilateral *ovarian cysts*. One a serous cystadenoma, one a papillary carcinoma. Widespread *Paget's disease* of bone.	+	ANF + Thyroid +
XXI, 35	F	45	Simultaneous onset of *thyrotoxicosis* and pelvic mass=bilateral carcinoma of ovaries and adenocarcinoma of endometrium. (Three malignancies).	+	RF + ANF + Thyroid +
XXI, 36	F	74	Aged 39 years hysterectomy for *fibroids*. Now well-marked *rheumatoid arthritic* deformities and carcinoma of right ovary.		Thyroid +
XXI, 37	F	73	*Raynaud's symptoms* as long as can remember. *Pernicious anaemia* for 8 years. Now cystic papillary carcinoma of the ovary of low grade.	+	ANF +
XXI, 38	F	86	Carcinoma of ovary.	+	
XXI, 39	F	68	Mother died of pernicious anaemia and father died of carcinoma, site unknown. Patient aged 42 years hysterectomy for *fibroids*. Aged 44 years thyroidectomy for *thyrotoxicosis*. Now moderate *rheumatoid arthritis* of hands and feet and carcinoma of ovaries.	+	ANF + RF + Thyroid + Gastric parietal cell +

Table XXI (continued)

XXI, 40	F	50	*Raynaud's phenomena* since aged 25 years. Aged 35 years *Hashimoto's thyroiditis*. Aged 40 years diagnosed *systemic lupus erythematosus* with *auto-immune haemolytic anaemia*. Under continuous treatment since. Now carcinoma of ovary.	+	Lupus erythematosus cells +, ANF +t, RF +t, Thyroid +t
XXI, 41	F	44	*Rheumatoid arthritis* for 6 years. Under continuous treatment. Now carcinoma of ovary.		
XXI, 42	F	52	Sero-positive *rheumatoid arthritis* for 8 years. Under continuous treatment. Now adenocarcinoma of both ovaries.		RF tt
XXI, 43	F	51	Chronic rhinitis since ter twenties and *allergic to many different drugs*. Now simultaneous carcinoma of the right ovary and right breast.		Thyroid +
XXI, 44	F	11	Father had a cholecystectomy for chronic cholecystitis and gall stones. Her mother had an operation for cystic mastitis. The patient has dysgerminoma of the right ovary.		Thyroid +
XXI, 45	F	52	Father suffered from diabetes. Twenty years previously patient treated for 5 years for pulmonary tuberculosis. *Diabetes 8 years*. Now cystadenocarcinoma of right ovary.		Thyroid +
XXI, 46	F	57	Aged 45 years onset of moderately severe *rheumatoid arthritis*, especially in hands, wrists and feet. Aged 40 years cholecystectomy for *chronic cholecystitis*. Aged 50 years removal of uterine polyp. Aged 55 years on set of *ulcerative colitis*. Presented with abdominal swelling. Laparotomy showed tumours in both ovaries, left=malignant pseudo-mucinous cystadenoma, right=secondary carcinoid from a primary in appendix.	+	Gastric parietal cell +

V. Vagina

XXI, 47	F	55	Recent onset of *exophthalmic ophthalmoplegia* and *thyrotoxicosis*. Carcinoma of vagina.		ANF +

345

Table XXII. Male genitalia

Case	Sex	Age	History	Presence of achlorhydria	Serum auto-antibodies
I. Testicular tumours					
XXII, 1	M	38	*Diabetes* for 17 years. Treated with insulin. Xow teratoma of right te;;tis.		Thyroid + Gastric parietal cell +
XXII, 2	M	29	For 6 years *alopecia universalis*. Now semiroma of testis.		Thyroid +‡
XXII, 3	M	38	*Diabetes* for 10 years. Now sem inoma of testis.		ANF +
XXII, 4	M	40	Indian immigrant. History of *rheumatic pains*. No physical signs. Now carcinoma of undescended testis.		
XXII, 5	M	36	Mother aged 62 years. Patient a mongol. Teratoma,eminoma of te3tis 8 years previously. Now disseminated. Mild *rheumatoid arthritic* change in llands.		
XXII, 6	M	30	Severe *rheumatoid arthritis* since age of 23 years. Now semJ10ma of te>tis.		RF ‡‡ Thyroid +
XXII, 6a	M	58	*Diabetes* since aged 33 years. Onset of testicular sem'noma aged 52 years.		Thyroid + ANF +
II. Prostate					
XXII, 7	M	60	Carcinoma of prostate.		ANF + Gastric parietal cell +
XXII, 8	M	72	Carcinoma of prostate.		RF +
XXII, 9	M	64	Carcinoma of prostate.		
XXII, 10	M	76	Very advanced carcinoma of prostate.		ANF +
XXII, 11	M	66	Carcinoma of prostate.		Thyroid ‡‡
XXII, 12	M	72	Very advanced carcinomatosis of prostate.		
XXII, 13	M	64	Carcinoma of prostate.		
XXII, 14	M	73	Carcinoma of prostate.	+	
XXII, 15	M	89	Severe *rheumatoid arthritis* of hands. Now carcinoma of prostate.	+	RF +

Table XXII (continued)

XXII, 16	M	89	Pre3ented with cardiac failure and carcinoma of prostate. *Paget's disease* of spine and pelvis pre3ent.			ANF + Thyroid +
XXII, 17	M	82	*Adhesive otitis.* Now carcinoma of prostate.	+		RF + Thyroid +
XXII, 18	M	70	Carcinomatosis of prostate and *rheumatoid arthritis.*			ANF +
XXII, 19	M	80	Carcinoma of prostate. I:amentia. Severe *ichthyosis acquisita.*		+	Thyroid +
XXII, 20	M	60	Carcinoma of prostate.		+	ANF +

Table XXIII. Unknown primaries

Case	Sex	Age	History	Presence of achlorhydria	Serum auto-antibodies
XXIII, 1	M	61	From aged 53-57 years recurrent painless swelling of parotid salivary gland of auto-immune nature. Now metastatic cancer of dorsal spine.		RF +
XXIII, 2	F	74	Aged 70 years metastatic colloid cancer in right axillary node? Primary in a sweat gland. Aged 72 years acute rheumatoid arthritis. Aged 74 year3 pernicious anaemia	+	RF + Gastric parietal cell +
XXIII, 3	M	74	Post-necrotic cirrhosis of liver. Liver metastases from unknown primary.	+	Thyroid +
XXIII, 4	M	75	On et of rheumatoid arthritis aged 24 years. Two years ago frozen shoulder and temporal arteritis. Very advanced carcinomatosis.	+	RF +
XXIII, 5	M	68	Paget's disease of bone. Collapsed verte ra due to metastase3. Primary unknown.		ANF +
XXIII, 6	F	60	Severe rheumatoid arthritis. Carcinomatosis. Unknown primary.		Thyroid +
XXIII, 7	F	48	Severe rheumatoid arthritis. Carcinomatosis. Primary unknown.		
XXIII, 8	M	55	Pre3ented with epilepsy and then parameoplastic neuropathy and dementia. Primary unknown.	+	ANF +
XXIII, 9	F	62	Abdominal mass. Rheumatoid arthritis of hands. Severe ichthyosis acquisita.	+	Thyroid + ANF +

Summary of the findings in the 643 cases of cancer

In the above cases associated collagen or auto-immune diseases have been underlined. Attention has already been drawn to the fact that with the development of malignant disease in a patient RF and auto-antibodies tend to disappear from the serum and to reappear with successful treatment of the tumour. Zeromski et al. (1975) in 86 patients with lung cancer as compared with 2 control groups found the incidence of several auto-antibodies higher in cancer cases than in controls, especially smooth muscle and gastric parietal cell antibodies and ANF. The majority of antibodies were in the IgG and IgM class of immunoglobulins. Twomey et al. (1976) found that in 85 per cent of cancer cases RF was present in the serum in certain circumstances, especially after successful treatment of the tumour by any method and especially in cancer of the lung and breast. Thus, the non-existence of auto-antibodies or RF and ANF in the serum of cancer cases is no indication that these were not present prior to the onset of the tumour and indicative of rheumatoid and auto-immune infections. From the detailed examination of the above cases of benign and malignant tumours it will be seen that:-

1) In almost all cases there is evidence of the a) pre-existence of auto-immune disease in the organ developing cancer or b) the presence of one or more manifestations of collagen and auto-immune disease elsewhere in the body in the past over many years or developing at the same time as the tumour as a so-called paraneoplastic condition. The evidence of the presence of Iimax amoebae infection may consist only in the presence of auto-antibodies of some kind in the serum or of aC'hlorhydria, usually indicative of the existence of atrophic gastritis when carcinoma of the stomach is not present.

2) Tumour formation may be the culminating event in a life in which various manifestations of collagen and auto-immune disease have occurred over a long period.

3) Manifestations of collagen and auto-immune disease are more likely to be present with cancer the older the patient, that is when manifestations of aging are present.

4) In younger subjects no such evidence of collagen and auto-immune disease may be found at the time of development of the tumour, but, if the latter is successfully treated, they may be found when the patient is examined shortly after.

5) In cases of lymphomata, leukaemia or myelomatosis serological evidence of collagen and auto-immune disease may be present prior to the onset of malignancy, but after the onset the auto-antibodies disappear from the serum.

6) In a number of cases of lymphoma and myeloma there was no evidence of past or present collagen or auto-immune disease, but the patient had suffered from chronic malaria.

7) Twelve cases with Sjogren-Mikulicz's syndrome with or without other manifestations of collagen and auto-immune disease developed malignant lymphoma or chronic lymphatic leukaemia and another case carcinoma of the antrum.

8) Cases of malignant lymphoma confined to the stomach or duodenum and adjacent lymph nodes may occur in young subjects without evidence of collagen or auto-immune disease. One case developed follicular lymphoma within the parotid gland and neighbouring lymph nodes, suggesting the causative infection entered by way of the parotid duct.

Such observations suggest that the aetiology of many malignancies may well be related to that of the accompanying collagen and auto-immune manifestations.

Chapter XI

Review of the relationship of different "collagen" and "auto-immune" diseases to malignancy

1) Disseminated eosinophilic collagen disease in tumour formation

Reference has been made to this form of collagen disease. Its features are very like those resulting from infections with known tissue parasites. It was pointed out that the condition may merge and develop into that of "eosinophilic leukaemia", granulocytic leukaemia with eosinophilia with or without the formation of chloroma and myeloblastic tumours of bone marrow or lymphomata (see above). A case of eosinophilic collagen disease lasting 13 years developing "acute paramyeloblastic leukaemia" was reported by Olmer et al. (1970). The development of a carcinoma of the colon in such cases has been recorded. This condition is to be distinguished from the occurrence of eosinophilia in the course of cases of cancer. In disseminated eosinophilic collagen disease, therefore, there is observed the direct development of myeloid or "eosinophilic" leukaemia, lymphoma, chloroma, myeloblastoma or cancer in subjects of collagen disease.

2) Rheumatoid arthritis and other collagen and auto-immune diseases, Waldenstrom's macroglobulinaemia and myelomatosis

There is increasing evidence that plasma cell dyscrasia with hypergammaglobulinaemia or monoclonal gammopathy may be induced by diverse forms of protracted reticulo-endothelial stimuli, such as by tuberculosis, syphilis and other chronic infections, including osteomyelitis (Osserman, 1971). This may be associated with monocytic leukaemia. It has been shown above that the prolonged cellular multi-an'itigenic stimulation present in collagen and auto-immune diseases, such as in cases of rheumatoid arthritis and Sjogren's syndrome, may in some cases result in the development of paraproteinaemia or Waldenstrom's macroglobulinaemia. RF activity is usually present in the macroglobulin (Ball, 1969). The last is true in cases of paraproteinaemia or Waldenstrom's macroglobulinaemia, whether there is obvious evidence of rheumatoid arthritis or not. This suggests that paraproteinaemia or macroglobulinaemia are commonly the result of chronic limax amoeba infection with its associated stimulation.

McNutt and Fudenberg (1973) mention that two or more anomalous immunoglobulins (M bands) may occasionally be found in the serum and that previously six patients have been described with co-existing Waldenstrom's macroglobulinaemia and IgG multiple myeloma. They add another such case as do Sankale et al. (1973) and Pruzanski et al. (1974) (4 cases).

Goldenburg et al. (1969) found that antecedent rheumatoid arthritis was presnt in 3 of 80 cases of plasma cell neoplasia and Waldenstrom's macroglobulinaemia. In 112 cases of plasma cell and lymphocytic neoplasms 3.6 per cent had rheumatoid arthritis. The authors report cases with the following features:– rheumatoid arthritis followed by multiple myeloma (2 cases); rheumatoid arthritis followed by Waldenstrom's macroglobulinaemia; a case with positive RF in the serum with reticu-

Jum cell sarcoma; a case of rheumatoid arthritis with a positive RF developing macroglobulinaemia: and a case of rheumatoid arthritis with positive RF and paraproteinaemia developing lymphosarcoma; Davis et al. (1957) (2 cases), Hamilton and Bywaters (1961), Strandberg and Jarlev (1961), Lucchelli and Beretta (1962) (2 cases), Mackenzie and Scherbel (1963), Moesmann (1969), Sauvezie et al. (1974), Garcin Morteo et al. (1971) and Kyle (1975) all describe cases of chronic rheumatoid arthritis in which myelomatosis appeared. Meijers (1969) reports 2 cases, one of rheumatoid arthritis and one of ankylosing spondylitis, which developed myelomatosis. RF is usually present in the IgM factor of the globulins. Rheumatoid arthritis terminating in plasmocytoma was reported by Galli and Chiti (1955) (1 case) and 5 cases of progressive rheumatoid arthritis developing myelomatosis and one developing a benign monoclonal gammopathy with marked plasma cell proliferation, but no evidence of myeloma were reported by Wegelius et al. (1970). The latter authors found that positive RF tests preceded by many years (usually 15-39 years) the appearance of paraproteinaemia and myelomatosis. During progression of the myelomatous process the joint symptoms may abate and the titre of RF in the serum tended to fall. One case developed allergic dermatitis and another diabetes, while a third also developed carcinoma of the bronchus. Holly et al. (1961) found RF absent in 27 cases of myelomatosis, but in 12 cases of Waldenstrom's macroglobulinaemia 8 gave positive reactions. In 2 cases of rheumatoid arthritis and macroglobulinaemia reported by Gothani et al. (1965) the RF titres were very high. Leng-Lvy et al. (1967) describe a patient with chronic rheumatoid arthritis and hypothyroidism who developed myelomatosis. Zawadski and Benedek (1969) report on 16 patients with rheumatoid arthritis and co-existent paraproteinaemia and 6 of these had multiple myelo-

rna, one Waldenstrom's macroglobulinaemia and one heavy-chain disease. Other primary neoplasms were present in 6 of the cases of rheumatoid arthritis. They included one cancer of the breast, one of the lung, two of the colon, one parathyroid adenoma and one with multiple cancers of kidney, prostate and bronchus. The patient with the three tumours also had myelomatosis. One patient developed lymphosarcoma. In 5 of the cases of rheumatoid arthritis developing paraproteinaemia and the one case in which lymphosarcoma developed the RF titre fell with the appearance of the abnormal protein and in the case of lymphosarcoma it disappeared. The authors review the literature on rheumatoid arthritis and monoclonal gammopathy and compare rheumatoid arthritis and immunoproliferative disorders. The symptoms of rheumatoid arthritis antedate the findings of paraproteinaemia by an average of 25 years (1-34 years). Their unexpected high incidence of second neoplasms among patients was noted. It was not possible to demonstrate when asymptomatic paraproteinaemia becomes transformed into overt disease (macroglobulinaemia or myelomatosis). The authors speculate on the possible relationship between rheumatoid arthritis, paraproteinaemia and neoplasms and suggest prolonged antigenic stimulation manifested by rheumatoid arthritis may be a pathogenic factor in the evolution of immunoproliferative disorders.

Other collagen and auto-immune diseases which may be followed by or associated with myelomatosis

Fateh Moghandam et al. (1971) describe a patient with Raynaud's phenomena and scleroderma who developed myelomatosis. Joseph et al. (1970) recorded the case of a patient whose disease extended over seven years in three distinct phases, a) an asymptomatic hypergammaglobulinaemia with a monoclonal element, b) an "auto-immune" phase with arthritis, pulmonary fibrosis, glomerulitis, anaemia, leucopenia, paraproteinaemia, ANF and lupus erythematosus cells in the blood and Bence-Jones proteinuria and c) a terminal acute leukaemia. In the review of the literature which follows there is mentioned myelomatosis associated with other collagen and auto-immune diseases, including vasculitis (Christianson et al., 1967; Sams et al., 1968); Paget's disease (Reich and Brodsky, 1948; Hanisch, 1950; Rosenkrantz et al., 1952; Layani et al., 1952; Hoo, 1954; Rosenkranitz and Gluckman, 1957; Serre and Simon, 1959; Klijn, 1961; Grader and Moynihan, 1961; Bedard and Uhthoff, 1964; Sherman, 1966; Scurr, 1972); atrophic gastritis with pernicious anaemia (Panders and Leeksma, 1963; Jacottet and Ramel, 1965; Galton, D.A.G., personal communication; Fraser, 1969; Hrncir, 1970); Larsson, (1962) (3 definite and 2 possible cases of pernicious anaemia in 69 cases of myeloma); Nordenson (1966) (3 cases of permcrous anaemia in 310 of myeloma); Twomey et al. (1971) (1 patient with pernicious anaemia and 2 with atrophic gastritis in 21 cases of myeloma); polycythaemia vera (Giersten, 1956; Lawrence and Donald, 1959; Spickard, 1960; Brody et al., 1964; Franzen et al., 1966; Heinle et al., 1966); myelofibrosis (Spickard, 1960; Brody et al., 1964); Sjogren's syndrome (see below); auto-immune haemolytic anaemia (Berliner et al., 1968); dermatomyositis (Holzmann and Herz, 1969); Hashimoto's thyroiditis (Saita et al., 1969); thymoma (Anderson and Vye, 1967; Lindstrom et al., 1968; Gilbert et al., 1968); thyrotoxicosis (Tourniaire et al., 1972); myasthenia gravis (Rowland et al., 1969); myasthenia, thymoma and pancytopenia (Lemenager et al., 1972); asthma (Imahori and Moore, 1972); fibrosing alveolitis (Holt et al., 1970); postnecrotic cirrhosis of the liver (Schneiderbauer, 1959); coeliac disease (Gilbert et al., 1968; Marano et al., 1970); ulcerative colitis (Nixon, 1964), and preceding diabetes (Vladutiv and Sielski, 1973).

In the South West Metropolitan Cancer Registry Series there were 3 cases of myelomatosis following long-standing rheumatoid arthritis, 1 case of rheumatoid arthritis and myxoedema and one of Paget's disease developing myelomatosis. In the author's own series there were 17 cases of myelomatosis and 14 showed clinical evidence of collagen and auto-immune disease in some form, including rheumatoid arthritis. One developed myelomatosis 19 years after the onset of rheumatoid arthritis. Four showed associated tumours (acute lymphoblastic anaemia, carcinoma of the breast, carcinoma of the thyroid and eosinophilic pituitary tumour).

Twomey et al. (1971) describe interesting family histories of patients with myelomata, 1) a 57 year old woman with myelomatosis had a mother with pernicious anaemia and hypothyroidism and a father who died of carcinoma of the stomach, 2) a 58 year old woman with myeloma had a maternal aunt who died from gastric carcinoma and both had heavy chain gammopathies, 3) a 64 year old woman with myeloma had a maternal aunt who suffered from pernicious anaemia and a sister with hypothyroidism, 4) a 59 year old woman with myeloma had a sister with hyperthyroidism and both had IgG monoclonal gammopathy and 5) two brothers had myelomatosis and their mother pernicious anaemia. Lohrmann et al. (1972) described a brother and sister with myelomatosis. The former also suffered from chronic lymphatic leukaemia and rectal carcinoma.

The long latent period in the develop.
ment of myelomatosis

Mention has been made above of the long period between the appearance of rheumatoid arthritis and the development of myelomatosis (up to 39 years). Norgaard (1971) studied 3 cases of myelomatosis with a preclinical phase of 15-24 years when a monoclonal gammopathy was present without symptoms or other features. He stresses that this disease

Addendum: Multiple myeloma in primary biliary cirrhosis. Blade J. Moserrat E, Brugnera Metal. Scand J. Haematol 1981; 26/1; 14;18. The authors point out that both conditions are the result of chronic stimulation of reticulo-endothelial system.
Addendum: Fine, J.M., Lambin, P., Derycke, C. et al., Rev. Fr. Transfus. Immuno-Haematol., 1978, 21, 973-979, record that in the serum of 36,015 blood donors an incidence of monoclonalgammopathies of 0.14 per cent, 86 per cent of which were asymptomatic and 14 per cent were malignant melanoma or Waldenstrom's macroglobulinaemia.

cannot be precluded in cases of so-called benign monoclonal gammopathy.

The tendency of cases of myelomatosis to develop other tumours

The tendency for cases of myelomatosis following rheumatoid arthritis to develop other tumours has been mentioned above. It has also been remarked on by Shanbrom (1963), who described 4 cases of myelomatosis which developed carcinoma of the colon, and found 5 others in the literature. Beevers (1972) reports another. Sparagana (1970) describes a case of myelomatosis developing bronchial carcinoma and Parolari (1963) one with basal cell carcinoma of the skin of the nose. Comes et al. (1961) also reported patients with myelomatosis and plasma cell disorders developing carcinomata and Warren and Gates (1932) malignant lymphoma, cancer of the uterus and breast and myelomatosis together. Osserman (1971) and others record an incidence of non-reticular neoplasms of 19-22 per cent in cases of myelomatosis, chiefly bowel, breast and biliary tract. Coils and Carrell (1970) studied 52 cases of monoclonal gammopathy of which 31 (59 per cent) were myelomata. In 8 of these cases a second malignancy was present. Like others, the authors point out that gammopathy may precede overt clinical disease by many years. In the large series of multiple malignancies considered above there are found cases of multiple myelomatosis combined with every other kind of tumour or leukaemia. Ito et al. (1968) report multiple myelomata with multiple cancers of the stomach; Mazzaferri et al. (1968) and Ettinger et al. (1975) with Kaposi's sarcoma; Dugois et al. (1967) and Rever et al. (1965) with multiple and extensive skin cancers; Stalewski et al. (1965) with lung cancers; Anderson and Vye (1967), Gilbert et al. (1968) and Lindestrom et al. (1968) with malignant thymoma; Stobbe (1962) and Sany et al. (1976) with chronic lymphatic leukaemia; Narasimham et al. (1975) with chronic lymphatic leukaemia and lymphosarcoma; and Lohrmann et al. (1972) with chronic lymphatic leukaemia and rectal carcinoma. Kyle (1975) in reviewing 869 cases of multiple myeloma at the Mayo Clinic found that 61 (7 per cent) had other cancers.

Tumour development in macroglobulinaemia

The later development of malignancy of various kinds in cases of macroglobulinaemia is also well recognized, especially in the frequent development of lymphomata and leukaemia. Thus, Wanebo and Clarkson (1965), Bosken and Noltenius (1968), Kellner et al. (1968) (2 cases), Cooper (1970), Meltzer and Franklin (1966), Bonomo et al. (1970), Osterberg and Ransing (1970) describe cases of Waldenstr◇m's macroglobulinaemia, which later developed reticulum cell sarcoma. Dreyfus et al. (1966) point to the relationship of lymphoma and macroglobulinaemia in families. Braunsteiner and Sailer (1960) and Jaeger and Lapp (1970) describe cases of macroglobulinaemia associated with chronic lymphatic leukaemia. A case of Waldenstr◇m's macroglobulinaemia developing acute leukaemia was reported by Gilly et al. (1969) and another developing Kaposi's sarcoma by Cohen et al. (1965). Sometimes Waldenstrom's macroglobulinaemia may terminate with the later development of myelomatosis. In addition to lymphomata and leukaemia Waldenstr◇m's macroglobulinaemia may be associated with the development of thymomata in patients exhibiting manifestations of collagen and auto-immune disease (see below). It may also precede the development of *carcinomata* (Schaub, 1953; Weitzel, 1958; Boudin, 1962; Paraf and Bragard, 1962; RMl et al., 1965; Lohmann and GHiser, 1965; Blatrix et al., 1968; Thrush, 1970; Solignac et al., 1972). These tumours include carcinoma of the larynx, skin, bronchus, bile ducts, ampulla of Vater, stomach, liver, kidney, rectum, body of uterus, cervix, ovary and

Addendum: Mandel E.M. et at. (Acta Haematol., 1977, 58, 120) describe multiple myeloma associated with Kaposi's sarcoma. Law, I.P. and Blom, J. (Oncology [base 1]), 1977, 34, 20) report 7 patients with myeloma, four of whom developed acute leukaemia, one renal cancer and 2 with combined adenocarcinoma of another organ and a carcinoma of the bronchus. Smith, A.G. and Cumming, R.L.S. (J. ctn, Path., 1977, 30, 1053) describe myelomatosis with oat-cell carcinoma of the bronchus and stress the linking of multiple myeloma with a higher incidence of other cancers than in the normal population.
Addendum: Parathyroid adenoma and tight chain myeloma. Chisholm RC, Weaver YJ, Chung EB and Townsend JL. J. Natl. Med. Assoc. 1981 73 875 880.

prostate. A case of Waldenstrom's macro-globulinaemia shown at a Clinico-Pathological Conference at Hammersmith Hospital in 1963 was found to have developed four neurolemmomata in the medulla of the right kidney. Coppala et al. (1969) describe both Hodgkin's disease and carcinoma of the stomach developing in a case of Waldenstrom's macroglobulinaemia. Osserman (1967) found that in 57 cases of macroglobulinaemia 15 developed non-reticular neoplasms. In all the long series of cases of multiple tumours considered above cases of Waldenstrom's macroglobulinaemia developing carcinoma are recorded. According to Kappeler et al. (1958) 10 per cent of cases of macroglobulinaemia are associated with cancer.

Conclusions

There are, thus, very many cases of myelomatosis and macroglobulinaemia in which a previous and often long history of rheumatoid arthritis or other collagen disease or some other form of auto-immune disease is present. Furthermore, RF is frequently present in the serum of cases of myelomatosis, even in the absence of obvious evidence of rheumatoid arthritis. Boyle and Buchanan (1971) report that in cases of myelomatosis not obviously associated with rheumatoid arthritis, rheumatoid granulomata (nodules) may be found in the region of the joints. It would appear that the causation of myelomatosis and macroglobulinaemia in the absence of obvious chronic infection is commonly closely bound up with that of long-standing collagen and auto-immune disease. Since antibodies are produced by lymphocytes and plasma cells, it would seem that the proliferation of these cells in collagen and auto-immune diseases, in Waldenstrom's macroglobulinaemia and in myelomatosis initially is a response to chronic antigenic stimulation, a conclusion also reached by Wegelius et al. (1970) This would appear to be derived from the chronic infective agent causing collagen

and auto-immune diseases, namely limax amoebae. In cases of paraproteinaemia and/or cryoglobulinaemia following known chronic infections the paraprotein or cryoglobulin contains the antibodies to the infection and in cases of collagen diseases, lymphomata and myelomatosis with paraproteinaemia the rheumatoid factor is also present in the paraproteins (Bonomo et al., 1970).

Moreover, paraproteinaemia, macroglobulinaemia and myelomatosis may be associated with the development of leukaemia, lymphoma or carcinoma. The same causation may apply to these conditions as to paraproteinaemia and myelomatosis. In favour of such an aetiology for myelomatosis is the finding that a blood eosinophilia of up to 25 per cent may occur in cases of myelomatosis (Osserman, 1971), that urticaria is common both in myelomatosis (personal observation and Thiers et al., 1969) and lymphoma and that patients with myelomatosis often present as cases of recurring pyrexia of unknown origin, suggesting the possibility of an allergic response to a parasite. The not infrequent finding of multiple clones of plasma cells as evidenced by several M bands in the electrophoretic pattern of cases of myelomatosis or paraproteinaemia points to multiple antigenic stimulation of the reticulo-endothelial system by the limax amoebae.

Myelomatosis and xanthomatosis

Xanthomatosis with hyperlipidaemia may precede and be associated with myelomatosis or hyperglobulinaemic purpura (Waldenstrom's) (Cohen et al., 1966; Salin, 1965). It, thus, appears that limax amoebae infection may result in hyperlipidaemia and xanthomatosis as well as in diabetes mellitus.

3) Paraproteinaemia, macroglobulinaemia, cryoglobulinaemia and Bence-Jones proteinuria in malignant disease other than myelomatosis

—354—

It has been seen that paraproteinaemia, macroglobulinaemia, cryoglobulinaemia and Bence-Jones proteinuria are often the late result of collagen and auto-immune disease. They have also been reported as preceding (primary) or associated with (secondary) malignant lymphomas and leukaemias and with some cancers (Kappeler et al., 1958; Owen et al., 1959; Lucchelli and Nathangelo, 1964; Radl et al., 1965; Lohmann and Glaser, 1965; Krauss and Sokal, 1966; Meltzer and Franklin, 1966; Wintrobe, 1967; Slotoft and Lind, 1968; Blatrix et al., 1968; Worlledge et al., 1968; Lynch and Joske, 1969; Wager and Rasanen, 1970; Bonomo et al., 1970; Balmes et al., 1970; Clinico-Pathological Conference, Brit. med. J. 1969, 3, 33; Cooper, 1970). Lohmann and Glaser (1965) examined the serum of 1,500 patients by electrophoresis. Of these 119 showed atypical monoclonal precipitin bands. Of these 40 had either plasma cell tumours or Waldenstrom's macroglobulinaemia and 22 carcinomata. Of 200 patients with carcinoma atypical monoclonal bands were found in 32. Of 5 patients with carcinoma of the kidney 4 showed them. The atypical bands were chiefly a-globulins, but sometimes (3-1 or (3-2 globulins. The cryoglobulins frequently exhibit ANF and RF activity like that found in chronic infections and collagen and auto-immune disease. Furthermore, both lymphomata and leukaemias and carcinomata may occur in a high proportion of cases associated with Waldenstrom's macroglobulinaemia and myelomatosis. This suggests that the occurrence of these abnormal proteins before or associated with malignant diseases, both of the lymphoid system and carcinomata, may be related to the previous existence of collagen and auto-immune disease, which could thus be causally related to the development of some reticuloses and cancers, or since the serum abnormalities may improve or disappear after treatment of the tumours, arise from the organisms present in the tumours.

4) Acquired immune deficiency states (acquired hypogammaglohulinaemia) and malignancies

Evidence has been adduced in Chapter II that rheumatoid disease may result not only in an increase in the immunoglobulins, but also in hypogammaglobulinaemia and immune paresis. Moreover, it was indicated that cases of acquired hypogam-. maglobulinaemia, like congenital cases, are predisposed to develop any manifestations of collagen or auto-immune diseases. It was suggested that in such acquired cases the hypogammaglobulinaemia was, in fact, the first manifestation of rheumatoid disease preceding other obvious manifestations of the condition. Cases of malignant disease; including lymphomas, leukaemia, myeloma, fulminating pelvic cancer, myasthenia and thymoma, and carcinoma, may be preceded by up to 10 years by, or be associated with hypogammaglobulinaemia (Ultman et al., 1959; Eastman and Yeoman, 1960; Fairley and Scott, 1961; Page et al., 1963; Wood, 1963; Green et al., 1963; Hoffbrand, 1964; Alexeieff, 1964; Godfrey, 1964; Jacob et al., 1964; Roe et al., 1966; Velde et al., 1966; Good et al., 1966; Metters, 1968; Harris et al., 1972; Heidelberger et al., 1974). Hermans and Huizenga (1972) described 3 cases of idiopathic late onset immunoglobulin deficiency who had gastric cancer and found two in the literature. One of the cases developed myxoedema. Lowe (1976) reported a case of rheumatoid arthritis with sprue-like diarrhoea, who developed hypogammaglobulinaemia, pernicious anaemia and later carcinomata of both urinary bladder and lung.

Harris et al. suggest that in such cases the immune-deficiency state, like the malignancies, results from ·the direct action of the carcinogenic agent. This is in accord with the possibility that both the malignancy and the immune deficiency are due to limax amoebae infection.

5) Sjogren's syndrome, Mikulicz's disease and malignant disease

Sjogren's syndrome and Mikulicz's disease appear to be the same condition and essentially a manifestation of rheumatoid disease. In some cases benign lympho-epithelial lesions (adenolymphoma, lymphocytic tumour or papillary cystadeno-lymphomatosum) appears in such salivary glands. As described above cases of Sjogren's syndrome or Mikulicz's disease may be complicated by Waldenstrom's macroglobulinaemia or other types of para-proteinaemia. Becq Girandon et al. (1976) report a case of Sjogren's syndrome with Waldenstrom's disease in which a double IgM M-band was present in the same. In addition they may also develop any type of lymphoma, such as follicular lymphosarcoma, lymphosarcoma, reticulosarcoma or Hodgkin's disease, or indeed myelomatosis. Rothman et al. (1951) described a case of rheumatoid arthritis with splenomegaly and Sjogren's syndrome which developed lymphoblasto-ma. Sjogren's syndrome associated with reticulosarcoma was also reported by Syman et al. (1957). Hench et al. (1962) mentions a case of Sjogren's syndrome which developed lymphoma and had lupus erythematosus cells in the blood. Tala! and Bunim (1964) followed 58 patients with Sjogren's syndrome over 4 years. In 3 cases reticulum cell sarcoma and in one Waldenstrom's macroglobulinaemia developed. Three of the cases had splenomegaly. They refer to two other cases. These authors also quote a case of Dr. H.C. Stolze seen at the Mayo Clinic, in which a patient with Sjogren's syndrome developed malignant lymphoma. In one of Tala! and Bunim's cases the RF and tissue auto-antibodies disappeared from the blood as reticulum cell sarcoma developed. Bloch et al. (1965) report 3 cases of Sjogren's syndrome which developed reticulum cell sarcoma in remote tissues and referred to a fourth case. A case of Sjogren's syn-drome which was complicated by nodular reticulum cell sarcoma was also reported by Hornbaker et al. (1966). They quote a case of Sjogren's syndrome of Dr. C.S. Hardison who developed Hodgkin's disease and one of Sjogren's syndrome in which giant follicular lymphoma appeared (Senti et al., 1964). Miller (1967) records Sjogren's syndrome preceding reticulosarcoma. Talal et al. (1967) report 8 patients with Sjogren's syndrome, two of which developed macroglobulinaemia, one reticulasarcoma and five a syndrome described as "pseudolymphoma". In all these cases there was lymphadenopathy. Other cases of Sjogren's syndrome developing malignant lymphoma have been reported by Maxwell (1960), Deutsch (1967), Abrahamson et al. (1968), Sage and Forbes (1968), Anderson and Tala! (1972), Haritopoulos et al. (1973) and Heckmayr et al. (1976). Ryan et al. (1974) report a case of rheumatoid arthritis, Felty's syndrome and Sjogren's syndrome developing malignant lymphoma. Gryminski and Szymanska (1970) described the case of a woman who developed Sjogren's syndrome and fibrosing alveolitis and 11 years later lymphadenopathy, which on biopsy showed Hodgkin's disease. She died soon after and autopsy showed widespread reticulosarcoma in the lymph nodes and left lung and changes characteristic of Sjogren's syndrome were found in salivary glands, buccal mucosa, trachea, bronchi, right lung and spleen. Shearn (1971) describes a case of Sjogren's syndrome with auto-immune haemolytic anaemia which developed reticulosarcoma. Grundy (1972) reports Sjogren's syndrome with widespread lymphoid deposits, including the vocal cord, macroglobulinaemia and cervical lymph node enlargement. Gumpel (1972) describes a case of Sjogren's syndrome in a woman of 72 years with salivary gland enlargement and with chronic lymphatic leukaemia, lymphadenopathy, hepatomegaly and splenomegaly. In the Case Records of the Massachusetts General Hospital, New England, J. Med., 1972, 286, 992, was described a patient with Sjogren's syndrome, pericarditis, myositis, silicosis, lymphocytic lymphoma and squamous cell carcinoma of the upper lobe of the right lung. Whaley et al. (1973, b) record four cases of Sjogren's syndrome developing malignant lymphoma, often beginning in a salivary gland, and give numerous other references to such cases. Nime et al. (1976) found 43 cases and added 4 new ones in which a malignant lymphoma arose initially in a salivary gland showing a pre-existing Iympho-epithelial lesion with or without Sjogren's syndrome.

Mikulicz's disease has been known for many years to precede or be associated with lymphadenoma, reticuloses or leukaemia (Aird, 1958; Bloch et al., 1965). Pinkus and Dekker (1970) reported a case of Sjogren's syndrome in which the parotid glands contained a benign lympho-epithelial lesion and which developed reticulosarcoma. Azzopardi and Evans (1971) describe 5 cases of benign lympho-epithelial lesions which were associated with or preceded the development of Hodgkin's disease or reticulosarcoma. In the Cancer Registry series, described above, there was one case of Sjogren's syndrome which developed malignant lymphoma.

In the author's own series cases of Sjogren-Mikulicz's syndrome with or without other manifestations of collagen or auto-immune disease were common. Six cases developed malignant lymphoma, one with paraproteinaemia and one with chronic lymphatic leukaemia, and one reticulosarcoma. In two cases a benign lympho-epithelial lesion was present in the parotid. Of considerable significance is the finding that in 3 of the cases the patient first developed Sjogren's syndrome and later a mass within the parotid gland, which proved on biopsy to be a lymphoma, suggesting that what caused the Sjogren's syndrome also caused the lymphoma.

Sjogren-Mikulicz's lesions may lead to

tumour formation other than benign lympho-epithelial lesions in the salivary glands. Stoltze et al. (1960) described the development of a mixed parotid tumour in a case of Sjogren's syndrome. Lloyd (1946) reported a syncytial reticulosarcoma arising in the stroma of one of his cases of the solid type of adenolymphoma. Pasqualini and Bazzocchi (1968) also described an adenolymphoma of the parotid developing into lympho-reticulosarcoma. In addition the epithelial element of the adenolymphoma may become malignant and spread to local lymph nodes. References to this change are given by StOhr and Riska and by Ssobelow, quoted by Plaut (1942), who tabulates the reported cases, and by Ruebner and Bramhall (1960) and de Ia Pava et al. (1962). Delaney and Balogh (1966) report a case of carcinoma of the parotid with benign lympho-epithelial lesions (Mikulicz's disease) developing in a case of SjBgren's syndrome and rheumatoid arthritis and mention a similar case. Cases of malignant change in a benign Iympho-epithelial lesion were also reported by Dobrossy et al. (1972), Larrauri et al. (1973) and Gradient and Kalfayan (1975), while Assor (1974) describes a case of bilateral carcinoma of the parotid, one cancer arising in a benign lympho-epithelial lesion, a manifestation of rheumatoid disease. Lumerman et al. (1975) record a single case and refer to 5 others in the literature, in which a lympho-epithelial lesion was accompa nied by a mixed parotid tumour. In all the large series of cases of multiple tumours mentioned above there are found cases of mixed parotid tumours or carcinoma of the parotid occurring in association with lymphomata or other cancers and, therefore, the former tumours are presumably produced by the same factor as produces the lymphomata, etc.

In one of the author's cases of Sjogren's syndrome with rheumatoid arthritis a carcinoma of the maxillary antrum developed. Cases of Sjogren's syndrome may also de-

Addendum: Familia I Warthin's tumour. NovekAM, Prilzker KPH, Greyson ND et al. J. Otolaryngeol., 1980, 90-96
The authors suggest that Wartin's tumour is suggested as a hypersensitivity disease.
Addendum: Squamous cell carcinoma arising in benign adenolymphoma (Warthin's tumour) of the parotid gland.
Baker M, Yuzon D and Baker BH. J. Surg. Oncol. 1980, 15/1, 1-10.

velop thymic tumours with or without hepatosplenomegaly. Such cases have been reported by Lattes (1962), Birch et al. (1964) and Hall (1968). A case of rheumatoid arthritis with Sjogren's syndrome developing adenoma of the adrenal cortex producing Cushing's syndrome, was reported by Gerardy (1959), while Shearn (1971) describes cases of Sjogren's syndrome in which a duct carcinoma of the breast and two in which carcinoma of the cervix later developed. In the Cancer Registry series described above a case of Sjogren's syndrome developed cancer of the male breast.

It appears that cases of Sjogren-Mikulicz's syndrome with or without rheumatoid arthritis are liable to develop malignant lymphomata, Waldenstrom's macroglobulinaemia and myelomatosis and they may also develop lymphoma or malignant disease in the salivary glands often preceded by adenolymphoma, thus directly relating malignant change and lymphoma formation and paraproteinaemia to the rheumatoid process.

6) Hashimoto's thyroiditis, myxoedema and thyrotoxicosis in relation to tumour formation

It has been seen that there is a close association between Hashimoto's thyroiditis and myxoedema, which is the end result of lymphocytic thyroiditis and these again with thyrotoxicosis, all of which are regarded as manifestations of collagen and auto-immune disease. The first two disturbances appear closely related to malignancy, both in the thyroid gland and elsewhere in the body. Thyrotoxicosis may well be primarily a manifestation of hypothalamic disturbance produced by limax amoebae infection.

a) Hashimoto's thyroiditis and lymphoma of the thyroid gland or elsewhere in the body

The histological picture of Hashimoto's disease may closely resemble and may merge into that of a reticulosarcoma or lymphosarcoma (Shaw and Smith, 1925; Welch et al., 1958; Metcalfe and Sclare, 1961; Graham and McCullagh, 1931; Cureton et al., 1957; Kellett and Sutherland, 1949; Dick and Kellett, 1951; Kenyon and Ackerman, 1955; Lindsay and Dailey, 1955 (7 cases); Walt et al., 1957; Ranstr5m, 1957 (8 cases); Mikal, 1964; Cox, 1964; Macak, 1975; Chesky et al. (1962) described 5 cases which developed a malignant lymphoma out of 452 cases of Hashimoto's thyroiditis. Woolner et ul. (1959) at the Mayo Clinic report 605 cases of Hashimoto's thyroiditis and related thyroidal disorders with lymphocytic infiltration of the gland and found 12 cases of local lymphosarcoma in which the lesion extended beyond the thyroid capsule. Woolner et al. (1966) report 5 cases of Hashimoto's thyroiditis present in 46 cases of primary malignant lymphoma of the thyroid. Gelbashstein and Nabakov (1968) studied 53 cases of Hashimoto's thyroiditis and in 10 (19 per cent) the changes of malignant lymphoma had developed (4 follicular lymphoblastoma, 6 reticulosarcoma). They concluded that Hashimoto's thyroiditis is a premalignant condition. Besbee and Thoeny (1975) report a similar case. In the Cancer Registry series above one patient with rheumatoid arthritis and Hashimoto's thyroiditis developed lymphoma of the gland.

Brewer and Orr (1953) were concerned with the long survival of cases of malignant lymphoma developing in Hashimoto's thyroiditis. They were impressed by the metastatic pattern of such cases, especially the occurrence of nodules in the gastrointestinal tract. They suggest the condition may be due to a granulomatous lesion exhibiting a predilection for thyroid and gastro-intestinal tract. The alleged association of thyroid lymphosarcoma with intestinal lesions cannot, however, be regarded as statistically significant (Evans, 1966). More et al. (1968) reporting on plasmocytoma of the thyroid, found it had many features in common with malignant lymphoma in this site, including an association with Hashimoto's thyroiditis in more than half of the reported cases. Saita et al. (1969) describe the case of a woman with Hashimoto's thyroiditis with thyroid auto-antibodies in the serum who developed myelomatosis and Leng-Levy et al. (1967) a case of rheumatoid arthritis with hypothyroidism who also developed myelomatosis. In the Cancer Registry series was described a case of rheumatoid arthritis with myxoedema who also developed myelomatosis.

Scheuer-Karpin and d'Heureuse-Gerhardt (1965) mention a female patient of 69 years who had suffered from Hashimoto's thyroiditis for 8 years and who developed splenomegaly, Hodgkin's disease, chronic lymphatic leukaemia and systemic lupus erythematosus. The liver was heavily infiltrated witn lymphocytes. Powell and Thomas (1968) described a case of diabetes mellitus and myxoedema in a patient who developed Hodgkin's disease. The author has observed 2 cases in which goitre due to Hashimoto's thyroiditis was associated with the development of Hodgkin's disease in the neighbouring lymph nodes (see also Case VIII, 42). Dr. A.M. Jeliffe of the Middlesex Hospital (personal communication) has seen one such case. The author also had under his care a case (Case VIII, 39) which developed reticulosarcoma of the tonsil treated by X-ray therapy. Ten years later she developed abdominal Hodgkin's disease and later myxoedema. No thyroid auto-antibodies, RF and ANF were found in the serum.

Goudie (1968, personal communication) has seen a case of Hashimoto's thyroiditis which developed chronic lymphatic leukaemia. Auto-immune thyroiditis rapidly merging into myxoedema was found in a patient with stem-cell leukaemia (Ando-fallo et al., 1963). At a Clinico-Pathologi-

cal Conference at Hammersmith Hospital held on 9.2.1966, there was shown a case of Hashimoto's thyroiditis which developed pancytopenia and then acute myeloid leukaemia. In the discussion which followed this case Dr. (now Professor) E.D. Williams mentioned 3 cases of myxoedema, presumably due to diffuse thyroiditis. The first developed aplastic anaemia, which later turned into acute leukaemia, the second developed leukopenia, which later developed into chronic lymphatic leukaemia and the third developed leukopenia, which later developed into acute leukaemia. Bitan et aL (1964) also record a case of myxoedema developing acute lymphoblastic leukaemia. A number of similar cases were present in the author's series.

b) Thyroiditis and carcinoma of the thyroid

Thyrotoxicosis and thyroid adenoma may develop in cases of pituitary ablation for carcinoma of the breast (Baron and Gurling, 1959), showing that the thyroid changes are independent of pituitary hormones. Again, cancer of the thyroid sometimes occurs in cases of Simmond's disease (Fraser, 1956), indicating that the development of thyroid cancer may be independent of the pituitary secretions.

Not only does Hashimoto's thyroiditis predispose to the development of malignant lymphoma in the thyroid, but also to carcinoma. Dube and Joyce (1971) draw attention to the appearance of squamous metaplasia in parts of the thyroid affected by Hashimoto's thyroiditis. Shands (1960) collected 66 cases from the literature of carcinoma of the thyroid developing in glands showing lymphocytic thyroiditis and added three of his own. Blackburn and O'Gorman (1961) described two such cases. Woolner et al. (1966) in their series of 605 cases of Hashimoto's thyroiditis and related thyroidal disorders with lymphocytic infiltration of the gland found 18 cases of carcinoma developing in such glands. Prior and Fairchild (1963) report a similar development of thyroid cancer in Hashimoto's thyroiditis. Crile and Fisher (1953), Dailey et al. (1955), Schlicke et al. (1960), Fowler et al. (1961) and Ratnakar et al. (1976) report similar cases. One such case occurred in the Cancer Registry series reported above. Chesky et al. (1962). found that of 453 patients with Hashimoto's thyroiditis in 49 (11 per cent) cancerous changes had occurred compared with 6.4 per cent of cases of cancer of the gland occurring without Hashimoto's thyroiditis. Hirabayashi and Lindsay (1965) found an incidence of cancer of the thyroid in glands affected by Hashimoto's thyroiditis as high as 22.5 per cent. Finally Ayala et al. (1968) report the case of an elderly female patient who developed a rapidly enlarging goitre, which at histological examination showed Hashimoto's thyroiditis and both lymphosarcoma and carcinoma. Glass et al. (1956) described a similar case.

Sclare and Nicol (1964) report 3 cases of cancer of the thyroid found at autopsy in 37 cases of myxoedema which is, of course, the end result of lymphocytic thyroiditis. The thyroid gland showed marked fibrosis with foci of lymphocytes and plasma cells and in one case three separate malignant tumours had formed.

In the author's series malignant disease of the thyroid occurred in patients suffering from:-

1) Chronic rhinitis, asthma, rheumatoid arthritis and myelomatosis.

2) Ulcerative colitis and rheumatoid arthritis.

3) Thyrotoxicosis with lymphocytic thyroiditis.

Thyroid auto-antibodies in cases of thyroid carcinoma

Stuart and Allen (1958) found that 3 of 6 cases of thyroid cancer had high titres of antibodies to thyroglobulin in the serum and 2 of the 3 showed the changes of lymphadenoid goitre. Doniach et al.

(1958) found thyroid auto-antibodies in 10 of 36 cases of thyroid cancer.

c) Hashimoto's thyroiditis and Hiirthle-cell tumours

In addition, the development of Hiirthle-cell tumours in glands showing Hashimoto's thyroiditis is recorded (Gardner, 1955; Dailey et al., 1955).

d) Lymphocytic thyroid disease and malignancy elsewhere in the body

Sommers (1955) found that in 85 per cent of cases of carcinoma of the breast the thyroid was atrophic and infiltrated with lymphocytes and plasma cells as compared with controls. Yakoleva (1958) found atrophy and sclerosis of the thyroid was frequent in cases of gastric and bronchial carcinoma. Brain and Hensen (1958) noted that 3 of 15 women in their series of cases of carcinomatous neuropathy had myxoedema and two of the cases showed extensive lymphocytic infiltration of the thyroid. Brain et al. (1951) described a similar case. In the case described in the Clinico-Pathological Conference (Brit. med. J., 1970, 1, 281) an oat-cell carcinoma of the lung was associated with bilateral adrenocortical hyperplasia and severe focal thyroiditis. Erez et al. (1965) report the case of a woman who had undergone partial thyroidectomy for chronic thyroiditis and later developed bilateral benign cystic teratomata of the ovary which contained thyroid tissue exhibiting Hashimoto's changes. Hilton and Whittaker (1972) described a patient with Hashimoto's thyroiditis and myxoedema occurring 20 years after successful treatment of carcinoma of the bladder. Itoh and Maruchi (1975) found that patients with Hashimoto's thyroiditis are a high risk population for breast cancer in Japan and that mild thyroid deficiency may predispose to breast cancer. In a case presented at a Medical Staff Round at the Post-Graduate Medical School, Hammersmith in 1963, a patient with Hashimoto's

Addendum: Yamashitta, N., Maruchi, N. and Mori, W. Hashimoto's thyroiditis: a possible risk factor for lung cancer among Japanese women. Cancer Lett. 1979, 7, 9·13. report an increased incidence of lung cancer among Japanese women with Hashimoto's thyroiditis, though the relationship with breast cancer was not significant.

thyroiditis and myxoedema developed a pituitary tumour. According to Lerman (1947) low thyroid function is linked with the development of cancer. Liechty et al. (1963) found a higher incidence of cancer in myxoedematous patients than in euthyroid or hyperthyroid patients attending a goitre clinic.

In the South West Metropolitan Cancer Registry Series Hashimoto's thyroiditis preceded or was associated with the onset of malignancy in 14 cases, 12 being in women. One was a carcinoma of the thyroid, two were of the bronchus in women and four of the senile breast in women. Two cases of rheumatoid arthritis with Hashimoto's thyroiditis developed malignancy, one a cancer of the thyroid, the other a malignant lymphoma. Myxoedema preceded or was associated with the development of malignancy in 29 cases. They included two cases of chronic lymphatic leukaemia and one of carcinoma of the senile breast in a woman. In 3 cases myxoedema associated with diabetes preceded the onset of cancer of the senile female breast, the uterine body or haemangio-endothelioma of the face. One case of rheumatoid arthritis and myxoedema developed myelomatosis. In the author's series hypothyroidism and/or Hashimoto's thyroiditis was found to be a very frequent accompaniment or followed the onset of successfully treated extrathyroid malignant disease.

Gemma et al. (1968) report the case of a lympho-epithelioma of the thymus developing in relation to aberrant thyroid tissue showing Hashimoto's changes.

e) Thyrotoxicosis and malignant disease

In cases of thyrotoxicosis, which is regarded as an auto-immune manifestation, the diffuse goitre does not usually show much evidence of lymphocytic infiltration, though the disease may complicate Hashimoto's thyroiditis.

Malignant change in the thyroid in cases of diffuse toxic goitre and not exhibiting lymphocytic infiltration is rare (Evans, 1966). Papillary carcinoma occurred in the thyroid in a case of thyrotoxicosis in the author's series. The gland was infiltrated with lymphocytes.

f) Thyrotoxicosis and malignant lymphoma

In cases of thyrotoxicosis it will be recalled that lymphadenopathy and splenomegaly occasionally occur. Long-standing cases of thyrotoxicosis may develop malignant lymphoma. Six such cases have been reported by Ultmann et al. (1963) and other cases were collected from the literature. The malignant lymphoma was either lymphoblastic lymphosarcoma, Hodgkin's disease, giant follicular lymphosarcoma or chronic lymphatic leukaemia. A number of such cases occurred in the author's series above. Moloney et al. (1970) describe a case of thyrotoxicosis with lymphosarcomatosis and heavy-chain disease with amyloid deposits. Biopsy at first showed chronic inflammatory change in the lymph nodes.

g) Thyrotoxicosis and extrathyroidal neoplasms

Wanebo et al. (1966) found that of 300 women with thyrotoxicosis 83 had neoplastic disease. Of these women (excluding thyroid and skin cancer) 56 per cent had breast primaries, which is significantly different from the 36 per cent incidence of breast cancer among all women with malignant neoplasms at the centre (Memorial Hospital. New York). A diagnosis of both diseases (thyrotoxicosis and breast cancer) was made in 21 of 40 women within the same year. The incidence of thyrotoxicosis was only 0.25 per cent in females without breast cancer. McDougall et al. (1971) described thyrotoxicosis developing in a woman of 46 years with bilateral ovarian cancers. Thymolipoma in patients with thyrotoxicosis were recorded by Beaton and Gerard (1966) and thyrotoxicosis with myelomatosis by

Addendum: Rose, D.P. and Davis, T.E. Plasma triiodothyronine concentration in breast cancer. Cancer (Philadelphia) 1979; 43, 1434-1438, found a proportion of breast cancer cases who were mildly hypothyroid.

Tourniaire et al. (1972). In a Clinico-Pathological Conference held at Hammersmith Hospital on 5.2.1966 there was reported the case of a patient who had suffered from thyrotoxicosis at the age of 38 years, who developed carcinoma of the cervix at the age of 49 years, of the breast at the age of 50 years, of the bronchus at the age of 57 years and chronic myeloid leukaemia at the age of 58 years.

In cases in the South West Metropolitan Cancer Registry series thyrotoxicosis preceded or coincided with the appearance of malignant disease in 77 cases, 16 males and 61 females. Two of these were thyroid carcinomata. There were two cases of Hodgkin's disease, one of reticulosarcoma and one of acute monocytic leukaemia and 20 cases of carcinoma of the bronchus, 11 in women. Of two cases of rheumatoid arthritis with thyrotoxicosis one developed reticulosarcoma and the other multiple basal cell carcinoma. In the author's series there were numerous examples of thyrotoxicosis preceding or accompanying malignant disease. Miller and Chodas (1966) and Leblay et al. (1969) regard thyrotoxicosis as a paraneoplastic condition.

h) Carcinoma. of the thyroid associated with other primary cancers

Cancer of the thyroid may be associated with other primary malignant tumours, more than in controls (Wyse et at. 1969) and see all reports of multiple primaries given above. Takenchi and Pickren (1967) found 14 such cases and 165 in the literature. Leukaemias were commonly the second malignancy. Chalstrey and Benjamin (1966) found a high incidence of breast cancer in thyroid cancer cases.

Conclusions

It seems, therefore, that lymphocytic thyroiditis of any degree predisposes to carcinoma in the gland, to malignant lymphoma in the gland and elsewhere, to myelomatosis and leukaemia and is especially associated with malignancy m other tissues. Thyrotoxicosis not infrequently precedes or is associated with malignant lymphomatosis, leukaemia or carcinoma and may be regarded as a paraneoplastic condition as well as a precursor of these diseases.

7) Collagen disease and parathyroid tumours

Howell (1972) described the case of a woman of 64 years who had suffered *from* rheumatoid arthritis for 27 years and who had developed a goitre with thyrotoxicosis and hyperparathyroidism due to a cystic adenoma of a parathyroid gland. Bergeret et a!. (1975) quote a case of a woman in which rheumatoid arthritis was present and parathyroid adenoma developed. They quote similar cases from the literature. Zawadski and Benedek (1969) report a case of rheumatoid arthritis and paraproteinaemia with a parathyroid adenoma. The author's had under his care a patient who developed parathyroid adenQma, thyroid adenoma at the age of 17 years and rheumatoid arthritis at the age of 19 years. Hajjar and Salti (1973) and Ackerman and Arribas (1976) describe the co-existence of thyrotoxicosis and hyperparathyroidism due to a parathyroid tumour. Due et al. (1973) recorded the case of a patient with thyrotoxicosis, acute myasthenia and a confusional syndrome with hypercalcaemia in which a parathyroid adenoma and lymphocytic thyroiditis was found at autopsy. Richards (1971) records the case of a patient who suffered from Raynaud's phenomena for years and who developed thyroid carcinoma and parathyroid adenoma with "pseudo-clubbing" of the fingers. This last was unaffected by removal of the parathyroid adenoma. The frequent association of parathyroid adenoma with thyroid carcinoma was described by Summers and Sisson (1972) and Petro and Hardy (1975). Dent et al. (1975) describe a case of coeliac disease who developed fibrosarcoma of the breast and a parathyroid adenoma. Again, in various lists of multiple tumours referred to previously parathyroid tumours, either benign or malignant, may occur in subjects who also exhibit tumours of other organs (Kaplan et al., 1971), including lymphomata, and these presumably are caused by the same factors. Such observations suggest a possible relationship of collagen and auto-immune disease to the development of a parathyroid adenoma or carcinoma.

8) Collagen b(auto-immune disease and thymic tumours

It has been concluded that thymic lesions form part of the manifestations of collagen and auto-immune disease. They are of two types. They consist of hypertrophy with the appearance of germinal centres in the medulla, *comparable to the changes of Hashimoto's thyroiditis,* with or without tumour formation. The latter may be a lymphoma, a lympho-epithelioma or a spindle-cell tumour (White and Marshall, 1962; Maldonado, 1964; Hall, 1968) or a thymolipoma (Benton and Gerard, 1966). Either condition may be associated with myasthenia gravis. Thus, the tumour formation in the thymus would appear to be a manifestation of collagen and auto-immune disease. An interesting case was reported by Gemma et al. (1968). The patient was a 28 year old woman with a seven year history of goitre and signs of thyrotoxicosis. The serum contained thyroid auto-antibodies in high titre. She developed a thymic lymphoepithelioma with metastases. Aberrant thyroid tissue with chronic Hashimoto's changes was found in the tumour mass and the tumour appeared to develop in relation to this lymphoid infiltration, suggesting it might be aetiologically related to it.

Thymic hypertrophy and tumour and extrathymic tumours

According to Blumenthal and Berns (1966) extra-thymic malignancies are not uncommonly found in auto-immune diseases. Co-existent thymoma and multiple myelomatosis was reported by Anderson and Vye (1967), Lindstrom et al. (1968), Gilbert et al. (1968) and Lemenaget et al. (1972). The blood contained RF. Thymic hypertrophy or tumour may also precede acute leukaemia (Cooke, 1932; Biebel, 1947; Kaplan, 1954; Adams, 1963; Anderson and Pederson, 1967). Acute leukaemia following resection of a malignant thymoma was reported by Santy et al. (1954). Thymoma associated with Kaposi's sarcoma was described by Mabery and Stone (1967). Sonadjian et al. (1968) reported an increased incidence of non-thymic cancers in subjects with thymomas (21 per cent of cases followed for up to 20 years). Thymic hypertrophy or tumour may be associated with acromegaly due to eosinophil adenoma of the pituitary (McEachern and Parnell, 1948; Irvine, 1964). Lapresle et al. (1976) describe a case of myasthenia with thymoma which developed a pituitary tumour associating heterogeneous adenomatous proliferation with ganglioneuroma. Pirofsky (1968) reports two cases of thymoma accompanied by auto-immune haemolytic anaemia. One also suffered from pernicious anaemia, thyroid adenoma, diabetes, systemic lupus erythematosus and adenocarcinoma of the prostate and the other from myelomatosis, thyroid adenoma and diabetes. Imaizumi et al. (1974) described a case in which a malignant thymoma was successfully removed and which 5 months later developed myasthenia gravis when a carcinoma of the stomach was found to be present. A case of thymoma associated with systemic lupus erythematosus which developed squamous carcinoma of the skiP.. was reported by Agus et al. (1975).

Thus, collagen and auto-immune disease appears to be the cause of thymic tumours and to be related to the development of extra-thymic tumours, including lymphomas, myelomatosis and leukaemias with which thymic lesions may be associated.

9) Myasthenia gravis and malignancy

Myasthenia gravis is also a manifestation of collagen and auto-immune disease. It's association with chronic myeloid leukaemia and an anterior mediastinal mass was described by Djaldetti et al. (1968) and myasthenia followed by chronic lymphatic leukaemia and auto-immune haemolytic anaemia by Cohen and Waxman (1967). Corino et al. (1971) report a case with pernicious anaemia and myasthenia which developed chronic myeloid leukaemia. Myasthenia gravis with myelomatosis was described by Rowland et al. (1969) and Lemenaget et al. (1972). Silberstein (1970) reported the case of a man aged 53 years, who 22 years previously was noticed to have splenomegaly and for 16 years suffered from myasthenia. He later developed hypersplenism. At splenectomy the organ showed islets of reticulum cells and six months later he showed generalized reticulosarcoma. RF and thyroid auto-antibodies were found in the blood. Simpson (1966) described a myasthenic patient who developed reticulum cell sarcoma and stated he knew of two similar unreported cases. Rowland (1971) states that myasthenics may develop cancer of any organ, though whether more frequently than controls is doubtful. Papatestas et al. (1971) in reviewing previous reports of the incidence of extrathymic tumours in cases of myasthenia state that these had varied between 1.4 and 2.5 per cent. Ferguson (1962) found 8 (5 per cent) of 145 cases of myasthenia developed extrathymic cancers (5 breast, 1 bronchus, 1 bladder, 1 gastro-intestinal tract). Papatestas et al. (1971) found that of 1,243 myasthenia patients of both sexes without thymectomy followed up 94 (7.5 per cent) developed extrathymic malignancies after the onset of myasthenia, that is about a *three-fold increase over the expected prevalence of all extra-thymic neoplasms,* especially of breast cancer (41 per cent). The primary site of the extra-thymic neoplasms, which occurred whether a thymic tumour was present or not, were breast 25 cases, genital organs 14 cases (prostate 5, ovary 3, uterus 4, other 2), digestive organs 12 (colon-rectum 6, pancreas 2, liver 1, stomach and small intestine 2, other 1), respiratory system 9 (lung 8, larynx 1), skin 7, brain and central nervous system 5, leukaemia 6, lymphoma-lymphosarcoma 4 and multiple myeloma 1. Of significance is that in 8 cases (10.5 per cent) there were multiple primary tumours. A myasthenic syndrome associated with a small cell carcinoma of the bronchus was reported by Kennedy and Jiminez-Paben (1968). Vessey and Doll (1972) followed up 382 patients undergoing thymectomy for myasthenia and found 10 who developed tumours after a varying period. In two of these a thymoma had been present. The tumours included cancer of the breast (2 cases), Hodgkin's disease, chronic lymphatic leukaemia, squamous cancer of the abdominal wall, metastatic cancer, cancer of the spine primary unknown, osteosarcoma of the sacrum, bronchial adenoma-carcinoid type, astrocytoma of the cord and pituitary adenoma. The authors found no evidence of increased incidence of neoplastic disease after thymectomy. Levo et al. (1975) described reticulosarcoma developing 14 years after myasthenia and remark on the increasing frequency of reports of patients with myasthenia developing malignancy.

Thus, the manifestation of collagen and auto-immune disease known as myasthenia often associated with thymoma appears to predispose to the development of various malignancies.

It has been seen that the *Eaton-Lambert syndrome* may be a manifestation of auto-immune disorders and presumably due to limax amoeba infection. This syndrome is also a common manifestation of carcinoma,

Addendum: Vogel J.M. et al. (N.Y. State J. Med. 1977, 72, 2255) report the occurrence of 5 cases of concomitant chronic lymphocytic leukaemia among 1300 myasthenics, coinciding with previous reports of a high overall incidence of extrathymic neoplasms in non-thymectomized patients with myasthenia gravis.
Addendum: Hassan, M.M. (Childs Brain, 1977, 3, 65) reports the case of a child aged 3 with myasthenia and ganglia-neuroblastoma of the mediastinum and mentions one similar report in the literature.

especially carcinoma of the bronchus. This suggests a connection of auto-immune disease with malignancy.

10) Dermatomyositis (polymyositis) and malignant disease

It is well recognized that dermatomyositis may be associated with malignant disease. This association was reviewed by Curtis et al. (1952) and by Williams (1959), who collected 92 cases from the literature. Since then many more have been reported (Heathfield and Williams, 1960; Klingmuller and Vorlaender, 1965; Katz and Digby, 1965; Hegewald and Hagemann, 1966; Szegedi et al., 1968; Gascard et al., 1969). Winkelmann et al. (1968) reported 16 cases. Holzmann and Herz (1969) reviewed 233 cases. They tend to occur in older subjects. The malignancies associated with dermatomyositis include lymphoma and leukaemia, retroperitoneal sarcoma, Hodgkin's disease, mycosis fungoides (Connor, 1972), myeloma, thymomas, malignant melanomas (Katz and Digby, 1965), carcinoma of the breast, stomach, lung (especially), ethmoid (Mackenzie and Scherbel, 1963), ovary, gall-bladder, oesophagus, colon, rectum, kidney, uterus, larynx, vocal cord (Mackenzie and Scherbel, 1963), cervix, vagina and chromophobe adenoma of the pituitary. Wilson et al. (1965) described a patient with dermatomyositis and three primary tumours of breast, rectum and transverse colon and whose daughter had chronic myeloid leukaemia. Koeppen et al. (1976) report a case of polymyositis associated with Kaposi's syndrome in which muscle biopsy showed plasma and eosinophil infiltration resembling the myopathy of Sjögren's syndrome. In Wilhams (1959) paper of 58 cases where details were available in 47 dermatomyositis preceded the recognition of the tumour and in 11 followed its discovery. In the latter case the tumour preceded the appearance of dermatomyo-

sitis at intervals of several years to several weeks. Heathfield and Williams (1960) report a number of significant cases. One woman developed carcinoma of the uterus three years after the polymyositis became inactive. She died five years later without reactivation of the muscle disease. Another case had systemic lupus erythematosus six years before developing fulminating dermatomyositis, later followed by carcinoma of the bronchus. Another case had muscular weakness for over 20 years and then developed carcinoma of the breast, while a further case had polymyositis and five years later developed adenosis of the cervix. Batschwarov and Minkov (1968) report dermatomyositis 3 years before any evidence of carcinoma of the bronchus. Chamberlain and Whittaker (1963) describe a case of Hashimoto's thyroiditis and dermatomyositis which many years later developed an ovarian carcinoma. Mescon and Clark (1964) reported an interesting case of a woman of 49 years who suffered from rheumatoid arthritis for 7 years. She then developed a goitre and signs of myxoedema, which biopsy showed was due to Hashimoto's thyroiditis. This was followed by the appearance of dermatomyositis and then by a carcinoma of the breast. The stroma of the cancer showed an appearance very like that of the Hashimoto's thyroiditis and contained much lymphoid tissue. In the South West Metropolitan Cancer Registry Series dermatomyositis preceded the onset of malignancy in 3 cases at intervals of 3 to 14 years and sclero-dermatomyositis in one case by 8 years. In the author's experience dermatomyositis has preceded the appearance of malignant disease in 4 cases by 8, 12, 9 and 8 years respectively, the malignant disease being Hodgkin's disease, chronic lymphatic leukaemia, carcinoma of the breast and lymphosarcoma respectively. In the last case (Case 5) described above the operation of hysterectomy for fibroids appeared to have precipitated the appearance of dermatomyositis, while subsequent gastrectomy caused it to disappear. A malignant lymphoma developed 8 years later without the reappearance of dermatomyositis.

The cases of Klingmuller and Vorleander (1965) and Szegedi et al. (1968) already mentioned are of interest. The former described two cases of systemic lupus erythematosus and in one dermatomyositis was also present. The patient developed Hodgkin's disease 12 years later. In the first case reported by Szegedi et al. the patient developed polyarthritis, dermatomyositis with lupus erythematosus cells, ANF and RF in the blood and five years later Hodgkin's disease. With the advent of the latter the skin lesions and blood changes disappeared.

On the other hand, Simpson (1953) reports a case of cancer of the breast occurring six years before evidence of dermatomyositis appeared without signs of recurrence of the cancer. In two of the cases of Heathfield and Williams polymyositis *followed* successful removal of a carcinoma of the cervix a year before. Wilson (1948) reported a case of cancer of the breast who developed dermatomyositis 9 years after successful treatment. Winkelmann et al. (1968) in their important paper on 289 cases of dermatomyositis found 16 patients developed malignancies and 8 of them died of these with associated dermatomyositis. Eight other patients with malignancy were in remission of the dermatomyositis at the onset of malignancy. One patient developed two carcinomas of the colon 8 years after remission of the dermatomyositis. They found that malignancy can be related in time to dermatomyositis, but a patient in remission of dermatomyositis may develop malignancy. Segura and Ziegler (1973) report the case of a patient in which a first attack of dermatomyositis preceded the onset of bronchial carcinoma by 12 years. Two attacks of polymyositis occurred three years after successful removal of the tumour. Development of malignancy is one

of many factors which may precipitate an exacerbation of dermatomyositis. As shown above the development of malignancy may likewise cause dermatomyositis to disappear.

There are many reports of cases in which dermatomyositis and malignancy have been associated in time in which successful treatment of the malignant disease has caused a regression of the dermatomyositis, which may return with a recurrence of the tumour. Grace and Dao (1959) reported on a case of dermatomyositis with breast carcinoma in which the patient showed hypersensitivity to an extract of her own tumour.

The relationship of dermatomyositis to the appearance of a tumour seems complex. In the first place dermatomyositis or polymyositis may precede the appearance of lymphoma or cancer by a very long interval of up to 18 years. During this time the dermatomyositis may come and go on several occasions and appears to be precipitated by various factors, such as operations, infections, etc. With the appearance of the tumour dermatomyositis may reappear or if already present it may disappear, but it seems that a past history of dermatomyositis appears to predispose to *the development of malignant disease or lymphoma*. In the second place dermatomyositis may occur at the same time as malignant disease or lymphoma. In this case the Rose-Waaler and latex fixation test in the blood may be positive (Mills, 1963). In these cases successful removal, radiation or chemotherapeutic treatment of the malignant disease may or may not cause a regression or disappearance of the dermatomyositis. In the third place dermatomyositis may appear years after successful removal or other treatment of a tumour.

It appears, therefore that subjects who suffer from dermatomyositis, apparently a manifestation of limax amoebae infection, are predisposed to the development of any type of malignancy, lymphoma or leukaemia at a later date or dermatomyositis may appear with or after the development of a tumour.

11) Scleroderma (systemic sclerosis) and malignant disease

It has been seen above that dermatomyositis may develop into scleroderma and cases intermediate between the two diseases are not uncommon. Moreover, scleroderma may be preceded or complicated by Raynaud's phenomenon. This being so, it would be expected that there would be a relationship between scleroderma and malignant disease and, in fact, cases of scleroderma may occasionally develop cancer or lymphoma (Montgomery et al., 1964); Willis, 1967). This is particularly so in the case of carcinoma of the lung. Weaver et al. (1967) found 11 cases in the literature in which systemic sclerosis affecting the lung developed alveolar cell carcinoma, 5 adenocarcinoma of the bronchus and 2 oat cell carcinoma. They reported a further case of adenocarcinoma. Basten (1968) collected 20 cases. Mackezie and Scherbel (1963), Petitjean et al. (1968), Tomkin (1969) and Seignon et al. (1972) each added single cases. Cavazzini et al. (1970) report a further case said to be the twenty-second described, Haggani and Holti (1973) another and Monti (1973) yet another. Twersky et al. (1976) add two more cases. Six cases are known to Dr. C. Gray of Toronto General Hospital (personal communication, 1970). In the lung affected by systemic sclerosis the development of the alveolar cell carcinoma is preceded by the heaping up and proliferation of the alveolar epithelium, which is atypical and accompanied by stratification of the epithelium. Similar changes can be seen in fibrosing alveolitis. Holzmann and Frisch (1970) in 99 patients with scleroderma found 73 had malignancies, 34 in the lungs followed in order of frequency by skin, breast, uterus, stomach and small intestine. Romey and Moskowitz (1973) describe a case of scleroderma which developed reticulum cell sarcoma of the lungs. Fateh Moghandam et al. (1971) described a case in which Raynaud's phenomenon and scleroderma were followed by the development of myelomatosis. Long-standing scleroderma leading to carcinoma of the oesophagus, which was affected by the sclerosing process, was reported by Matzner et al. (1963) and by Kilton and Gottlieb (1971). Sandstrom (1976) recorded a case of sclerosis of oesophagus and lungs complicated by thymic lymphoepithelioma. Neto et al. (1968) describe a case of scleroderma of hands, arms and chest, which developed cancer of the underlying breast and Barlow (1939) a case of scleroderma in which an adrenal adenoma was found. In the South West Metropolitan Cancer Registry series were found 3 cases of long-standing scleroderma developing malignant disease up to 9 years after the onset of the skin disease. The cancer involved the pancreas, bronchus and the senile breast affected by scleroderma. Razis et al. (1959) found 3 cases of Hodgkin's disease developing in cases of scleroderma.

In contrast to such cases of long-standing scleroderma developing malignant disease there exist cases of malignant disease which develop scleroderma during the course of the former illness. Colomb et al. (1973) report patch-like scleroderma developing in the course of Hodgkin's disease of the stomach. Christiansen et al. (1956) described 4 patients with *localized* scleroderma and associated malignancy. In 2 cases adenocarcinoma of the breast and in one adenocarcinoma of the thyroid preceded the appearance of scleroderma. In one case scleroderma preceded the appearance of carcinoma of the ovary. In 8 cases *generalized* scleroderma was associated with malignancy. The cancer preceded the scleroderma by 4 months to 3 years in 4 cases. In one case the disease appeared simultaneously and in 3 the symptoms of cancer followed the appearance of scleroderma by one month to two years. Panizo et al. (1974) reported a similar association of scleroderma and ovarian cancer. Generalized scleroderma associated with the development of plasmocytoma was reported by Schnack and Stefenelli (1954). Scleroderma developing malignant carcinoid syndrome was reported by Hay (1964) and Asboe-Hansen (1959).

It appears, therefore, that in cases of long-standing scleroderma malignant disease, particularly of the lung, may develop. Since scleroderma and dermatomyositis appear to be the same condition this is no more than to be expected. As in the case of dermatomyositis in which the development of malignancy may precipitate the appearance of the former, so it appears that the development of malignancy may also precipitate the appearance of scleroderma. These observations suggest that the factor which causes scleroderma, namely limax amoebae infection, predisposes to malignant change.

12) Raynaud's phenomenon as a manifestation of malignancy

It has been seen that Raynaud's phenomenon is frequently a manifestation of collagen disease or rheumatoid arthritis. Hawley et al. (1967) reviewed the literature and described 6 cases, all women, in which malignant disease and Raynaud's phenomenon developed together. In one case Raynaud's phenomenon was associated with carcinoma of the antrum, the second had had a cholecystectomy previously and developed Raynaud's phenomenon in association with hypernephroma. Another patient had a cancer of the rectum removed ten years before and then developed Raynaud's phenomenon in association with cancer of the splenic flexure, a left ovarian cyst and primary carcinoma of the body of the uterus. A third patient

showed Raynaud's phenomenon and malignant ovarian cyst. A fourth woman developed Raynaud's phenomenon and cancer of the pancreas and/or ovary. A further patient developed Hodgkin's disease of the parotid and lung and later Raynaud's phenomenon and cryoglobulinaemia. Previously reported cases include Raynaud's phenomenon developing in association with carcinoma of the breast, stomach, oesophagus and colon and in association in one case with myelomatosis, cryoglobulinaemia and carcinoma of the lung. Palmer (1974) reports 3 cases of this association with reticulum cell sarcoma gastric cancer and abdominal cancer. In the author's series several cases of Raynaud's phenomenon with malignancy were found. In all such cases it seems that the development of malignancy results in the appearance of Raynaud's phenomenon, a manifestation of collagen and auto-immune disease.

13) (Peri) arteritis and malignant disease

(Peri-) arteritis may be found in association with malignant disease. Razis et al. (1959) report 2 cases of peri-arteritis with Hodgkin's disease and Hench et al. (1962) arteritis in 2 cases of malignant lymphoma. Necrotizing vasculitis associated with leukaemia, malignant lymphoma or multiple myelomatosis was described by Christiansen et al. (1967) and Sams et al. (1967). Scheuer-Karpin (1972) and Michlmayer et al. (1973) also mention arteritis as preceding the onset of malignant lymphoma. McCombs (1965) reviews 72 patients with vasculitis of which 12 had rheumatoid arthritis and 5 developed lymphoproliferative disease. Godeau et al. (1975) report two cases of peri-arteritis, one with bronchial carcinoma and the other with rectal carcinoma. Newcastle and Tom (1962) described a case of granulomatous angeitis of the central nervous system preceding the appearance of Hodgkin's disease and demyelination in anatomical relationship to the angeitis. Examples of periarteritis with Hodgkin's disease taken from a large collection of over 2,000 cases of lymphoma considered in the author's book (Wyburn-Mason, 1964) are the following: -

Case 97 Male. At the age of 22 years onset of seborrhoeic dermatitis, which persisted. Four years later swelling of the cervical nodes occurred following an attack of tonsillitis. Later lymph nodes in the axillae and the tonsils enlarged. Nodal biopsy showed Hodgkin's disease. The enlarged nodes disappeared spontaneously. After a further year he developed an acute illness with high swinging temperature, severe headaches, rigors, drenching night sweats, prostration and vomiting. Enlarged nodes reappeared in the neck and the spleen enlarged. Biopsy again showed Hodgkin's disease and the blood vessels showed peri-arteritis.

Case 98 In 1947 he suffered from bronchopneumonia and five weeks later developed pyrexia, sweating and pain in the left flank and shoulder and both big toes. The spleen was found palpable. A diagnosis of acute Hodgkin's disease was made. He died eight weeks after the pyrexial onset. At autopsy the mesentery was found almost solid with tumour tissue. The liver and spleen were enlarged. The spleen was adherent to all the organs around it and to the diaphragm. The pleura was thickened, the hilar nodes enlarged. *Tumours and swellings were found along the coronary vessels* and beneath the epithelium of the ureters.

Histology. The lymph node changes were those of acute Hodgkin's disease with no eosinophils, but marked proliferation of reticulum cells, macrophages and lymphocytes and plasma cells. The portal tracts were infiltrated with the same cells. The lungs showed thickened pleura, which contained many mononuclears and the alveoli thickened walls infiltrated with many lymphocytes. The bronchial walls were also infiltrated with lymphocytes. Many of the smaller arteries showed the changes of peri-arteritis.

Gerber et al. (1972) describe peri-arteritis associated with lymphatic leukaemia. Rouzaud et al. (1969) report a case of acute aleukaemic erythraemic monocytosis with diffuse arteritis. O'Neill (1961) refers to 2 cases, one in a woman who had peri-arteritis associated with recurrence of a cancer of the colon, which had been removed 9 years previously. The other showed peri-arteritis with a large bowel cancer.

It appears that peri-arteritis, a manifestation of collagen disease, may sometimes accompany malignant disease, especially lymphoma.

14) The relationship of rheumatoid arthritis and systemic lupus erythematosus to malignant lymphoma and carcinoma

That there may be a relationship between collagen and auto-immune disease, especially rheumatoid arthritis, and the subsequent development of cancer is shown by the condition of congenital or primary acquired agammaglobulinaemia in which both types of disease are abnormally frequent. Again, it has been shown that cases of disseminated eosinophilic collagen disease develop both leukaemias, lymphomas and cancers and the same applies to cases of dermatomyositis and scleroderma. Attention has been drawn to the fact that rheumatoid arthritis and/or Sjögren's syndrome, of which it is a part, may be complicated by the development of Waldenström's macroglobulinaemia and myelomatosis. Cases of Waldenström's macroglobulinaemia may subsequently develop lymphoma, leukaemia and/or carcinoma and cases of myeloma often develop carcinoma and/or leukaemia. Thus, it would be expected that in cases of rheumatoid arthritis and systemic lupus erythematosus there would be an increased tendency to the development of lymphomata and cancer. It will be recalled that, when a lymphoma, myelomatosis or leukaemia develops, RF, ANF and auto-antibodies tend to disappear from the serum and then serological evidence of pre-existing collagen and auto-immune disease may not be found in such cases. Furthermore, every gradation between the various forms of lymphoma and combinations of lymphoma with leukaemia exist, while clinically myelomata (plasmocytoma) appear to shade into various forms of lymphoma.

In Chapter X attention was drawn to the existence of a familial relationship between collagen and auto-immune disease, including rheumatoid arthritis, and cancer. Malignant disease and rheumatoid arthritis are so common that they are bound to be associated with one another frequently and this could be purely by chance. However, mention has been made in Chapter X that a number of authors have failed to establish a statistical relationship between the diseases, while others have found a high incidence of malignancy in cases of rheumatoid arthritis. Any statistics on such an association depend to a large extent on what is taken to constitute rheumatoid arthritis, *which in itself is only one manifestation of a generalized disease.* Also reference has been made already to the fact that attempts to correlate the occurrence of lymphomata and cancer with pre-existing rheumatoid arthritis by comparison of the incidence of malignancy in cases of rheumatoid arthritis as compared with controls not suffering from rheumatoid arthritis are quite unacceptable, since it is impossible to find controls unaffected with the causative organism of collagen and auto-immune disease. The high incidence of cancer in cases of rheumatoid arthritis is, however, shown by the author's geriatric series and the series of Strandberg and Jarl<w (1961), Gardner (1969) and Moesmann (1969) and of signs of

rheumatoid arthritis of varying degree m many cases of lymphoma and cancer in the author's large series of cancer cases.

A number of reports on the association of rheumatoid arthritis or systemic lupus erythematosus and lymphoma or cancer have appeared. The lymph nodes and spleen are frequently enlarged in the collagen diseases. Motulsky et al. (1952) described a series of cases in which the changes in the lymph nodes in cases of rheumatoid arthritis varied from reactive hyperplasia to giant follicular hyperplasia and closely resembled or were identical with the changes of lymphosarcoma, Hodgkin's disease or giant follicular lymphadenopathy. Harvey et al. (1954) in cases of systemic lupus erythematosus described lymph node enlargement which histologically looked like Hodgkin's disease or reticulosarcoma. In other cases it seems a true lymphoma has co-existed with one or other of the collagen diseases. Ogryzlo (1956) reports the presence of lupus erythematosus cells in the blood in cases of Hodgkin's disease. Lee (1955) described a case of systemic lupus erythematosus which developed acute myeloblastic leukaemia after a number of years. Sinclair and Cruikshank (1956) in a study of 16 cases of rheumatoid arthritis with extensive visceral involvement found one case with malignant lymphoma and another with carcinoma and chronic lymphatic leukaemia. Beickert (1958) describes the development of Hodgkin's disease in a case of systemic lupus erythematosus and Monto **(1961)** likewise the occurrence of lupus erythematosus cells in the blood in cases of Hodgkin's disease. Etcheverry et al. (1959) found that in 103 cases of lymphosarcoma 20 had polyarthritis and 2 of these were cases of rheumatoid arthritis. In 147 cases of Hodgkin's disease 8 had polyarthritis and one frank rheumatoid arthritis. In 40 cases of chronic lymphatic leukaemia 5 had arthralgias and one rheumatoid arthritis. The authors considered there was an association between lymphoma and rheumatoid arthritis. Sperling (1961) drew attention to a relationship between rheumatoid arthritis and malignant lymphoma. Hench et al. (1962) in reviewing 1,000 cases of lymphoma found significant rheumatic complaints, including rheumatoid arthritis, systemic lupus erythematosus and polyarteritis in many cases, and these were the presenting symptoms in 22 of the cases. Rheumatoid arthritis was diagnosed in 5 cases, systemic lupus erythematosus in 4, polyarteritis in 2 and rheumatoid spondylitis in 1. In one case Sjogren's syndrome was the first manifestation of any disease. Hargraves (1962) reported the occurrence of lupus erythematosus cells in the blood in a number of cases of Hodgkin's disease. Holman (1963) mentions that Dr. M.N. Hargraves of the Mayo Clinic had a collection of nearly 100 cases of collagen disease and malignant lymphoma occurring in the same patient. Mackenzie and Scherbel (1963) describe 18 cases of rheumatoid arthritis and two of systemic lupus erythematosus associated with cancer. These included one case of Hodgkin's disease and one of reticulosarcoma, while Moesmann (1969) records cases of rheumatoid arthritis followed by Hodgkin's disease and by myeloma or plasmocytoma. Cammarata et al. (1963) described 4 cases in which a lymphoma was associated with a collagen disease. In one case Hodgkin's disease and systemic lupus erythematosus were found together and lupus erythematosus cells were present in the blood, which showed an eosinophilia. In the second case a lymphosarcoma was present in a case of systemic lupus erythematosus, while in a third reticulosarcoma was associated with systemic lupus erythematosus, the case presenting as one of polyarthritis and in the fourth case rheumatoid arthritis and giant follicular lymphadenopathy occurred together, the rheumatoid arthritis being present for Ilf2 years before the lymphadenopathy appeared. These authors postulated some immunological abnormality

operating in the development of both diseases. Howqua and Mackay (1963) reported 2 cases. In the first, a case of lymphosarcoma, an atypical rash and evidence of liver involvement were present and the blood showed lupus erythematosus cells, RF and thyroid auto-antibodies. The second case of Hodgkin's disease exhibited an arthritis like rheumatoid arthritis and lupus erythematosus cells in the blood. Kataria and Rao (1964) described a case of polyarthritis and Hodgkin's disease occurring together. Macsween (1965) reported a case of a patient with XY/XXY/ XXXY chromosomes, Klinefelter's syndrome and normal intelligence in which rheumatoid arthritis developed and was followed by reticulum cell sarcoma. Wybum-Mason (1964) in a series of over 2,000 cases of reticulosis found 40 began as acute polyarthritis or rheumatoid arthritis. In 3 cases systemic lupus erythematosus was followed by Hodgkin's disease or malignant lymphoma. Scheuer-Karpin and d'Heureuse-Gerhardt (1965) mention the case of a woman aged 69 years who suffered from Hashimoto's thyroiditis for 8 years and then developed systemic lupus erythematosus and finally Hodgkin's disease and chronic lymphatic leukaemia. Scheuer-Karpin (1972) also mentions 2 cases of systemic lupus erythematosus with Hodgkin's disease in men of 24 and 41 years. Klingmtiller and Vorlaender (1965) describe 2 cases of systemic lupus erythematosus. In the first dermatomyositis was also present. The systemic lupus erythematosus began 12 years before the development of Hodgkin's disease. In the second case systemic lupus erythematosus was diagnosed and she later developed joint swelling and several years later Hodgkin's disease. Meyer zum Buschenfelde et al. (1965) also ::::tudied a case of systemic lupus erythematosus with lymphosarcoma. Bernard (1965) reported a case of acute lymphoblastic leukaemia in which complete remission was induced by mercaptopurine and 5 years later systemic lupus erythematosus developed. Napiorskowska (1966) described lupus erythematosus cells occurring in the blood in the course of Hodgkin's disease. McDonald and Hill (1967) also reported malignant lymphoma developing in cases of collagen disease. Deaton and Levin (1967) recorded a case of systemic lupus erythematosus in a boy present at least five and possibly fifteen years before the onset of acute myeloblastic leukaemia. Klein et al. (1974) describe Kaposi's sarcoma developing in systemic lupus erythematosus. Miller (1967) reports a number of cases in which "auto-immune disease" and malignant lymphoma occurred in the same patient. In three chronic lymphatic leukaemia and systemic lupus erythematosus, lymphosarcoma and rheumatoid arthritis and Hodgkin's disease and dermatomyositis occurred simultaneously. In the rest the two diseases occurred at different times.

They include Hodgkin's disease with systemic lupus erythematosus, Hodgkin's disease with discoid lupus erythematosus, reticulum cell sarcoma and Sjogren's syndrome, chronic lymphatic leukaemia and rheumatoid arthritis, reticulosarcoma and rheumatoid arthritis, follicular lymphosarcoma and systemic lupus erythematosus, and Hodgkin's disease and systemic lupus erythematosus. In this group of cases the interval between the appearance of the two diseases was 1-30 years. In 4 cases lymphoma occurred after and in 5 before the "auto-immune" disease. In one case Hodgkin's disease developed in the skin at the site of healed discoid lupus erythematosus. The author concludes that the same patients may be susceptible to the two types of disease which were not necessarily related. Oleinick (1967) quoted the case of a 44 year old woman with a seven year history of systemic lupus erythematosus who died of Hodgkin's disease and another case of systemic lupus erythematosus, who died six years later of reticulum cell sarcoma. In considering the relationship of the two diseases he

came to no definite conclusion. Nilsen et al. (1967) recorded the case of a 51 year old woman, who suffered from systemic lupus erythematosus for ten years before she developed lymphadenopathy and died two years later of Hodgkin's disease. An interesting observation was made in this case. All clinical and laboratory signs of systemic lupus erythematosus disappeared with the onset of Hodgkin's disease and none were found at autopsy. Fernandez-Herlihy and Kott (1967) report the case of a boy of 5 years, who developed migrating arthralgias, fever and haematuria found to be due to systemic lupus erythematosus. He was given plaquenil and prednisolone and improved, but a butterfly rash and mild episodes of generalized arthralgias persisted and later cranial neuropathy appeared. At the age of 15 years he developed lymphadenopathy, which on biopsy proved to be due to lymphosarcoma. In this case again all the laboratory tests for systemic lupus erythematosus reverted to normal with the onset of the lymphosarcoma. Schmidt and Gebhardt (1969) report the case of a 37 year old man who had suffered from discoid lupus for 10 years, and who developed Hodgkin's disease and then the lupus healed. Schaison et al. (1969) record the case of a woman of 21 years with acute lymphoblastic leukaemia treated with cortisone and 6-mercaptopurine, who 4 years later developed systemic lupus erythematosus. Haslock et al. (1970) in a series of 34 cases of rheumatoid arthritis with neuromuscular disorders record a case which developed lymphoma. Goldenburg et al. (1969) found that 1 of 32 patients with lymphoma had rheumatoid arthritis and report a case of reticulosarcoma with RF in the serum and a case of rheumatoid arthritis with positive RF in the serum and paraproteinaemia, which developed lymphosarcoma. Druet et al. (1969) in a long paper discuss the relationship of rheumatoid arthritis to chronic lymphatic leukaemia and reticuloses. They describe 7 cases of rheumatoid arthritis in whom chronic lymphatic leukaemia developed and compared the incidence of leukaemia in cases of rheumatoid arthritis and the general population. They conclude that the association was not fortuitous. They also reported several other cases. One, a woman of 36 years, developed carcinoma of the breast and at the age of 44 years rheumatoid arthritis and reticulosarcoma. In another case systemic lupus erythematosus with articular symptoms was followed by acute leukaemia. In a further case of seropositive rheumatoid arthritis with ANF and thyroid auto-antibodies in the blood developed what appeared to be Brill-Symmer's disease. In another case a woman developed subacute rheumatoid arthritis at the age of 64 years and at the age of 70 years a lymphoplasmocytic proliferation was present in the blood. Zawadski and Benedek (1969) report on 16 patients with rheumatoid arthritis and co-existent paraproteinaemia which developed malignant lymphosarcoma. Acute leukaemia developing in a 13 year old patient suffering from juvenile rheumatoid arthritis showing cystic osseous lesions was reported by Saatci and Pirner (1970). Garcin Morteo et al. (1971) described two cases with classical rheumatoid arthritis who developed chronic lymphatic leukaemia. . One showed lupus erythematosus cells ·and RF in the blood. The other had high titre of RF, hypergammaglobulinaemia, IgG Kappa type monoclonal paraproteinaemia and cryoglobulinaemia. Joint involvement preceded the blood changes by many years. The authors suggested that both the arthritis and the blood changes were due to the same cause. Cooper (1970) describes 2 cases of rheumatoid arthritis which developed reticulosarcoma. Smith et al. (1970) report 8 cases in which systemic lupus erythematosus and malignant lymphoma were associated. Sadiewicz et al. (1970) described a case of rheumatoid arthritis developing Hodgkin's disease and Abdala and Roland (1970) a case of rheu-

matoid arthritis developing Brill-Symmer's disease in the Argentine. Louyot et a!. (1971) report 2 cases of polyarthritis associated with malignancy. In one case of lymphosarcomatosis sero-negative polyarthritis developed 20 weeks after the onset and in the second acute polyarthritis with pyrexia developed followed by a cancer of the oesophagus. Cudworth and Ellis (1972) report a case of a woman of 79 years, who developed a maculo-papular rash, fever, weakness, lymphadenopathy due to Hodgkin's disease, hepatomegaly, an auto-immune haemolytic anaemia, blood eosinophilia and RF in high concentration and lupus erythematosus cells in the blood. Lipsmeyer (1972) reported a case of systemic lupus erythematosus treated with azathioprine, who developed cerebral lymphoma. Evers (1976) describes a case of rheumatoid arthritis developing vasculitis and lymphoma, Nilsen (1976) one of connective tissue disturbance developing Hodgkin's disease and Gumpel and Crow (1976) one of rheumatoid arthritis with ic'hthyosis followed by lymphoma, hepatomegaly and splenomegaly.

In the series from the South West Metropolitan Cancer Registry rheumatoid arthritis was followed by the development of reticulosarcoma in 5 cases, of malignant lymphoma in 1 case, of Hodgkin's disease in 3 cases, of chronic lymphatic leukaemia in 3 cases, of chronic myeloid leukaemia in 1 case, of acute lymphoblastic leukaemia in 2 cases, of acute monocytic leukaemia in 1 case and of erythromyeloblastic leukaemia in one case. One of these cases of acute lymphoblastic leukaemia was noteworthy. It occurred in a boy of 6 years, who one year before had developed juvenile rheumatoid arthritis. One case of rheumatoid arthritis with Hashimoto's thyroiditis developed malignant lymphoma; six cases of rheumatoid arthritis with long-standing diabetes and one case of rheumatoid arthritis with long-standing diabetes and pernicious anaemia

Addendum: Cohen, S.R., Landing, B.H., Isaacs, H., et al. Ann. Otol. Rhinol. Laryngol., 1978, 87, H. Supple. 52. 11. report the case of a soltary plasmocytoma of the larynx and upper trachea developing in a patient with systemic lupus erythematosus of nine years standing.
Addendum: Wallach, H.W., Arch. Intern. Med., 1977, 137, 532-535 reported 2 patients with locally advanced cancer of the breast treated with radio-therapy which was followed in a year by the lupus syndrome.

also ended in malignant lymphoma. Acute monocytic leukaemia developed in one case of systemic lupus erythematosus. In the author's series of cases of cancer rheumatoid arthritis, systemic lupus erythematosus and jor Sjogren's syndrome was followed by or associated with malignant lymphoma on numerous occasions.

In Chapter X consideration was given to the numerous papers in which the development of cancer, as opposed to lymphoma, in cases of rheumatoid arthritis is described. It was concluded that the incidence is probably high. Hollander et at. (1957) describe cases of rheumatoid arthritis which developed carcinoma of the stomach or prostate. Sperling (1961) draws attention to the occurrence of rheumatoid arthritis before or with cancer of the bronchus, carcinoid and other malignant tumours. Cobb (1967), in considering 583 cases of rheumatoid arthritis, found 15 died of cancer. Mackenzie and Scherbel (1963) describe 18 cases of rheumatoid arthritis in old people followed by cancer. These involved prostate (8 cases), breast (3), bladder (2), kidney (1), bronchus (1), colon (1), cervix (1), malignant hepatoma (1), Hodgkin's disease (1) and reticulosarcoma (1). Moesmann (1969) likewise reported rheumatoid arthritis in old subjects followed by cancer of pancreas, stomach, bronchus (3), breast (5), ovary (1), unknown primary (1), bladder (1), pleura (1), caecum (1), skin (1), uterus (2), malignant melanoma (1), Hodgkin's disease (1), plasmocytoma or myelomatosis (2). Siurala et al. (1965) in their 71 cases of collagen disease found one case with carcinoma of the colon. Karten and Bertfield (1962) described early rheumatoid arthritis preceding carcinoma of the bronchus. Strandberg and Jarlφv (1961), however, in the paper mentioned above found that 26 of 53 patients with rheumatoid arthritis developed cancer, lymphoma or leukaemia. They included reticulosarcoma (2), lymphosarcoma (1), myelomatosis (1), myelogenic

leukaemia (1), lymphatic leukaemia (1), cancer of the breast (1), uterine body (2), cervix (2), stomach (3), colon (1), bronchus (4), kidney (2), pleura (1), osteosarcoma of the tibia (1), sarcoma of the sacrum (1) and melanotic sarcoma of the jaw (1). Pallis and Scott (1965) describe rheumatoid arthritis followed by carcinoma of the stomach and Gardner's (1969) series will also be recalled. In all these series any form of benign or malignant tumour has been found to develop in cases of rheumatoid arthritis. Strandberg (1974) found that in a 10 year follow-up of 394 cases of rheumatoid arthritis 50 (13%) developed carcinoma. One of the author's patients suffering from rheumatoid arthritis had two children. The first died with bilateral retinoblastoma at the age of three years. The second is now sixteen years old and has juvenile rheumatoid arthritis and unilateral retinoblastoma. As regards systemic lupus erythematosus sometimes malignant tumours develop directly out of the lupus lesions. Thus, verrucose plaques of chronic discoid lupus erythematosus may develop into rodent ulcer or squamous cell carcinoma (Pringle, 1900; Beeson and Elbert, 1934; Salzburger and Wolf, 1940; Bechet (1942). Sklarz (1955), Simonelli (1971), Miezynska (1972) and Gwiezdzinski and Szyszymar (1972) describe cases of chronic discoid lupus erythematosus who developed a basal or squamous cell epithelioma in the scar. Rich (1951) described systemic lupus erythematosus associated with various malignant tumours, Lansbury (1953) a case in which testicular seminoma preceded the development of systemic lupus erythematosus. Heathfield and Williams (1960) mention a patient who suffered from systemic lupus erythematosus for 6 years, then developed fulminating dermatomyositis and later carcinoma of the bronchus. Mills (1963) mentions a case of systemic lupus erythematosus who was found at autopsy to have a meningioma. Miller (1967) reports cases of rheumatoid arthritis and systemic lupus erythematosus with solid tumours of the breast, genital tract, gastro-intestinal tract or of the head and neck. Rahn et al. (1966) describe a case of systemic lupus erythematosus and ovarian dysgerminoma occurring simultaneously. Removal of the tumour caused disappearance of both clinical and histological features of systemic lupus erythematosus. Sumner and Dwek (1976) report a very similar case with carcinoma of the lung. Tripp (1967) described a patient who developed vitiligo and then chronic discoid lupus erythematosus and later systemic sclerosis. Eleven years later a squamous carcinoma of one labium majus and leukoplakia of the other appeared. The liver was enlarged, lupus erythematosus cells and ANF were present in the blood and atrophy of the gastro-intestinal mucosa was present. Biopsy of the skin showed the changes of systemic lupus erythematosus. Sharland (1971) described a patient of 80 years who had a carcinoma of the colon removed 11 years previously and now had systemic lupus erythematosus. Joseph and Zarafonetis (1967) and Rotman et al. (1972) report the association of systemic lupus erythematosus and malignancy. Nyman (1972) described a case of rheumatoid arthritis with carcinoma of the bronchus and Manny et al. (1972) a case of systemic lupus erythematosus treated with azathioprine which developed a malignant melanoma. A case of disseminated eosinophilic colla- .gen disease developing carcinoma of the colon was reported by Boone (1969). In 1977 Mrs. Betty Hull of the American Lupus Society kindly supplied the author with the following information. Of 300 unselected patients suffering from systemic lupus erythematosus 14 developed malignant tumours of the uterus, 7 of the ovary, 5 of the pharynx, 1 each of parotid, vagina, rectum and skin of the temple.

In the South West Metropolitan Cancer Registry series there were 3 cases of systemic lupus erythematosus, all in females, in whom cancer of the cervix, kidney and bronchus later appeared. In the severe cases of rheumatoid arthritis cancer of practically every organ of the body was recorded as developing later. In a patient with rheumatoid arthritis and thyrotoxicosis multiple basal cell carcinoma was recorded and in a number of cases of rheumatoid arthritis with long-standing diabetes developed carcinoma of the senile breast.

Some cases appear very significant. In the Clinico-Pathological Conference held at the Royal Post-Graduate Medical School on 1.2.1965 there was reported the case of a 68 year old woman with an 8 years history of rheumatoid arthritis with Sjogren's syndrome and hypertension, but no symptoms of malignant disease. At autopsy there were found bilateral renal carcinomata of different types (hypernephroma and adenocarcinoma), a carcinoid tumour of the jejunum, a parasaggital meningioma of the left frontal lobe, a pituitary mucoid adenoma, an adenomatous colonic polyp, an endometrial polyp, myopathy and subacute cerebellar atrophy. In another case shown on 23.11.1966, a man, aged 49 years, developed rheumatoid arthritis, neuropathy and RF in the serum. Two years later he was found to have multiple polyposis of the colon and rectum, a malignant tumour in the first part of the duodenum and a polyp in the third part. One of the author's patients (Case XVI, 23), a woman aged 59 years, who had suffered from rheumatoid arthritis since the age of 40 years and had Sj5gren's syndrome, Hashimoto's thyroiditis and Paget's disease was found at autopsy to have five malignancies, of both ovaries, stomach and two colonic cancers. Such cases suggest strongly that rheumatoid disease is a premalignant condition.

Biebel et al. (1957) studying the Rose-Waaler test in 271 cancer patients found it positive in only 8 and 2 of those were suffering from rheumatoid arthritis. They found 70 per cent of 17 cases of cancer without rheumatoid arthritis showed a

375

positive Rose-Waaler test in the serum. It will be recalled that the presence of a malignancy in the body depresses the formation of RF and auto-antibodies if these have previously been present. Twomey et al. (1976) found that in 85 per cent of cancer cases RF was positive in certain circumstances, especially after treatment of the tumour, but its incidence in untreated cases was less. Burnham (1972) found ANF positive in 19 per cent of 432 patients with a variety of malignancies compared with 0.99 per cent of 201 blood donors. In the former there was no evidence of connective tissue disease, drug reactions or a family history of connective tissue disease. The author suggested that this might be used as a screening test for cancer. Zeromski et al. (1972) confirmed that 13 per cent of cases of malignant disease had ANF in the serum and suggested that in the absence of connective tissue disease a patient with ANF in the serum should be thoroughly examined for malignancy. Zeromski et al. (1975) found in 86 patients with lung cancer as compared with two series of control groups, that the incidence of auto-antibodies was significantly higher in the cancer cases, especially ANF, gastric parietal and smooth muscle antibodies. Whitehouse and Holborow (1971) found smooth muscle antibodies at a titre of 1/10 or more of 67.5 per cent of patients with cancer as compared with 20 per cent of controls. Yamamoto et al. (1970) in 74 cases of stomach cancer in Japanese in Hawaii found that the sera showed a higher incidence of thyroid auto-antibodies and RF and a lower incidence of ANF and gastric parietal cell auto-antibodies than normal controls.

Lansbury (1953) and Mackenzie and Scherbel (1963) have reported the condition of *carcinoma polyarthritis,* a condition indistinguishable from rheumatoid arthritis and associated with cancer, but in which the polyarthritis tends to be asymmetrical and of later onset in life. There is sparing of the wrists and fingers and nodules are absent. Joint manifestations preceded those of the neoplasm by an average of 10 months in 11 of 18 patients. RF was present in 1 of 18 cases. The arthritis responded to therapy. Courcy (1964) reported the condition in 5 per cent of cases of lung cancer. Scherbel et al. (1964) describe the case of a 42 year old man who developed rheumatoid arthritis with a strongly positive latex fixation test. The condition was well controlled under treatment for 4 years. He then developed an adenocarcinnoma of the bronchus and this was accompanied by a marked increase in the joint symptoms and titre of RF. The joint symptoms were unrelieved by intensive therapy until the time of his death 6 months later. Litwin et al. (1966) report a three year study of a 43 year old woman in whom the appearance of a carcinoma of the bronchus was accompanied by the development of rheumatoid arthritis with an uniquely high titre of RF in the blood and an eosinophil count of over 50 per cent. After resection of the lung lesion clinical remission of rheumatoid arthritis and rheumatoid nodules occurred and then eosinophilia and RF disappeared from the blood. There was a terminal relapse resulting in the return of RF in the blood. Mantovani and Netri (1973) report a similar case, Virschup and Sliwinski (1973) describe the case of a man of 52 years who developed subcutaneous rheumatoid nodules and polyarthritis in association with an acinar cell carcinoma of the pancreas. The arthritis did not respond to phenylbutazone, indomethacin or corticosteroids.

In conclusion, the evidence suggests a close relationship between rheumatoid arthritis, systemic lupus erythematosus and leukaemias, lymphomas, myelomatosis, benign tumours and cancer of any organ in some subjects. Rheumatoid arthritis and systemic lupus erythematosus, as do other manifestations of collagen disease, such as dermatomyositis or scleroderma, may pre-

-376-

cede by a long period, coincide with or follow the appearance of lymphoma or cancer. If rheumatoid arthritis is already present, the development of cancer may cause a severe exaggeration of the arthritis and a great increase in the titre of RF in the serum. Removal of the tumour may then cause amelioration in the joint symptoms. Since rheumatoid arthritis and other types of collagen disease appear to be due to infection with limax amoeba, which are present in large numbers in malignant tumours the simultaneous occurrence of the two conditions in one subject is readily explained.

15) Paget's disease of bone and malignancy

It appears that Paget's disease of bone is part of the collagen and auto-immune complex of diseases. It has been seen to be common over the age of 55 years. The relationship of Paget's disease to the later development of malignant tumours of bone is well established. Summey and Pressley (1946) suggested that it may occur in 2-4 per cent of cases of Paget's disease. Malignant change may appear after the disease has been present for many years. It often involves many bones at the same time, but only those affected by Paget's disease are liable to such a change. The disease appears responsible for all malignant bone tumours in later life. Most growths are osteogenic sarcomata, fibrosarcoma or chondrosarcoma, but giant-cell sarcoma or reticulosarcoma (Vignon et al., 1969) also occur. Myelomatosis is also well-known to develop in association with Paget's disease (Reich and Brodsky, 1948; Hanisch, 1950; Rosenkrantz et al., 1952; Layani et al., 1952; Hoo, 1954; Heilman, 1957; Rosenkrantz and Glickman, 1957; Serre and Simon, 1959; Klijn, 1961; Bedard and Uhthoff, 1964; Sherman, 1966; Scurr, 1972; Bouvenot et al., 1974. Grader and Moynihan (1961) reported a significant case of

Paget's disease in which both osteogenic sarcoma and multiple myeloma developed. Paget's disease with macroglobulinaemia was reported by Jacottet and Ramel (1965) and Osserman (1958) and plasma cell leukaemia associated with Paget's disease by Kassai et al. (1959).

While the relationship of Paget's disease to the development of sarcomatous change in bone or myelomatosis is well recognized, the disease may also be accompanied by the development of malignancy in extra-osseous tissues, though whether this is more frequent than in normal subjects is not clear. Thus, Davis (1960) described Paget's disease with Hodgkin's disease; Serre and Simon (1959) and Lauchlan and Walsh (1963) with reticulosarcomatosis; Duverne et al. (1967) with lymphoma; Cazeilles et al. (1953) with chronic lymphatic leukaemia; Kintner (1951) with both sarcoma of bone and a malignant mixed salivary gland tumour; Turner and Nigrisoli (1957) with sarcoma of bone and carcinoma of both oesophagus and prostate. Paget's disease with underlying intracranial glioma was reported by Wolfe and Black (1941), Estridge (1950), Gal (1957) and Legre et al. (1959). Paget's disease with pituitary tumour was described by Pond (1940); with thyroid carcinoma and lymphatic leukaemia by Varja et al. (1962); with parotid gland tumour by Del Castillo and Trucco (1959); with salivary gland tumour of the middle ear by Novak (1947); with hyperparathyroidism due to parathyroid adenoma by Martin et al. (1964) and others; with epithelioma of the bladder by Trabucco and Marquez (1947); with epidermoid carcinoma of the maxilla by Szlezak and Przynora (1957); with carcinoma of the colon (4 cases) by Shanbrom (1963), who reviewed other reported cases; and with carcinoma of the bronchus by Stalewski et al. (1965) Wilmer and Sherman (1966) record the association of Paget's disease with reticulasarcoma of bone and other tissues (2 cases), with multiple myeloma (I case) and

Addendum: Carassone, Y., Bonvenot, G., Gastant, J.A. and Sebahour, G. The association of myeloma and Paget's disease. Ann. Med. Interne., 1979; 130, 177-184, remark on the frequent association of Paget's disease and myeloma in recent reports and emphasize that the former may also be associated with macroglobulinaemias or other monoclonal gammapathies.

with two cases each of carcinoma of the prostate, colon and kidney and one each of carcinoma of the breast and bronchus.

Of 150 consecutive cases of Paget's disease studied by the author (Wyburn-Mason, 1964) 2 had bony sarcomata, 2 generalized lymphosarcoma, 1 acute myeloid leukaemia, 1 both carcinoma of the bronchus and of the bladder and there were single cases of carcinoma of the oesophagus, squamous carcinoma of the pyriform fossa and carcinoma of the bronchus, stomach, colon, rectum and kidney. In the author's series of cases of Paget's disease, described in a previous section, one patient with Hashimoto's thyroiditis and Paget's disease developed melanoma of the eye and reticulosarcoma of thyroid and lung. Another case of Paget's disease of the vertebrae and skull developed a cerebral glioma underlying the affected skull. In another case an adenomatous polyp of the colon was found and yet another case complicated by rheumatoid arthritis developed carcinoma of the pancreas. In a further case bilateral ovarian cysts appeared and one of these was malignant; another had multiple rodent ulcers of the trunk; yet another developed carcinoma of the bronchus; another case of Paget's disease with rheumatoid arthritis was found to have a benign adenoma of the bronchus and yet another carcinoma of the prostate.

In cases at the South West Metropolitan Cancer Registry 37 were found in which Paget's disease was associated with malignancy. Of these 4 were bone sarcomata, 2 reticulosarcomata, 1 Hodgkin's disease, 1 lymphoblastic leukaemia and 1 multiple myelomatosis. There were 4 cases of cancer of the bronchus, 2 of the oesophagus, 2 of the stomach, 1 of the gall bladder, 2 of the pancreas, 5 of the large intestine, 1 of the kidney, 5 of the prostate, 2 of the bladder, 3 of the female breast and 1 of the nostril.

While it is conceivable that, since both cancer and Paget's disease are common in later life, the association of extra-osseous cancers and Paget's disease could be mere chance, yet a number of the cases described would seem of significance. Thus, Kintner's case of Paget's disease developing both sarcoma of bone and a malignant mixed salivary gland tumour and the case of Paget's disease developing both sarcoma of bone and carcinoma of oesophagus and prostate would seem to indicate that the existence of Paget's disease was related aetiologically both to the bony tumour and the accompanying extra-osseous tumours. Again, since myelomatosis and macroglobulinaemia are regarded as related to Paget's disease and myelomatosis and macroglobulinaemia are histologically and clinically related to malignant lymphoma, the number of cases of lymphoma and leukaemia reported as complicating Paget's disease of bone would suggest that the two diseases are related. Also of significance is the development of glioma of the brain in the neighbourhood of Paget's disease of the overlying skull, which again suggests an aetiological relationship between the two. It would seem highly probable that in many cases the occurrence of extra-osseous cancers in association with Paget's disease is not fortuitous and that the probable factor causing the appearance of Paget's disease namely limax amoebae infection, is responsible for the malignant change in bone and also for the leukaemia, myeloma, lymphoma and cancer with which Paget's disease may be associated.

16) Fibrosing alveolitis and malignant change

Collagen disease may produce various changes in the lung ranging from nodule formation to fibrosing alveolitis. Haddad and Massaro (1968) described the atypical epithelial proliferation seen in the air spaces in cases of fibrosing alveolitis with the appearance of cuboidal and columnar epithelium, squamous metaplasia or stratification and then malignant change. Histologically fibrosing alveolitis appears to be closely similar *to* the lung changes in systemic sclerosis and both to predispose to malignant change. Arnoff et al. (1955) describe a case of rheumatoid arthritis with fibrosing alveolitis who developed squamous carcinoma of the lung. Spain (1957) and Lee and Brain (1962) also described similar cases. In the 8 cases of fibrosing alveolitis of Haddad and Massaro (1968) 3 developed carcinoma, either peripheral or central, 2 being peripheral-an adenocarcinoma and an epidermoid carcinoma, and a third an oat-cell carcinoma. Fox and Risdon (1968) report 2 cases of fibrosing alveolitis, one of which was associated with rheumatoid arthritis and which developed malignant pulmonary adenomata. The other developed bronchial carcinoma. The author had similar cases in his series. Drissen and Scherpenisse (1970) describe fibrosing alveolitis in two brothers, who both died of alveolar cell carcinoma. A cousin also suffered from fibrosing alveolitis. Lutwyche (1976) describes a similar case. Haddad and Massaro (1968) conclude that fibrosing alveolitis is a premalignant condition. Meyer and Liebow (1965) point out that fibrosis of the lung is often associated with proliferation of the epithelium leading to malignant change. Rheumatoid arthritis, scleroderma and other collagen disease with the formation of rheumatoid nodules are among the causes of fibrosis.

Scadding (1967) described a case of Hodgkin's disease developing in the mediastinal lymph nodes and infiltrating the lung supervening on a case of antecedent fibrosing alveolitis. Andret al. (1967) also report a case of Hodgkin's disease treated for 6 years, who died with fibrosing alveolitis (? due to Endoxan). In a case demonstrated in a Medical Staff Round at Hammersmith Hospital Professor Scadding also mentioned a case of fibrosing alveolitis which developed chronic lymphatic leukaemia. In the South West Metropolitan Cancer Registry series was recorded a case of fibrosing alveolitis developing generalized lymphosarcomatosis after 15 months. Holt et al. (1970) describe a patient which presented with fibrosing alveolitis and who developed myelomatosis. In the author's series a number of cases of fibrosing alveolitis with or without other signs of collagen and auto-immune disease developed lymphoma or malignancies.

Since fibrosing alveolitis is a collagen and auto-immune disease, its presence seems to predispose to the development of lung cancer and lymphomata.

17) Lesions of the skin in internal malignant disease

In Chapter II consideration was given to the skin lesions which may occur in various collagen and auto-immunne diseases, that is those due to limax amoebae infections. These included pruritus, eczema, urticaria, ichthyosis acquisita, psoriasis, parapsonasts, dermatitis herpetiformis, lupus erythematosus, pemphigus, papular and annular eruptions, alopecia areata and universalis, light sensitivity, dermatomyositis, vitiligo, melanoderma, acanthosis nigricans, figurate erythema and purpura.

In cases of malignant lymphoma and leukaemias the skin may exhibit disturbances months or years before the appearance of specific tumours or blood changes. In the case of chronic lymphatic leukaemia reported by Pophristov and Cesmedziev (1959) the patient, aged 62 years, had suffered from pruritus, lichenification and hyperpigmentation since the age of 20 years. Parapsoriasis preceded Hodgkin's disease and reticulosarcoma by 18 years in a case reported by Kawada (1969). In the course of Hodgkin's disease it has been stated that 2o-40 per cent of patients exhibit symptoms referable to the skin (Hoster and Dratman, 1948).

Addendum: Horton, L.W.L., Chappell, A.G. and Powell, D.E.R. (Brit. J. Dis. Chest., 1977, 71, 44) report a case of fibrosing alveolitis with Hodgkin's disease.
Addendum: Cryptogenic fibrosing alveolitis and lung cancer Turner-Warwick, M,. Lebowtz M. Burrows B., Johnson A. Thorax, 1980 35/7 496-499 Of 205 cases of cryptogenic fibrosing alveolitis 12.9% died of cancer of the lung which is significantly higher than the number for controls matched for age and sex.
Addendum: Carcinoid tumour of the thymus. A clincio-pathologic report of 7 cases wth a review of the literature. Wick MR, Scott RE, Li Cy, Carney JA. Mayo. Clin. Proc. 1980 55/4 246-254.

The skin lesions associated with lymphoma and leukaemia include:-

1) Pruritus, local, segmental or general (Boyd, 1950).

2) Urticarial wheals, which may appear several years before other manifestations.

3) A localized or generalized brown pigmentation or vitiligo.

4) Toxic erythemas, which may be generalized (homme rouge).

5) Figurate erythemas (erythema marginatum or gyratum repens) (Balus and Gogonea, 1971; Summerley, 1964).

6) A macular, scarlatiniform or morbilliform eruption.

7) Eczema, seborrhoeic eczema.

8) Psoriasis, parapsoriasis.

9) Dermatitis herpetiformis.

10) Papules, vesicles, bullae, licheniform eruptions, cheiropompholyx and impetiginous lesions.

11) Lupus erythematosus.

12) Pemphigus and pemphigoid lesions.

13) The lesions of dermatomyositis.

14) Acanthosis nigricans.

15) Ichthyosis acquisita.

16) Light sensitivity (Wyburn-Mason, 1964). (Compare disseminated lupus erythematosus and dermatomyositis).

In malignant disease other than lymphomata and leukaemias skin lesions may also occur. Reference to these has been made by Rothman (1925), Becker et al. (1942), Wiener (1947), Peterkin and McMillan (1959), Sneddon (1963) and Boyd (1964). Again skin lesions may be present long before signs of cancer are manifest. Such lesions include:-

1) Simple pruritus.

2) Prurigo-like eruptions with hyperpigmentation.

3) Bullous erythema multiforme.

4) Eczematous rashes.

5) Figurate erythema (erythema marginatum or gyratum repens).

6) Erythema multiforme (Davis, 1922; Urbach, 1942).

7) Typical dermatitis herpetiformis.

8) Lupus erythematosus.

9) Exfoliative dermatitis (McGaw and McGovern, 1956).

10) Generalized urticaria (Davis, 1922; Urbach, 1942).

11) Purpura or purpuric dermatitis with widespread necrosis.

12) Psoriasis (Wiener, 1947) or parapsoriasis.

13) Seborrhoeic dermatitis or warts (Gougerat and Duperrat, 1942; Jousserand et al., 1948).

14) Acanthosis nigricans.

15) Leucoderma and melanoderma.

16) Pyoderma gangrenosum (Jablonska et al., 1967).

Some of these skin lesions persist even after X-irradiation or removal of the tumours. Others, however, disappear. The skin shows well-marked eosinophilia in these conditions.

Among the author's experience are the following cases:- a case of long-standing eczema in a patient who developed both carcinoma of the bronchus and bladder; and a patient with severe long-standing eczema, who developed carcinoma of the body of the uterus. Another woman aged 48 years had been subject all her life to urticarial rashes when excited. The skin showed a marked sensitivity to sunlight. She had also developed dermatitis from contact with rubber and with her suspenders. Two years before being seen large bullous eruptions appeared on the hands and feet and her nails were affected. This lasted a month and recurred again after a year and during the second attack she developed a black mole on the inner side of her heel, which proved to be a melanotic sarcoma.

The following case reports are taken from the author's book (Wyburn-Mason, 1964):-

Addendum: Cairns et al., (Brit. med. J., 1978, ii, 474) report 2 cases of Henoch- Schtinlein purpura with polyarthritis who later developed squamous carcinoma of the bronchus. Maurice, T.R. and also Hoffbrand (Ibid p. 831) report similar cases clearing after tumour resection.

Table XXIV Skin rashes with leukemia

Case XXIV, 1   Male, aged 20 years at onset, he had an attack of *dermatitis*, which recurred at iiTt'gl.llar intervals, without cause, over the next 19 years. A year after the onset he suffered an attack of *polyarthritis* lasting six months and 5 years later he had an attack of enteritis, which recurred over a year and for which no obvious cause was found. At the end of 19 years he developed acute myeloid leukaemia.

Case XXIV, 2   Male, aged 25 years, he began to suffer from severe *seborrhoeic dermatitis* which persisted for 2 years when a diagnosis of chronic myeloid leukaemia was made.

Case XXIV, 3   Male, aged 26 years. He began to suffer from *chronic seborrhoeic dermatitis*, which persisted for 8 years when a diagnosis of chronic lymphatic leukaemia was made.

Case XXIV, 4   Male, aged 20 years at the onset of an itching rash on the penis, later affecting the face and hands. The glans penis sloughed. Three months later the tonsils and cervical lymph nodes enlarged and a blood count showed the presence of chronic myeloid leukaemia.

Case XXIV, 5   Male, aged 45 years when he developed bouts of *urticaria* and then an attack of herpes zoster. A year later he had an attack of "influenl.al pneumonia", which recurred over the next ten months, the last attack being followed by a sore throat, an *erythematous* rash, swelling of a lymph node below the angle of the jaw and pain and swelling over the left scapula. A blood count now showed the changes of acute lymphatic leukaemia.

Table XXV Skin rashes with lymphoma

Case XXV, 1   Male, aged 30 years, when he developed *cheiropompholyx*, which persisted and this was followed by the development of sweating, tachycardia, loss of weight and a year later the signs of lymphosarcoma of the mediastinum appeared.

Case XXV, 2   Male, aged 31 years, when he developed *parapsoriasis*, which was followed by chronic lymph node enlargement and after by slight general malaise and indigestion. Nine months after the onset enlarged lymph nodes were found in the left groin, which on biopsy showed the changes of Hodgkin's disease.

Case XXV, 3   Female, aged 26 years. Onset with *cheiropompholyx* and marked *generalized pruritus* with the appearance of *urticarial* wheals. This was followed by sweating and "anxiety symptoms". Three years later she developed enlarged cervical lymph nodes. Biopsy showed the changes of Hodgkin's disease.

Case XXV, 4   At the age of 40 years he developed *dermatitis* of the hands and feet, which persisted through the rest of his life. He became tired and suffered repeated bouts of vomiting, pyrexia, profuse sweating and the cervical lymph nodes enlarged. He died a year later. Autopsy showed the changes of acute Hodgkin's disease.

Case XXV, 5   Male, aged 20 years at the onset of an irritating *dryness of the skin*, which became so severe as to constitute *ichthyosis acquisita*. This persisted and later patchy *erythema* appeared in various parts of the body. Four years later he began to lose weight and developed oedema of the left side of the face, ann and leg and enlarged lymph nodes in the left groin. Biopsy showed the changes of Hodgkin's disease.

—381—

Table XXV (continued)

Case **XXV**, 6   Male, aged 28 years at the onset of *seborrhoeic dermatitis,* which persisted. Four years later the cervical lymph nodes swelled following an attack of tonsillitis and enlarged nodes later appeared in the axillae. Biopsy showed the changes of Hodgkin's disease. The enlarged nodes disappeared spontaneously. A year later he developed an acute illness with a high swinging temperature, severe headaches, rigors, drenching night sweats, prostration and frequent vomiting. Enlarged nodes reappeared in the neck and the spleen also enlarged. Nodal biopsy again showed the changes of Hodgkin's disease and the blood vessels showed marked periarteritis.

Case **XXV**, 7   Male, at the age of 20 years onset of *chronic eczema,* which showed a marked exacerbation 10 years later. After a further year he developed recurrent *chronic conjunctw!tzs.* Aged 31 years the cervical lymph nodes enlarged and biopsy showed the changes of Hodgkin's disease.

Case **XXV**, 8   Male, aged 32 years at onset of *seborrhoeic dermatitis and psortaslS,* which persisted. A year later he had two attacks of painless jaundice of toxic type with pyrexia. The psoriasis persisted and became extremely severe when 9 years after the onset of the dermatitis he developed a generalized lymphadenopathy. Biopsy showed the changes of Hodgkin's disease.

Case **XXV**, 9   Male, aged 35 years. He gave a 16 year history of *eczema* of the arms and hands and for the last 2 years of the legs also, when he developed acute pneumonic symptoms. Five months later abdominal pains and ascites developed followed by enlarged cervical lymph nodes. Biopsy showed the changes of Hodgkin's disease.

Case **XXV**, 10   Male, aged 26 years at the onset of *swelling* and *pruritus of the right leg.* This was followed by generalized boils and by the appearance of blepharitis and six months later of folliculitis of both legs, which became severe enough to require hospitalization. Eleven months after the onset he developed *coryza* and "toxic" *jaundice* followed by swelling of the right cervical and hilar lymph nodes and oedema of the right leg. Biopsy showed the changes of Hodgkin's disease.

Case **XXV**, 11   Male, aged 20 years when he developed *seborrhoeic dermatitis* and patches of *ichthyosis acquisita* appeared and persisted. A year later the inguinal nodes became swollen and tender and later the left leg swelled and he developed diarrhoea. This was followed by generalized lymphadenopathy. Biopsy of a node showed the changes of a reticulosarcoma.

Case **XXV**, 12   Male, aged 30 years when he began to suffer from *recurrent boils* which persisted for the next 3 years. At the end of this period the axillary lymph nodes enlarged accompanied by sweating and by pyrexia of 103°F. The lymphadenopathy disappeared spontaneously. From that time he was subject to periodk attacks of diarrhoea with pale watery stools and 18 months later the axillary lymph nodes again enlarged and the spleen and liver were also found enlarged. Biopsy showed the changes of Hodgkin's disease.

Case **XXV**, 13   Male, aged 28 years, when *eczema* appeared over the body, arms and legs and a year later the axillary and inguinal lymph nodes enlarged and an impetiginous area appeared over various parts of the body. Biopsy showed the changes of Hodgkin's disease.

Case **XXV**, 14   Male, aged 29 years at the onset of *dermatitis* of the legs and thighs and later of the forearms, which persisted. Three years later the left inguinal nodes enlarged and biopsy showed the changes of Hodgkin's disease.

Case **XXV**, 15   Male, aged 26 years when he gave a four year history of *giant urticaria* appearing at intervals. He then developed loss of energy, night sweats, backache and fever and enlarged nodes appeared in the neck. Biopsy showed the changes of Hodgkin's disease.

Table XXV (continued)

Case XXV, 16   Male, aged 50 years. From the age of 21 years he had suffered from *chronic irritation, desquamation and generalized erythema of the skin of the whole body.* Biopsy of the skin now showed thinning of the epidermis and infiltration of the dermis by lymphocytes, plasma cells and eosinophils. A blood count was normal. Six months later blisters and tender lumps appeared in the scalp and other parts of the skin, became inflamed and more scaly and then enlarged lymph nodes appeared in the neck, axillae and groins. The condition was diagnosed as *exfoliative erythroderma* with thickening, oedema and infiltration of the skin. The condition persisted. Two years later the white blood count was 11,600 per cu. mm., of which 12 per cent were eosinophils. The lymph nodes now enlarged and biopsy showed the changes of Hodgkin's disease. A chest X-ray revealed diffuse streaking of the lung fields considered to be due to involvement of the peribronchial lymphatics.

Case XXV, 17   Male, aged 22 years when he developed furunculosis of the axillae. A year later enlarged nodes appeared in the left axilla and regressed spontaneously. After a further two years he burned his right foot. This was followed by *dermatitis* of the foot and later of the face. This was impetiginous in type. Soon afterwards he dew-loped abdominal pain and vomiting, which died down spontaneously. Three years later the left axillary nodes again enlarged and biopsy showed the changes of Hodgkin's disease.

Dermatitis herpetiformis and cancer

Sneddon (1963), Bayo (1964) and Reinert Dilthey (1970) refer to cases of dermatitis herpetiformis associated with neoplasia, including lymphoma, cancer of the bronchus, stomach, kidney, pancreas, ovary, uterus, labia, chorionepithelioma or hydatidiform mole. Gjore and Nordoy (1970) describe two cases of dermatitis herpetiformis and steatorrhoea, one of which developed lymphom of the jejunum and one carcinoma of the kidney. Fry (1971) and Goodwin and Fry (1973) mention a patient with dermatitis herpetiformis and enteropathy who developed lymphoma of the small bowel. Johnson (1965) recorded a case of mycosis fungoides with dermatitis herpetiformis or pemphigus. Mansson (1971) reported on 9 patients with dermatitis herpetiformis examined for gastro-intestinal abnormalities, of whom 5 developed malignancies during 3 years observation. The malignant change was not confined to those commonly associated with coeliac disease. Fowler and Thomas (1976) describe a case of dermatitis herpetiformis which developed lymphoma of the skin and fibrosing alveolitis. Balus and Gogonea (1971) also record dermatitis herpetiformis with various internal malignancies and regard it as a paraneoplastic condition. Its presence may lead to the diagnosis of a clinically silent malignancy.

Ichthyosis acquisita and cancer

Ichthyosis acquisita has been regarded as a paraneoplastic phenomenon (Welch and Epstein, 1952, Bureau et al., 1958; Steva novic et al., 1960, Leading Article, Lancet, 1961, ii, 1203; Brun et al., 1965; Michel et al., 1970; Dugois et al., 1970). It is most frequently found in cases of Hodgkin's disease (26 of 32 cases), but may occur with any type of malignancy. Michel et al. (1970) reported a case of ichthyosis acquisita which developed squamous carcinoma of the right temple and bronchial carcinoma. Barnes (1974) described a similar case. Rusciani and Amerio (1971) reported the association of the skin lesion with carcinoma of the stomach. Brookes and Harrington (1977) report a patient with malabsorption and subtotal villous atrophy of the jejunum responding to a gluten-free diet, who relapsed and developed generalized ichthyosis and finally reticulosarcoma in the mesentery. In the author's large series of cancer cases ichthyosis acquisita was often found when sought, especially in cases of advanced cancer. In one case the condition preceded by many years the development of carcinoma of the colon (Case XVI, 43). It was shown that the administration of copper sulphate or bile salts to these cases caused the skin lesion to disappear rapidly. It is presumably a manifestation of rheumatoid disease, which is uncovered by or precedes the appearance of malignancy.

Vitiligo and hyperpigmentation (leucoderma and melanoderma) and cancer

Leucoderma and melanoderma appear to be associated with cancer in some subjects. Stahano (1933) described vitiligo as common in cases of cancer of the vulva. Franklin (1960) reported vitiligo and melanoderma associated with Hodgkin's disease and visceral cancer. Tripp (1967) described a patient who developed vitiligo and then chronic discoid lupus erythematosus and later systemic sclerosis. Eleven years later a squamous carcinoma of one labia majus and leukoplakia of the other appeared. The liver was enlarged, lupus erythematosus cells and ANF were present in the blood with atrophy of the gastrointestinal mucosa. Biopsy of the skin showed the changes of lupus erythematosus. A patient with vitiligo who developed malignant melanoma of the skin was reported by Balabanov et al. (1969), Fodor and Bodrogi (1975) and Gregor (1976) and others are mentioned in Leading Article (Lancet, 1971, 2, 1298). In two of the author's cases of cancer (Cases XVI, 75 and VII, 20) patches of melanoderma appeared years before the appearance of cancer. The first case developed cancer of the pancreas and the second lymphosarcoma. Such pigmentary disturbances 'lay, therefore, be regarded as paraneo-astic in nature. Their occurrence years

before the appearance of malignancy suggests that pre-existing collagen and auto-immune disease predisposes to malignancy.

Acanthosis nigricans and malignant disease

In about 50 per cent of cases of acanthosis nigricans developing later in life and even in some juvenile cases followed for some years malignant disease may develop. (For a review see Curth et al., 1962). This commonly involves the stomach, but may affect almost any other organ, especially intra-abdominal, or the growth may be a sarcoma, Hodgkin's disease (Ackerman and Lantis, 1967), lymphosarcoma, choriocarcinoma or pinealoma (Brown et al., 1961). In one case in the author's series (Case X, 23) acanthosis nigricans preceded the diagnosis of chronic lymphatic leukaemia by 10 years. In other cases acanthosis nigricans may be associated with a pituitary tumour of any type (Brown et al., 1966) or an adrenocortical tumour or hyperplasia producing Cushing's syndrome (Robinson and Tasker, 1947; Rothman, 1954; Curth et al., 1967; Wheeler, 1971). In most instances the two conditions occur synchronously, but in about one fifth of the reported cases the skin lesions antedate the malignancy by several years (up to 18 years in one reported case) and in the author's own experience by 10 years in a case of pituitary tumour and 7 years in a case of pancreatic tumour. In another fifth of the cases the skin changes develop after the cancer has been detected. Occasionally the skin changes may disappear after removal of the cancer and recur with recurrence of the latter.

The author has observed three cases of acanthosis nigricans, one case as mentioned associated with chronic lymphatic leukaemia, one with carcinoma of the stomach and one with carcinoma of the ovary, in all of which RF and other auto-antibodies were found in the serum. A number of cases have been described in which the mother of a patient suffering from the

Addendum: Another case of vitiligenous achromia developing malignant melanoma was reported by Perrot, H., Ortonna, J.P. and Schmitt, D. (Arch. Dermatol. Res., 1977, 357·273).
Addendum: Albert D.M., Sober, A.J., Fitzpatrick, T.b. Arch. Ophthalmol (Chicago), 1978, 96, 2081·4 described two patients with vitiligo, malignant melanoma and uveitis.

benign type of acanthosis had died of cancer some years after the birth of the offspring.

The relationship of acanthosis nigricans to tumour formation is exactly parallel to that of dermatomyositis and cancer. A number of authors have suggested that a common cause for acanthosis nigricans and tumour formation exists and this is transmitted transplacentally. Since the skin lesion appears to be a manifestation of collagen and auto-immune disease and may precede the development of malignancy by many years, it further suggests that the former condition predisposes to cancer or benign tumour formation.

Pemphigus and pemphigoid and malignancy

Pemphigoid is a senile form of dermatitis herpetiformis and may occur in cases of carcinoma of varying sites, such as pancreas, breast, bronchus or malignant melanoma (Boyd, 1964; Kilby, 1965; Krain, 1974; Krain and Bierman, 1974). Pemphigus vulgaris preceded Kaposi's sarcoma in a patient reported by Rosenmann (1966). Tagami et al. (1976) describe a case of peculiar pemphigoid like dermatitis herpetiformis, which occurred with myasthenia and malignant lymphoma.

Photosensitivity and malignant disease

Photosensitivity is a feature of dermatomyositis and disseminated lupus erythematosus. In some cases it may precede the appearance of lymphoma or leukaemia. This is exemplified by the following cases Table XXVI:-

Table XXVI

Case XXVI, 1   Male, aged 32 years when he experienced a severe reaction on the face and hands following exposure to the sun. This recurred every summer for the rest of his life. The affected skin showed erythema, scaling of the face and tender induration of the neck. Ten years later following an attack he experienced prolonged malaise and six months afterwards cough, headache, pyrexia, aching in the limbs, lassitude and a purulent discharge from the gums appeared. A blood count showed the changes of acute myeloid leukaemia.

Case XXVI, 2   Male. He had been subject to swollen cervical lymph nodes in the neck as a child and these were treated by X-rays at the age of 17 years. Soon afterwards he continued to develop severe solar dermatitis from which he suffered every spring for some years. At the age of 29 years seborrhoeic dermatitis appeared and soon after oedema of the ankles. A year later he developed pains in the neck, pyrexia, exertional dyspnoea and the spleen was found enlarged. A blood count showed the changes of aleukaemic leukaemia.

Case XXVI, 3   Male, aged 32 years when, following exposure to the sun, he developed alopecia arcata and acute eczema of the head and neck lasting 3 months. This recurred after a further 3 months and was accompanied by pyrexia. The eczema was now of seborrhoeic type and became generalized. A white blood count showed 12,400 cells per cu. mm. of which 21.5 per cent were eosinophils. The cervical lymph nodes now enlarged. Biopsy showed hyperplasia with active lymphoid centres. Many of the sinuses were filled with eosinophil cells. There was no evidence of Hodgkin's disease. The seborrhoeic dermatitis and the lymph node enlargement regressed, but two years later the skin lesions reappeared and painless enlarged lymph nodes were present in the groin. Biopsy of a node now showed the changes of Hodgkin's disease. A white blood cell count showed 10,000 per cu. mm. 64 per cent being small lymphocytes, 12 per cent large lymphocytes and 1 per cent lymphoblasts, that is the changes of chronic lymphatic leukaemia.

385

Addendum: Maddin W.S. and Wood W.S. Multiple Keratoacanthomas and squamous cell carcinomas occurring at psoriatic treatment sites. J. Cutaneous Pathol. 1979, 6, 96-100.

Balding and malignancy

Generalized or localised baldness (alopecia areata) may be a feature of collagen and auto-immune disease and may be a feature also of reticuloses. Bleehen (1963) reports a case with generalized thickening of the skin, generalized alopecia, enlarged axillary and inguinal lymph nodes, oedema of the left arm and a high eosinophilia in the blood. Biopsy of a lymph node showed it to be markedly infiltrated with plasma cells. Personal cases are exemplified by the following:-

Table XXVII

Case XXVII, 1   Male, aged 35 years when there was a sudden appearance of marked alopecia followed two years later by generalized lymph node enlargement. Nodal biopsy showed the changes of Hodgkin's disease.

Case XXVII, 2   Male. *At* the age of 20 years he developed over the course of one year a marked alopecia and in the next six months the cervical nodes swelled. He died following a haematcmesis. Autopsy showed the presence of a lymphosarcoma of the stomach.

Case XXVII, 3   Male, aged 22 years. He developed a pyrexial illness in which the hair came out in patches. One month later there was enlargement of the submandibular lymph nodes which persisted. Biopsy showed the changes of Hodgkin's disease.

See also Case XXVI, 3.

Reticulohistiocytosis (lipoid dermato-arthritis or lipoid rheumatism) and malignancy

This skin lesion is usually preceded by RF positive rheumatoid arthritis in two thirds or more of cases or arthritis may occur with or after the rash. It is considered by Rooney et al. (1975) and Hall-Smith (1976). In 25 per cent of cases of the skin disease and arthritis an associated neoplasm is found. In the case of Hall-Smith it was an ovarian carcinoma.

Conclusion

Thus, all the skin changes which may be associated with malignancy have been seen to be manifestations of collagen and auto-immune disease. They may exist for long periods prior to or occur in association with malignant disease pointing to a relationship between the aetiology of the two.

18)   Paraneoplastic neurological and psychical disturbances, lymphoma, leukaemia and cancer

Collagen and auto-immune disease may involve the peripheral nerves, muscles and central nervous system. In man, in the absence of direct involvement of the peripheral or central nervous system by growth various neurological and psychotic dis?urbances, so-called paraneoplastic manifestations, may be associated with malignant disease of any type, including carcinoma, lymphoma, myeloma and leukaemia. These conditions include peripheral neuropathy, myopathy and myasthenia or elements of all these, motoneurone disease (Brain et al., 1965), cerebellar degeneration, dementia and psychoses of all types. The peripheral neuropathy is more or less symmetrical. The autonomic nervous system may be involved (Lhermitte et al., 1970; Park et al., 1972). This may result in orthostatic hypotension, which may be reversed by radiotherapy to the tumour, showing the changes are not permanent. The peripheral nerves may show perivascular lymphocytic cuffing and in t me destruction of root ganglia and Wallerian degeneration of the nerves appears. Their cause is unknown, though it has been suggested they are due to auto-immune disease (Posner, 1971). The Guillain-Barre syndrome, that is ascending polyneuropathy, may also complicate carcinoma, Hodgkin's disease, leukaemia or myeloma (Klingen, 1965; Rowles and Malpas, 1967; Gravano et al., 1970; Posner, 1971). The incidence of neuropathy or myopathy in cancer cases has been reported to be as high as 16 per cent in men with carcinoma of the bronchus, 16 per cent in women with carcinoma of the ovary and 4 per cent of cases with carcinoma of the breast (Hills, 1967). The onset of the neurological disturbances may coincide with the evolution of the cancer, may *antedate the appearance* of the cancer by as long as *five years* (Croft and Wilkinson, 1969; Thrush, 1970) or it may follow successful treatment of the cancer. In a personally observed case of chronic progressive peripheral neuropathy Hodgkin's disease developed after six years, and in a patient who developed carcinoma of the ovary, motoneurone disease preceded the diagnosis by 65 months. Treatment of the cancer usually has no effect on the neurological disease, the course *of which seems independent of that of the cancer.*

Peripheral neuropathy in association with malignancy is commonly associated with cerebellar disturbances, psychotic symptoms and dementia and, if prolonged, is accompanied by degenerative changes in the brain, cerebellum, hypothalamus and spinal cord. Paraneoplastic psychic symptoms of any type may occur in association with malignancy in the absence of cerebral metastases (Gal and Liszka, 1970). Brown et al. (1974) remark on the high frequency of cases in which an underlying non-cerebral malignant disease presents as a functional psychiatric illness, usually depression, many years before the appearance of a malignancy. The dramatic effect of anti-amoebic substances on the neuropathic and psychic changes in cases of malignant disease described above shows that these changes appear to be the result of intoxication with substances produced by limax amoebae infection and in early cases is reversible. These *neurological and psychical changes appear* identical *in nature, distribution and pathology with* those seen in *collagen and auto-immune disease.* The long period by which the generalized neurological and psychical disturbance may precede the onset of signs of malignant disease suggests that 1) malignant disease may not be present at the onset of such disturbances, 2) some *general* bodily disturbance exists to produce the neurological and psychical change, and 3) both the neurological and psychical disease and the malignancy are due to the same cause, namely limax amoebae present generally in the body and in the tumour. The occurrence of the psychical disease as a paraneoplastic manifestation of malignancy is just what would be expected if the conclusions on the identi al causation of psychoses and maligancy made above are correct.

Paralysis agitans and malignancy

It has been suggested above that paralysis agitans is produced in many cases by limax amoeba infection. Pritchard and Netsky (1973) found that malignant disease is twice as common in subjects of paralysis agitans as compared with controls. In one case of the disease there were three primary tumours. Paralysis agitans may thus be regarded as being a paraneoplastic lesion at times.

19) Blood diseases predisposing to malignancy

a) Polycythaemia vera (erythraemia) and malignant disease

It has been seen that polycythaemia vera appears to be a manifestation of auto-immune disease. Cases of polycythaemia vera may be found associated with or developing into chronic lymphatic leukaemia, chronic myeloid leukaemia, Hodgkin's disease often with paraproteinaemia or multiple myeloma or may terminate in acute leukaemia or myelofibrosis (Lawrence and Donald, 1959; Badella, 1962; Zographov, 1962; Brownstein and Scherl, 1966; Heinle et al., 1966; Wintrobe, 1967; Vianna and Essman, 1971), even in the absence of treatment with radiation. Spickard (1960) (1 case), Giertsen (1956) (1 case), Franzen et al. (1966) (3 cases) and Heinle et al. (1966) report cases of polycythaemia developing myelomatosis. A case of pernicious anaemia developing polycythaemia ana then acute leukaemia was described by Zarafonetis et al. (1957). In some cases other forms of cancer are seen. These include epithelioma of the skin, bronchial carcinoma and cancer of the rectum (Bernadou et al., 1968). Lawrence and Donald (1959) studying 871 patients with polycythaemia vera in the literature found 61 (7.0 per cent) had tumours. Apart from 1 case of lymphosarcoma, 2 of reticulum cell sarcoma, 1 of Hodgkin's disease and 1 of multiple myelomatosis, they found that 7 developed carcinoma of the skin, 1 of the oesophagus, 4 of the stomach, 4 of the colon and rectum, 1 of the pancreas, 16 of the kidney, 1 fibromyoma of the kidney, 1 carcinoma of the bladder, 3 of the prostate, 1 of the cervix, 1 of the ovary, 4 of the breast, 3 of the thyroid, 5 intracranial tumours and 3 malignant melanomata. They suggested that in this disease the liability to develop malignant disease of any type was increased. Cases of polycythaemia developing cerebral tumour were reported by Perlmutter and Strain (1954) and developing carcinoma of the bronchus was described by Garrod and Clarke (1966) and 2 such cases were shown at a Medical Staff Round at Ham-mersmith Hospital in 1965-6. Two similar cases were present in the author's own series reported above. Such associations of polycythaemia with cancer have been regarded as fortuitous (Fauvert et al., 1961).

Such examples as the above where pre-existing polycythaemia is followed by the development of malignancy are to be distinguished from cases in which malignancy is followed by polycythaemia resulting from the secretion by the tumour of an erythropoietin-like substance. In these successful removal of the tumour may cause the polycythaemia to disappear. It may well be that the presence of polycythaemia vera, apparently a manifestation of limax amoebae infection, predisposes to the development of lymphoma, leukaemia, myelomatosis and other tumours at a later date.

b) Myelofibrosis and leukaemia or reticuloses

In cases of myelofibrosis a rise in the number of leucocytes and the presence of immature cells in the circulating blood may cause confusion with myeloid leukaemia. In some cases, however, a true acute or chronic myelocytic leukaemia or reticulosarcoma (Lewis and Szur, 1963; Cooper, 1970) or multiple myelomatosis (Spickard, 1960) have developed in cases of myelofibrosis. Galnick et al. (1971) found in 181 patients with chronic granulocytic leukaemia 39 showed myelofibrosis at some stage. This manifestation of collagen and auto-immune disease appears to predispose to the development of leukaemia or lymphoma.

c) Auto-immune haemolytic anaemias and malignant disease

Auto-immune haemolytic anaemia and thrombocytopenic purpura are sometimes seen in collagen diseases (Wintrobe, 1967). They may antedate the appearance of the collagen diseases by a significant period. An auto-immune haemolytic anaemia and sometimes thrombocytopenic purpura are also occasionally features of various malignant diseases, including Hodgkin's disease, malignant lymphoma, chronic lymphatic leukaemia, multiple myeloma and carcinoma of many organs, especially the stomach and ovary (Wintrobe). This may be associated with cryoglobulinaemia (Cooper, 1926). A most significant observation is that manifestations of the anaemia or thrombocytopenic purpura may antedate the development of malignant lymphoma or cancer by months or up to 13 years (Cooper, 1926; Rosenthal et al., 1955; Dacie, 1962; Young, 1966; Wintrobe, 1967; Pirofsky, 1968). Dameshek (1963) reports a patient with auto-immune haemolytic anaemia for several years who eventually developed chronic lymphatic leukaemia. Marchal and Duhamel (1965) describe a case of auto-immune haemolytic anaemia which two years later developed leukoblastic anaemia. Bawdier and Glick (1966) record auto-immune haemolytic anaemia preceding by more than three years the onset of Hodgkin's disease. Becker (1964) reports a similar case developing lymphoma after two years and Ben-Ishay et al. (1963) one developing leukaemia after 17 years. Boccardi et al. (1968) describe a similar case of auto-immune haemolytic anaell).ia of apparently idiopathic type ending in lymphosarcoma. Occasionally removal or treatment of the malignancy abolishes the haemolytic anaemia. At a Clinico-Pathological Conference (Brit. med. J., 1969, 3, 33) a case of Hodgkin's disease with cold agglutinins was described and was preceded for a long period by auto-immune haemolytic anaemia. It was stressed that the auto-antibodies appear to arise in normal lymphocytes or plasma cells and not in the tumour. Fischer et al. (1974) described the development of an auto-immune haemolytic anaemia three years after successful treatment of a malignant thymoma.

Pirofsky (1968) concludes that auto-immune haemolytic anaemias may accompany, follow or precede the development of neoplasia of the reticulo-endothelial system and that *both appear* to *be due* to *the same common* cause. He cites seven interesting cases of auto-immune haemolytic anaemia 1) associated with acute monocytic leukaemia and Raynaud's phenomena, 2) associated with acute monocytic leukaemia, carcinoma of the cervix and chronic tuberculosis, 3) associated with reticulosarcoma and an aplastic bone marrow, 4) associated with myelomatosis, 5) associated with thymoma, myelomatosis, thyroid adenoma and diabetes, 6) associated with thymoma and red cell aplasia and 7) associated with thymoma, pernicious anaemia, thyroid adenoma, diabetes, systemic lupus erythematosus and adenocarcinoma of the prostate.

Such observations suggest that both the auto-immune haemolytic anaemia and various malignancies may be due to limax amoebae infection.

d) Pure red cell aplasia and malignancy

As shown above pure red cell aplasia either with or without thymoma appears to be a collagen or auto-immune disease. Of cases occurring without thymoma 10 per cent terminate in leukaemia (Wintrobe, 1967) or may be associated with carcinoma of the bronchus (Entwistle et al., 1964; Fentem and Jacobs, 1964).

e) Thrombocytopenia and thrombocytae.mia and malignancy

Both *thrombocytopenia* and *thrombocytosis* may be manifestations of collagen and auto-immune disease. Thrombocytopenia may occur with or precede the onset of acute and chronic leukaemias, Hodgkin's disease, lymphosarcoma, macroglobulinaemia and multiple myeloma. *Thrombocytosis* also occurs in case of chronic myeloid leukaemia, Hodgkin's disease and in many cases (40 per cent) of malignant disease (Wintrobe, 1967). These findings could be explained if thrombocytopenia, thrombocytosis and their associated malignancies were due to the same cause, namely limax amoebae infection.

f) Pancytopenia and malignancy

Pancytopenia may be caused by collagen and auto-immune disease and also precedes the development of many cases of aleukaemic leukaemia (Wintrobe, 1967). Both could be due to the same 'cause.

20) Atrophy of the buccal pharyngeal and oesophageal mucosa and malignant disease

It has been seen that atrophy of the pharyngeal and oesophageal mucosa may occur in the collagen diseases and in Sjogren's syndrome and often in association with atrophy of the buccal mucosa. In the Plummer-Vinson syndrome atrophy of the gastric mucosa is accompanied by an atrophic inflammatory state of the oesophagus, pharynx and tongue and by angular stomatitis. This is often coupled with hypothyroidism (Jacobs and Kilpatrick, 1965). Post-cricoid webs are commonly found. Of 55 patients studied 5 had upper oesophageal (post-cricoid) carcinoma, 1 lower oesophageal cancer, 1 patient had had cancer of the thyroid and another cancer of the stomach. Carcinoma of the pharynx may also occur in this syndrome (Sleisenger, 1967). Evans (1966) observes that this post-cricoid cancer is sometimes associated with cancer of the lip, larynx, buccal mucosa and oral cancer is frequently multicentric. Chisholm et al. (1971) found there is high incidence of malignant disease in the upper gastro-intestinal tract (12 per cent) in association with Plummer-Vinson syndrome and post-cricoid webs. Moreover, such malignancies are frequently found in relatives of the patient. It would seem that collagen and auto-immune disease affecting the fore part of the gut is a highly pre-malignant condition.

21) Atrophic gastritis and malignant disease

Atrophic gastritis has been shown to form part of the spectrum of the collagen and auto-immune diseases. Whether other causes exist is not known. The condition is associated with achlorhydria and often with pernicious or iron-deficiency anaemia. There was formerly some difference of opinion as to whether atrophic gastritis alone predisposes to cancer of the stomach (see Willis, 1967). Wilkinson (1945, 1950) denied that atrophic gastritis combined with pernicious anaemia did so. It is, now considered, however, that atrophic gastritis combined with pernicious anaemia is pre-malignant to a marked degree (Kaplan and Rigler, 1945; Mosbech, 1953; Siurala and Seppala, 1960; Siurala et al., 1961; Evans, 1966; Wintrobe, 1967; Peterson, 1967; Blackburn et al., 1968; Leading Article, Brit. med. J., 1972, ii, 3097. Freytes and Carii, 1973; Siurala et al., 1974). According to Wintrobe (1967) 12 per cent of cases of pernicious anaemia develop carcinoma of the stomach and there is a high incidence of gastric cancer in their relatives. Wright et al. (1970) reported the case of a man of 46 years who developed thyrotoxicosis and 8 years later was found to have pernicious anaemia, vitiligo and cancer of the stomach with a low gastric acidity and gastric parietal cell auto-antibodies in the serum, but no thyroid antibodies or ANF. The gastric mucosa was not atrophic.

Moreover, atrophic gastritis predisposes to the development of the Paterson-Kelly (Plummer-Vinson) syndrome with atrophic changes higher up in the digestive tract, which itself predisposes to the development of post-cricoid carcinoma and other cancers of the foregut (Jacobs, 1962, 1963; Jacobs and Kilpatrick, 1964). Wilkinson (1950) in 1,820 cases of pernicious anaemia found 34 cases developing carcinoma of the stomach and 47 of other organs, 11 of the buccal cavity, pharynx

Addendum: Borochowitz D., Dutz W., Kohont E. and Vessal, K. Isr. J. Med. Sci., 1979, 15, 397-404 Gastro-intestinal mucosa and primary gastro-intestinal lymphoma. The authors report that in Shiraz (Iran) gastro-intestinal lymphoma affects the upper duodeno-jejunal area and is associated with atrophy of the surrounding non-lymphomatous area and formation of lymph follicles. This is frequently linked to repeated gastro-enteritis leading to mucosal atrophy, mutation of plasma cell precursors and secretion of alpha-heavy chain proteins. In USA gastro-intestinal lymphoma affects the stomach and is accompanied by superficial perifovealar plasma cell gastritis of the surrounding mucosa or in preformed lymphoid tissue of the ileo-colon surrounded usually by normal mucosa. In both areas the lesions are suggestive of a parasitic infection.

and oesophagus, II of the large intestine, 3 of epithelial tissues, 5 of the cervix and vagina, 2 myelomata, 3 of the pancreas, 6 of the breast, 2 of the prostate and I each of liver, bladder andbronchus. Nine cases of pernicious anaemia developing reticulosarcoma were reported by Larsson (1962) and others by Cooper (1970). Cases of pernicious anaemia followed by lymphosarcoma or myelomatosis were described by Blackburn et al. (1968). Pauders and Leeksma (1963) reported 3 cases of pernicious anaemia developing multiple myelomatosis, one Waldenstrom's macroglobulinaemia and one Hodgkin's disease and paraproteinaemia. Cases of pernicious anaemia developing Hodgkin's disease were also described by Steinbrinck (1941) and Cieza Rodriguez and Tau (1943). A case of pernicious anaemia followed by plasmocytoma and liver cirrhosis was reported by Jacottet and Ramel (1965). Dr. D.A.G. Galton of the Royal Marsden Hospital (personal communication) has seen cases of pernicious anaemia developing into lymphocytic lymphoma or myelomatosis. Other cases of myelomatosis appearing in cases of pernicious anaemia were described by Fraser (1969) and Hrncir et al. (1970). Twomey et al. (1971) report a case of pernicious anaemia with myelomatosis, two others with atrophic gastritis and myelomatosis and· two patients with atrophic gastritis and lympho-proliferative disease.

Moreover, the atrophic gastritis associated with pernicious anaemia predisposes to the development of acute myeloblastic leukaemia or chronic lymphoid leukaemia (Rich and Schiff, 1936; Sterne et al., 1941; Wooley, 1944; Videbaek, 1947; Townsend, 1949; Talley et al., 1952; Mosbech, 1959; Blackburn et al., 1968), or to chronic myeloid leukaemia (Tawast and Siurala, 1956; Hitzenberger, 1958). Corcino et al. (1971) reported a case of pernicious anaemia and myasthenia gravis which subsequently developed chronic myeloid leukaemia. Siurala and Ikkala (1965) found that of 31

patients with leukaemia, lymphoma or myeloma 70 per cent had atrophic gastritis.

In the South West Metropolitan Cancer Registry series there were two cases of rheumatoid arthritis with long-standing diabetes and pernicious anaemia, both in females. One developed malignant lymphoma, the other carcinoma of the stomach. Four cases of pernicious anaemia developed malignancies, one a malignant lymphoma and one each of the prostate, bronchus and skin cancers. There were 8 cases of pernicious anaemia combined with diabetes. One developed chronic lymphatic leukaemia, two malignant lymphoma, one myelomatosis and one each cancer of the pancreas, colon and malignant melanoma.

In the author's series there were cases of pernicious anaemia developing chronic lymphatic leukaemia and carcinoma of the bronchus; carcinoma of the stomach; carcinoma of the bronchus; malignant lymphoma; and carcinoma of the ovary. Moreover in very many cases atrophic gastritis as shown by the presence of achlorhydria was found in cancerous subjects.

Clearly the "auto-immune" disease, atrophic gastritis may predispose to malignancies of the stomach, foregut and elsewhere and also to lymphoma, leukaemias and myelomatosis.

22) Subtotal or total villous atrophy of the small intestine and malignant disease

It has been shown that at least some cases of villous atrophy of the small intestine are probably part of the spectrum of collagen and auto-immune disease. It results in coeliac disease. The submucosa is heavily infiltrated :with lymphocytes. This often is associated with atrophic gastritis with a similar infiltration. Such cases frequently develop malignancy of various kinds years after the appearance of the steatorrhoea. Malignant lymphoma developing after idiopathic steatorrhoea has been described by many workers (Fairley and Mackie, 1937; Badenoch, 1950; Schlesinger et al., 1953; Best and Cook, 1961; Gough et al., 1962; Spracklen, 1963; Kent, 1964; Creamer, 1964; Eakins et al., 1964; Barratt, 1964; Jandle and Creamer, 1965; Siurala and Ikkala, 1965; Dymock, 1966; Missen, 1966; Clinico-Pathological Conference, Brit. med. J., 1966, 1, 1104; Austed et al., 1967; Hoskins, 1967). Harris and Cooke (1967) in 202 cases of this condition followed for a mean period of 10.4 years found 34 developed malignancy. Of these 27 involved the gut and 15 were lymphomas. The lymphoma may develop in the affected mucosa. There were 14 gastro-intestinal carcinomas (6 of oesophagus, 3 of stomach and one each of tongue, hypopharynx, colon, rectum and anus) and 5 other malignancies (one each of lung, ovary, bladder and one not biopsied). Gupte et al. (1971) report a case of coeliac disease in a girl who developed acute myeloid leukaemia. Wright and Richardson (1967) describe 4 cases of coeliac disease who developed carcinoma of the oesophagus. Fry and Russell (1968) report the case of a patient with gluten-sensitive steatorrhoea and exfoliative dermatitis who developed carcinoma of the tongue and multiple skin malignancies. Goldstein and Poker (1966), Gilbert et al. (1968) and Marano et al. (1970) describe cases of malabsorption which were associated with myelomatosis and in which villous atrophy of the mucosa of the small bowel was present and there was conspicuous infiltration of the mucosa by lympho-monocytoid cells, plasma cells and eosinophils and paraproteinaemia. In the case of Gilbert et al. a thymoma was also present. In Case 18, described above, a man suffered from typical sero-positive rheumatoid arthritis associated with lymphadenopathy from an early age. He afterwards developed coeliac disease which was gluten-sensitive and years later Hodgkin's disease. One of the author's

patients with coeliac disease developed meningioma. It is now estimated that about 10 per cent of cases of coeliac disease develop abdominal lymphoma.

In the South West Metropolitan Cancer Registry series were reported 6 cases following coeliac disease, 3 of malignant lymphoma and 3 of carcinoma elsewhere. In one case the onset of lymphoma was 15 years after the discovery of coeliac disease.

Thus, the "auto-immune" condition, coeliac disease, appears to predispose to lymphoma and to carcinoma other than in the affected bowel.

23) Ulcerative colitis and malignancy

It has long been known that ulcerative colitis is a locally pre-malignant condition (Councell and Dukes, 1952; Welch and Hedberg, 1965). Morson (1971) reports that the development of cancer is preceded by a phase of epithelial dysplasia or carcinoma in-situ, comparable to pre-cancer in the cervix and other organs. An increased incidence of cancer of the alimentary tract apart from the large bowel in cases of ulcerative colitis was reported by Edwards and Truelove (1964). Ulcerative colitis may be accompanied by cancer of the bile duct (Almy, 1961; Rankin et al., 1966). Fusco et al. (1971) report a case of ulcerative colitis treated with azathioprine, which developed sarcoma of the pancreas. In addition Comes et al. (1960) report two patients and refer to five in the literature in which lymphosarcoma of the large bowel developed after long-standing ulcerative colitis. Similar changes were present in the neighbouring lymph nodes. Warren (1959) reported two such cases developing 15 and 16 years after the onset of colitis. Similar cases have since been reported by Walker and Weaver (1964) and Federman et al. (1963). Friedman et al. (1968) state that 11 such cases have been reported since

1928 and add 4 more of their own. Bargen (1928) described 1 case of ulcerative colitis which developed lymphosarcoma, 1 lymphatic leukaemia and 1 Hodgkin's disease. Nugent et al. (1972) stated that up till their paper 13 cases of malignant lymphoma developing locally in cases of ulcerative colitis were known. They reported four further cases (3 of reticulum cell sarcoma and one of Hodgkin's disease). Swenson and Orne! (1974) described a case of lymphosarcoma of the small and large bowel associated with ulcerative colitis. Vieta and Delgado (1976) report a case of ulcerative colitis complicated by colonic lymphoma. A local development of Kaposi's sarcoma of the bowel in a case of ulcerative colitis was reported by Gordon and Rywlin (1966). Rosen and Teplitz (1965) describe the association of ulcerative colitis with chronic granulocytic leukaemia and Cattell and Bochine (1947) a case of ulcerative colitis with both adenocarcinoma of the rectum and reticulum cell sarcoma. Novis et al. (1971) record a case of ulcerative colitis and lymphoma of the gut, while Fadem (1952) and Bernstein and Nixon (1964) described cases of ulcerative colitis developing myelomatosis.

In the South West Metropolitan Cancer Registry series were found cases of ulcerative colitis which developed cancer of the stomah. breast, pancreas, bronchus and bladder and one case developed chronic lymphatic leukaemia. In the author's series multiple basal cell carcinoma developed in one case of ulcerative colitis and chromophobe adenoma of the pituitary in another.

Thus, ulcerative colitis, part of the collagen and auto-immune spectrum, may predispose to carcinoma and lymphoma of the large bowel and perhaps to carcinoma elsewhere and to myelomatosis.

24) Diabetes and cancer

It has been shown that the majority of cases of non-pancreatic diabetes appear to result from the action of secretions of Iimax amoebae on the hypothalamus or as an anti-insulin. *Hyperglycaemia and diabetic glucose tolerance curves are very frequent in neoplastic disease* (33 of 60 cases reported by Garijo et al., 1973) and may disappear with successful treatment of the cancer. Furthermore, this development of malignancy in a known diabetic may increase the insulin requirements or make the diabetes unmanageable. *Such findings are readily explicable on the identity of the organism producing the diabetes and with that present in most cancers.*

Diabetics may be more liable to cancer than normal subjects. This problem is considered in part by Oakley et al. (1968) and Malins (1968). It may be divided into the liability of cases of dia betes to develop a) cancer of the pancreas and b) cancer of other organs. As regards the former there are 1) patients with pancreatic cancer who subsequently develop symptomatic diabetes and 2) patients in whom idiopathic diabetes preceded the onset of cancer of the pancreas often by many years and in such cases the incidence of cancer is about twice as great as in the general population (Bell, 1957; Cohen, 1965; Warren et al., 1966; Kessler, 1970, 1971). The pancreatic islets in such diabetics may exhibit lymphocytic infiltration and in some cases they appear to undergo adenomatous hypertrophy (Evans, 1966) or even tumour formation (Howard et al., 1950). A number of cases of pancreatic insulinomas developing in known diabetics have been reported (Bielchowski, 1932; Bickel et al., 1935; Van der Sar et al., 1956; Gittler et al., 1958; Knight, 1967). In addition diabetes may develop after the removal of insulinomas (Dunn, 1971, Lit.). Conn (1946) s peculated as to *whether the diabetes and t.he insulinomas have a common cause.*

As regards the liability of diabetics to develop cancer of organs other than the pancreas there are conflicting reports. Some authors can find no difference in the incidence of cancer in diabetics from that in the general population (Joslin et al., 1959), while others report a four-fold increase. Porto and Saldanha (1969) regard diabetes as a paraneoplastic condition and predisposing to cancer. Williams (1962) and Kessler (1971) conclude that the clinical evidence in the aggregate suggests a relationship between diabetes and subsequent development of malignancy in tissues other than the pancreas and especially between diabetes and the later development of cancer of the pancreas. Possibly a special association exists between pre-existing diabetes and cancer of the body of the uterus (see Haldemann, 1970), diabetes being present in 11 per cent of cases of cancer of the uterine body. Hoffman et al. (1969) describe a marked liability to cancer of the female genitalia in diabetics. In elderly diabetics there often occurs carcinoma of the body of the uterus associated with fibroids and a hyperplastic endometritis, which is precancerous (Leading Article, Brit. med. J., 1966, i, 247). Lender et al. (1977), remarking on the fact that diabetes appears to be an auto-immune disease often associated with similar conditions in other organs, stress that it is accompanied by increased incidence of fibrocystic disease and cancer of the breast.

In the South West Metropolitan Cancer Registry series 1,979 cases of diabetes accompanied or preceded the signs of cancer often by many years. In 60 cases it was a symptom of cancer of the pancreas. In 58 cases of long-standing diabetes cancer of the pancreas developed. Of the rest in 87 cases malignant lymphoma appeared. These included Hodgkin's disease and leukaemia. The rest comprised cancer of almost every organ. The 14 cases of cancer following rheumatoid arthritis and long-standing diabetes comprised 6 cases of malignant lymphoma and 4 cases of cancer of the senile breast. In very many cases

diabetes appeared *with* the malignancy.

The presence of diabetes, a manifestation of collagen and auto-immune disease, thus seems to favour the later development of malignancy of any tissue and with it an exaggeration of the diabetes, or, if diabetes was not present before, the development of a tumour causes diabetes to appear.

25) Collagen and auto-immune disease of the liver and carcinoma or lymphoma

Primary biliary cirrhosis, active chronic hepatitis progressing to post-necrotic cirrhosis and cryptogenic cirrhosis appear to be manifestations of collagen and auto-immune diseases and predispose to malignant change in the liver in some cases. Sagebel et al. (1963) at the Massachusetts General Hospital studied 89 cases of hepatoma and found that in 66 livers the primary neoplasm was associated with cirrhosis. In 47 it was post-hepatitic and in 19 post-necrotic. Spinivasa and Sharma (1968) found that in 31 cases of primary cancer of the liver 29 were hepatocellular in type, 74 per cent of these were associated with cirrhosis, of which 87 per cent were post-necrotic. Mori (1967) found a significant relationship between post-necrotic and post-hepatitic cirrhosis and the development of liver cancer. In the Leading Article (Brit. med. J., 1972, i, 261.) it is stated that virus hepatitis is an unimportant cause of cancer of the liver. Thus, it appears that auto-immune liver disease predisposes to hepatoma.

Heiman (1971), Paton (1971) and Wetherley-Mein and Cottom (1956) describe non-alcoholic fibrosis, portal cirrhosis or simply unspecified cirrhosis as associated with lymphoproliferative disorders or acute leukaemia. Rosenberg et al. (1961) in 1,269 cases of lymphosarcoma found this tumour associated with cirrhosis on two occasions, cirrhosis and hepatitis and cirrhosis and liver tumour each on one occasion and hepatitis on four occasions, one of which was associated with liver tumour. Post-necrotic cirrhosis may be associated with Brill-Symmer's disease (Bassler, 1959); with Hodgkin's disease (Tichy et al., 1962) (11 cases); and with malignant lymphoma (Steiner, 1937; Fraisse et al., 1952; Rosenberg et al., 1961; D'Antuono et al., 1961). In one of the cases of Fraisse et al. (1952) a man of 50 years had suffered from acute rheumatoid arthritis at the age of 20 years and developed hepatomegaly and jaundice with collateral venous anastomatic channels. He was found to have cirrhosis and chronic myeloid leukaemia. In the other case there was generalized lymphadenopathy due to reticulosis and the liver showed active chronic hepatitis. Hodgkin's disease developed in the course of active chronic hepatitis reported by Pirotte (1974). Bagley et al. (1972) in discussing the findings at liver autopsy in 127 patients with Hodgkin's disease found not only changes of Hodgkin's disease, but in other cases cellular infiltrates, mononuclear or mixed, or atypical reticulum cells, liver fibrosis or granulomata. The author has seen post-necrotic cirrhosis of the liver in two cases of Hodgkin's disease, in one of lymphosarcomatosis and another of both lymphosarcoma and carcinoma of the stomach in a woman from whom a carcinoma of the breast had been removed 10 years previously (Wyburn-Mason, 1964). In the author's series of cases of cancer recorded above chronic active hepatitis was found in association with myxoedema and chronic lymphatic leukaemia, in a case of lymphosarcoma of the spleen, and in a patient with hepatoma, acute monocytic leukaemia and auto-antibodies in the serum. Cirrhosis with multiple myeloma was reported by Schneiderbauer (1959).

Cirrhosis is said to be associated with an increased incidence of malignancy not only in the liver, but also in the skin or other organs (Weglanka, 1966).

Thus, it appears that collagen and autoimmune disease of the liver may be associated with a tendency to local formation of an hepatoma and also occurs in association with lymphoma and possibly cancers of extrahepatic tissues. This suggests both the liver disease and the malignancies arise from a single cause. In some parts of the world, however, aflatoxin or HBAg cause both cirrhosis and hepatoma (Leading Article, Brit. med. J., 1975, ii, 647).

26) Chronic cholecystitis and carcinoma of the gall-bladder

Evidence has been adduced to show that chronic cholecystitis is commonly a manifestation of rheumatoid disease involving the mucosa of the gall-bladder. Marked proliferation of the mucosa leads to the formation of deep clefts which penetrate down to or even through the muscularis like carcinoma (Rokitansky-Aschoff sinuses) and polypoid and adenomatoid change of the mucosa may be found. This is well-recognized as accompanying malignant change (Evans, 1966; Willis, 1967) and is a premalignant condition.

27) Chronic pancreatitis and carcinoma of the pancreas

As shown above chronic (relapsing) pancreatitis unassociated with disease of the bile passages or gall stones may be a manifestation of collagen and autoimmune disease. It eventually results in cirrhosis and perhaps calcification of the organ. It often leads to steatorrhoea and diabetes. Cirrhosis of the pancreas may be associated with cirrhosis of the liver. There has been some difference of opinion as to whether chronic pancreatitis is a premalignant condition. According to Ewing (1940), Willis (1967) and Oberling and Guerin (quoted by Ewing) many cases of cancer of the pancreas occur in cirrhotic organs. According to Bailey and Love (1962) pancreatic carcinoma develops in patients with pancreatic calcinosis with such frequency as to warrant the assumption that such calcinosis is a pre-malignant condition. Pauline-Netto et al. (1960) report that 6 per cent of cases of chronic pancreatitis develop carcinoma and that pancreatic carcinoma develops in 25 per cent of cases of pancreatic calcification.

Moderate to severe pancreatitis was associated with cancer of the pancreas in 26 of 255 (10 per cent) cases of carcinoma examined histologically at the Mayo Clinic (Gambill, 1970). In a paper at the 51st. Annual Session of the American College of Physicians at Philadelphia, April 12-17th. Grozinger et al. (1969) investigated 169 cases of pancreatic cancer and found chronic pancreatitis present in 60 per cent of cases. They state that in more than 50 per cent of cases of pancreatic cancer the growth is the consequence of the fibrotic inflammatory change and chronic disease in neighbouring organs does not contribute to this development. In 20 per cent of cases only biliary disease was also present. Mikhailichenko et al. (1974) also stress the relationship between pre-existing chronic pancreatitis and the subsequent development of cancer. Evans (1966), however, states that the onset of carcinoma is unrelated to pre-existing chronic pancreatitis.

In the South West Metropolitan Cancer Registry series 3 cases of chronic (relapsing) pancreatitis developing malignancy were recorded, one of carcinoma of the pancreas and two of the bronchus.

It seems possible that a chronic pancreatitis arising in the absence of diseases of the bile passages and as a manifestation of collagen and auto-immune disease is a locally pre-malignant condition.

28) Idiopathic Addison's disease preceding malignancy

The development of Hodgkin's disease in a case of Addison's disease was described by Porcellini et al. (1971). In the South West Metropolitan Cancer Registry series malignancy developed in 6 cases of idiopathic Addison's disease, in 1 case 15 years after its onset. Three of these were cases of malignant lymphoma. Perlmutter et al. (1956) described the case of a patient with atrophy of adrenals and parathyroids and thyroiditis and who had a history of recurrent giant cell tumour of the tibia. Two patients in the author's series suffered from idiopathic Addison's disease, one of whom had had a hysterectomy for fibroids and developed carcinoma of the bladder.

29) Rheumatic epididymo-orchitis and cancer

An acute epididymo-orchitis may be a manifestation of collagen and auto-immune disease, including rheumatoid arthritis or Paget's disease. Seddon (1960) describes spontaneously occurring acute epididymo-orchitis as preceding teratoma of the testis in two cases. In one this preceded signs of the tumour by five months. In the other a right inguinal hernia had been repaired two years previous to the onset of acute epididymo-orchitis and the tumour developed five months later. In the series of Hodgkin's disease reported by the author (Wyburn-Mason, 1964) the first manifestation of Hodgkin's disease was preceded by an acute funiculitis or epididymo-orchitis in a number of cases or the latter appeared in the course of the disease. In other cases under the author's care acute epididymo-orchitis preceded cancer of the bronchus or cancer of the bladder by a number of months. The RF was positive in both sera.

Chapter XII

Conclusions as to the aetiology of many human cancers

In cases of multiple malignancies, as described above, every kind of malignancy, myelomatosis, lymphoma or leukaemia, adenomata of endocrine glands, benign or malignant ovarian cysts and fibroids occur in every conceivable combination and up to six malignancies in the same subject have been described. Furthermore, two different types of cancer or cancer and lymphoma may affect a single organ and every transition from one type of lymphoma to another or to myelomatosis may occur in a particular case. Such considerations indicate a single aetiology for many different cancers and benign tumours.

From an analysis of the author's own series of cases and of cases quoted from the literature it appears that:–

1) Various manifestations of collagen and auto-immune disease may coincide with the appearance of evidence of malignancy, when they are called *paraneoplastic manifestations*. The latter include rheumatoid arthritis, systemic lupus erythematosus, dermatomyositis, scleroderma, polyarteritis, carcinomatous peripheral neuropathy or other neurological and mental disturbances, thyrotoxicosis, leukoderma or melanoderma, ichthyosis acquisita, acanthosis nigricans, Raynaud's phenomena, dermatitis herpetiformis and diabetes or, if pre-existing diabetes or rheumatoid arthritis are present, these may be exaggerated. Removal or other treatment of the tumour may or may not cause regression of these paraneoplastic disturbances. Many of these disturbances unassociated with cancer have been shown to disappear or lessen when the patient is treated with anti-amoebic drugs or bile or copper salts. Now it has been shown in man that malignant tumours contain large numbers of such amoebae. In many advanced cases of leukaemia, lymphoma or carcinoma the state of "toxicity" with pyrexia, sweats, rigors and coma is identical with that which occurs in cases of disseminated eosinophilic collagen disease or acute rheumatoid disease and can also be relieved by anti-amoebic substances. Again, in guinea pigs experimental infections with free-living amoebae have been seen to produce a state closely resembling that of advanced malignant disease in man. Thus, it seems that with the development of cancer in any form there appear the effects of infection with limax amoebae contained in the tumour. Successful treatment of the tumour and, thus, removal of the *collection* of limax amoebae may cause the paraneoplastic phenomena to lessen or disappear.

2) any form of collagen or auto-immune disease, including rheumatoid arthritis, systemic lupus erythematosus, dermatomyositis (polymyositis), scleroderma or polyarteritis, disseminated eosinophilic collagen disease, Sjogren-Mikulicz's syndrome, thymic hypertrophy and thymoma, myasthenia, lymphocytic thyroid disease, thyrotoxicosis, Paget's disease, atrophic gastritis, coeliac disease, tibrosing alveolitis, ulcerative colitis, auto-immune liver disease or haemolytic anaemia or diabetes may be *followed after years* by the development of any type of tumourous disease, whether it is carcinoma or benign tumour, lymphoma, leukaemia, myelomatosis (in which various other malignancies, often multiple, tend to develop), or Walden-

strom's macroglobulinaemia (in which lymphoma, leukaemia or any other malignancy also occur).

3) any localized manifestations of collagen and auto-immune disease, such as Sjogren's syndrome, thymic hyperplasia or tumour, Hashimoto's thyroiditis or myxoedema, atrophic gastritis with or without pernicious anaemia, atrophic stomatitis, chronic cholecystitis, coeliac disease, ulcerative colitis, Paget's disease of bone, fibrosing alveolitis, chronic active hepatitis and post-necrotic cirrhosis of the liver are premalignant and may be followed by the development of

a) cancer or lymphoma or both developing in the primarily affected organ after a long latent period.

b) generalized lymphoma, including Hodgkin's disease, leukaemia or myelomatosis,

c) cancer of other organs,

d) multiple malignancies of any tissue of the body.

Thus, in the *majority of* cases *of cancer of all kinds in* Western *Countries the tumour* is *preceded by many years by* evidence *of collagen and auto-immune disease* or its *presence results in the* appearance *of such disturbances in the patient.*

It has been seen that in animals malignant lymphoma can be produced experimentally by chronic antigenic stimulation induced by the injection of foreign cells in early life, while lymphoma and other cancers occur in man with undue frequency after organ transplants. In both situations there exists a chronic antigenic stimulation in the organism. A similar state also exists in cases of collagen and auto-immune diseases in man, which are apparently caused by limax amoebae infection and which so frequently pre-exist or accompany human cancer. Cases of congenital hypogammaglobulinaemia are especially liable to both collagen and auto-immune disease and to malignancies, sometimes multiple and including lymphoma. Moreover, families exist in which

different members exhibit either collagen and auto-immune disease or malignancy. Are most human cancers due, in fact, to the same infection as causes collagen and auto-immune diseases or are they coincidental? The evidence favours the former. Thus, it has been seen that many cases of myelomatosis and lymphomata, which are often associated with other malignancies, follow long-standing clinical collagen or auto-immune disease and exhibit evidence of long-continued antigenic stimulation and RF, ANF and other auto-antibodies in the serum, indicative of limax amoebae infection. Again, lesions of collagen and auto-immune disease affecting a specific organ have been seen to be premalignant and to be followed frequently by local malignant change. Furthermore, the trophozoites of limax: amoebae are destroyed by deconjugated bile salts in the strength found in the small intestine. Such deconjugated salts are present throughout the duodenum and small intestine, whereas conjugated salts are found in the bile passages and gall-bladder. The deconjugated bile salts are gradually reabsorbed into the circulation during their descent throughout the small intestine. Absorption is complete by the time the bowel contents reach the ileo-caecal valve. It is highly significant that, while primary malignancies occur in the bile passages and large intestine and gastric ulcers become malignant, very rarely do primary tumours develop in the duodenum or small intestine and duodenal ulcers rarely become malignant. This is readily explained if it is assumed that limax amoebae cause malignancy and are destroyed by the deconjugated bile salts in the small intestine. Again, there is an increase in the incidence of both collagen and auto-immune disease and tumours, both benign and malignant, with age. Both are part of the "aging process" and, therefore, both could be due to the same cause. All the evidence is completely in accord with the conclusion that *limax amoebae infection not only causes collagen and auto-immune diseases, but also in susceptible subjects many benign and malignant tumours in man in many parts of the world* (see also Friov, 1974). The reason why the organism has not been demonstrated previously in tumours has already been explained. They appear as macrophages.

It seems that the blood changes in leukaemias, the lymph node changes in lymphomata and plasma cell proliferations in the marrow are initially the response of the reticulo-endothelial system of individuals sensitive to chronic stimulation by the antigens of Iimax amoebae and are comparable to similar responses produced by other infections. It has been shown above that the administration of substances which inhibit limax amoebae may cause a complete regression of the changes of some cases of chronic lymphatic or monocytic leukaemia, while the blood count in other cases of chronic lymphatic and other types of leukaemia, the lesions of lymphomata and the plasma cell proliferation in the marrow in cases of myelomatosis are unaffected. Some cases of *chronic lymphatic leukaemia thus appear to be the direct response* to *infection with limax amoebae.* In other cases of *leukaemias, lymphomata and* myelomatosis *somatic mutation has taken place in white cell precursors, cells of the lymph nodes* or *plasma cells in the bone marrow or elsewhere* in response to the stimulation by the infection, so that treatment against limax amoebae has no beneficial effect.

The role of lymphocytic infiltration in relation to malignant change

Limax amoebae infection causes lymphocytic and often plasma cell and eosinophil infiltration in affected tissues. This may be associated with the formation of germinal centres. In cases of Hashimoto's thyroiditis and myxoedema the thyroid gland exhibits such changes. This predisposes to the development of both lympho-

rna and malignant change in the thyroid gland. The case of Mescon and Clark (1964) cited already is of considerable interest. This patient previously developed rheumatoid arthritis, Hashimoto's thyroiditis and then dermatomyositis followed by a carcinoma of the breast. The stroma of the breast cancer appeared identical with the lesion of the thyroid gland, that is Hashimoto's thyroiditis, and it would seem that the malignant change in the breast developed in relation to this lymphocytic lesion. The patient reported by Gemma et al. (1968) was also significant. In this case a woman with a seven year history of goitre and signs of thyrotoxicosis developed a thymic neoplasm and at operation aberrant thyroid tissue with the changes of Hashimoto's thyroiditis was found in the tumour mass, which appeared to develop in relation to this lymphoid infiltration. Again, in cases of Sjogren-Mikulicz's syndrome there may develop local malignant tumours in the salivary gland or local or generalized lymphoma. In cases of atrophic gastritis the mucous membrane is infiltrated with lymphocytes with the formation of germ follicles and this predisposes to the development of gastric carcinoma. Likewise, atrophic pharyngitis and oesophagitis with the same mucosal changes predisposes to the development of local cancers, while the mucous membrane in cases of ulcerative colitis is also predisposed to the development of local carcinoma. The same is true of chronic pancreatitis with its small round cell infiltration which in a proportion of cases results in the development of carcinoma of the organ. Again, the infiltration of the alveolar walls of the lung in cases of fibrosing alveolitis predisposes to the development of carcinoma of the bronchioles. In cases of thymic hypertrophy with germ follicle formation associated with collagen or auto-immune disease there is a predisposition to the formation of lympho-epithelioma, sarcoma or lymphoma in the gland. In auto-immune disease of the liver there is also an infiltration of the portal tracts with lymphocytes and a tendency to the development of hepatoma. In cases of cystic mastitis occurs a pronounced lymphocytic infiltration around the affected acini and ducts which may later show epithelial malignancy. In one case of rheumatoid arthritis in the author's series and another in the literature a malignant synovioma developed in an affected joint. From such observations it would seem that *chronic infiltration of an organ with lymphocytes induced by the* presence *of limax amoebae* over a *long period often results in the development of a local malignancy in susceptible subjects.* In this respect Hernandez Perez (1975) described 6 cases of cancer developing in genital amoebiasis lesions due to E. histolytica.

A lymphocytic and plasma cell infiltration is a notable feature of certain growths, such as basal cell carcinoma or squamous cell carcinoma of the skin or cancer of the oral cavity. The same is true of carcinoma of the tongue, tonsils, pharyngeal wall, pyriform recess, nasal mucosa, gastro-intestinal tract, cervix, penis and vulva and some cases of carcinoma of the breast and in such cases it may resemble Hashimoto's thyroiditis or reticula- or lympho-sarcoma (Evans, 1966; Willis, 1967). In cancers arising in the alimentary tract the stroma may contain so many lymphocytes as to resemble subacute or chronic inflammation. This stromal lymphocytic reaction present in cancers was formally regarded by Murphy (1921) as a bodily reaction to the growth and this idea has recently been revived by some workers, such as Fairley, as an indication that lymphocytes are conveying antibodies against the malignant cells. Most workers do not, however, credit this (Evans, 1966; Willis, 1967) and they point out that these cells are present in the precancerous state and their presence around can ers is explained by their persistence after malignant change has developed. It

seems very probable that these changes are, in fact, evidence of the tissue reaction to the presence of the limax amoebae which caused and are present in the neoplasm. They cause not only this chronic inflammatory response with its lymphocytic and plasma cell infiltration, but often also changes like lymphoma in the stroma of both the primary and metastatic carcinomata. Highly malignant tumours, such as the inflammatory cancer of the breast, are very vascular and contain very large numbers of lymphocytes in the stroma, while slowly growing scirrhous cancers are avascular and exhibit very little lymphocyte response (see Willis, 1967), the opposite of what would be expected if lymphocytes were opposing tumour growth. The rate of growth of a tumour thus appears to vary with the chronic inflammatory response, vascularity and the degree of lymphocytic infiltration. As shown above the administration of bile salts and other substances which kill limax amoebae often slows or stops the growth of cancers. Moreover, the small bowel mucosa where deconjugated bile salts, which **kill** limax amoebae, are present is resistent to infiltration by growths from other sites. The significance of this infiltration of the stroma by lymphocytes and plasma cells in relation to the growth of basal cell carcinoma may be elucidated by the work of Van Scott and Reinertson (1961). They found that transplantation of basal cell carcinoma into extracutaneous situations was only possible if the stroma of the growth, presumably containing limax amoebae, lymphocytes and plasma cells, was included in the transplant as well as the epithelial parenchyma. *This suggests that the limax amoebae within a human tumour and resultant chronic inflammation and the lymphocytic infiltration is largely essential for the continued growth of malignant cells.* This suggestion is borne out by the effect of clotrimazole on the inflammation and growth of metastases in the case described already.

The genetic state of cancerous cells

Chromosome abnormalities of many kinds are described in the cells of various malignancies, while the other cells of the body are normal. These are, however, inconstant. For a review see Gottlieb (1969). Whether these are important in the initiation of neoplasia is uncertain, but they indicate that malignant cells differ from normal. They are perhaps secondary to the neoplastic change, except in the case of the Philadelphia chromosome of chronic myeloid leukaemia. Willis (1967) states "there is at present no evidence that nuclear or extrachromosomal mutations are a feature of malignant tissue".

One theory of cancer, the "deletion theory", postulates that cancer cells progressively lose specialized enzymes. This is exemplified by their inability to synthesize asparagine, suggesting some genetic change has taken place in these cells. The author (Wyburn-Mason, 1958) showed, that, while normally growing foetal tissue and normal adult tissue under repair attract macrophages and growing nerve ends, during the growth of cancerous tissue this power is lost. This attraction is dependent on genetically controlled antigen-antibody-like reactions between cells and again suggests that some genetic change has occurred in cancerous cells. In addition, it is now known that cancer cells not only lose functions, but in some cases acquire them. Thus, bronchial carcinoma cells quite often produce pituitary-like hormones, although normal bronchial epithelial cells never do. Filipe and Cooke (1974) also found that changes in the composition of mucin as compared with normal occurred adjacent to carcinoma of the colon. It has also been found that a new antigen resembling embryonic protein (carcino-embryonic antigen) is produced by many cancer cells, but not by normal adult cells. Again, the cells of congenital anomalies, which appear to be genetically different from those of the host, are especially liable to malignant change (see below). Such observations suggest the existence in cancer cells of some kind of *"malditferentiation"*, in which the normal orderly utilization of genetic information is disturbed. In the author's opinion the evidence points to some genetic difference as existing between normal and cancerous cells. Pitot (1974) reviews the evidence as to whether neoplasia is a somatic mutation in cells or a heritable change in their cytoplasmic membranes. Harnden (1976) concludes that chromosomal changes are important both in progression and as a predisposing factor in cancerous change.

The processes of tumour formation

Willis (1967) in reviewing the nature of tumour formation quoted Nicholson "We are beginning to see that tumour formation is ..... reaction to excitation, , ... consequent acquisition of characters, maintenance and transmission to future cell generations of the characters thus acquired", and Haddow on the genesis of tumours by carcinogenic substances "these agents inhibit the growth and metabolism of cells; the cells react by alteration of metabolism which has survival value and in effect confers a biological advantage"; there thus appears "a new type with an increased rate of growth" ..... "It i important to emphasize that the alteration does not consist in the acquisition of a new function, so much as in variation in the property of growth which is normally possessed by the majority of cells". Willis has emphasized that *neoplastic change tends to occur multicentrically* or *diffusely over smaller or larger fields* of *tissue and also by progressive neoplastic conversion of tissue within these fields.* "Neoplastic change does not take place suddenly, but in a gradual and cumulative manner, long-standing hyperplasia often passing insensibly into neoplasia or an early benign or non-invasive tumour by progressive stages into a malignant invasive one without any sudden change in cellular characters, the degree of differentiation or rate of growth. This neoplastic change takes place either simultaneously or successively in vast numbers of cells over more or less extensive fields of tissue. Benign and malignant tumours are not sharply distinct. In many tumour classes every possible gradation of structure and behaviour is to be found, from the most malignant to the most benign".

The conclusions reached above on the relationship of limax amoebae infection to malignant change completely fulfill Nicholson's and Willis' postulates on the nature of the aetiological agent of cancer as acting over a prolonged period over "fields" and producing both benign and malignant tumours. Malignant *"mutation" or "maldifferentiation" in the cells of a tissue* is *thus an expression of the adaptibility of these cells to a new cell climate modified from the normal by the presence of limax amoebae and lymphocytes in the tissues. It is a manifestation of the evolutionary tendency of adaption of cells to environment. It is indeed part of nature itself.*

Since limax amoebae infection appears to be universal after a certain age, why does not every person die of cancer? It has been seen that lymphomata may be familial and occur in families other members of which have collagen and auto-immune disease. Now, as already mentioned, sensitivity of an individual to the antigens of an infecting organism, that is the ability of the latter to cause a cellular and humoral reaction in the host, is genetically controlled and, thus, the constant stimulation of antibody-producing cells (plasma cells and lymphocytes) and the eventual production of lymphomata, myelomata and plasmocytoma and the lymphocytic and plasma cell tissue reaction which may eventually lead to the tendency to cancerous change, must also be genetically determined. Furthermore, since certain families appear prone to cancer in general rather than of a specific organ, there must

be some kind of *genetically controlled predisposition* to *develop the change from normal* to cancerous cells, that is the "maldifferentiation" or "mutation" evidently indicating an *instability of the genetic make-up of such individuals.* The apparent genetic susceptibility of certain organs to collagen and auto-immune disease could explain the familial liability to cancer generally or in certain organs.

Previous description of protozoa in cases of cancer

Old observers, such as Korotneff (1893), Eisen (1900) and Clarke (1912) regarded certain of the tumour cells in a growth as parasitic amoebae, because of their bizarre forms and long pseudopodia, which stretched between cells. These were the Rhopalocephalus carcinomatosus of Korotneff and Cancriamoeba macroglossia of Eisen. The descriptions are highly fanciful and never confirmed and quite unlike limax amoebae. Moreover, as pointed out the protozoal disease is a generalized one and the amoebae are not confined to the growth.

The effect of spread of limax amoebae infection from the mouth or respiratory tract to other tissues

Limax amoebae enter the body by way of the nose, nasopharynx and bronchi or by way of the mouth and gastro-intestinal tract. Spores may enter and lodge in the conjunctivae. The organism may be non-pathogenic, but may become so if there is a lowering of resistance or a pathogenic strain of the organism invades the tissue, producing local stomatitis, gingivitis and tonsillitis or the appropriate HLA antigens are present. Spread from here may result in:-
1) Atrophic local changes in the buccal mucosa extending to nose and pharynx with or without malignancy.

Addendum: Reference was made earlier to the fact that infectious organisms introduced into the body tend to localize in areas of trauma or chronic inflammation. This applies to free-living amoebae and readily explains the fact that malignant disease may begin at the site of trauma or chronic inflammation, an observation to which reference has been made previously. Obviously this only occurs in subjects with a labile genetic state.

Addendum: Feingold, N., Bull, Cancer (Paris), 1978, 65, 79-82 in considering the relationship of the HLA system to malignant diseases found a significant geographical association between some cancers and specific HLA antigens and considered this evidence for a genetic background of susceptibility or resistance to cancer.

2) Deafness with or without malignancy of the middle ear.

3) Up the salivary and lacrimal gland ducts to cause Sjogren-Mikulicz's disease with or without malignancy.

4) Lymphoma and plasmocytoma in tonsil, adenoids, the lymphoid tissue of the base of the tongue and the cervical lymph nodes (cervical collar).

5) Thymic hypertrophy or tumour or mediastinal lymphoma (nodes and thymus).

6) Lymphocytic thyroid disease with or without malignant change and with or without parathyroid disease.

7) Spread to larynx, bronchi and lungs leading to bronchitis, asthma and bronchial malignancy and endochonchial Hodgkin's disease.

8) Atrophic oesophagitis and gastritis with or without cancer and localized lymphoma.

9) Fibrositis of the neck.

10) Rheumatoid arthritis and other collagen and auto-immune diseases in any part of the body.

11) Cancer elsewhere.

12) Leukaemias.

1 3) Generalized malignant lymphoma and myelomatosis.

Systemic amyloidosis and malignancy

It will be recalled that the infection of collagen and auto-immune disease may result in systemic amyloidosis in long-standing cases. Cases of Hodgkin's disease may likewise be complicated by systemic amyloidosis. Azzopardi and Lehner (1966) in 8,758 necropsies found 93 cases with systemic amyloidosis, of which 14 were associated with malignancy, 7 of these were cases of myelomatosis or malignant lymphoma and 7 of carcinoma (uterus, bronchus, stomach, bladder, ovary, biliary tract). They review the literature. Amyloidosis seems to occur in 10 per cent of cases of myelomatosis, 4 per cent of cases of Hodgkin's disease, less than 1 per cent

of lymphosarcoma, in a much higher proportion of cases of macroglobulinaemia and in 1 in 375 cases of carcinoma. The amyloidosis may have a "primary" or "secondary" distribution. It is a product of the reticulo-endothelial cells. It may well be that it is associated with the antibody response of the body to the antigens of the causative organism of the malignancy.

Collagen and auto-immune diseases, aging, immunosurveillance and cancer

Walford (1969) argues that the key process in aging is the accumulation of mutations in immunocytic clones. Aberrant immunocytes are ideally placed to cause havoc. If their antigenic properties are changed, they are thought to attack healthy body cells, generating auto-immune disease, while at the same time they may themselves be attacked by unmutated immunocytes-civil war within the body's defence forces. Burnet (1967) argues that the prime function of the thymus-dependent immune system is "immunological surveillance"-the quality control of cell manufacture, whereby mutant cells are weeded out. He has put forward the theory that a decline in the efficiency of "immunosurveillance" is the cause of many malignant tumours. For him throughout life many tissue cells capable of division do so and may produce aberrant mutant clones of cells which are, however, destroyed or held in check by the normal thymus-producing lymphocytes (immunocytes) of the body. Burnet suggests that with age the production of such cells by the thymus falls off and with this there is a breakdown of "immunosurveillance", so that the abnormal mutant cells proliferate and clinical cancer appears. In this regard Maclaurin (1971) reports the presence in the serum of cases of rheumatoid arthritis of a substance which diminished lymphocytic responsiveness to allogenic and tumour cell stimulation. This could give rise to impaired immunosurveillance. Doll and Kinlen (1970), however, have found that the evidence at present forthcoming provides only weak support for the idea that the appearance of clinical cancer is generally due to the breakdown of immunological surveillance.

If the author's deductions about the nature of so-called collagen and "auto-immune" disease are correct, such theories as Burnet's and Walford's are untenable. The collagen and auto-immune phenomena appear to result from an infection with limax amoebae, which occurs either transplacentally or early in and throughout life. As life progresses there is an increased incidence of the various manifestations of collagen and auto-immune disease and various benign and malignant tumours, all presumably due to decreased resistance or reinfection with different strains of limax amoebae.

In favour of this is the finding that there is an accelerated aging process in young mothers of children with mongolism as suggested by Emanuel et al. (1972). It has been suggested above that such mothers are infected with and react to limax amoebae and exhibit thyroid and other auto-antibodies in the serum more commonly than controls. Furthermore, there is an increased frequency of diabetes and malignancy in the ·families of mongols (Zsako and Kaplan, 1968). Such findings are readily explicable on the basis of the conclusions reached that aging, diabetes, mongolism and cancer are all due to the same cause. These conclusions as to the role of the protozoon in causing human disease would appear to cast serious doubt on the validity of the auto-immune theory put forward by Burnet, including his ideas on aging.

The prenatal origins of cancer in man

Miller (1973) has considered the prenatal origins of human cancer from epidemiological evidence. He concludes:-

1) At least one cancer, namely adenocarcinoma of the vagina, has been induced in the child by synthetic oestrogen therapy during the mother's pregnancy.

2) Prezygotic (genetic) determinants may be submicroscopic mutants as in retinoblastoma and chromosomal aberrations as in mongolism with leukaemia.

3) Specific cancers may be associated with congenital malformations (dysplasias), suggesting that both arise from the same origin during embryogenesis.

4) Early peaks in the occurrence of childhood cancers suggest they arise in utero.

5) Cancers can reach lethal size during intrauterine life.

The liability of congenital anomalies (dysplasias) to malignant change after birth

Evidence has been adduced to suggest that many congenital anomalies result from the effects of limax amoebae infection in the foetus causing mutation and an abnormal clone of cells in the embryo, differing genetically from the normal and which develops into the anomalous tissue. Such foetuses and embryos harbour limax amoebae. The process by which limax amoebae cause congenital growth anomalies or benign tumours seems identical with that which produces benign or malignant tumours in later life. From the earliest studies of malignant disease the common association between congenital abnormalities or malformations (dysplasias) and malignant change in the tissues of an anomaly has been commented on. This is observed in respect of numerous tumours (Willis, 1967; Fraumeni and Glass, 1968). Kobayashi et al. (1968) found congenital anomalies, especially heart disease, harelip, cleft palate, were more frequent in cases of childhood malignancies, including leukaemia, than in children without malignancies, especially in cases of Wilm's tumour, embryonal and teratomatous tu-

-404-

mour and neuroblastomata. Minor anomalies were more frequent in leukaemia and lymphoma. *Neuroblastomata* may be associated with developmental anomalies occurring elsewhere in the body in some cases (see Willis, 1958). These include cleft lip and palate, microcephaly, defective corpus callosum and patent ductus arteriosus, hydrocephalus, extensive spina bifida, coarctation of the aorta, absence of the left ureter and a malformed rib in a premature foetus or vascular anomalies and a thymic cyst, polydactyly, Meckel's diverticulum and other visceral anomalies. Wilm's tumour may be associated with developmental anomalies occurring elsewhere in the body, such as aniridia, hemihypertrophy, microcephaly, pigmented and vascular naevi, mental and growth retardation and pseudo-hermaphroditism (Scarabicchi et al., 1960; Wilson and Orten, 1965; Boxer and Smith, 1970; Canale and Muecke, 1974) and genito-urinary defects (Miller et al., 1964). Perlman et al. (1975) describe a child with foetal gigantism, renal hamartomas and nephroblastomatosis with Wilm's tumour and Carney (1975) a case of Wilm's tumour and renal carcinoma in a retroperitoneal teratoma. Meadows et al. (1974) report a family in which the mother had congenital hemihypertrophy and three of her four children developed Wilm's tumour and the fourth urinary tract anomalies, while Kaufman et al. (1974) describe Wilm's tumour in a father and son. *Retinoblastomata* may be accompanied by developmental anomalies of the affected eye, such as microphthalmos or persistent embryonal vessels. In a case under the author's care a mother had two children. The first died at the age of 5 years of bilateral retinoblastoma and the second developed a unilateral tumour and rheumatoid arthritis at the age of 14 years. Melanomata of the eye may be associated with congenital anomalies of the eye and orbit, such as oculo-dermal melanosis (Jay, 1965). Arnesen and Nemes (1975) report that in 78 per cent

of 95 cases of malignant choroidal melanoma elements of pre-existing benign naevus were found suggesting malignant change usually occurs as a gradual change from a dysplasia.

Malignant change may occur in sequestrated portions of the breast or in supernumerary breasts, aberrant portions of the thyroid, thymus, pancreas, uterus, ovary and adrenal (Ewing, 1940). Malignant change in the thyroglossal duct remnants is reviewed by Keeling and Ochsner (1959). The development of malignant change in branchogenic cysts is well recognized. Renal carcinoma tends to develop in polycystic kidneys in adults and sarcomata in infants in kidneys showing other growth anomalies (Hogan and Simons, 1957). Congenital vascular tumours and malformations involving the urinary tract were described by Hamsher et al. (1958). Carcinoma tends to develop in extrophic bladders (see Cordonnier and Spjut, 1957). Malignant testicular tumours tend to affect undescended testicles. Didelphic uterus with carcinoma in situ in both cervices was recorded by Wall (1958). Uterus bicornis unicollis with rudimentary horn and bilateral carcinoma and carcinoma of the Fallopian tube was reported by Shemwell (1971). Malignant tumours of the jaws (adamantinomata and squamous cell carcinomata) may arise in paradental remains. Malignant tumours may develop in the urachus or in the remains of the notochord (chordoma). Gastric type carcinoma arising in duplication of the small intestine is mentioned by Micolonghi and Meissner (1958). *Congenital pigmented* or *vascular naevi* may become malignant (Potter, 1952; Pack and Davis, 1961; Borello and Gorlin, 1966) and melanosis oculi affecting one eye may develop malignant melanoma (Jay, 1005). Cases of naevus unius lateralis may develop cerebral tumour (Meyerson et al., 1967). Congenital lipomata often associated with growth anomalies may become malignant (liposarcomata) (Adair et al., 1932).

Addendum: Mueller, 5. et at., (J. Pediat, 1978, 127, 219) describe a case of hemihypertrophy and hamartomas with Wilma's tumour and adrenocorticalcarcinoma.

Kaplan (1935) recorded the case of a patient with a segmental naevus associated with an extradural haemangioblastoma and Devic and Tolot (1906) that of a patient with multiple congenital anomalies and an angioma of the left breast becoming malignant. Multiple naevoid basal cell carcinomata associated with congenital anomalies was described by Davidson (1962). *Benign teratomata* are commonly associated with congenital developmental anomalies, including buphthalmos, and may undergo malignant change (Wyburn-Mason, 1958). Teratoma or glioma of the central nervous system may likewise be associated with developmental errors and may undergo malignant change (Davidson and Small, 1960).

It, thus, appears that malignant tumours, other than lymphomata or leukaemia, often arise in dysplastic tissues with a genetic make-up different from the rest of the body and that the occurrence of this abnormal tissue is often due to limax amoebae infection in the embryo. Such genetically abnormal tissues seem predisposed to a further "maldifferentiation" or malignant change (see also Harnden, 1976). The tendency for congenital anomalous (dysplastic) tissues to become malignant appears to depend on the same process as that which produces both benign or malignant tumours later in life. The liability to the latter may be inherited.

Generalized chromosomal abnorntalities and cancers

Generalized chromosomal abnormalities present before the initiation of the neoplastic process makes it more likely that such initiation will take place or having taken place will be more likely to progress to malignancy. This is seen in the predisposition of diseases like mongolism, Klinefelter's and Turner's syndromes to malignancies (Harden, 1976).

Congenital malignant tumours

It has been shown previously that almost all foetal tissues contain free-living amoebae and the serum of all human new-borns contains antibodies against antigens of free-living amoebae. It has been deduced that growth anomalies and benign tumours in the foetus and new-born are commonly the result of limax amoebae infection in causing somatic mutations and the production of abnormal clones of cells, the process being identical with that causing many benign tumours in later life. Congenital benign tumours appear to consist of tissues genetically different from the rest of the body. Just as in later life these benign tumours or growth anomalies may become maiignant, so the same processes may occur in the foetus. Thus, malignant tumours may also be present at birth. The classical paper on these is that of Wells (1940). These are also described by Potter (1952) and Willis (1958). Among such malignant tumours the largest group are the sarcomata. These may be spindle cell sarcomata, embryonic sarcomata, fibrosarcomata or myxosarcomata. Adrenal and extra-adrenal neuroblastomata are the next group and Wilm's tumour the third in order of frequency. Among other tumours are neuro-epitheliomata and gliomas of the retina, malignant renal and testicular tumours, malignant teratoma, cerebral glioma, embryonic malignant tumours of the liver of various kinds, carcinoma, malignant melanoma, malignant thyroid tumours, chorionepitheliomata, congenital leukaemia (Potter, 1952; Brescia et al., 1955; Brodie and Henderson, 1960; Yoshikawa et al., 1960; Anastassea-Vlachou et al., 1961; Bernard et al., 1964), adamantinoma, schwannoina (Potter, 1952), gastric teratoma (Keeley et al., 1963), lymphomata and Hodgkin's disease (Sacrez et al., 1954) and myeloma (Suzuki et al., 1960). Sometimes Hodgkin's disease, reticulosarcoma or lymphosarcoma may be present at birth in infants born of an apparently healthy mother and occasionally of a mother suffering from a reticulosis (see Berghinz, 1900; Branch, 1933, Wells, 1940; Hoster and Dratman, 1948; Kasdon, 1949; Sacrez et al., 1954; Wintrobe, 1956; Zaidi and de Bellefeuille, 1960; Leading Article, Lancet, 1972, 2, 907). Such cases point to the factor which causes reticuloses and leukaemias and other tumours as being present in the mother, in whom it may or may not cause a reaction and tumours, and its being transmitted across the placenta to cause congenital anomalies, benign tumours or malignant disease in a susceptible foetus. Congenital malignant tumours differ in no way from those occurring in post-natal life. Their similar features suggest a similar aetiology.

Placental tumours

The author found limax amoebae in many placentae, especially when the foetus was abnormal. The placenta forms an integral part of the foetus and may be affected by benign tumours or hamartomata, to which reference has already been made. For an account of these tumours see Potter (1952). Hydatidiform mole, choriocarcinoma and teratoma may develop in the placenta. The last-named would appear to have the same origin as that of teratomata in the rest of the foetus. Hydatidiform mole is usually associated with a macerated foetus, the cells of which often show chromosomal abnormalities causing non-viability. In other cases the foetus may exhibit hamartomata of blood and lymph vessels and foetal hydrops and is aborted. This suggests that not only the congenital abnormalities and the chromosomal abnormalities, but also the mole may perhaps result from limax amo bae infection of the foetus.

Choriocarcinoma in the uterus follows an hydat idiform mole in half the cases, abortions in a quarter and in a quarter of pregnancies with a viable foetus (Potter,

1952). It may be associated with a dysgerminoma in the mother. Suggestions have been made that its development and spread may be related to immunological factors. This again may perhaps result from limax amoebae infection in the placental part of the foetus.

Conclusions on the relationship of development of congenital anomalies and malignant change

Thus, it seems that the development of human benign or malignant tumours in tissues exhibiting lymphocytic infiltration as a response to limax amoebae infection is not due to the incorporation of a virus into the cell mechanism, but is a slow adaptation of the cells of a tissue, over a smaller or larger area to a new environment induced by the amoebae infection. The malignant change is "induced" by the climatic changes around the cell. This is akin to the induction of changes in normally developing foetal tissues by neighbouring cells and tissues. When foetal tissues are infected with limax amoebae and the resulting collection of lymphocytes occurs, it has been seen that a "malinduction" of the development of tissues arises, producing either a congenital growth anomaly or a hamartoma, essentially a benign tumour, or congenital malignant change. Such observations recall the close relationship between embryological growth disturbances and malignancy (see Willis, 1958). The tendency for malignant change or benign tumour development to occur either in the foetus or after birth, is, in fact, part of the natural tendency of cells and organisms to adjust their metabolism to a new environment, a property dependent on genetic factors, which would explain a familial tendency to cancer. This property is an essential one for normal evolution and cancer and evolution are, in fact, manifestations of the same characters of living cells.

Cancer due to trauma or chronic irritation

It is now accepted that trauma may play a part in the causation of skin cancers, meningiomas, glioma and fibrosarcoma, possibly bone sarcoma, testicular tumour and malignant melanoma (Evans, 1966). Tumour as a sequel to an accident was considered by Becker (1960) and meningioma after head injury by Walshe (1961). This is well-known after surgical intervention in cases of Von Recklinghausen's disease. Injury to bone affected by Paget's disease may lead to sarcomatous change (Semple, 1969). Injury of the cervix uteri by childbirth may likewise predispose to cancer. Trauma is especially well-known to play a part in initiating malignant change in congenital growth anomalies, such as cryptorchidism, after surgical interference.

Furthermore, chronic irritation, such as by a denture or a jagged tooth in the mouth, of the cervix, in varicose ulcers, by the pressure of a truss or calculi in the bile passages or renal pelvis, or of a gastric ulcer may result in cancerous changes in the involved area. Cancerous change may occur in the scars of pulmonary tuberculosis, in chronic sinuses or areas of osteomyelitis. Cancer of the middle ear in 50 per cent of cases follows chronic infection (Fairman, 1972). Actinic rays or exposure to weather have a similar effect on the skin. Trauma of mouth, pharynx, larynx and lung by smoking may have a similar effect, unrelated to any special effect of tobacco.

It has been shown that such an irritation or injury may cause the localization of any organism, including protozoal infections, to the affected area. Such observations raise the possibility that chronic irritation and trauma lead to malignant change because they induce the localization of limax amoebae to this area and thus a liability to malignant change in genetically susceptible subjects. It may well be that known carcinogenic agents also act in part by causing local irritation and localizing amoebae to the irritated area. Virchow's chronic irritation hypothesis of the cause of cancer may have some basis in certain cases, but the mechanism is not as simple as he suggested.

Malignant disease in animals

It is well known that malignant disease in some lower mammals and birds may result from viral infections. However, growths occur in invertebrates, fishes, amphibia and reptiles and probably in all mammals, but the cause of these remains unknown. It has been seen that small amoebae may be parasitic on invertebrates, fish and reptiles and they were found in ordinary butclier's meat and tumours of horses. It could well be that these organisms are causative of some of the tumours in these animals.

Chapter XIII

Humoral changes in the blood in cases of malignant disease explained on the basis of limax amoebae infection

It has been concluded that in many manifestations of collagen and auto-immune disease there must be some abnormal substance circulating in the blood to produce such disturbances as Kohner's phef?Omenon, Henoch-Schonlein purpura and various disturbances of the hypothalamus, such as mental disease, paralysis agitans, thyrotoxicosis, diabetes, etc. Limax amoebae infection appears to be responsible for many of the bodily disturbances associated with malignancy and substances derived from the organism must exist in the blood in such circumstances. Nakahara and Fukuoka (1950) isolated from tumours a substance they called "toxohormone", apparently protein-like and heat stable, which affected the liver catalase in mice and disturbed protein metabolism. This could well be derived from limax amoebae in the tumour. Again, in many cases of leukaemia there may be abnormal bleeding and petechial haemorrhages with a positive cuff test (symptomatic purpura). Allen et al. (1949), Barnard (1948) and others found these phenomena resembled the effects of heparin administration and the bleeding time was prolonged and the clotting time decreased. They found that the bleeding tendency ceases and the bleeding and clotting times may return to normal after intravenous administration of an antiheparin, such as toluidine blue or protamine sulphate. The author confirmed this as in the following case:-

Case 99 Female, aged 50 years, suffering from chronic myeloid leukaemia with severe generalized petechiae and bleeding from nasal mucosa and gums. The bleed-

ing and clotting time were determined before and two hours after the slow intravenous injection of 1 mi. of 1 per cent protamine solution. On the first occasion the readings were as follows:–

Bleeding time (Dukes method)	Before injection	2 hours later
Normal 2-5 minutes	9 minutes	5 minutes 10 seconds
Clotting time (Wrights method)		
Normal 6-12 minutes	5 minutes 20 seconds	9 minutes

There was immediate cessation of the bleeding and appearance of petechiae for 8 days, when both returned. The injection was repeated with the following result:–

	Before injection	2 hours after
Bleeding time	9 mins. 35 secs.	4 mins.
Clotting time	3 mins. 50 secs.	6 mins. 15 secs.

Since protamine and toluidine blue neutralize mucopolysaccharides like heparin, this suggests that such a substance exists in the blood in this condition. It will be recalled that limax amoebae give a strongly positive PAS stain indicative of the presence of mucopolysaccharides in the cytoplasm. It may well be that the substance in the blood in the above situation is a mucopolysaccharide derived from limax amoebae.

Intravascular clotting and cancer

Earlier it was pointed out that a tendency to intravascular thromboses was a feature of rheumatoid disease, that is limax amoebae infection, while in advanced cases of malignant disease there exists in the blood a mucopolysaccharide heparin-like substance, which decreases the clotting time and must tend to favour the occurring of spontaneous intravascular clotting in such circumstances. A tendency to recurrent thrombophlebitis of various vessels may be observed in cases of lymphomata, leukaemia and myelomatosis and malignant disease of various organs (Wintrobe, 1967) including carcinoma of the pancreas, bronchus, gall-bladder, stomach, ovaries, uterus, etc. (see Evans, 1966; Wintrobe, 1967; Willis, 1967). The tendency for thrombophlebitis to affect a number of vessels in succession has been given the name thrombophlebitis migrans, but this is unsatisfactory as not only are veins subject to thromboses, but there is also a widespread thrombotic occlusion of small arteries, friable vegetations on the heart valves, later giving rise to verrucose endocarditis and infarctions of various organs (Smith and Yates, 1955; Rohner et al., 1966; Zuffa et al., 1972). The endocarditis may eventually be indistinguishable from that occurring in rheumatic heart disease. Histologically the affected vessels exhibit an inflammatory change in their walls with numerous lymphocytes and often giant cells and often with well-marked periphlebitis. There may be considerable proliferation of the endothelium. The changes may be related to the vasa vasorum and the accompanying nerve bundles may also be affected. It is tempting to suppose that this phenomenon could be due to the heparin-like substance derived from limax amoebae in the tumours and elsewhere.

Chapter XIV

Conditions in which there is a known lowered resistance to infection and an increased liability to both "collagen" and "auto-immune" diseases and malignancy

The depression of immune mechanisms with the development of lymphoma and other malignancies

In cases in which lymphoma, myelomatosis and chronic lymphatic leukaemia develop in subjects suffering from rheumatoid arthritis or other manifestations of rheumatoid disease, RF and organ specific antibodies may disappear from the blood. Tala! and Bunim (1964) describe a case of Sjogren's syndrome which developed malignant lymphoma, RF and organ specific antibodies, previously present, disappeared from the serum with the development of the reticulosarcoma. Nilsen et al. (1967) recorded a case of systemic lupus erythematosus which developed Hodgkin's disease ten years later. All clinical and serological signs of systemic lupus erythematosus then disappeared. Fernandez·Herlihy and Kott (1967), Schmidt and Gebhardt (1969), Szegedi et al. (1968) and Klingmuller and Voelander (1965) also record similar cases. In one case successful treatment of the Hodgkin's di·sease caused a reappearance of the serological changes and antibodies in the blood. Zawadski and Benedek (1969) describe a case of rheumatoid arthritis with RF in the blood, which disappeared with the development of lymphosarcoma, and five cases of seropositive rheumatoid arthritis in which myelomatosis developed and in which the RF titre fell markedly with the onset of the malignancy. In the author's experience, described above, with cases of rheumatoid arthritis developing lymphoma or lymphatic leukaemia and sometimes carcinoma, this phenomenon

has also been noted. Alexander and Fairley (1968) report that in reticuloses, including leukaemia, circulating antibody formation is usually impaired, especially in disease of lymphocytic and plasma cells (chronic lymphatic leukaemia, lymphosarcoma and myelomatosis) . In other reticuloses and carcinoma variable results are obtained, but usually only the primary response to antigenic stimulation is impaired. Arenberg (1964) and Hughes and MacKay (1965) point out that in cases of cancer and lymphoma there develops depression of immune mechanisms and tissue anergy, which may return to normal with successful treatment of the tumour. Southam (1968) reports that in cases of non-lymphomatous cancer many patients show impaired immune responses, especially those requiring mediation of cells rather than the production of serum antibodies. Lee et al. (1970) report similar findings of depressed antibody-producing capacity in cases of human cancer. It has been shown that limax amoebae infection which exists in cancer cases may depress the formation of immunoglobulins and the humoral mechanisms resisting the growth of cancer cells and thus a cancerous process gains momentum. That this does occur was shown by Dostalova et al. (1970), who found a progressive decrease in IgG and IgM in the serum with advancing cancer. The loss of the immune mechanisms in advanced c;ancer not only explains the rapid progress of malignant disease after it has appeared, but also why intercurrent infections, which further depress immune mechanisms, may cause a sudden growth of hitherto stationary secondaries (Gordon-Taylor, 1959; Willis, 1967) or the sudden appearance of Hodgkin's disease (Hoster and Dratman, 1946).

In a number of conditions in man there occurs a depression of bodily resistance to infections and in these there appears to be a special liability to both collagen and auto-immune diseases and to lymphomata and cancer. Among these are:-

1) Congenital agamm:<globulinaemia, already considered.

2) Increasing age, already considered.

3) Generalized sarcoidosis.

4) The effects of administration of hydantoins.

5) The effects of organ transplants and administering immunosuppressive drugs.

6) The effects of generalized irradiation.

a) Sarcoidosis and malignant lymphoma and carcinoma

In cases of sarcoidosis with its partial failure of cellular immunity there appears to be an increased susceptibility to the manifestations of collagen and auto-immune disease (see above). There are a number of reports in which disseminated sarcoido10is has been associated with or followed by the development of malignant lymphoma or leukaemia (Poutier, 1934, quoted by Raben et al., 1962; Craver, quoted by Hoster and Dratman, 1948; Lamache et al., 1954, quoted by Raben et al., 1962; Moertel and Hagedorn, 1957; Razis et al., 1959 a; Raben et al., 1962). Buckle (1960) described a patient with sarcoidosis of the lungs who developed generalized reticulosarcoma as the former was regressing. Kissel et al. (1961) reported the case of a patient with lymphoma in which the histological changes of sarcoidosis were present in some of the lymph nodes and the changes of lymphatic leukaemia appeared terminally. Atwood et al. (1966) described the case of a 49 year old negro with generalized sarcoidosis who developed mycosis fungoides and fatal malignant lymphoma. They found 14 previously reported cases of this association. Two cases of co-existent disseminated sarcoidosis and Hodgkin's disease were described by Goldfarb and Cohen (1970) and another in which sarcoidosis was followed by lymphosarcoma by Silver et al. (1967). Five cases of sarcoidosis followed by Hodgkin's disease or chronic lymphatic leukaemia were reported by Brincker (1972), of which one case had both Hodgkin's disease, squamous carcinoma of the lip and leukoplakia of one vocal cord and the other chronic lymphatic leukaemia and carcinoma of the cervix. Sarcoidosis always comes first.

Gresham and Ackerley (1958) and Gregorie et al. (1962) record sarcoid-like lesions within neoplasms and in regional lymph nodes and these have been reported in association with a variety of tumours, for example, tumours of the breast, skin, bronchus, bile ducts, ovaries and neurocytoma. Generalized sarcoidosis may also occur. The former authors report a case of carcinoma of the stomach with sarcoid lesions in the lymph nodes whether or not these were affected by metastases. They were also present in the lung and liver, and Gresham and Ackerley mention ten cases of carcinomatosis in which regional lymph nodes showed diffuse granulomata and giant cell reaction. Granulomatous lesions like sarcoidosis are also described in ovarian dysgerminomata and granulosa cell tumours. In such cases of "sarcoid" in local lymph nodes draining a malignant tumour it seems that the sarcoid changes are a reaction to substances produced by the tumour.

Carcinoma may also exhibit a relationship to disseminated sarcoidosis. Sarcoidosis associated with bronchial carcinoma has also been described by Jefferson et al. (1954) and Sakula (1963). Warner (1962) reports sarcoidosis and malignant teratoma of the lung. Badmaeva (1970) reports a case of sarcoidosis which developed angio-sarcomatosis and Jahn et al. (1969) the case of a patient with generalized sarcoidosis, ulcerative colitis and carcinoma of the terminal ileum. In n case known to the author multiple shadows were present in both lungs radiologically and a carcinoma of the pylorus was found at operation. Total gastrectomy and splenectomy were performed and histologically the spleen showed the changes of sarcoidosis.

In cases in which generalized sarcoidosis preceded or accompanies the manifestations of malignant lymphoma it may well be that the liability of patients with sarcoidosis to develop the manifestations of rheumatoid disease is related to the subsequent development of lymphoma or carcinoma. As regards the association of generalized sarcoidosis with various malignant tumours this may be ambivalent. It may be that the development of malignant disease with its associated loss of resistance to infection may favour the development of sarcoidosis or vice versa.

b) The effects of administration of hydantoins

It has been suggested that some cases of idiopathic epilepsy may result from limax amoebae infection. Hydantoins are, of course, widely used in its treatment. Attention has already been drawn to observations suggesting that .they depress both cellular and humoral immunity mechanisms.

Hydantoins and lymphomata

It has been seen that hydantoins may result in the appearance of collagen diseases, including benign lymphadenopathy. A condition closely mimicking malignant lymphoma, clinically and pathologically, following taking of various hydantoins over a prolonged period was described by Saltzstein and Ackerman (1959). The syndrome included lymphadenopathy, fever, exanthemata, eosinophilia in the blood and bone marrow and less often hepato- and spleno-megaly. Pathologically the lymph nodes showed obliteration of their normal architecture, hyperplasia of reticulum cells and other elements, frequent mitoses, infiltration with eosinophils, focal necrosis and phagocytosis, but no Reed-Sternberg cells or a picture like Hodgkin's disease or reticulosarcoma, or only chronic inflammation. One patient, and another quoted from the literature, showed persistent plasmacytosis in the bone marrow and resected nodes abnormal serum proteins. There was no conclusive evidence of myeloma. Hyman and Sommers (1966), however, report six cases of true Hodgkin's disease and lymphoma developing during anticonvulsant therapy and Rausing and Trell (1971) another. Brown (1971) reports that there is a spectrum of lymphadenopathies varying from hyperplasia to neoplasm with Reed-Sternberg cells. It may be that depression of resistance to limax amoebae by the drug is responsible for the appearance of both collagen disease and lymphoma in such circumstances.

c) Human organ transplants and cancer

In cases of human organ transplants in which therapeutic immunosuppresion is used there are now over 40 reported cases of the development of malignant lymphoma (Doll and Kinlen, 1970). Fairley (1971) reports that in about 4,000 renal transplants there occurred 12 reticulum cell sarcomas, 3 other lymphomas, 2 carcinoma of the gastro-intestinal tract, 9 of the lip or skin, 2 of carcinomatosis and 4 of other organs. Inadequate information was available in 5 cases and carcinoma-in-situ of the cervix occurred in 5 cases. Walder et al. (1971) report skin cancer, often multiple, as developing in 7 of 71 cases of kidney allograft recipients receiving immunosuppressive drugs. Tallent et al. (1971) describes a case which developed a carcinoma of the cervix and Hyun-Hank and Williams (1972) the development of endometrioid carcinoma of the uterus and bilateral ovarian carcinoma in a subject of renal transplantation and immunosuppression. Pierce et al. (1972) found 3 cases of reticulum cell sarcoma in 151 cases of renal transplants, more than 100 times greater than expected. In the Leading Article (Brit. med. J., 1972, 3, 713) it is stated that in about 5,000 organ transplant recipients on immunosuppressive drugs there have been recorded 17 cases of reticulum cell sarcoma and two of unclassified lymphoma. In 9 cases the brain has been involved (normally a rare occurrence) and in 6 cases exclusively. This incidence of lymphoma is perhaps 50 times the normal. In addition there have been 2 cases of Kaposi's sarcoma, 2 leiomyosarcoma and at least 28 other tumours and probably 7 further tumours have been reported from Australia. The authors state that this could be due to either 1) a breakdown in immunosurveillance, 2) proliferation of oncongenic viruses (or other causative organisms), 3) direct induction of neoplastic change by immunosuppressive drugs (for which there is little evidence) or 4) a continuous antigenic stimulation by the presence of the graft. Myking (1971) in discussing the appearance of malignant lymphomata in these circumstances suggested that they arise from chronic antigenic stimulation by the transplanted organ. That this is so seems proved by the case reported by Brown et al. (1974) who describe a reticulum cell sarcoma of host origin arising in a transplanted kidney. This may also apply to the development of non-lymphomatous tumours.

Relationship of radiation injury to malignancy

Exposure to radiation may result in acute radiation injury or if the dosage is less to late radiation effects (see Hempelmann, 1971). In either case there occurs cell damage and death most extensive in rapidly proliferating tissues, such as blood-forming tissues and intestinal and germinal epithelium, which soon become depleted of all radio-sensitive cells. This leads to granulocytopenia and depression of formation of immune bodies by lymphocytes and plasma cells with resultant impaired resistance to infection, which may persist indefinitely. Later any kind of malignancy may occur in locally exposed tissues as a direct effect on the constituent cells. In other cases there may develop the late manifestations of whole body irradiation, such as premature aging, acute or chronic myeloid leukaemia and other myeloproliferative disorders or malignant lymphomata, including Hodgkin's disease. These are found without evidence of previous radiation effects and differ in no way from those occurring spontaneously. These later developments could be explained as the result of depression of resistence to limax amoebae infection.

—414 —

Chapter XV

Other types of chronic antigenic stimulation as possible causes of malignancy

The geographical distribution of cancer

Comparisons of the incidence of cancer in different organs in different parts of the world indicate that differences in the environment, in diet, surroundings, socio-economic status and personal habits must play a part in the occurrence of many human cancers. In Africa and India the disease appears to be caused by a varying number of agents, not only in different countries, but even in different parts of the same country. Its incidence ultimately seems to depend on the degree of carcinogenicity of individual agents or a combination of them and on the amount of environmental and other contaminants to which a particular population is exposed, both at the general and personal levels. In many cases the causation is probably multifactorial and since limax amoebae are world-wide in distribution they may Constitute one factor in the causation of many cancers in all parts of the world. Cook (1971) in considering the high incidence of cancer of the oesophagus in different African races suggests that the use of maize as a major ingredient of alcoholic drinks is important in this respect. The similar incidence of different cancers in negroes and whites in the United States of America suggests that race and thus genetic factors are not important in their causation. However, it has been argued above that both the response of the human body to limax amoebae infection and the occurrence of lymphomata and cancer in response to this infection may depend on genetic factors. That this is so is shown by the fact that limax amoebae are world-wide in distribution, but it will be recalled that rheumatoid arthritis and "auto-immune" diseases in general occur only rarely in certain parts of Africa. This may be due to genetic and immunological factors responsible for different responses to the organisms in different races of man or perhaps to different species of amoebae or variations of their virulence in different parts of the world. Such differences would perhaps be reflected in different incidences of malignancy in different places.

It could also be that chronic antigenic stimulation from causes other than limax amoebae infection plays a part in causing lymphoma in some parts of the world. Among chronic infections leading to prolonged antigenic stimulation are:–
a) Chronic malaria.
b) Leprosy.
c) Tuberculosis.

a) Chronic malaria in relation to the development of malignant lymphoma, myelomatosis and leukaemia

Mention has been made above to the finding of M-antiglobulins (RF-like globulins) in high titre in the blood in infections with certain protozoa in Central Africa in the absence of rheumatoid arthritis. These infections include trypanosomiasis, malaria and kala-azar. In Uganda in the indiginous population there are found in the serum a high titre of malarial antibody and high levels of IgM, RF and circulating auto-antibodies to heart, thyroid and gastric parietal cells (see above). The levels of the latter and of RF were related to that of the malarial antibody titre.

The immunological syndrome was related to malarial infection. It disappears after a period of treatment with antiprotozoal drugs.

Beale et al. (1972) found that in cases of acute malaria there occurred a rapid, but temporary rise in the IgM content of the serum in the attack. After repeated malarial infections permanent increases in IgG and IgM in the serum appear in response to the chronic antigenic stimulation. It has been shown (Jerusalem, 1968; Leading Article, Lancet, 1970, 2, 1121) that mice repeatedly infected with the protozoon, Plasmodium berghei, develop a non-leukaemic malignant lymphoma, the incidence of which seems to depend on the severity of the primary infection. In long-standing cases of malaria in man severe qualitative and quantitative changes occur in the reticuloendothelial system (Marsden, 1971). There may be an eosinophilia in the blood. The lymphoid-macrophage system of spleen, liver and marrow responds to the infection by intense phagocytic activity destroying large numbers of parasitized cells with enlargement of the respective organs. Hyperaemia, haemorrhages and thromboses in the various organs, centro-lobular necrosis of hepatic cells and diffuse cellular hyperplasia of the spleen may all be found. Similar, but less pronounced, changes in other organs are described.

Watson-Williams and Allan (1968), Marsden and Hamilton (1969), Ziegler et al. (1969), Sagoe (1970). Marsden (1971) and Ziegler and Stuvier (1972) discuss the condition known as tropical splenomegaly syndrome found in tropical Africa, New Guinea and elsewhere where malaria is hyperendemic. This is ascribed to an abnormal immunological response to malarial infection, but not apparently to P. malaria. This may be genetically determined (Ziegler and Stuvier, 1972). The splenomegaly is associated with anaemia, in part due to splenic pooling of blood, and is often accompanied by hepatomegaly. Lym-phocytic and plasma cell infiltration of the hepatic sinusoids, portal tracts and spleen may be seen and there may be an increase in the lymphocytes in the upper abdominal lymph nodes, marrow and blood and an increase in the fixed phagocytic cells of the tissues (Kupffer cells and histiocytes). The condition is considered as a reactive *"lymphoreticular proliferative* disorder". Cases show a high fluorescent malarial antibody titre and RF in the blood, hyper-gammaglobulinaemia and often cryoglobu-linaemia. The IgM (macroglobulin) level in the blood is raised. It is thought that the malarial antibodies reside in this fraction. The condition generally responds, often slowly, to prolonged administration of antimalarial drugs, such as chloroquine or proguanil.

There is mounting evidence that the reactive proliferation of lymphocytes, "the lymphoreticular proliferative disorder" in this manifestation of chronic malarial infection may, in some cases, become neoplastic with the resultant development of chronic lymphatic leukaemia or lymphoma of various types (Hildts and Shaw, 1958; Lowenthal and Hutt, 1968; Watson-Williams and Allan, 1968; Ziegler et al., 1969; Sagoe, 1970). Watson-Williams and Allan described a case ending in reticulosarcomatosis and point out that in Nigeria tropical splenomegaly and chronic lymphatic leukaemia are two ends of a spectrum of diseases differing only in the white cell count and both respond to antimalarial drugs. Sagoe (1970) investigated 43 cases of tropical splenomegaly, of which 11 were clinically identical with the other 32, but failed to respond to treatment with proguanil. Like those that did respond 3 of these cases showed hepatic sinusoidal lymphocytosis and 3 lymphocytosis in the portal tracts. They were, therefore, similar histologically to the responders to proguanil. These differed only in the fact that the level of IgM in the blood was not raised or was below normal. Of these 11 cases 3 were lost to follow up. Of the others three developed chronic lymphatic leukaemia, one Hodgkin's sarcoma and one malignant lymphoma, while the other three developed anaemia, in two of which this was auto-immune in type and possibly associated with malignant lymphoma. As in cases of malignant lymphoma and lymphatic leukaemia occurring in this country it may well be that antibodies disappear from the blood in cases of chronic malarial infection with the development of such malignancies.

In this regard some cases in the author's series above are of interest. One, a white woman, aged 57 years, had lived in Central Africa until four years before hospital attendance and had suffered from many attacks of malaria and two attacks of trypanosomiasis. She had now developed lymphosarcoma. The other, a Jamaican male aged 41 years, had suffered from severe and long-standing malaria in childhood until his twenties and was now found to be suffering from myelomatosis. Another case in the author's series was as follows:-

Case 100 Male, aged 55 years, had Dengue fever 11, 10 and 8 years before admission and he had suffered recurrent malaria in India and Malaysia. Each attack was accompanied by swelling of the right inguinal and axillary nodes, which later subsided. After an attack 6 months before admission glandular swelling persisted, but diminished in size after taking a mixture containing arsenic. Six weeks before admission to hospital he developed indigestion and later jaundice. Examination showed enlarged lymph nodes in the right posterior triangle of the neck, right axilla and both groins and hepatomegaly. Post mortem showed also enlarged mediastinal and para-aortic nodes, splenomegaly, hepatomegaly and ascites. Histologically these were typical of Hodgkin's disease.

These cases and the above considerations suggest that chronic antigenic stimulation from chronic malarial infection may

be responsible for the development of some cases of malignant lymphoma, chronic lymphatic leukaemia and myelomatosis. This would apply to the endemic areas of malarial infection which include the Mediterranean, littoral Spain, Corsica, Sardinia, Italy, the Balkans, South Russia, the Middle East, Afganistan, Arabia, India, South China, Indo-China, Indonesia, New Guinea, Northern Australia, Tropical and South Africa, Southern North America and Northern South America.

b) Leprosy and cancer in man

As mentioned already in cases of leprosy ANF, RF and thyroid and other auto-antibodies may occur in the blood and vitiligo in the skin. Malignant disease may develop in cases of leprosy. This was discussed and reviewed by Keil (1965) and Michalany (1966). The former described 539 cases of skin cancer in cases of leprosy among 60,000 histological examinations and added 94 previously unreported cases. He estimated that one per cent of cases of leprosy developed skin cancer. The type of leprosy was always lepromatous and the leproma and cancer associated was evident in the same section. The author has personally observed three such cases. Mailloux (1959) described a case of leprosy developing melanoma-sarcoma. Rodriguez et al. (1968) collected six cases of leprosy developing malignant lymphoma 10-22 years after the onset of leprosy. Clinically they showed the normal evolution of each disease. Oleineck (1969) reported two cases of leprosy developing leukaemia /lymphoma. He found no evidence that chronic intense stimulation of the reticulo-endothelial system by leprous infection leads to lymphomatous transformation. He regarded the association of the two diseases as fortuitious. Nevertheless the possibility remains that the chronic antigenic stimulation and the cellular reaction in the tissues which occurs in cases of leprosy may perhaps result in the development of malignancy in the same way as does limax amoebae infection. Alternatively the chronic irritation of the leprosy infection may localize limax amoebae to the area and this may be the ultimate cause of the malignant change.

c) Chronic antigenic stimulation by tuberculosis and tumour formation

Tuberculosis frequently occurs in cases of Hodgkin's disease and other lymphomata and a "leukaemoid" reaction is well known in the blood in this disease (Wintrobe, 1967). Tuberculosis infection has been reported in as many as 20 per cent of cases of Hodgkin's disease (Hoster and Dratman, 1948). This has usually been attributed to secondary infection and regarded as causatively unrelated to Hodgkin's disease. Several workers have postulated a relationship between tuberculosis and cancer (see Willis, 1967). Carcinoma may develop in the neighbourhood of old pulmonary tuberculous lesions or sinuses (Willis, 1967) and explained as due to "chronic irritation". Tuberculosis and cancer of the breast may co-exist (Bundschuh, 1914). Tuberculosis and cancer of the Fallopian tube, endometrium and testis have also been reported as occurring in association. In view of what has already been said it would seem possible that the chronic antigenic stimulation of tuberculous infection may perhaps cause lymphoma in susceptible subjects or local cancer in infected areas. Alternatively it may cause localization of limax amoebae infection to the inflamed area.

d) Chronic antigenic stimulation in cases of osteomyelitis and malignancy

The bacterial infection causing chronic osteomyelitis may lead to local malignant change in the walls of the sinuses (Schiewe, 1966; Browne, 1966; Schiewe and Koch, 1967; Cervenansky, 1970; Buachidze and Onoprienko, 1970). The tumour is usually a squamous cell carcinoma. According to Schiewe (1966) there are 266 cases of this change on record with an incidence of 0.38 per cent of malignancy in chronic osteomyelitic cases. The malignancy develops 13-46 years after the onset of the bone condition. Baitz and Kyle (1964) describe a case of chronic osteomyelitis of 40 years duration which developed a solitary myeloma in the sinus tract. Scheuer-Karpin and d'Heureuse-Gerhardt (1965) suggest that reticuloses and leukaemia may result from chronic osteomyelitis. In these cases it may be that the squamous carcinoma results from the chronic infection and lymphoma and myeloma from chronic antigenic stimulation by the causative bacteria. Alternatively, localization of limax amoebae to the inflamed area may be responsible for these changes.

418-

Leukaemoid blood pictures and leukaemia

Leukaemoid blood pictures are considered by Wintrobe (1967). They may occur as a result of certain infections and in some cases are associated with anaemia, fever, splenomegaly and changes identical with those of true leukaemia, *from which they sometimes cannot be differentiated even at autopsy.* They are differentiated from leukaemia by the fact that they disappear with successful treatment of the causative infection. The infections known to cause leukaemoid reactions are:-

1) Bacterial, for example pneumococcal, meningococcal, tuberculous, diphtherial, plague and streptococcal septicaemia.

2) Spirochaetal, especially congenital syphilis.

3) Viral.

4) Protozoal, includinamoebiasis histolytica and malaria (Hildts and Shaw, 1958; Gard, 1964).

The response may be myelocytic, myeloblastic, lymphocytic or monocytic. This pathological response to such infections has been thought to be due to immunological disturbances or possibly due to collapse of cellular defense mechanisms.

In true leukaemias, as has been stated, the same bodily changes are found as with leukaemoid blood pictures resulting from known infections. True leukaemias could thus often be a response to an unknown infection. Osserman (1971) points out that chronic infections, such as tuberculosis, syphilis and osteomyelitis, may lead both to plasma cell dyscrasia, hypergammaglobulinaemia, monoclonal gammopathy and to monocytic leukaemia. Reference has also been made to the occurrence of chronic lymphatic leukaemia in cases of tropical splenomegaly due to malaria and its disappearance on giving antimalarial drugs. Scheuer-Karpin (1959, 1972) describes cases of chronic lymphatic leukaemia associated with chronic antigenic stimulation by bacterial infections, such as active chronic tuberculosis, repeated malarial attacks, osteomyelitis, bronchiectasis, urinary infections and otitis media. In the majority of cases of leukaemias no history of exposure to known leukaemogens is found, but evidence of limax amoebae infection is present and the leukaemic changes appear to result from this. This is shown by the following:-

1) Mention has already been made of the finding of limax amoebae in all the tissues of all cases of leukaemia examined.

2) In the acute disease features, such as fever, sweating, rigors, lymphadenopathy and splenomegaly, are like those associated with acute limax amoebae infection.

3) It has been shown that the acute or chronic manifestations of leukaemia may be partly relieved or in cases of chronic lymphatic leukaemia abolished by antiamoebic drugs.

4) Cases of disseminated eosinophilic collagen disease may develop imperceptibly into chronic myeloid leukaemia with eosinophilia or into eosinophilic leukaemia.

5) Every form of collagen or "auto-immune" disease may develop any type of leukaemia. Such cases were among the series from the South West Metropolitan

Cancer Registry and in the author's own series. Among the former was the case of a boy of five years with Still's disease, who developed acute leukaemia a year later. Saatci and Pirnar (1970) reported the case of a boy of 13 years suffering from juvenile rheumatoid arthritis, who developed acute leukaemia and Balthazar et al. (1973) a similar case. Patients may develop acute myelogenic leukaemia some time after an initial blood picture of anaemia, neutropenia or thrombocytopenia or all three (pancytopenia), often a manifestation of collagen disease (Kumas and Bhargave, 1970). Cases of childhood leukaemia often present as polyarthritis. Fink et al. (1972) described such cases in which the blood studies were normal when the case first presented and the joints showed increase in synovial fluid and synovial thickening. Spilsberg and Meyer (1972) reporting on 74 cases of arthritis in childhood leukaemia found that 10 presented with arthritis prior to the leukaemia. RF and other auto-antibodies were present in 11 per cent of cases. Schaller (1972) described ten children with acute lymphoblastic leukaemia who presented with arthritis at a rheumatic clinic.

6) Acute or chronic leukaemia of any type may also occur in association with any type of lymphoma, myelomatosis, any type of carcinoma· or even in multiple cancers.

7) Paraproteinaemia and cryoglobulinaemia may be a feature of collagen and "auto-immune" disease due to limax amoebae infection and they also occur in association with any form of leukaemia.

8) Eosinophilia, a response to a parasite, may occur in association with myeloid leukaemia and may form 20 per cent of the total white blood count (Wintrobe, 1967). This suggests a parasitic aetiology of the leukaemia.

9) Auto-antibodies tend to disappear from the blood in cases of leukaemia. However, Innis (1963) reported the presence of a positive rheumatoid arthritic latex fixation test in 7 of 17 patients with acute myeloid leukaemia, in 4 of 8 with subacute and in 1 of 3 with chronic myeloid leukaemia. Innis and Ferguson (1964) in 14 cases of chronic lymphatic leukaemia found 5 gave a positive latex fixation test. Sherry (1968) found a positive latex fixation test for RF in 43 per cent of patients with acute and 22 per cent of patients with chronic leukaemia. Druet et al. (1969) found that in 37 cases of chronic lymphatic leukaemia 7 gave a positive RF in the blood. Kaplan (1963) found 74 per cent of 23 patients with myelo-proliferative diseases have positive latex tests. Cannat and Seligmann (1973) found that in 24 children with juvenile myelo-monocytic leukaemia ANF was present in 52 per cent of cases and antihuman IgG antibodies in 43 per cent.

Thus, all the evidence points to true leukaemias as being in most cases the result of limax amoebae infection. However, different types of leukaemia appear to be of different nature. Chronic lymphatic leukaemia may, in malarial areas, be a response to chronic malarial infection and disappears with prolonged anti-malarial drug treatment. In the Western World chronic lymphatic leukaemia differs from other types of leukaemia in the slowness of its progression, in the lack of associated symptoms and its lack of response to drugs which are helpful in other forms of leukaemia. Prolonged remission in cases of chronic lymphatic leukaemia has been reported by Walter et al. (1958) and spontaneous remission by Chervenick et al. (1967). It has been shown above that some cases may respond remarkably to anti-protozoal drugs and copper and bile salts with a return of the blood count to normal, while these have no effect on the blood picture of other types of leukaemia, though they may relieve the toxic symptoms. It appears, therefore, that some cases of *chronic lymphatic leukaemia are the "leukaemoid" response to limax* amoebae infection, just as it may be to chronic malaria and other chronic infections. The same conclusion may apply to some monocytic leukaemias. In other types of leukaemia mutation has taken place in the various white cell precursors, producing changes like the appearance of the Philadelphia chromosome, and the conditions appear to be true cancers and are unresponsive to anti-amoebic drugs. Such conclusions would explain leukaemia "clusters" or "houses" or conjugal cases, where a virulent strain of limax amoebae perhaps exists in a locality.

The family association of mongolism and leukaemia

Heath and Moloney (1965) report acute leukaemia in five members of three generations of a family, one member of which was a mongol. Eddin et al. (1968) described a case of leukaemia in a child who had a sib and three other relatives who were mongols and three of the latter showed G21 trisomy. Kucera (1971) found 21 leukaemia subjects in 801 families of children with mongolism, appreciably more frequently in the families of mothers than of fathers. Miller (1961) describes a family with an XXXXY male, a leukaemic male and two 21 trisomic mongoloid females.

These observations are explicable on the same causation for mongolism, viz coHagen disease in the motherS' ovary, and leukaemia in the affected offspring of infected mothers.

Chapter XVII

Features of reticuloses, including Hodgkin's disease, suggestive of limax amoebae aetiology

Transitions of different types of lymphoma

Mention has been made above of transitional cases of various types of lymphoma, including Hodgkin's disease, to one another and to myelomatosis, to the occurrence of various histological types of lymphoma in the same patient, to any type of lymphoma or myelomatosis or leukaemia following collagen and auto-immune disease and to any type of lymphoma being combined together or with any type of carcinoma. Cooper (1970) in considering 80 cases of reticulosarcoma found that:-

1) Some cases presented with histological features of another type of lymphoma, for example follicular lymphoma, Hodgkin's disease, lymphosarcoma or chronic lymphatic leukaemia.

2) Some developed from myelofibrosis, chronic myeloid leukaemia, multiple myelomatosis or macroglobulinaemia or from long-standing cases of auto-immune haemolytic anaemia and/or cryoglobulinaemia present up to thirteen years before. This suggests an identical aetiology for all these conditions.

The early lymph node lesions in lymphoma

The earliest lesions in the lymph nodes in lymphomas are those of a simple inflammation or reactive hyperplasia. This may be true of the more easily accessible nodes overlying the main mass (Ackermann and Del Regato, 1954). The nodes may be surrounded by peri-adenitis. Such changes are typical of an infection. Later the changes in the nodes vary from giant follicular lymphadenopathy to those of a granuloma (Hodgkin's disease) or a malignant lymphoma. The appearances in different parts of the same node, in different nodes of the same group or in nodes taken at different times from the same patient may show all gradations from reactive hyperplasia to those of a granuloma or lymphoma. The reactive hyperplasic appearance strongly favours the infective nature of the conditions.

Familial lymphoma

Occasionally familial cases of Hodgkin's disease or lymphoma occur (Zachau-Christiansen and Christensen, 1966; Gunz et al., 1966; Robbins et al., 1966; Vettori and Erie, 1967; Lindmark et al., 1967; Hambleton, 1969). Razis et al. (1959) from their study conclude that familial Hodgkin's disease occurs more often than one would expect from co-incidence. They could not determine whether the familial occurrence was a consequence of heredity or environmental similarity for members within a family, but suggest the latter to be the significant factor. Mazar and Strauss (1951) review cases of marital Hodgkin's disease from the literature and also suggest an infective origin.

Vianna et al. (1971 a) point out that all the evidence seems to indicate that Hodgkin's disease is an acquired condition as indicated by the very low familial incidence, the lack of association with any congenital defects or with any preceding

Addendum: Cutaneous granulomas in malignant lymphnoma. Randle HW, Banks PM, Winkelmann RK. Arch. Dermatol 1980, 116/4, 441-443 Two patients wth massive localized dermal and subcutaneous epithlioid granulomatous masses were finally diagnosed after a years investigation as Hodgkin's disease by lymph node biopsy

immunological deficiency, the normal immune responses prior to the onset of the disease, the lack of history of maternal exposure to irradiation or of premature delivery and subsequent abnormal growth and development. Vianna et al. (1971 b) report on an extended epidemic of Hodgkin's disease in high school students in the United States. Four students in a class developed Hodgkin's disease. Twelve cases showed an interrelationship in more than two generations, suggesting an infective disease with a carrier state and a long incubation period. In the Leading Article (Lancet, 1972, 1, 242) there is reported an epidemic of lymphoma in rhesus monkeys in a centre in the United States.

Lymphomata and collagen and auto. immune diseases

It has been shown above that Hodgkin's disease and other lymphomata may follow or be associated with any form of collagen or auto-immune disease and with leukaemias a nd they may be preceded or accompanied by paraneoplastic neuropathies, recurrent thrombophlebitis, leucoderma and melanoderma, alopecia or ichthyosis acq uisita, all features of collagen and auto-immune disease. They may also be preceded or accompanied by paraprotein-aemia, macroglobulinaemia or cryoglobu-linaemia, Bence-Jones proteinuria and many cases of Hodgkin's disease may develop amyloid changes. All are features of rheumatoid disease. Cases of lymphoma, Hodgkin's disease or myelomatosis may be associated with any form of leukaemia and any type of carcinoma, suggesting they often arise from the same cause as leukaemia or myelomatosis, namely limax amoebae infection.

The serum RF in cases of lymphoma

Innis and Ferguson (1964) found a rheumatoid factor (RF) in the serum in one case of reticulosarcoma and a negative test in one case of lymphosarcoma. Sherry (1968) found a negative test in all cases of Hodgkin's disease tested. Kaplan (1963) found a negative test in 40 cases of lymphoma of which 12 were chronic lymphatic leukaemia. Hoffbrand (1965) in 39 patients with Hodgkin's disease described one patient with preceding thyrotoxicosis, but none showed thyroid auto-antibodies, and one each exhibited gastric parietal cell antibodies, ANF or RF in their blood, a proportion no higher than in controls. However, it has been shown above that in advanced cases of malignant disease, particularly in malignant lymphomata and lymphatic leukaemia, antibody production by the immunocytes is depressed and, therefore, such investigations as are recorded above cannot be taken to indicate the pre-existence of RF and other auto-antibodies in the serum. As seen above serological evidence of systemic lupus erythematosus or rheumatoid arthritis may disappear when lymphoma develops in a case of collagen disease and the connection between the diseases is overlooked.

Extra-nodal lesions in cases of lymphoma

In all cases of malignant lymphoma, including myelomatosis and Hodgkin's disease, extra-nodal primaries are present in one third of cases. Single extra-nodal primary lesions occurring in gut, bladder, gall bladder, bone, breast, skin, lung, thyroid, orbit, mouth, tonsil, thymus, ovary, spermatic cord, epididymis and testicle have been recorded, indicating that the causative factor is generalized, as in rheumatoid disease. Extra-nodal primaries may develop in any tissue so affected. In Case 98 the patient exhibited fibrosing alveolitis, portal tract infiltration with lymphocytes in the liver and tumours were present along the coronary vessels, suggesting they may arise from a peri-arteritic lesion at the site of exit of limax amoebae from the vessels.

-423-

"Sarcoid" reaction in lymphoma

"Sarcoid" reactions in the tissues of cases of Hodgkin's disease and other malignant lymphomas were described and previous cases reviewed by Kadin et al. (1970), Stoker (1971) and Brincker (1972). The last-named describes 14 such cases of a "sarcoid reaction", that is noncaseating epithelioid cell granulomata (NCECG), associated with malignant lymphoma. In two cases the lymphoma was Hodgkin's disease and a carcinoma of the colon and a carcinoma of the cervix respectively were also found. In another case rheumatoid arthritis and Hodgkin's disease were present with the granulomata. The sarcoid reaction always precedes the lymphoma. It appears that this "sarcoid" reaction, which is found in tissues both affected and unaffected by lymphoma, is essentially the rheumatoid nodule. It appears to be identical with the rheumatoid nodules described around the joints in cases of myelomatosis by Boyle and Buchanan (1971).

Amoebae in the tissues of lymphomata

The author (Wyburn-Mason, 1964) showed that all the tissues of the body as well as the lesions themselves in cases of lymphoma, including Hodgkin's disease, contain limax amoebae. Kofoid and Swezy (1922) also found an amoeba in the lymph nodes of cases of Hodgkin's disease and McDonald and Moore (1965) reported the case of a patient who had a reticulum cell sarcoma confined to the stomach and neighbouring lymph nodes, which contained amoebae in the growth and lymph nodes, but not elsewhere in the body. It has been shown above that many of the manifestations of Hodgkin's disease and other lymphomata are those of limax amoebic infection, and they are abolished by anti-amoebic substances. Culbertson et al. (1972) showed that experimental infection with Naegleria in guinea pigs causes splenomegaly and lymphadeno-

pathy, the lymph nodes showing changes like those in Hodgkin's disease with multinucleated giant cells and the animal presented a picture like that of malignant disease. *All the above observations are in accord with the aetiology of malignant lymphoma as being due to infection with the parasite limax amoebae in many cases.* Hoster and Dratman (1946), in fact, in their long review of Hodgkin's disease conclude "Many of the manifestations of Hodgkin's disease, such as eosinophilia, relapsing fever, adenopathy and fatal termination, may be explained on the basis of a fungal, yeast or *protozoal* aetiologic agent, since organisms of this variety cause granulomatous lesions". Kaplan (1971) puts forward the hypothesis that Hodgkin's disease may evolve from a chronic immunologic reaction analogous to that of graft versus host. This could be a response to a parasite. Lymphomata are to be compared with the effects of filarial infection.

Filariasis and "lymphoma"

Many of the features of filariasis are allergic responses to the presence of the worm in the tissues, as shown by pruritus, fever, sweating, urticaria, asthmatic attacks, eosinophilia and lymphadenopathy and splenomegaly. Some cases of filariasis exhibit a condition closely resembling Hodgkin's disease or other lymphomas. For example, Galliard and Mallann(1955) described a case under the title of a pseudo-Hodgkin's form of filaria resembling tropical eosinophilia. The patient was a man of 27 years who developed painless swelling of the lymph nodes followed by asthenia, loss of weight, fever, pruritus and sweating. Clinically the nodes felt typical of Hodgkin's disease. The blood count showed 56,000 W.B.C. per cu. mm., 72 per cent being eosinophils. The lymph nodes showed the picture of a granuloma with lymphocytes, plasma cells and histiocytes, proliferation of large macrophages accompanied by many eosinophils, but no Reed-Sternberg cells. A microfilaria was found in the material aspirated from the nodes and the patient was cured with the drug, diethylcarbamazine. Such cases strongly resemble some cases of Hodgkin's disease which also exhibit eosinophilia, pruritus, fever, anorexia and sweating and again suggests that Hodgkin's disease may result from a reaction to chronic antigenic stimulation by the presence of a parasite.

The "lymphomatous" stroma of many carcinomata

Mention has already been made of the fact that carcinomata, whether primary or secondary, exhibit a lymphocytic infiltration of the stroma which appears to be a response to the limax amoebae in the tumour. In some cases this may be so marked as to resemble closely or be identical with the changes of a lymphoma or reticulosarcoma. This change appears to be the local response to the presence of limax amoebae in the tumour.

The explanation of certain clinical features of cases of lymphoma

Certain clinical features of cases of lymphomata are readily explained by the above conclusions. They · are:-

1) In cases of lymphomata and Hodgkin's disease the skin may exhibit recurrent *urticaria* and especially *pruritus,* suggestive of a parasitic infection.

2) Cases of reticuloses invariably exhibit *recurrent pyrexial bouts* at some time. This is well-known in the case of Hodgkin's disease (Hoster and Dratman, 1948), but occurs in all other forms of reticuloses. Accompanying the pyrexia there are often general malaise, headache, which may be intense, severe or drenching *night sweats,* as well as **pruritus** or urticarial wheals and sometimes muscle pains and cramps. Not infrequently *rigors* occur. This is a common manner

of onset. Such features are highly suggestive of a parasitic infection. In tropical countries the symptoms are often attributed to malaria or sand-fly fever, but no malarial parasites are demonstrable in the blood. The symptoms may persist for several weeks and may be recurrent over long periods of up to several years before other manifestations of the disease occur. They are exemplified by the following cases described by Wyburn-Mason (1964).

Case 101 Male, aged 30 years. Acute onset in India with shivering, drenching night sweats and pyrexia lasting two days. This was thought to be malaria, but no malaria parasites were demonstrable in the blood. The symptoms recurred at intervals over the next ten years, at the end of which time the cervical lymph nodes enlarged during an attack. These disappeared without treatment. After a further five years they again enlarged. This was accompanied by mediastinal lymphadenopathy. Nodal biopsy showed Hodgkin's disease.

Case 102 Male, aged 40 years. The disease was ushered in by sudden pyrexia, malaise, headache, night sweats, intense rigors and pruritus. Three months later painless generalized lymph node enlargement occurred and biopsy showed Hodgkin's disease.

Case 103 Male, aged 52 years. A Baghdadi. He began to suffer from bouts of fever, drenching night sweats and lack of energy lasting up to three weeks. He commenced to lose weight and his skin to itch. Fifteen months after the onset a painless enlargement of the right cervical lymph nodes occurred during one of the bouts. Biopsy showed typical Hodgkin's disease. A white blood count showed II per cent of eosinophils.

Case 98 Male, aged 26 years. His illness began with an attack of cough, sputum, pyrexia and severe night sweats. X-rays showed diffuse shadowing in various parts of both lungs. The symptoms gradually died down, but five weeks later the pyrexia and sweating returned and he developed pain in the left flank, shoulder and both big toes. The spleen was palpable. A diagnosis of acute Hodgkin's disease was made. He died three months after the onset. At autopsy the mesentery was almost solid with tumour. The liver and spleen were enlarged. The spleen was adherent to all the surrounding tissues, including the diaphragm. The pleura was thickened and thickenings were present in various parts of the lungs. The hilar nodes were enlarged. Small tumours were found along the coronary vessels and beneath the epithelium of both ureters. Histologically the changes were those of acute Hodgkin's disease without eosinophils, but with marked proliferation of reticulum cells, macrophages and lymphocytes. The portal tracts of the liver were infiltrated with macrophages, lymphocytes and plasma cells. In the lungs the thickened pleura contained many mononuclears and the alveolar walls and alveoli contained many lymphocytes and plasma cells consistent with the diagnosis of fibrosing alveolitis. The bronchiole walls were infiltrated with the same cells.

3) A blood *eosinophilia* is not uncommon in cases of Hodgkin's disease, in which it may appear and disappear in the course of the disease. It has been stated that this eosinophilia occurs especially at times of acute exacerbations of the symptoms. Fifteen to twenty per cent of patients are said to show an eosinophilia of some degree (Wintrobe, 1967). Occasionally, however, extreme degrees of eosinophilia as high as 90 per cent of a total of 200,000 W.B.C. per cu. mm. have been recorded (Wintrobe, 1967). Such cases have been described by Sibley (1915), Sears (1932), Baker and Mann (1939), Major and Leger (1939), Koide and Kogure (1959), Giacovazzo et al. (1967) and Felman et al. (1969). The author has observed three such cases (see Case 114). A significant point is that the blood usually does not show any eosinophil precursor cells.

Cases of lymphoma other than Hodgkin's disease do not exhibit an eosinophilia in the blood so frequently or to such a degree (Rosenberg et al., 1961). Bailey and Campbell (1973) described a case of lymphosarcoma in a child which was preceded by Loffler's syndrome (eosinophilic lung) with a high blood eosinophilia which recurred with the onset of the malignancy. Henderson and Mefia (1969) reported lymphosarcoma with a high blood eosinophilia and eosinophilic pleursy and pericarditis and a blood eosinophilia may occur in cases of mycosis fungoides (Wintrobe, 1967) and eosinophilic granuloma. As seen already cases of disseminated eosinophilic collagen disease or "eosinophilic leukaemia" may also develop lymphoma, chloroma or myeloblastoma (Benvenisti and Ultmann, 1969).

Such an eosinophilia is consistent with a parasitic aetiology of these diseases and occurs in other protozoal infections, such as trypanosomiasis, etc.

4) The lesions in cases of Hodgkin's disease frequently show an eosinophilia. Fossgren (1962) described the case of a woman of 36 years with itching, symptomatic sprue and eosinophilic infiltration and granulomata of many organs, which the author considered a form of Hodgkin's disease. Gemme (1963) reported a case of Hodgkin's disease in a child with marked leucocytosis and eosinophilia in the blood and tissues and with Charcot-Leyden crystals in the granulomatous tissue.

Reticulosarcomata also commonly contain areas of eosinophilic infiltration and may look like "eosinophilic granulomata". Such a lesion in the mesentery was described by Rogier et al. (1956). Hansen (1949) reports a case with eosinophilic granuloma and reticulum cell sarcoma at different sites. Christofferson and Nielsen (1964) described the case of a 35 years old woman, who developed an eosinophil granuloma of the right humerus. After treatment this recurred in the soft tissues around the original lesion and now showed the changes of a reticulosarcoma. Knoth (1954) recorded eosinophilic granuloma of the skin associated with reticulosis and Sannicaudro (1963) one with mycosis fungoides. In fact, eosinophilic granuloma of the skin of the face is thought to be a reticulosarcoma (Steigleder, 1955). Lupovitch et al. (1965) described a case of malignant lymphoma presenting as necrotizing eosinophilic granulomata with eosinophilia in the blood, fever and leukaemic changes. The lesions were thought to be allergic in nature and related to a vasculitis. In a personally observed case an ulcerated swelling of the jejunum produced intestinal obstruction and was removed and showed an eosinophilic granulomatous lesion in the mucosa, submucosa and muscularis. The lesion recurred and was then found to have the structure of a reticulosarcoma. Another patient with the symptoms of coeliac disease developed small intestinal obstruction due to a mass in the mucosa which showed a gross eosinophil infiltration and scattered lymphocytes and histiocytes. The tumour later recurred as a typical reticulosarcoma. Such tissue eosinophilia in lymphomata is explicable on the basis of a parasitic causation.

5) Urticaria, allergic swelling and oedemas are very common signs of parasitic infection, such as filariasis, amoebiasis and trypanosomiasis. In the reticuloses *unexplained oedemas, itching and allergic swellings of* soft tissues may *occur in any part of* the *body*, both during the course of the disease and also preceding the onset of other evidence of reticuloses by many years. These symptoms may be accompanied by eosinophilia in the tissues and in the blood. Limper (1939) described the case of a child, who suffered from asthma, purpura and angioneurotic oedema and Hodgkin's disease developed following an attack of herpes zoster. Another patient suffered from hives from childhood and developed Hodgkin's disease at 26 years of age (Hoster and Dratman, 1948). Oedemas, allergic swelling and urticaria occurred frequently in cases of reticuloses in the author's series and those of Diamond (1958). This was also seen in a case of Mikulicz's disease followed by malignant lymphoma reported by Azzopardi and Evans (1971). They were features of the following cases from the author's book (Wyburn-Mason, 1964):–

Case **104** Male, at the age of 24 years he woke up one morning with an "allergic" itching swelling of the face in the parotid region and eyelids and swollen, puffy, sweating hands, lasting one week. The condition returned six weeks later, lasting three weeks on this occasion. He remained well for 5 years when he developed a sore throat, "allergic" swelling of the face and hands with enlarged cervical lymph nodes, which slowly subsided. After a further five years he began to lose weight and a mass of enlarged nodes appeared on the left side of the neck. The liver and spleen enlarged and he ran a temperature of 103°F. At autopsy the changes of Hodgkin's disease with acute yellow atrophy of the liver were found.

Case **105** Female, aged 38 years. At the age of 30 years she developed acute oedema and itching of the right side of the face and parotid region lasting one month. This disappeared and then returned for another two weeks or so. Eight years later it again appeared and she noticed swelling of the nodes on the right side of the neck and the right trapezius muscle became infiltrated. Biopsy of a lymph node showed the changes of Hodgkin's disease.

Case **106** Female, aged 30 years. Five years before the onset of other symptoms she suddenly developed a severe urticarial rash over the whole body with swelling of the eyes and face lasting one month. Five years later this returned, the symptoms and signs of abdominal Hodgkin's disease then appeared.

Case **107** Male, aged 24 years. He suddenly developed intense unilateral right frontal headache with profuse watering, redness and oedema of the same eye and orbit, lasting about six weeks. After this he suffered from a fine impetiginous rash over the whole body. Thirteen months after the onset of the headache enlarged lymph nodes appeared on the same side of the neck and biopsy showed the changes of Hodgkin's disease.

Case 108   Male, aged 28 years. The onset of the disease was with acute swelling and itching of the right side of the face and behind the angle of the jaw lasting some six weeks, at the end of which time enlarged axillary nodes appeared. Biopsy showed the presence of a lympho-sarcoma.

Case 109   Male, at the age of 22 years he developed acute painful itching and swelling of the left parotid region and side of the face lasting about a month. Aged 26 years he had two recurrences of this condition accompanied by painful enlarged nodes on the same side of the neck. Aged 32 years the left parotid swelling recurred and persisted and a mixed parotid tumour was removed. Aged 39 years the left cervical nodes again enlarged and biopsy showed the changes of Hodgkin's disease.

Case 110   Male, aged 43 years. Following a "cold" he noticed swelling and itching of the right side of the face, lasting about five months. This was followed by swelling of the right cervical nodes, biopsy of which showed the changes of Hodgkin's granuloma. The symptoms regressed without treatment, but reappeared two years later. They were followed by diffuse enlargement of the right arm and shoulder and some oedema of the hand. A year later dermatitis appeared in the scalp. A further glandular biopsy again showed the changes of Hodgkin's disease.

Case 111   Female, aged 23 years. Onset with three attacks of angioneurotic oedema of the face each lasting about a week and occurring over two months. Six years later, after the birth of her first child, she experienced similar oedema and then noticed painless enlargement of the cervical lymph nodes, biopsy of which showed the changes of Hodgkin's disease.

Case 112   Male, aged 19 years. Onset with an attack of swelling of the face lasting ten days. This was followed by a painful swelling of the left spermatic cord and epididymis lasting some seven weeks. Two years later he noticed painful swollen left cervical lymph nodes followed two months later by swelling of the right cervical, axillary and inguinal nodes. Two nodal biopsies showed the changes of "chronic inflammation". The enlarged nodes regressed spontaneously. After a further year he developed nasal blockage and the adenoids were found very enlarged, the spleen palpable and masses could be felt in the mesentery. The eyelids became swollen and the right side of the face numb. Six months later he was found to have a mass below the sphenoidal bone, which infiltrated the nasal mucosa and a radiograph showed enlargement of the mediastinal nodes. The right 5th and the left 6th and 7th cranial nerves were involved and left perceptive deafness was present. He then developed a generalized papular rash and confluent urticarial areas. Biopsy of lymphoid tissue now showed the changes of Hodgkin's disease.

Case 113   Male, aged 26 years. The disease began with swelling of the feet and wheezing dyspnoea. Examination showed the presence of generalized rhonchi in the chest, which persisted. Two months later enlarged lymph nodes appeared in the neck, but regressed spontaneously. A year later he developed generalized rheumatic pains, recurrence of bronchitis and generalized lymphadenopathy and pyrexia appeared. He passed into delirium. Biopsy of a lymph node showed the changes of Hodgkin's disease.

Case 114   Male, aged 35 years at onset of illness. He was taken ill while visiting Brazil. From that time to his death 9 years later he was subject to intermittent swellings of different parts of the body and a recurrent swelling of the left side of the face, eyelids and orbit. Five years after the onset there appeared enlarged painless lymph nodes, first in the right groin and later in the left, and in the neck and axilla on both sides, pallor and oedema of the feet. Biopsy of the nodes showed initially the changes of a chronic inflammation (reactive hyperplasia) later changing to a follicular lymphadenopathy. A blood count showed anaemia and a total W.B.C. of 17,000 per cu. mm., of which 34 per cent were lymphocytes and 42 per cent eosinophils. He became subject to persistent and severe pruritus and severe sweating, an extensive maculopapular rash and recurrent oedemas. Nine months before he died herpes zoster appeared over the left 07-8 dermatomes and soon after pains in the limbs and back with marked muscular cramps, weakness and wasting making walking difficult, paraesthesiaes in the hands and feet and drooping of the left eyelid. The tendon reflexes disappeared. The muscles were very tender and exhibited contractures. Asthmatic symptoms were present and the liver and spleen enlarged. He developed marked confusion and other mental disturbances. Throughout his illness he ran an irregular temperature reaching 103°F ai times. In the last three years of his life the W.B.C. count gradually rose and reached 79,200 per cu. mm. and the eosinophilia remained marked, at one time as much as 32.5 per cent of a total of 58,000 per cu. mm. Towards the end the blood urea gradually rose. He died suddenly of coronary infarction. Autopsy showed generalized lymphadenopathy and muscular atrophy. The peripheral nerves and nerve roots were also atrophic. Sections of the lymph nodes showed the changes of Hodgkin's disease with marked eosinophilia. Lymphocytes, plasma cells, eosinophils and macrophages infiltrated the peripheral nerves and nerve roots and many other tissues.

Case 115 Male, aged 26 years. Onset with diarrhoea followed by shivering and headache lasting one week. One month later painless enlargement of the right axillary lymph nodes occurred and was followed by enlargement of the right supraclavicular nodes, colicky lower abdominal pain, constipation and weight loss. He was found to have marked oedema of the whole of the right shoulder, pectoral and upper arm regions and tenderness and enlarged nodes in the epigastrium. Biopsy of a node showed the changes of lymphosarcoma. He died three months after the onset in delirium and a moribund state.

Case 116 Male, aged 25 years. He suffered from recurrent haemoptyses for which no cause could be found and began to run an irregular temperature over six weeks. He then developed an acute painful swelling and itching of the right eyelids and orbit followed by enlargement of the right cervical lymph nodes. Nodal biopsy showed the changes of lymphosarcoma.

Case 11'7 Male, aged 30 years. The illness began with an attack of "influenza", which was followed by prolonged debility, cough, expectoration, severe headache and injected conjunctivae. He was diagnosed as suffering from chronic bronchitis. He then became tremulous and experienced insomnia and during the next year had attacks of unexplained abdominal discomfort and diarrhoea. Two years after the onset he developed a "cold" lasting two weeks to be followed by oedema of the face, which later spread to the neck, arms and legs over the course of a week. This gradually disappeared, except in the forearms. Investigations showed a severe anaemia and the W.B.C. count was 1,600 per cu. mm. with relative depression of polymorphs. Six weeks later an enlarged node appeared in the left axilla and the liver and spleen were also found enlarged. A biopsy showed the changes of Hodgkin's disease. He then developed an acute lymphangitis of the left leg. He was given X-ray therapy with improvement, but later developed ascites and slight icterus. These symptoms disappeared spontaneously. He remained well for 5 years when the liver, spleen and lymph nodes again enlarged with generalized oedema and anaemia. He again improved under chemotherapy, but the symptoms returned and he died nine years after the beginning of the illness.

6) Skin lesions preceding lymphomata

Reference has already been given to the finding that psoriasis, dermatitis, dermatitis herpetiformis, leucoderma, melanoderma, acanthosis nigricans, ichthyosis acquisita and light sensitivity, all manifestations of collagen and auto-immune disease, may precede the appearance of or be associated with malignant lymphoma. This is indicative of a common aetiology.

7) Hay-fever, asthma, bronchitis and reticuloses

Hay-fever may sometimes be a feature of Hodgkin's disease and may precede the onset of the latter by some years (Hoster and Dratman, 1948). Sometimes the onset of clinical evidence of a reticulosis is preceded by recurrent attacks of asthma and bronchitis. Thus, chronic bronchitis preceded the appearance of lymphoma in two of the cases described by Krueger and Meyer (1936). The onset of Hodgkin's disease was marked by severe upper respiratory disease. A child, who had been an asthmatic since the age of seven years, developed Hodgkin's disease and the blood showed a marked eosinophilia (Stewart, 1929). Limper (1939) described the case of a child who suffered from asthma, purpura and angioneurotic oedema and in whom Hodgkin's disease developed after an attack of herpes zoster. Scheuer-Karpin and d'Heureuse-Gerhardt (1965) mention a patient with allergic asthma for 25 years who developed cirrhosis and Hodgkin's disease and Scheuer-Karpin (1959) cases of lymphoma and chronic lymphatic leukaemia who had previously suffered from asthma and allergic bronchitis. In the large series of cases of lymphoma described by the author (Wyburn-Mason, 1964) several gave a history of asthma prior to the onset of Hodgkin's disease. These are as follows:-

Case 118 Male, aged 22 years, developed acute asthmatic attacks with drenching night sweats. Chest X-rays were normal. Blood counts showed a high eosinophilia. The attacks continued irregularly for a year, when, during one of these, generalized lymphadenopathy appeared. Biopsy of a lymph node showed the changes of Hodgkin's disease.

Case 119 Male, aged 42 years. Aged 26 years onset of asthmatic attacks which continued and four years later cervical laminectomy for extradual reticulosarcoma was carried out. Aged 42 years onset of retroperitoneal Hodgkin's disease with ascites. Treated with chloroquine when both asthma and abdominal masses disappeared dramatically to return later in spite of continuation of treatment.

Case 120 Male, suffered from asthma from childhood. At the age of 20 years onset of severe asthmatic attack with pyrexia, sweating and loss of weight. The attack persisted for 6 weeks, when lymphadenopathy appeared. Biopsy of a node showed the changes of Hodgkin's disease.

Case 121 Male, at the age of 20 years a patch of lupus erythematosus appeared in front of the left ear and persisted. At the age of 40 years he had an attack of bronchial asthma, which recurred repeatedly over the next five years. In several attacks blood counts showed an eosinophilia of up to 25 per cent. In one attack the cervical lymph nodes and the lupus lesion enlarged. Biopsy of a node showed the changes of Hodgkin's disease.

Case 122 Male, aged 25 years. Suffered from recurrent "malarial" attacks and then developed spasms of acute dyspnoea and cough. Chest X-rays were normal. These spasms persisted over the next year. At the end of this time in one bout he became pyrexial and the left cervical and mediastinal lymph nodes enlarged and the left side of the face swelled. Biopsy of a lymph node showed the changes of Hodgkin's disease.

Case 123 Male, aged 30 years. He suffered from recurrent asthma and bronchitis which began when aged 15 years and continued until aged 34 years, when he developed acute epididymo-orchitis and funiculitis, gradually subsiding. Later enlarged nodes appeared in the cervical region and the liver was enlarged. Nodal biopsy showed the changes of Hodgkin's disease.

Case 124 Male, aged 40 years at onset of right epididymo-orchitis and three years later enlarged tender nodes in the right groin and the epitrochlear nodes also enlarged and later regressed. One month later itching of the toes and dermatitis of the legs appeared. After a further three months he developed boils on the thighs. Four years later enlarged nodes appeared in the left axilla. Biopsy showed the changes of a reticulosarcoma.

Case 125 Male. At the age of 30 years he developed a sudden attack of cough, dyspnoea, fever and cyanosis with generalized rhonchi and r:iles in the chest. This lasted for 8 days and recurred after two weeks. Chest X-rays were normal. The pyrexia persisted irregularly and seven months later the spleen and liver were found enlarged and tender. Chest X-rays now showed enlargement of the hilar nodes. He died a month later and autopsy revealed Hodgkin's disease.

Case 126 Male, aged 34 years. Suffered from recurrent hay-fever and asthma since the age of 8 years. At 26 years he developed enlarged inguinal lymph nodes. Biopsy showed the changes of Hodgkin's disease. Treated with 4-aminoquinolines (antrycide), intravenously 300 mgms. daily for 6 weeks with disappearance of all symptoms and signs both of the Hodgkin's disease and of asthma and hay-fever over the next two years.

Case 127 Male, aged 16 years. Suffered from eczema and asthma from the age of

5 years. The former disappeared after three years. At the age of 16 years, during a bout of asthma, blisters appeared over the hands, forearms, feet and shins followed by enlargement of the right cervical lymph nodes. Biopsy showed the changes of Hodgkin's disease. He was treated with chloroquine 300 mgms. intravenously daily for six weeks with cessation of asthma and disappearance of lymphadenopathy.

rn one of the author's large series of cases of malignancy recorded above, a man developed generalized urticaria at the age of 17 years, especially after exercise, and Hodgkin's disease at the age of 32 years. Another patient, a doctor aged 40 years, and his three sisters, suffered from eczema, hay-fever and intrinsic asthma from an early age. At the age of 21 years he noticed an enlarged node in the axilla following an attack of asthma. Then at the age of 40 years after a further attack the node enlarged and a biopsy showed the changes of Hodgkin's disease.

All the above observations are readily explicable on the basis that they are due to a parasitic infection with limax amoebae.

Amyloidosis and Hodgkin's disease

Amyloidosis is well-known to occur in some cases of Hodgkin's disease (see Wintrobe, 1967) as in cases of rheumatoid disease. It is presumably of the same nature in the two conditions and the result of a chronic antigenic stimulation.

Non-tropical splenomegaly and malignant lymphoma

In Britain Dacie et al. (1969) report on the condition of massive non-tropical splenomegaly, which has similar histological features both to tropical splenomegaly due to malarial infection and to the changes found in *Felty's syndrome,* a manifestation of collagen disease. The same histological features are found in the liver and spleen in all three conditions. Of the ten cases of non-tropical splenomegaly described by Dade et al., one developed auto-immune haemolytic anaemia and in another case possible rheumatoid arthritis developed three years after splenectomy, suggesting that the condition might be related to collagen disease. The authors suggested that in both non-tropical and tropical splenomegaly the changes are the response to an antigenic stimulus and an abnormality in the host response to infection. In the case of tropical splenomegaly the antigenic stimulus appears to arise from chronic malarial infection. The similarity of the changes in Felty's syndrome to those in non-tropical splenomegaly and the relationship of the latter to collagen disease suggests, in fact, that Felty's syndrome and non-tropical splenomegaly are the same condition and a manifestation of collagen and auto-immune disease.

Of the ten cases described by Dade et al. two developed lymphosarcoma and one oat cell carcinoma of the lung. This tendency to lymphosarcomatous change has been reported by others. The splenomegaly may precede the malignant change by many years. In Case 261231 considered at a Clinico-Pathological Conference at Hammersmith Hospital, a man presented with a massively enlarged spleen at the age of 25 years. He died at the age of 62 years of generalized lymphosarcoma involving the enlarged spleen. Thus, tropical splenomegaly is a manifestation of infection with the malarial parasite and appears to predispose to lymphomatous change. Felty's syndrome, which appears identical with non-tropical splenomegaly, appears likewise to be a manifestation of infection with another protozoon, limax amoebae, and likewise predisposes to the development of lymphoma.

Site of entry of causative organism in lymphomata

Binnie et al. (1971) call attention to the primary oral symptoms, periodontitis and toothache occurring in cases of lymphosarcoma, while Cook (1961) remarks that many cases of malignant lymphoma begin in the mouth. Vianna et al. (1971) suggest the infection in Hodgkin's disease enters through the oral and respiratory tract portals. Parant et al. (1971) report a case of reticulum cell sarcoma preceded by multiple lesions in the mouth of benign type. Again, cases of Hodgkin's disease may follow dental sepsis (Hoster and Dratman, 1948). This was so in one of the author's patients, a doctor aged 40 years. In these cases the cervical nodes enlarge first. A large number of cases have been mentioned above in which Sjogren's syndrome or Mikulicz's disease have preceded the development of a malignant lymphoma. Recurrent unilateral facial oedema and itching of mouth or pharyngeal infection have often preceded the development of a lymphoma (Hoster and Dratman, 1948; and see cases cited above). There are many cases of Hodgkin's disease, malignant lymphoma or plasmocytoma (Wiltshaw, 1971) which begin in the tonsil, adenoids (Stewart and Stuart, 1971), upper respiratory tract and back of the tongue (Waldeyer's ring) and may be multifocal (Friedberg et al., 1957; Wiltshaw, 1971). Such observations indicate that the infection commonly gains entrance to the body from the mouth, nose or nasopharynx. This explains why the cervical nodes are usually the lymph nodes first affected. Sometimes Hodgkin's disease begins in the endobronchial tissues (Vaughan, 1958; and one of the author's own series). Infection of the salivary glands must occur by ascent of the ducts of the salivary glands from the mouth. A number of cases of primary lymphoma at the base of the brain (Gereb, 1953) have been reported. Such cases indicate that limax amoebae entered through the cribriform plate and closely resemble those cases of amoebic meningo-encephalitis due to free-living amoebae (Naegleria fowleri) already described. However, again it is not infrequent to find malignant lymphoma beginning in the stomach or upper small intestine with locally involved nodes, but none elsewhere, suggesting the causative organism entered the body by this route. McDonald and Moore (1965), in fact, and others describe lymphomata in the stomach and neighbouring nodes in which amoebae were seen in the growth and nodes. Occasionally lymphoma begin in the conjunctivae, where it must be presumed that limax amoebae spores have settled. In some cases Hodgkin's disease is limited to the lung and then takes a cavernous course (Steel, 1964; Bernard et al., 1966). It then resembles pulmonary tuberculosis. Such cases are readily explicable as due to inhalation of limax amoebae spores from the air.

The possibility of cure of malignant lymphoma

All the above observations are in accord with the conclusion that malignant lymphomata in Western Countries are caused by infection with limax amoebae and are,

in fact, a response to long-standing antigenic stimulation from the organism in subjects sensitive to some or all strains of this protozoon. Is the lymphadenopathy and extranodal lesions merely a tissue response to the organism, which will disappear if the causative organism is inhibited or killed or have the affected tissues become autonomous? In the former case if the organism could be killed, it is conceivable that the lymphomatous response to it would disappear. As seen already some cases of malignant lymphoma may apparently be cured (Case VII, 3.), when treated with chloroquine. A ten year cure of Hodgkin's disease was claimed by Easson and Russell (1963) and Papillon et al. (1971), and a benign form of the condition was described by Dawson and Harrison (1961). This suggests that in some cases at least lymphomata are not autonomous tumours. In such cases the treatment of malignant lymphoma by radiotherapy to enlarged lymph nodes or splenectomy would appear to be irrational, since it merely treats the lymphadenopathic response to an infection. Radiotherapy probably lowers the resistance to this infection. It is tempting to suppose that cytotoxic drugs act not on the cells of the lymphoma, but on the causative limax amoebae. This explains why they have little beneficial effect on carcinomata, once somatic mutation has occurred.

-433-

Chapter XVIII

Limax amoebae and carcinoma

It has been deduced that a large proportion of both benign and malignant tumours of all tissues occurring both before and after birth, at any rate in Western countries, may be due to infection with limax amoebae, and are usually accompanied by evidence of collagen or auto-immune disease. Both the latter diseases and benign and malignant tumours particularly occur in genetically disposed individuals. In this chapter some special features of certain benign and malignant tumours of different types in relation to their causation by limax amoebae infection will be considered.

Eosinophilia in the tumours and blood in cases of carcinoma

It has been shown that most malignant tumours contain limax amoebae and it has been suggested that their presence is responsible for the lymphocytic and lymphomatous reaction seen in the stroma of many carcinomata. The stroma of many cancers also contain eosinophils in large numbers and in some cases there also occurs a high blood eosinophilia and the bone marrow may be heavily infiltrated with these cells (Willis, 1952). It is tempting to suppose that these local and generalized reactions are evidence of an allergic response to the amoebae in the growths and elsewhere and are identical with reactions which may occur in cases of lymphoma.

1) Skin tumours

a) Limax amoebae and skin cancer

Genetic factors, as in cases of xeroderma pigmentosum and Gorlin's syndrome, may occasionally be important in the aetiology of these tumours. Occasionally arsenical poisoning plays a part. The incidence of both basal cell carcinoma (rodent ulcer) and squamous carcinoma of the skin increases with age and these tumours occur especially in the fifth to seventh decades (Evans, 1966). Skin cancer often develops in senile keratoses which have been seen to be a common manifestation of collagen and auto-immune disease. It has been seen that basal cell carcinoma and squamous carcinoma of the skin both in unexposed and exposed areas may often be accompanied by evidence of collagen and auto-immune disease. When such cancers arise in multiple foci, this is an excellent example of malignant change occurring in a precancerous field, namely the skin, which is known to be affected over large areas in cases of collagen and auto-immune disease.

These tumours are most common in the exposed parts of the skin, where environmental factors, such as thermic, actinic, radio-active, trauma and specific chemical influences, such as tar, play a part. Fifty per cent of basal cell carcinomata cases occur on the face and neck, showing the importance of such factors. It may well be that some of these factors act by localizing limax amoebae at sites of trauma or irritation.

2) The eye

a) Melanoma of the eye

Rheumatoid disease in the eye affects all the coats, but especially the uveal tract, choroid and sclera, resulting in iridocyclitis and episcleritis. These conditions may precede the onset of rheumatoid arthritis by many years or, in fact, may occur without other evidence of collagen disease. It is just the uveal tract, choroid and sclera which may develop malignant melanoma, the most common intra-ocular malignant tumour. The appearance of such tumours may be preceded by iridocyclitis (Duke-Elder, 1954; Willis, 1967), as occurred in two of the author's cases. The above deductions suggest a common aetiology with most other cancers. Thus, ocular melanoma and other tumours of adults appear aetiologically related to limax amoebae infection.

b) Limax amoebae and malignant melanoma of the skin

Clark et al. (1969) classify malignant melanomata into:-

1) Lentigo, a flat pigmented patch occurring on the face of elderly people, which slowly advances to tumour formation.

2) The superficial spreading type, normally slowly growing and metastasizing.

3) The actively growing nodular type of tumour.

4) Malignant change occurring in pigmented naevi (moles) or congenital anomalies.

Levene (1972) discusses the pathology of moles and melanomata.. Whether arising in a mole or de novo, the underlying processes of malignant development appear the same. There is an increasing incidence of malignant melanoma with age. Evidence has been adduced to show that limax amoebae infection is the usual cause of malignant melanoma, including such change in pigmented naevi. This appears to be the unknown endogenous factor postulated as important in causing malignant melanoma in unexposed areas (Leading Article, Lancet, 1971, i, 172).

As with basal cell and squamous cell tumours, sunlight appears to play a part in the aetiology of melanomata of the skin in exposed areas (Leading Article, Lancet, 1971, i, 172), where it may localize limax amoebae.

3) Limax amoebae infection and connective tissue tumours

a) Lipomata

Many lipomata are, in fact, congenital hamartomata and may be associated with other congenital growth anomalies and occur in unusual positions, such as intracranially. Lipomata of the thyroid and parathyroid glands may be present from birth and the gland shows the changes of chronic thyroiditis. Some lipomata in adults may have arisen on a congenital basis. As seen in Chapter XII such congenital lipomata would appear to result from limax amoebae infection of the foetus.

Multiple lipomata developing after birth may be an heredo-familial condition. Acquired solitary lipomata consist of fatty tissue, but, in addition, there is usually found an infiltration of this tissue with lymphocytes and plasma cells and often the formation of lymph follicles and germinal centres, so-called adenolipomatosis. Such changes recall those of collagen and auto-immune disease. Sometimes there is an admixture with myxomatous or angiomatous tissue. Cases of rheumatoid arthritis frequently develop lipomata in the region of the affected joints. The lipomata may develop from rheumatoid nodules (see Case 12). Lipomata may occur in the synovia of joints affected by rheumatoid disease (lipomata arborescens). One of the author's patients, with no family history of lipomata, developed a number of lipomata in her twenties and thirties, rheumatoid .disease at the age of 49 years and at the age of 70 years was found to have diabetes as well as marked rheumatoid changes. Solitary lipomas were recorded in association with malignant tumours in the author's own large series of cancers (Chapter X). Lipoma may be associated with an adjacent malignant tumour, such as a thymolipoma occurring in cases of thyrotoxicosis (Beaton and Gerard, 1966) or with underlying breast cancer (Behan, 1966; Shucksmith and Dossett, 1966). These tumours may also occur in association with thyroid disease in which focal or diffuse thyroiditis is found (Ewing, 1940). Lipomata may also occur at sites of trauma. It would seem that cases of acquired lipomata, other than those of familial nature, are also the result of limax amoebae infection.

b) Sarcoma of muscle and bone

The muscles are involved in the collagen diseases, especially in cases of polymyositis and scleroderma, while the bones may exhibit the changes of Paget's disease or rheumatoid nodules on the periosteum. Collagen and auto-immune disease is observed in many cases of sarcoma of muscle and bone. Thus, Strandberg and Jarl.pv (1961) reported cases of rheumatoid arthritis which developed osteosarcoma of the tibia and sarcoma of the sacrum respectively. Gardner (1967) found one case of osteosarcoma in his 25 tumours present in 142 cases of rheumatoid arthritis. As seen above dermatomyositis or acanthosis nigricans may both be associated with sarcoma. Sarcoma of bone in subjects over middle age is said to be confined to bones affected by Paget's disease. In one case in the South West Metropolitan Cancer Registry series rheumatoid arthritis preceded the development of a fibrosarcoma of muscle. It also occurred in two of the cases in the author's series. In one, a man of 50 years suffering from moderately severe rheumatoid arthritis, a very malignant sarcoma of the muscles of the right upper arm developed. The serum contained RF. In the other, a woman aged 72 years showing mild rheumatoid deformities of the hand, there developed almost simultaneously a fibrosarcoma of the right upper arm and a carcinoma of the breast. The serum contained ANF, RF and thyroid auto-antibodies. Another case, an Indian of 20 years, who had lived all his life in Kuala Lumpur, Malaya, developed an osteogenic sarcoma of the right tibia. There was no history of rheumatoid arthritis or other collagen or auto-immune disease, but the serum contained a moderate concentration of thyroid auto-antibodies. In cases of multiple malignancy lymphoma, leukaemia or any other cancer has been associated with sarcoma. It appears that sarcomata are usually due to limax amoebae infection. Local trauma has been reported as preceding the development of sarcoma in normal bone or bone affected by Paget's disease. It could cause localization of the organism to the damaged area and thus malignancy in susceptible subjects.

c) Malignant synovioma

Bywaters and Ansell (1969) report the case of a malignant synovioma arising in the elbow joint in a patient with rheumatoid arthritis starting apparently as a flare-up in a previously affected elbow and ultimately leading to death from lung metastases. There was one case in the author's series beginning in the big toe joint affected by rheumatoid arthritis. This suggests that synovioma is often the result of limax amoebae infection.

d) Tumours of the heart and blood vessels

The pericardium, myocardium, endocardium and vessel walls may be affected in cases of collagen diseases. The involvement of the blood vessels appears related to the presence of limax amoebae passing through the blood vessel walls. As would be expected the heart may sometimes be affected by lymphomata and sarcomata, the latter being sometimes congenital. In Case 98 it was found that the Hodgkin's nodules were present along the coronary vessels as well as elsewhere. Heilmann et al. (1971) reported an interesting case of a 42 year old woman who underwent hysterectomy for multiple fibroids and 3 months later developed symptoms suggesting a right atrial myxoma. She died soon after operation. At autopsy the cardiac tumour proved to be an extension of multiple polytopic angiomyofibromas of the veins of the small pelvis, the ovarian veins

Adden435dum: Salisbury, R. and Marshall, A., Brit. med. J., 19 ,435

8, report the case of a 53 year old woman with a

and inferior vena cava. This case suggests that all the tumours were due to limax amoebae infection of the vessel walls.

4) Limax amoebae infection and carcinoma of the bronchus

As with all other human malignancies it has been concluded that carcinoma of the bronchus is often produced by infection with limax amoebae. Thus, in the various series of multiple tumours cases of lymphoma or leukaemia or other cancers have frequently been associated with carcinoma of the bronchus (Chapter VIII). Moertel et al. (1959) found that in 1,588 cases of bronchial carcinoma 25 (4.1 per cent) had one or more other primary neoplasms, 4 of these being leukaemia or lymphoma and 17 of cancer of the skin or lips, suggesting in some cases a generalized rather than a local cause of bronchial carcinoma, irrespective of whether they smoke or not. Cases of carcinoma of the bronchus, even if there is no other evidence of collagen or auto-immune disease at the onset, frequently develop paraneoplastic peripheral neuropathy (16 per cent) prior to or with evidence of malignancy, indicating the existence of limax amoebae in the tumour in these cases. Furthermore, it was shown directly by fluorescent antibody staining techniques as well as by using thermotropism that bronchial cancer tissue contains limax amoebae.

Reference has already been made to the fact that systemic sclerosis affecting the lung, fibrosing alveolitis and also rheumatoid nodules leading to fibrosis in the lungs markedly predispose to the development of carcinoma of the bronchus. This suggests that the lung involvement leading to carcinoma in such cases of rheumatoid disease is part of the generalized disease. Limax amoebae could invade the lung, however, by direct inhalation of spores from the air in some subjects.

Various causative factors of cancer of the bronchus have been identified (see Willis, 1967). These include exposure to radio-active ores, chromates, nickel fumes, tuberculous infection and tobacco smoking. That chronic bronchitis, with of without asthma, arising from any cause predisposes to the development of carcinoma of the bronchus has frequently been suggested (Denoix et al., 1958; Case and Lea, 1959; Van der Wal et al., 1960; Leading Article, Brit. med. J., 1963, ii, 1144; Campbell and Lee, 1963; Meyer and Liebow, 1965; Van der Wal et al., 1966 a, b; Dobrynin, 1966; Miczoch, 1969), and to some it is a prerequisite for malignant change. In cases of chronic bronchitis, asthma and diffuse bronchiectasis, as with other premalignant lesions, the bronchial mucosa is infiltrated with lymphocytes and often plasma cells and its covering epithelium proliferates and may show metaplasia. Asthma and chronic rhinitis may precede or accompany the changes of chronic bronchitis and all have been seen to be features of many cases of collagen and auto-immune disease resulting from limax amoebae infection. Smoking undoubtedly plays a part in causing chronic bronchitis and thus a major role in the aetiology of carcinoma of the bronchus, but both chronic bronchitis and lung cancer may develop in subjects who have never smoked. It may be that smoking and other inhalations cause chronic trauma to the pharyngeal, laryngeal and bronchial mucosa and thus localize the almost universal infection with limax amoebae in these areas, resulting in a chronic inflammation. In what proportion of cases of carcinoma of the bronchus does smoking play a part remains to be determined.

5) Mesotheliomata

It has been seen that rheumatoid disease predisposes to the development of pneumoconiosis in miners (Caplan's syndrome). Turner Warwick and Parkes (1970) found that of 80 patients subject to asbestos exposure ANF and RF were found in 28 and 27 per cent respectively, at least a four fold increase over the incidence in a random population. Their presence was related to the extent of radiographic changes in the lungs. They remark on the similarity of asbestosis change to cryptogenic fibrosing alveolitis. These observations suggest the possibility that rheumatoid disease plays a part in the response to asbestos, including the subsequent development of mesothelioma.

6) Limax amoebae infection and breast cancer

In mice genetic factors are concerned with the development of breast cancer and a virus is concerned with its aetiology. Reference has already been made to the fact that no such virus has been found in cases of human breast cancer and indeed the evidence is against such an aetiology. Campbell (1972) has reviewed the known facts concerned with the genesis of human breast cancer. Its incidence increases with age, with a sharp increase in the years just preceding the menopause. It is rare in men. It shows geographical variations and its incidence is low in Eastern Asia, probably due to genetic factors. There is an increased incidence in single women. Its incidence falls with increased parity and early pregnancy lowers the risk, as does hysterectomy and bilateral oophorectomy before the age of 40 years. Its incidence is increased in subjects of cancer of the ovary and of the body of the uterus and there is a marked association with cystic mastitis, all effects of limax amoebae infections. The hypothesis most favoured to explain the onset of the condition is that of "le milieu interieur", which envisages a carcinogenic agent or an environment favourable to the growth of abnormal clones of cells initiated by chance.

It has been concluded that cystic mastitis occurring in women up to and beyond the menopause is a manifestation of collagen and auto-immune disease and this is certainly a highly premalignant condi-

tion (Evans, 1966; Willis, 1967). There is, however, much conclusive evidence already adduced that involvement of the breast in collagen and auto-immune disease is concerned with the development of most cases of malignancy of the breast. In all series of cases of multiple cancer there are found cases of cancer of the breast in association with other cancers, lymphoma or leukaemia (Chapter VIII), suggesting an aetiology for breast cancer the same as for other malignancies. It seems that "le milieu interieur" mentioned above and favouring the development of cancer of the breast could well be limax amoebae infection. Hormonal disturbances, however, may play a minor role.

Primary lymphoma of the breast appears to "develop in the same conditions as carcinoma. Wiseman and Liao (1972) describe the development of primary lymphoma of the breast from the changes of cystic mastitis and also following carcinoma

7) Parotid tumours

The parotid gland is often involved in collagen and auto-immune disease. Adena-lymphoma (benign lympho-epithelial lesion) of the parotid commonly develops in such cases, but lymphoma, mixed parotid tumours a nd carcinoma are also recorded. They are also recorded in association with lymphoma and leukaemia in the large series of cases of multiple malignancies already mentioned (Chapter VIII). Berg et al. (1968) found a unique association between salivary gland cancer and breast cancer existed. The evidence indicates that collagen and auto-immune disease is responsible for many cases of parotid cancer, lymphoma or mixed tumours.

8) Limax amoebae infection and cancer of the stomach

Cancer of the stomach may occasionally be familial, shows geographical variations and affects especially the lower social

—438

Addendum: Risberg B. Nickels J, Wagermark J. Familial clustering of malignant mesothelioma. Cancer 1980, 45(9) 2422-2427. The authors report malignant mesothelioma in a father, 3 sons and a daughter suggesting herdity is an important predisposing factor in the genesis of this tumour.

classes. As already mentioned its relationship to pre-existing atrophic gastritis with or without pernicious anaemia is now well recognized. Its occurrence in association with various other manifestations of collagen and auto-immune diseases has been shown. Carcinoma of the stomach appears to be commonly a result of limax amoebae infection of the gastric mucosa. Its association with other malignancies, including lymphoma and leukaemia, is recorded in all large series of cases of multiple tumours (Chapter VIII).

9) Limax amoebae infection and tumours of the kidney

It has been shown that collagen and auto-immune disease may lead at first to diffuse interstitial lymphocytic and plasma cell infiltration of the kidney, especially the glomeruli, and later to fibrosis and the changes of chronic interstitial nephritis affecting both kidneys and often associated with hypertension or other disturbances of renal function, such as renal tubular acidosis. In cases of adenoma and carcinoma of the kidney the tumours are frequently multiple and bilateral and the unaffected parts of the kidneys almost always show distinct evidence of the above changes (Willis, 1967). Both adenoma and carcinoma arise in hyperplastic convoluted tubules and cysts in the damaged kidney. The adenomata and carcinomata are closely related and a sharp distinction between the two is impossible in many cases. The two conditions may be present together.

In the literature and the author's series of cases described above various forms of collagen and auto-immune disease have preceded or accompanied the development of carcinoma of the kidney. Again, in cases of multiple malignancy; lymphomata and leukaemia and other cancers may also be combined with cancers of the kidney, suggesting a similar aetiology of the two conditions. Thus, a major cause of cancer of the kidney appears to be limax

amoebae infection.

10) Limax amoebae infection and endocrine tumours

a) Pituitary tumours

It has been seen that, like other endocrine glands, the anterior pituitary may be involved in collagen and auto-immune disease leading to hypofunction. In a case described above the subject of a Clinico-Pathological Conference at Hammersmith Hospital on 1.12.65 a 68 year old woman with an 8 year history of rheumatoid arthritis and Sjogren's syndrome developed among several other tumours a mucoid pituitary adenoma. In a Medical Staff Round at Hammersmith Hospital in 1962 there was shown a case of Hashimota's thyroiditis with myxoedema, which developed a pituitary tumour. McEachern and Parnell (1948) and Irvine (1964) found that in cases of acromegaly resulting from an eosinophil adenoma there was found lymph follicle formation and hypertrophy of the thymus, which has been seen to be evidence of a collagen and auto-immune disease. A case of dermatomyositis developing a pituitary tumour has been described (Chapter XI), while a case of Paget's disease developing a pituitary tumour was recorded by Pond (1940). Hyperthyroidism associated with chromophobe adenoma was reported by Werner and Stewart (1958). Acanthosis nigricans associated with pituitary tumour has also been described (Brown et al., 1966; Curth et al., 1967). In the author's series of ten cases of pituitary tumour of various types there was evidence of collagen and auto-immune disease in each. In the series of multiple cancers, described above in Chapter VIII, lymphoma and leukaemia and other cancers have been associated with pituitary tumours. Thus, pituitary tumours of any kind appear to result from limax amoebae infection.

b) Thyroid tumours

Hashimoto's thyroiditis may be followed by irregular fibrosis in the gland with the formation of nodular goitre or adenomata.

It has been held that thyroid cancer develops in many cases as a result of over-stimulation of the gland by excess of TSH. However, there occasionally occur cases in which carcinoma of the thyroid develops in cases of Simmond's disease (Professor Russell Fraser, personal communication). Professor Fraser has seen two such cases and found others in the literature. Ibbertson and Fraser (1956) reported such a case and this was associated with haemolytic anaemia and TSH was absent from the serum. Mason (1956) reported a similar case. This suggests that over-production of TSH is not concerned with the aetiology of thyroid cancer. Carcinoma of the thyroid is, however, prone to develop in a gland affected by Hashimoto's thyroiditis or in myxoedema (see Chapter XI). It also seems to appear in cases of collagen and auto-immune disease of any type in which the thyroid is usually affected. Again, thyroid cancer may be found in association with any other cancers, lymphoma and leukaemia (Chapter VIII), indicating an aetiology identical with that of other cancers and due to limax amoebae infection in such cases.

c) Cortical adrenal tumours

The adrenal cortex is frequently involved in collagen and auto-immune disease and usually exhibits lymphocytic and plasma cell infiltration, fibrosis and atrophy. Moreover, in infections, such as the collagen and auto-immune diseases, there is generally a stimulation of adrenal cortical secretion. It might, therefore, be expected that in these circumstances hyperplasia of the adrenal cortex might occur. In the Clinico-Pathological Conference (Brit. med. J., 1966, 1, 1027) a case of rheumatoid arthritis with arteritis exhibiting enlarged and nodular adrenal glands was described. Gerardy (1959) described a case of rheumatoid arthritis with Sjögren's syndrome, which developed

a cortical adrenal adenoma and Barlow (1939) a case of scleroderma developing a similar tumour. Again, acanthosis nigricans, may be found in association with cortical adrenal tumours (Curth et al., 1967). In one case in the author's series (Case X, 25), suffering from rheumatoid arthritis, thyrotoxicosis and diabetes, there developed chronic lymphatic leukaemia and bilateral cortical adrenal adenomata were found at autopsy. Weglenka et al. (1966) in a case of Cushing's syndrome found one adrenal enlarged and the whole gland infiltrated with lymphocytes and plasma cells (a feature of collagen and auto-immune disease). The blood corticotrophin level was not raised, but adrenal and thyroid auto-antibodies were present in the serum. They found a similar infiltration in the adrenal gland in 15 per cent of cases of Cushing's syndrome.

It would appear that cortical adrenal tumours are commonly the result of limax amoebae infection. They occur in about 10 per cent of autopsies (Brody, 1967).

d) Phaeochromocytoma

Phaeochromocytoma may be associated with Von Recklinghausen's disease or with medullary carcinoma of the thyroid gland and arise on a genetic basis. In one case of the author's series a woman, who had a long history of psoriasis and mild rheumatoid symptoms, a malignant phaeochromocytoma developed. The serum contained ANF. This suggests some cases of this tumour are due to limax amoebae infection.

e) Insulinomata

In the five cases in the author's series all showed evidence of collagen and auto-immune disease, suggesting this tumour results from limax amoebae infection.

11) Limax amoebae infection and gliomata, meningiomata and solitary neurofibromata

In the collagen diseases and Sjogren's syndrome the central nervous system may be involved by arteritis or cuffing of the vessels with lymphocytes and various neurological and mental disturbances may occur in these diseases. The meninges may also be involved and exhibit rheumatoid nodules in cases of rheumatoid arthritis (see Chapter II). The peripheral nerves may also exhibit local lymphocytic infiltration and vasculitis.

In the large series of cases of multiple tumours lymphomata, leukaemia or other cancers, have been reported as associated with glioma, fibromata or meningioma (Chapter VIII). Thus, it seems that gliomata, meningiomata and solitary neurofibromata are usually the result of limax amoebae infection. Trauma which sometimes appears to play a part in causing these tumours could be a factor in localizing limax amoebae to the damaged area. Some pertinent observations in support of these suggestions are recorded below.

a) Glioma

There are now a considerable number of cases of Paget's disease affecting the skull in which a glioma has developed in the underlying brain (see Chapter XI). Polycythaemia may be complicated by the development of cerebral tumour (Perlmutter and Strain, 1954). In the South West Metropolitan Cancer Registry series in separate cases severe rheumatoid arthritis preceded the development of an haemangioblastoma of the cerebellum and an ependymoma of the cauda equina. In the author's series there were 17 cases of glioma of the cerebrum, in two of these in young women of 29 and 30 years no evidence of collagen or auto-immune disease was present and the serum contained no ANF, RF or auto-antibodies. In all the others, usually occurring in older subjects, evidence of collagen and auto-immune disease was present.

b) Meningioma

Mills (1963) records a case of systemic lupus erythematosus found at autopsy to have a meningioma. In the Clinico-Pathological Conference held at the Royal Post-graduate Medical School on 1.12.65. a patient with rheumatoid arthritis and Sjogren's syndrome of 8 years duration developed multiple tumours, including a parasaggital meningioma. A patient under the author's care had coeliac disease and a meningioma. In another case in the author's series which developed a parasaggital meningioma marked hypothyroidism was present and the serum contained a high concentration of thyroid auto-antibodies (Case XIX, 22). In other cases in the author's series a patient suffering from rheumatoid arthritis developed an intracranial meningioma and another patient suffering from myxoedema with Paget's disease involving the skull developed an underlying meningioma. There are many cases in the literature of gliomata developing in relation to overlying Paget's disease, suggesting an aetiological relationship between the two. In a further case in the author's series thyrotoxicosis developed simultaneously with a spinal meningioma. Tanaka et al. (1975) report the late appearance of a meningioma at the site of a partially removed oligodendroglioma, showing that both tumours probably have a similar causation.

In many neuropathological reference books in the descriptions of various types of meningiomata are found references to the presence of areas of lymphocytic and plasma cell collections and even germinal centres. A subfrontal subdural tumour showing 1) areas of lymphocytes and germinal follicles, 2) an area of plasmocytoma and 3) areas of meningioma was reported by Banerjee and Blackwood (1971). This strongly suggests the relationship of meningioma formation to limax amoebae infection causing the lymphocytic and plasma cell reaction and germinal centre formation.

c) Neurofibroma

In a further case a large trigeminal neurofibroma was followed years later by Hashimoto's thyroiditis and after some years by rheumatoid arthritis and another case of auditory neurofibroma had signs of rheumatoid arthritis.

12) Limax amoebae infection and cancers of the female genitalia

The female genitalia may be involved in collagen and auto-immune disease and may lead to premature gonadal failure and atrophic vulvovaginitis, fibroids and benign ovarian cysts, while the latter tumours not infrequently become malignant.

Malignant change in the female genitalia has been attributed to hormonal disturbance and of the cervix has been related to poor sexual hygiene, to parity, frequency of sexual intercourse, herpetic infection and venereal disease.

Benign or malignant tumours of the female genitalia tend to involve several sex organs simultaneously. This is well exemplified by fibroids and benign ovarian cysts already considered in Chapter II. In the Leading Article (Brit. med. J., 1966, 1, 247) it is emphasized that cancer of the body of the uterus occurs in association with fibroids (leiomyomata), with hyperplastic endometritis and also in elderly diabetics, all of which appear to be manifestations of collagen and auto-immune diseases. Muzzioni and Giannone (1969) consider the same subject and describe a case with leiomyosarcoma and adenosarcoma of the uterus. Meyer et al. (1970) report the case of a woman of 62 years with a granulosa cell tumour of the ovary, an adenocarcinoma of the endometrium and a leiomyosarcoma of the myometrium. Jimerson and Merrill (1970) call attention to multiple malignancies in the cervix, vagina, vulva and perianal skin. Schottenfeld and Berg (1971) describe the positive association of multiple primary cancers of breast, ovary and endometrium, suggesting aetiological factors common to all three. Granulosa-cell, theca-cell and luteal tumours of the ovary may be associated with uterine abnormalities other than endometrial overgrowth. These include fibroids, adenomyosis al.ld

carcinoma of the endometrium (Willis, 1967). Silverman et al. (1972) reported on 413 patients with primary carcinoma of the ovary, especially endometrioid and granulosa-cell. Thirty-seven (8.9 per cent) had multiple primary malignancies, especially endometrial and breast. Cabera et al. (1966) found that women with anal cancer tended to develop multiple primary cancers in the urogenital tract at the same time, suggesting the action of a local agent. Watson (1972) described the case of a woman who had a myomectomy for fibroids at the age of 32 years and then a benign cystic ovarian teratoma was removed. Hashimoto's changes were present in the thyroid component of the teratoma. Erez et al. (1965) describe the case of a woman who had undergone partial thyroidectomy for chronic thyroiditis and later developed bilateral cystic ovarian teratomas. The thyroid tissue in the tumours showed Hashimoto's changes. In neither case were thyroid auto-antibodies present in the blood.

Such observations suggest an aetiological cause common to all such tumours and to fibroids and breast cancers. Again benign and malignant tumours of all kinds of the female genitalia occurring alone or in combination are reported as present in multiple tumour cases associated with lymphoma, leukaemia and other cancers (Chapter VIII). Arguments have been put forward above which indicate that all types of tumour of the female genitalia, benign or malignant, single or multiple, arise as a result of limax amoebae infection. In the case of cancer of the cervix certain other factors mentioned above may be important in causing local irritation and could act by localization of limax amoebae in the irritated and traumatized area.

13) Limax amoebae infection and cancer of the male genitalia

a) Testis and epididymis

The testis and epididymis may be involved in rheumatoid disease. The aetiology of malignant disease in these organs is unknown. Trauma appears to be important in some cases. Mention has been made that a rheumatoid epididymo-orchitis may precede teratoma or reticulosis of the testis. In the South West Metropolitan Cancer Registry and the author's series collagen and auto-immune disease in various forms were recorded in association with various malignancies of the testis. Furthermore, such malignancies may be found in association with any lymphoma, leukaemia or other cancer. Such observations indicate that testicular malignancies are in many cases aetiologically related to limax amoebae infection.

b) Prostate

It has been suggested by Burnet (1965) that nodular (benign) hyperplasia of the prostate may be a manifestation of auto-immune disease. Most observers, however, regard it as due to hormonal imbalance. It is stated (Evans, 1966) that the condition is present in 50-60 per cent of cases of prostatic cancer. However, a direct relationship between hyperplasia and the later development of cancer is uncertain and probably does not exist (Evans). Carcinoma and nodular hyperplasia of the prostate appear to be different diseases.

As with other glands, the P,rostate may be affected by collagen and auto-immune disease. Cancer arises from the outer true glands of the prostate, whereas hyperplasia affects chiefly the inner mucosal or submucosal glands. If nodular hyperplasia is the result of hormonal disturbance, then cancer is not so. The incidence of cancer of the prostate increases rapidly with age in men over 50 years and is present in almost 100 per cent of men over the age of 90 years (see Evans). It may be latent. Carcinoma of the prostate may thus result from the same cause as collagen or auto-immune disease and to constitute part of the aging process.

Limax amoebae infection as the possible cause of multiple sclerosis and related demyelinating diseases

Scheinberg (1971) points out that central demyelination must be considered a fundamental disorder of the oligodendrocyte, which, like the Schwann cell in the peripheral nerves, controls myelin metabolism. The demyelinating disorders have been grouped into two types, "myelinoclastic" and "dysmyelinative". The former includes the common demyelinating disease, multiple sclerosis and the related disease progressive multifocal leuko-encephalopathy. The latter is presumed to be an inborn error of metabolism. Most workers support an allergic basis for the first type. *Demyelination is the typical response of white matter to noxious stimuli* not severe enough to cause complete necrosis of tissue.

Now, as seen above, rheumatoid disease may lead to segmental demyelination in peripheral nerves by action on Schwann cells, the equivalent of the oligodendrocytes. Might it also lead to damage to the similarly functioning oligodendrocytes? This would be in accord with the general view of the infective nature of multiple sclerosis and with the fact that massive demyelination in the central nervous system may occur in association with malignant lymphomata, leukaemias and carcinomata, so-called progressive multifocal leuko-encephalopathy, with the appearance of demyelination in relation to the cerebral angeitis and Hodgkin's lesions in the case reported by Rewcastle and Tom (1962) and with the development of gliomata directly out of areas of demyelination in cases of multiple sclerosis reported by Scherer (1938), Ulrich and Wuthrich (1974), by Russell and Rubinstein (1959), Currie and Urich (1974) (3 cases) and by Lynch (1974). In these papers reference is made by the authors to the fact that the two conditions may be aetiologically related.

443

These observations suggest the possibility that infection with limax amoebae may be responsible for demyelinating processes, a suggestion put forward by Stamm (1972). The problem will be considered in a later publication.

Epilogue

In the foregoing pages it seems to have been shown that the presence of limax amoebae in the body and tissues controls our destiny and the quality of our life, not just from the cradle to the grave, but literally from the ovum to the grave. It may cause errors in gametogenesis and thus abortions, mongolism, Klinefelter's and Turner's syndromes or errors of implantation of the ovum and ectopic pregnancies. The organism may affect the foetus transplacentally and produce congenital anomalies or collagen or auto-immune disease. A subject may be born with cancer or congenital anomalies caused by limax amoebae may become cancerous by the further effect of the infection. A subject affected may be born mentally deficient. As age increases, so different manifestations of collagen or auto-immune disease appear. The reticulo-endothelial system may react to the presence of the organism and leukaemia, lymphoma or myelomatosis result. Various psychotic or psychoneurotic disturbances may develop. Any of these auto-immune manifestations may be fatal, for example diabetes and myxoedema. If the cells of the tissues tend to adapt to the new "climate" in which they find themselves malignant disease develops. In old age the subject exhibits a collection of manifestations of collagen and auto-immune disease, which may involve all tissues. His tissues exhibit senile amyloidosis and the E.S.R. is often raised, probably the result of the chronic infection and antigenic stimulation. Response or lack of response to the infection is apparently genetically controlled and in the latter case longevity runs in families. The tendency to malignant change is also probably genetically controlled and is a reflection of the natural tendency of all cells in nature to adapt to changed surroundings and of the very essence of evolution.

Limax amoebae infection in fact constitutes-

This long disease, my life.

(Alexander Pope, Epistles and Satires of Horace Imitated.

Prologue Epistle to Dr. Arbuthnot 1, 132).

Man and animals are the victims of their environment born to be killed by free-living amoebae derived from it.

The possibility of preventing or curing cancer and collagen and auto-immune diseases

Collagen and auto-immune diseases or some cases of chronic lymphatic leukaemia could be cured and the aging process slowed, if it were possible to kill limax amoebae completely. This can be accomplished by administering antiprotozoal drugs. However, reinfection may occur easily and repeated courses of treatment would be necessary. In cases of malignant disease, however, apart from some cases of chronic lymphatic leukaemia, permanent genetic changes in the affected cells have occurred and treatment of limax amoebae infection will not reverse these. The possibility of a fundamental cure of malignant disease seems remote.

Your Notes

Your Notes

References

A8BATT, J.D. and LEA, A.J.: Lancet, 1958, ii, 880.

ABDALA, J. and RoLAND, V.A.: Rev. Fac. Cienc. Med. Univ. Cordoba, 1970, 28, 55.

ABo-RABBO, H., et al.: J. Trop. Med. Hyg., 1969, 72, 287.

ABD-RABBO, H., ABAZA, H., HILLAL, G., Moo-HAZY, M. and AssER, L.: J. Trop. Med. Hyg., 1972, 75, 64.

ABERG, A., JoHANSSON, H. and WERNER, I.: Lancet, 1972, ii, 381.

ABRAHAMs, A.: In "French's Index of Differential Diagnosis," 8th. Edit., J. Wright and Sons, 1960, Bristol.

ABRAHAMS, C., SAFRO, I., LITHIGOW, D., GRAHAM, S., SHIR. MA. and CoPE, S.: Lancet, 1972, 1, 498.

ABRAHAMSON• A.L., GOODMAN, M. and KoLODNY, H.: Arch. Otolaryng., 1968, 88, 91.

AcKERMAN, A.B. and LANTIS, L.R.: Arch. Dermatol., 1967, 95, 202.

AcKERMAN, L.V. and DEL REGATO, J.A.: Cancer, 2nd. Edit., 1954, Kimpton, London.

ADAIR, F.E., PACK, G.T. and FARRIOR, J.H.: Amer. J. Cancer, 1932, 16, 1104.

ADA fs, D.D.: Hospital Medicine, 1967, 1, 676.

ADAMS, J.A.: Amer. J. din. Path., 1963, 40, 173.

ADENYI- JoNES, C.: Lancet, 1967, i, 188.

d'AcNosTINo.A.N. and BALIN, R.C.: Diabetes, 1963, 12, 327.

d 'AcoSTINo, A.N., PEASE, G.L. and KERNOHAN, J.W.: J. Neuropath. exp. Neurol., 1963, 22, 138.

AtRD, I.: "A Companion to Surgical Studies", 1958, 2nd. Edit., Livingstone, Edinburgh.

AISENBERc, A.C.: New Eng. J. Med., 1964, 270, 565 and 617.

ALARCN-SEcoviA, D., GALBRAITH, R.F., MAL· DONADO, J.E. and HowARD, F.M. Jr.: Lancet, 1963, ii, 662.

ALAR t;ON-SEGOVIA, D., HERSKOVIC, T., DEARING, W.H., BARTHOLOMEW, L.G., CAIN, J.C. and SHORTER, R.G.: Gut, 1965, 6, 39.

ALEXEIEFF, G.: Nouv. Rev. fran. d'Hematol., 1964, 4, 725.

ALEXANDER, P. and FAIRLEY, G.H.: In "Clinical Aspects of Immunology", 1968, 2nd. Edit., Edit. by Gell, P.G.H. and Coombs, R.R.A., Blackwell, Oxford.

AuEv, S.A.: Vopr. Onkol., 1964, 10, 81.

ALLAN, J.M. and MERCER, J.O.: J. Neurol. Psychiat., 1936, 17, 1.

ALLAN, N.C. and WATSON-WILLIAMs, E.J.: In Proc. 9th. Congress of European Soc. of Haematology, p. 906.

ALLEN, J.G., GROSSMAN, B.J., ELGHAMMER, R.M., MouLDER, P.U., McKEEN, C.L., JAcOB-soN, L.O., PIERCE, M., SMITH, T.R. and CRosBIE, J.M.: J. Amer. Med. Ass., 1949, 139, 1251.

ALMY, T.P.: Gastroenterology, 1961, 41, 391.

AMos, D.A., WELLMAN, W.E., BowiE, E.J.W. and LINMAN, J.W.: Mayo Clin. Proc., 1967, 42, 468.

ANASTASSEA-VI.ACHou, C., CAssrMos, C., MEs-SARITAKis, J. and PAPADAKI, E.: Ann. Pediat. (Basel), 1961, 196, 310.

ANDERSON, D.E.: In "Genetic Concepts and Neoplasia", Williams and Wilkins, Baltimore, 1970, 85, 109.

ANDERSON, E.T. and VYE, M.V.: Ann. intern. Med., 1967, 66, 141.

ANor::asoN, J.R., BucHANAN, W.W. and GouDIE, R.B.: Quoted by Asherson, G.L. Abstr. World Med., 1965, 37, 289.

ANDERSoN, K. and jAMIESON, A.: Lancet, 1972, ii, 379.

ANDERSON, L.G. and TALAL, N.: Clin. Exp. Immunol., 1972, 10, 199.

ANDERSON, V. and PEDERSEN, H.: Acta. Med. Scand., 1967, 182, 581.

ANDERSON; W.A.D.: "Pathology", 1957, 3rd. Edit., Kimpton, London.

ANDOLFALLO, Z.G., ZILIOTTO, D. and PAGLIAN, R.: Acta. med. Patov., 1963, 23, 347.

ANDRE, R., RocHANT, H., DREYFus, B., DuHA-MEL, G. and PE:cHERE, J.C.: Bull. Soc. Med. Hop. Paris, 1967, 118, 1133.

ANscoMB£, A.R., Fox, H. and GUNN, A.D.G.: Brit. J. Surg., 1967, 54, 525.

ANsELL, B.M. and LAWRENcE, J.S.: Arth. Rheum., 1963, 6, 260.

d'ANTONI, J.S.: Amer. J. trop. Med., 1952, 1, 146.

d'ANTUONO, G., PrERAGNOLI, E., TuRA, S. and ZAMPA, G.A.: Acta. hepato-planologica, 1961, 7, 375.

APLEY, J., CLARKE, S.K.R., RooME, A.P.C., SAN-DRY, S.A., SAYCI, G., SILK, B. and WARHURST, D.C.: Brit. med. J., 1970, i, 596.

ARMsTRONG, J.A. and PEREIRA, M.S.: Brit. med. J., 1967, i, 212.

ARNESEN, K. and NoRNES• M.: Acta Ophthal (Kbh.), 1975, 53, 139.

ARNOFF, A., BYWATERS, E.G.L. and FEARN LEY, G.R.: Brit. med. J., 1955, 2, 228.

AsBOE-HANSEN, G.: Acta. Derm-venerol. {Stockh.) , .1959, 39, 270.

AsHERsON, G.L.: Abstr. World Medicine, 1965, 37, 289 and 38, 145.

AsHERSON, G.L.: Case shown at Clinical Meeting of the Royal Society of Medicine, London, March 12th., 1973.

AsHURST, P.A.: Brit. med. J., 1968, 2, 647.

AsKANAzY, M.: Veri. Dtsch. path. Ges., 1921,

18, 78.

AsTRoM, K-E, MANCALL, E.L. and RicHARDSON, E.P. Jr.: Brain·, 1958, 81, 93.

AsQUITH, P., THOMPSON, R.A. and CooKE, W.T.: Lancet, 1969, 2, 129.

AssEIN, E.SX., TROTTER, W.R. and BELYAVIN, G.: Immunology, 1965, 9, 21.

AssENBERG, A.C.: New Engl. J. Med., 1964, 270, 565 and 617.

AssoR, D.: Amer. J. din. Path., 1974, 61, 270.

ATwooD, W.G., MILLER, R.C. and NELSON, C.T.: Arch. Derm., 1966, 94, 144.

AUGUST, P.J.: Proc. R. Soc. Med., 1974, 67, 1238.

AusTAD, W.I., CaRNEs, J.S., GouGH, I.C.R. Mc-CARTHY, C.F. and READ, A.E.: Amer. J. dig. Dis., 1967, 1235, 475.

AusTEN, K.F.: In Cecil-Loeb "Textbook of Medicine", 1971 13th. Edit., Edit. by Beeson, P.B. and McDermott, W., Saunders, Philadelphia.

AuTO-IMMUNITY and GENETics, 1968, Blackwell Scientific Publications, Oxford.

AYALA, A., SLOANE, J. and WoLMA, K.J.: J. Amer. med. Ass., 1968, 204, 829.

AzzoPARDI, J.G. and EvANS, D.J.: J. din. Path., 1971, 24, 774.

AzzOPARDI, J.G. and LEHNER, T.: J. din. Path., 1966, 19, 539.

BABES, V.: Ztschr. Bakr. Orig., 1906, 42, 541.

BAcHuus, B.E. and WILLIAMS, R.D.: Arch. Surg., 1966, 92, 537.

BADELLA, M.: Pedia t. int. (Roma), 1962, 12, 155.

BADENOCH, J.: Brit. med. J., 1960, ii, 879 and 963.

BADMAEVA, V.V.: Arkh. pat. (Mask.), 1970, 32, 67.

BAGLEY, C.M. Jr., RoTH, J.A., THOMAS, L.B. and DEVITA, V.J. Jr.: Ann. intern. Med., 1972, 76, 219.

BAGNELL, A.W.: Canad. Med. Ass. J., 1957, 77, 182.

BAGREN, J A.: Arch. Surg. Chicago, 1928, 17, 561.

BAILEY, C.C. and CAMPBELL, R.H.A.: Brit. med. J., 1973, 1, 460.

BAILEY, H. and LoVE, M.: "A Short Practice of Surgery", 1962, 12th. Edit., Lewis, London.

BAIN, A.D. and BouLD, I.K.: Lancet, 1963, ii, 304.

BAITZ, T. and KYLE, R.A.: Arch. intern. Med., 1964, 113, 872.

BAKER, A.B. and ADAMs, J.M.: Amer. J. Cancer, 1938, 34, 214.

BAKER, C. and MANN, W.N.: Guy's Hasp. Rep., 1939, 89, 83.

BAKKER, P.M. and TJON, A.J.S.S.: Dermatologica (Basel), 1971, 142, 50.

BALABANov, K., ANDREEN, V.C. and TcHERNO·ZEMSKr, I.: Dermatologica (Basal), 1969, 139, 211.

BALDWIN, J.N. and WrsNER, R.: Amer. J. Surg., 1966, 111, 230.

BALL, J.: Bull. J. Ann. Rheum. Dis., 1954, 13, 277.

BALL, J.: In "Textbook of Rheumatic Diseases", Edit. W.S.C. Copeman, 4th. Edit., 1969, Livingstone, London.

BALL, J.: Ann. Rheum. Dis., 1971, 30, 213.

BALL, J. and S!iARP, J.: In "Modem Trends in Rheumatology", 1971, Vol. 2 pp. 117-138. Edit. by Hill, A.G.S., Butterworth, London.

BALMEs. A., DAUVERCHAIN, J., RoBINET, M., et al.: Concburs med., 1970, 92, 6637.

BALTH:AZAR, P.A., CoRDEIRO, E.N., BARRETO, O.C. et al.: Rtfv. Hasp. Fac. Med. S. Paulo, 1973, 28, 25.

BANATVALA, J.E., BEsT. J. and WALLER, O.K.: Lancet, 1972, i, 1205.

BANERJEE, A.K.: Med. J. Malaya, 1972, 26, 173.

BANERJEE, A.K. and BLACKWOOD, W.: Acta. Neuropath. (Berl.), 1971, 18, 84.

BANERJEE, A.K. and CHOWDHURY, D. Sur Roy,: Lancet, 1965, i, 1276.

BARCLAY, J.A.: Brit. med. J., 1969, 1, 765.

BARLOW, G.W.: Arch. Derm. Syph., 1939, 39, 1021.

BARR, M.L, SaAvER, E.L., CARR, D.H. and PLUNKETT, E.R.: J. Ment. defic. Res., 1960, 4, 89.

BARNARD, R.D.: Science, 1948. 107, 571.

BARNES, H.M.: Proc. R. Soc. Med., 1974, 67, 28.

BARON, D.N. and GuRLING, K.J.: J. din. Endocrinol., 1959, 18, Proc. XX.

BARON. J.H. and LENNARD-JNEs, J.E.: Brit. J. Hasp. Med., 1971, 6, 303.

BARRATT. G.M.: Lancet, 1964, i, 723.

BARTHOLOMEW, L.G., CAIN, J.C. and SHORTER, R.G.: Gut, 1965, 6, 39.

BARTHOLOMEW, L.G., CAIN, J.C., WINKELMAN N, R.K. and BAGGENSTOSS, A.H.: Amer. J. Dig. Dis., 1964, 9, 43.

Von BAsEoow, GA.: Wschr. Heilk., Berlin, 1840.

BXssLER, R.: Arch. Path. path. Anat., 1959, 332, 335.

BAsTEN, A.: Med. J. Austral., 1968, 1, 452.

BASTENI.E, P.A., VANH:AELST. L., BoNNYNS, M., NEvE, P. and STAGNET, M.: Lancet, 1971, i, 203.

BATEMAN. O.J., SQUJRES, G. and TANNHAUSER, S.J.: Ann. int. Med., 1945, 22, 426.

-449-

BATSCHWAROZ, B. and MrNKOV, D.: Brit. J. Derm., 1968, 80, 84.

BAUMER, A.: Z. Rheumforsch., 1961, 20, 270.

BAWDLER, A.J. and GLicK, I.W.: Ann. intern. Med., 1961, 65, 761.

BEALE, P.J., CoRMACK, J.D. and OLDREY, T.B.N.: Brit. med. J., 1972, 1, 345.

BEATON, C. and GERARD, P.: J. thor. cardiavase. Surg., 1966, 51, 428.

BEARN, A.G.: In Cecil-Loeb "Textbook of Medicine", 1971. 13th. Edit. Saunders, Philadelphia.

BecHET, P.E.: Arch. Derm. Syph., 1942, 45, 33.

BEcK, J.S. and RowELL, N.R,: Lancet. 1963, i, 134.

BEcKER, F.P.: New York J. Med., 1964, 64, 1211.

BECKER, T.: Zbl. Chir., 1960, 85/17, a/suppl., 946.

BecKER, K.L., FeRGUsoN, R.H. and McCoNAHEY, W.M.: New Eng. J. Med., 1963, 268, 277.

BECKER, K.L., TILUS, J., WooLER, L. and McCoNAHEY, W.M.: Ann. int. Med., 1965. 62, 1134.

BECKER, S.W., KAHN, D. and ROTHMAN, S.: Arch. Derm. Syph., 1942, 45, 1069.

BECKETT, V.L. and DrNN, J.J.: Quart. J. Med., 1972, 41, 71.

BEDARD, P. and DHTHOFF, H.Q.: Un. med. Cane., 1964, 93, 45.

BEER, T.C.: Proc. R. Soc. Med., 1973, 66, 910.

BEESON, B.B. and ELBERT, M.H.: Urol. Cutan. Rev., 1934, 38, 785.

BEEVERS, D.G.: Brit. med. J. 1972, 4, 275.

BErCKERT, A.: Xrztl. Wschr., 1958, 13, 438.

BELL, E.T.: Amer. J. Path., 1957, 33, 499.

BEN -ISHAY, D., FREUND, M. and GRoEN, J.J.: Blood, 1963, 22, 100.

BENToN, C. and GERARD, P.: J. thor. cardiavase. Surg., 1966, 51, 428.

BENVENJSTI, D.S. and ULTMANN, J.E.: Ann. int. Med., 1969, 71, 731.

BERNARDELLI, J.L., HYMAN, C.J., CAMPBELL, E.E. and FIREMAN, P. : J. Pediat., 1972, 81, 751.

BERG, J.W.: J. nat. Cancer Inst., 1967, 38, 741.

BERG, J.W., HUTTER. R.V.P. and FooTE, F.W.: J. Amer. med. Ass., 1968, 204, 771.

BERGHINZ, G.: Gazz. Osp. Milano, 1900, 21, 606.

BERLINER, G.B. et al.: Klin. Med. (Moskva), 1968, 46, 139.

BERMUTH, G. Von, MINELLY, J.A., LoGAN, G.B. and GLEICH, G.J.: Pediatrics, 1970, 45, 792.

BERNADou, A., CLAUVEL, J.P., ANTEBI, L. and BILSKI-PASQUIER, G.: Sem. Hop. Paris, 1968, 44, 2101.

BERNARD, E., SAGRESTAN, J.M., RENAULT, P. and WEIL, J.: Poumon. Coeur, 1966, 22, 63.

BERNARD, J.: Israel J. med. Sci., 1965, i, 1316.

BERNARD, J., CHAVELET, F. and }ACQUILLAL, C.: Nouv. Rev. frano. Hemat., 1964, 4, 125.

BERNSTEIN, J.S. and NrxoN, D.D.: Amer. J. dig. Dis., 1964, 9, 625.

BERTRAM, U.: Acta Odont. Scand., 1967. 25, Suppl. 49.

BESANCON, L.T., PEGNIGNOT, H., ETIENNE, J.P., DEML, R. and PELITE, J.P.: Sem. Hop. Paris. 1966, 42, 2595.

BEsT, C.M. and CooK, P.B.: Brit. med. J., 1961' ii, 496.

BEUTNER, E.H., JoRDON, R.E. and CaoRZELSKr, T.P.: J. invest. Derm., 1969, 5, 63.

BEUTNER. E.H., CHORZELSKI, T.P., HALE, W.L. and HAUSMANOVA-PETRUSEWICZ, I.: J. Amer. med. Ass., 1968, 203, 845.

BrcHEL, J.: Acta. radio!., 1947, 28, 81.

SicHEL, J., HoLTEN, C., JENSEN, K.B. and CHRISTENSEN, A.S.: Acta. med. Scand., 1957, 158, 352.

BICKET, G., MozEL, J.J. and JAUNDRY, R.: Bull. Mem. Soc. Hop. Paris, 1935, 51, 12.

BrcKs, R.O., GoLDGRABOR, M.B. and KIRSNER, J.B.: Amer. J. Med., 1958, 24, 447.

BIELSCHOWSKI, F.: Klin. Wschr., 1932, 11, 1491.

BrEDER, L. and WIGLEY, R.D.: N.Z. J. Med., 1964, 63, 375.

BtNG, R..: "Textbook of Nervous Diseases", 1939, Kimpton, London.

BINNIE, W.H., BRETDAY, R.C. and LYNN, A.H.: Brit. Dent. J., 1971, 130, 235.

BIRCH, C.A., CooKE, K.B. DREW, C.E., LoNDON, D.R. MACKANZIE, D.H. and MrLNE, M.D.: ·Lancet, 1964, i, 693.

BIRCH, P.R.J. and RowELL, N.R.: Amer. J. Med., 1965, 38, 793.

BISBEE, A.C. and THoENY, R.H.: Cancer (Philad.), 1976, 35, 1296.

BrrAN• A., CHIMENES, H., MARTIN, E. and KLOTZ, H.P.: Press Med., 1964, 72, 1293.

BL-\ JCHMAN, M.A., DAcrE, J.V., HoBBS, J.R., PETTIT, J.E. and WoRLLEDGE, S.M.: Lancet, 1969, 2, 340.

BLACKBURN, E.K. et al.: Int. J. Cancer, 1968, 3, 16, 3.

BLAcKBURN, G. and O'GoRMAN, B.: Guy's Hosp. Rep., 1961, 110, 379.

BLATRIX, C., DEMASSIEUX, J.L., NEBUT, M. and FrNE, J.M.: Rev. fran<. Transfusion, 1968, 11, 145.

BLEEHEN, S.S.: Proc. R. Soc. Med., 1963, 56, 730.

BLE Nors, L.M., PARKINSON, M.C., SHr LKIN, K.B. and WILLIAMS, R.: Quart. J. Med., 1974,

43, 25.

BLENDrs, L.M., ANsELL, I.D., LLoYD, JoNEs, K., HAMILTO N, E. and WILLIAMS, R.: Brit. med. J., 1970, 1, 131.

BuzzARD, R.M.: In "Textbook of Immunopathology", 1969 Edit. by Miescher, P.A. and Miiller-Eberhard, H.J., Grune and Stratton, New York.

BLUMENTHAL, H.T. and BERNS, A.W.: Adv. Geromtological Res., 1964, 1, 289.

BLocH, K.J.: In "Textbook of Immunopathology", 1969 Edit. by Miescher, P.A. and Miiller-Eberhard, H.J., Grune and Stratton, New York.

BLOCH· K.J., BucHANAN, W.W., WoHL, N.J. and BuNIM, J.T.: Medicine (Baltimore), 1965, 44, 187.

BLOOMFIELD, A.L. and POLLAND, W.S.: "Gastric Anacidity. Its Relations to Disease". Macmillan Company, 1933, London.

BoccARDI, V., GRAsso, A. and DoLCE, V.: Haemat. Lab. (Milano), 1968, 11, 239.

BocHENEK, Z., Ku s, J. and DABSKA, M.: Mschr. Ohrenheilk., 1973, 107, 306.

BoMERS-MARREs, A.J.M.L.: Lancet, 1964, ii, 364.

BooNE, A.W.: Dis. Chest, 1969, 55, 341.

BooTH, C.C.: Brit. med. J., 1970, 3, 725. and 4, 14.

BoNDUELLE, M., BoRDER, F., BouYGUES, P. and CHARLES, F.: Rev. neurol. (Paris), 1955, 92, 551.

BoNDY, P.K.: In Cecil-Loeb, 1967, "Textbook of Medicine", 12th. Edit., Saunders, Philadelphia.

BoNOMO, L., DAMMACEO, F., PrNTO, L. and BAR· BIERI, G.: Lancet, 1963, ii, 807.

BoNOMO, L., DAMMACEo, T., TuRsi, A. and TRIZIO, D.: Clin. exp. 'Immunol., 1970, 6, 531.

BoNOMO, L., DAMMACEo, T., TuRSI, A. and TRIZIO, D.: Proc. Int. Symposium on Immune Complex Diseases. 1971, p. 122, Carlo Erba Foundation, Milan.

BoNOMO, L., TuRsi, A., TRoMrouozzr, G. and DAMMACEo, F.: Brit. med. J., 1965, ii, 689.

BoRELLO, E.D. and GoRLIN, R.J.: Cancer, 1966, 19, 196.

BosKEN, W. and NoLTENms, H.: Zbl. Allg. path. Anat., 1968, 111, 407.

BoTTAZZO, G.F., PouPLARD, A., FLORIN-CHRISTENSEN, A. and DoNIACH, D.: Lancet, 1975, ii, 97.

BorrcH.ER, E.: A.M.A. Arch. Path., 1959, 68, 419.

BoTTOMLEY, R.H. and CoNDrr, P.T.: Cancer Bull., 1968, 20, 22.

BouDIN, G.: Concours Md., 1962, 84, 301,

447, 777 and 943.

BouR NE, C. and SANDOROUND, J.H.: Amer. J. Cancer, 1939, 37, 173.

BoussER, J.: Sang, 1957, 28, 553.

BoussER, J., CRISTOL, D. and ZrTTOUN, R.: Sem. Hop. Paris, 1961, 37, 2531.

BouvENOT, G., PAILLAS, J.E. and CARCAssoNNE, Y.: Cah. Med., 1974, 10, 273.

BowrE, E.J.W., THOMPSON, J.H., PAscuzzi, C.A. and OwEN, C.A.: J. Lab. din. Med., 1963, 62, 416.

BoxER, L.A. and SMrrH. D.L.: Amer. J. Dis. Child, 1970, 120, 564.

BovD, R.V.: Brit. med. J., 1964, i, 1092.

BovD, W.: "A Textbook of Pathology", 1961 7th. Edit., Kimpton, London.

BoYLAND, E.: Progress in Experimental Tumour Research, 1969, 11, 222.

BovLE, J.A. and BucHANAN, W.W.: "Clinical Rheumatology", Blackwell Scientific Publications, 1971, Oxford.

BoYLE, J.A. and McGIRR, E.M.: Brit. med. J., 1965, i, 1170.

BRAILSFORD, J.: "The Radiology of Bones and Joints", 1953 5th. Edit., Churchill, London.

BRAIN, W.R.: Lancet, 1959, i, 109.

BRAIN, W.R.: Lancet, 1963, i, 179.

BRAIN, W.R., CRoFT, P.B. and WILKINSON, M.: Brain, 1965, 88, 479.

BRAIN, W.R., DANIEL, P.M. and GREENFIELD, J.G.: J. Neurol. Psychiat., 1951, 14, 59.

BRAIN, W.R. and HENsEN, R.A.: Lancet, 1958, ii, 971.

IIR'I.NDRORO, L L., GoLDBERG, S.B. and BREmEN· B..CH, W.C.: New Eng. J. Med., 1970, 283, 1306.

BRAUNSTEINER, H. and SAILER, S.: Acta. haemat. (Basel), 1960, 23, 306.

BREARLEY, K.S. and SPIERS, A.S.D.: Med. J. Aust., 1962, 1, 789.

BRESCIA, M.A., SANTORA, E. and SARNATORO, V.F.: J. Pediat., 1959, 55, 35.

BREWER, D.B. and ORR, J.W.: J. Path. Bact., 1953, 65, 193.

BREY, O., GARNER, E.P.R. and WELLS, D.: Brit. med. J., 1963, 3, 397.

BRIEF, D.K., GoPALAKRJSHNAN, A. and YouNo, M.K.: J. med. Soc. N.J., 1972, 69, 419.

BRINCKER, H.: Brit. J. Cancer, 1972, 26, 120.

BRODIE, J. and HENDERSON, A.: Scot. med. J., 1960, 5, 313.

BRODY, J.I., BEIZER, L.H. and ScHWARTz. S.: Amer. J. Med., 1964, 36, 315.

BRODY, P.K.: In Cecil-Loeb "Textbook of Medicine", 1971, 13th. Edit., Edit. by Beeson, P.B. and McDermott, W., Saunders, Philadelphia.

BROSTOFF, J, BoR, S. and FEIWEL, M.: Lancet,

1961, ii, 177.

BROWN, J.M.: Med. J. Aust., 1971, 1, 3V5.

BROWN, J. and WINKELMANN, R.K.: Mddicine (Baltimore), 1968, 47, 33.

BROWN, R.S., ScHIFF, M. and MITCHELL, M.S.: Ann. intern. Med., 1974, 80, 459.

BROWN, J.H., VARS...Mts, J., ToEws, J. and SHANE, M.: Canad. Psychiat. Ass. J., 1974, 19, 219.

BROWNE, H.J.: Surg. Gynec. Obstet., 1966, 123, 1252.

BROWNSTEIN, M.H. and SCHERL, B.A.: Arch. intern. Med., 1966, 117, 689.

BRUBAKER, M.M. et al.: Arch. Derma tol., 1965, 91, 320.

BRUCE, D.H., BERNARD, W. and BLAcKARD, W.G.: Amer. J. Med., 1970, 48, 768,

BRUN, J., MouLIN, G., QutNEAU, P. and MouuNIER, J.: Bull. Soc. franc;. Derm. Syph., 1965, 72, 92.

BRYANT, W.M. and RusH, B.F.: Ann. Surg., 1967, 166, 837.

BUACHIDZE, O.S. and ONoPRIENKo, G.A.: Ortop. Travm. Protez., 1970, 11, 19.

BucHANAN, W.W.: Geriatrics; 1965, 20, 941.

BucHANAN, W.W., CRooKs, J., ALEXANDER, W.D., KoUTAAs, D.A., WAYNE, c:t. and GRAY, K.G.: Lancet, 1961, i, 245.

BucKLE, R.: Tubercle (London), 1960, 41, 213.

BuEHLER, S.K., FIRME, F., FoDOR, G., FRASER, G.R., MARSHALL, W.H. and VAZE, P.: Lancet, 1975, 1, 195.

BuLLOCK, F.D. and CuRTIS, M.R.: J. Cancer Res., 1925, 9, 425.

BuNDSCHUH, E.: Beitr. path. Anat., 1914, 57, 65.

BUNIM, J.J.: Ann. Rheum. Dis., 1961, 20, 1.

BuNIM, J.J., BucHANAN, W.W., WERTLAKE, P.T., SoKOLOFF, L., BLOCH, K.L., BEcK, J.S. and ALEPA, F.P.: Ann. intern. Med., 1964, 61, 509.

BURCH, P.R.J.: Nature, 1963, 197, 1145.

BuRcH, P.R.J.: Lancet, 1963, (a), i, 1253.

BURCH, P.R.J.: Lancet, 1963, (b), ii, 200.

BuRCH, P.R.J.: Brit. J. Psychiat., 1964 (a), 110, 808.

BuRcH, P.R.J.: Brit. J. Psychiat., 1964 (b), 110, 818.

BuRcH, P.R.J.: Brit. J. Psychiat., 1964 (c), 110, 825.

BuRcH, P.R.J., BuRwELL, R.G. and RowELL, N.R.: Lancet, 1964, i, 720.

BuRCH, P.R.J. and RowELL, N.R.: Lancet, 1963, i, 507.

BuRCHENAL, J.H.: Cancer (Philad.), 1968, 21, 595.

BuRT, A.S., REINER, L., CoHEN, R.B. and SNrF-

FEN, R.C.: J. Clin. Endocrinol., 1954, 14, 79.

BuRKITT, D.P.: J. Nat. Cancer Aust., 1969, 42, 19.

BuRKITT, D.P.: Lancet, 1970, ii, 1237.

BuRKITT, D.P.: Brit. med. J. 1970, 4, 424.

BuRNET, F.M.: Lancet, 1967, i, 1171.

BuRNET, F.M.: Brit. med. J., 1965, i, 338.

BURNHAM, T.K.: Lancet, 1972, 2, 436. BuRRows, H.: "The Localization of Disease",
1932, Bailliere, Tindall and Cox, London.

BusooRFF, B. VoN: Acta. med. Scand., 1939, 100, 320.

BussE, K. and PAULYN, W.: Med. Welt. (Stuttg.), 1965, 13, 638.

BYWATERs, E.G.L. and ANSELL, B.: In "Textbook of the Rheumatic Diseases", 1969. Edit. by Copeman, W.S.C., 4th. Edit., Livingstone, London.

CABRERA, A., TsuKADA, PrcKREN, J.W., MooRE, R. and BRoss; I.D.J.: Cancer (Philad.), 1966, 19, 470.

CAMMARATA, R.J., RoDNAN, G.P. and JENSON, W.N.: Arch. intern. Med., 1963, III, 330. CAMPBELL, H.: Proc. R. Soc. Med., 1972, 65,
64.

CAMPBELL, A.H. and LEE, E.J.: Brit. J. Dis. Chest, 1963, 57, 113.

CANALE, V.C. and MuECKE, E.C.: CA (N.Y.), 1974, 24, 66.

CANEV, K.: Lit. Bioi. Med., 1960, 3/4, No. 868.

CANNAT, A. and SELIGMANN, M.: Brit. med. J., 1973, 1, 71.

CARNEY, J.A.: Cancer, 1975, 35, 1179.

CARPENTER, C.C.J., SoLOMON, N., SILVERBERG, S.G., BLEDsoe, T., WoRTHCUTT, R.C., KuNENBERG, J.R., BENNET, I.L. Jr. and HARVEY, A. Me. G.: Medicine (Baltimore), 1964, 43, 153.

CARRYER, H.M., SHERRICK, D.W. and GASTINEAU, C.F.: J. Amer. med. Ass, 1960, 172, 1356.

CARTER, C.O.: Brit. med. Bull., 1969, 25, 52.

CARTER, R.F.: Trans. R. Soc trop. Med. Hyg., 1972, 66, 193.

CAsE, R.A.M. and LEA, A.J.: Brit. J. Prev Soc. Med., 1955, 9, 62

CASSIRER, R. and HIRSCHFELD, R.: "Handbuch der Neurologic". Edit. by Humke, O. and Foerster, O.J. Springer, Berlin, 1935, Vol. 7, p. 312.

CASTAtGNE, P., HuGE, A., EseouROLLE, R. and BERGER, B.: Rev. neurol., 1965, 112, 143.

CAsTILLO, DEL E.B. and TRucco, E.: Semana med. (Buenos Aires), 1959, 115, 547; 549.

CATHCART, E.S., WILLIAMS, R.D., Ross, H. and

CAtKINs, E.: Amer. J. Med., 1961, 31, 758.

CATTELL, R.D. and BocHINE, E.J.: Gastro-enterology, 1947, 8, 695.

CAVANAGH, J.B., GREENBAUM, D., MARSHALL, A.H.E. and RuBINSTEIN, L.J.: Lancet, 1959, ii, 521.

C.wAZZINI, L., BEARZI, I. and FABRIS, G.: Riv. Pat. Clin. Sper., 1970, 11, 109.

CAzEILLES, M., CoRNET, L., JAVE, R. and PiNE, J.: J. Med., Bordeaux, 1953, 130, 1012.

CEciL, R.L. and KAMMERer, W.H.: Amer. J. Med., 1951, 10, 439.

CHRISTENSEN, E. and FoG, M.: Acta. Psychiat. KBH., 1955, 30, 141.

CHRISTENSEN, E. and RossEL, I.: Acta. neurol. Scand., 1964, 40, 150.

CHRISTIANSON, H.B., BRUNSTING, LA. and PERRY, H.O.: Arch. Derm., 1956, 74, 581.

CHrusTIANSON, H.B. et al.: Southern Med. J., 1967, 66, 567.

CHRISTOFFERsEN, P. and NIELSEN, A.R.: Acta. path. Microbiol. Scand., 1964, 60, 334.

CHRISTY, N.P.: In Cecil-Loeb "Textbook of Medicine", 1967 12th. Edit., Edit. by Beeson, P.B. and McDermott, W., Saunders, Philadelphia.

CERVENANSKY, J., 0l'ATIK, J. and HoasKY, I.: Acta. chir. Orthop. Trauma. Cech., 1970. 37, 236.

CHALSTREY, L.J. and BENJAMIN, B.: Brit. J. Cancer, 1966, 20, 670.

CHAMBERLAIN, M.A. and BRUCKNER, F.E.: Ann. Rheum. Dis., 1970, 29, 609.

CHAMBERLAIN, M.J. and WHITTAKER, S.R.F.: Lancet, 1963, i, 1398.

CHANDA&, K., MAIR, H.J. and MAIR, N.S.: Brit. med. J., 1968, i, 158.

CHAVEs-CARBALLO, E. and HAYES, A.B.: Mayo Clin. Proc., 1966, 41, 843.

CHERVENICK, P.A., BOGGS, D.R. and WrNTROBE, M.M.: Ann. intern. Med., 1967, 67, 1239.

CHESKY, V.E., HELLWIG, C.A. and WELCH, J.W.: Amer. J. Surg., 1962, 28, 678.

CHISHOLM, M., ADRAN, G.M., CALLENDER, S. and WRIGHT, R.: Quart. J. Med., 1971, 40, 421.

CHORZELSKI, T. and jABL6NsKA, S.: Acta. Dermatovenercolagica (Stockholm), 1970, 50, 81.

CrEzA RoDRIGUEZ, L.F. and TAu, R.: Dia Med., 1943, 15, 1322.

CLARK, W.H., FROM, L., BERNARDINO, E.A. and NrHM, M.C.: Cancer Res., 1969, 29, 705.

CLARKE, J.J.: "Protozoa and Disease. Part III, The cause of Cancer", 1912, Balliere, Tindall and Cox, London.

CoBB, S., ANDERSON, F. and BAUER, N.: New Eng. J. Med., 1953, 249, 553.

CoEuR, P.: Lyon Med., 1969, 221, 772.

COHEN, F.B., KANNERSTEIN, M. and KLOSK, E.: J. Newark Beth. Israel Hosp., 1965, 11, 30.

CoHEN, G.F.: Lancet, 1965, ii, 267.

CoHEN, H., RuBINs, S. and EISENMANN, G.: Cancer N.Y., 1958, 11, 1247.

CoHEN, L. et al.: Amer. J. Med., 1966, 40, 299.

CoHEN, S.M. and WAXMAN, R.S.: Arch. int. Med., 1967, 120, 717.

CoLLDAHL, H.: Acta Allerg. KBE, 1960, 15, 124.

CoLLIN, D.H.: Lancet, 1956, 2, 51.

CoFFMAN, J.D.: In Cecil-Loeb "Textbook of Medicine", 1971, 13th. Edit., Edit. by Beeson, P.B. and McDermott, W., Saunders, Philadelphia.

CoLLINs, J.P.: Brit. med. J., 1962, i, 947.

CoLLs, B.M. and CARRELL, R.W.: NZ. med. J., 1970, 72, 383.

CoLOMB, D., VACHOR, A. and CLAuov, A.: Bull. Soc. franc;. Derm. Syph., 1973, 80, 32.

CoMINGS, D.E.: Arch. intern. Med., 1965, 115, 79.

CONN, H.O., ScHREIBER, W. and ELKINGTON, S.G.: Amer. J. Dig. Dis., 1971, 16, 227.

CoNN, J.W.: Proc Diabetes Ass., 1946, 5, 79.

CoNNoR, B.: Proc. R. Soc. Med., 1972, 65, 251.

CooK, P.: Brit. J. Cancer, 1971, 25, 853.

CooK, P.: Oral Surg., 1961, 14, 690.

CooKE, J.V.: Amer. J. Dis. Child, 1933, 44, 1153.

CooPER, IA.: Med. J. Australia, 1970, 57, 697.

CoPEMAN, W.S.C.: "Textbook of Rheumatic Diseases", 1969 Edit. by Copeman, W.S.C., 4th. Edit., Livingstone, London.

CoPPoLA, A., YERMAKOV, V. and CAGGIANO, V.: Cancer (Philad.), 1969, 23, 576.

CoRCINO, J.J., ZALUSKY, R., GREENBERG, M. and HERBERT, V.: Brit. J. Haemat., 1971, 20, 511.

CoRDONNIER, J.J. and SPJUT, H.J.: J. Urol., 1957, 78, 242.

CoRNES, J.S.: J. Clin. Path., 1960, 13, 483.

CoRNES, J.S., JoNEs, T.G. and FrsHER, G.B.: Brit. J. Cancer, 1961, 15, 200.

CosTA, Da L.R.: Brit. med. J., 1971, 3, 281.

CosTELLO, J.F.: Proc. R. Soc. Med., 1972, 65, 751.

CouRcv, C.: Sem. Hop. Paris, 1964, 40, 2095.

CoUNSELL, P.B. and DuKEs, C.E.: Brit. J. Surg., 1952, 39, 1.

CouRVIILE, C.B.: "Pathology of the Central Nervous System", 1945, 2nd. Edit., Pacific Press Pub. Ass., Mountain View, California.

Cox, M.T.: J. Clin. Path., 1964, 17, 591.

CRAIG and FAusT: "Clinical Parasitology", 1970, 8th. Edit., Edit. by Faust, E.C., Russell,

P.T. and Jung, R.C., Lea and Fibiger, Philadelphia.

CRAwFORD, B.G.R.: Brit. med. J, 1936, i, 751.

CRAwFORD, M. d'A. : Lancet, 1961, ii, 22.

CREAOAN, E.T. and FRAUMENI, J.F. Jr.: Cancer (Philad.), 1973, 32, 1325.

CREAM, J.J., GUMPEL, J.M. and PEACHEY, R.D.G.: Quart. J. Med., 1970, 39, 461.

CREAMER, B.: Brit. med. J., 1964, ii, 1435.

CREAMER, B.: Gut, 1966, 7, 569.

CREAMER, B. and PINK, I.J.: Lancet, 1967, i, 304.

CRILE, G. and FisHER, E.R.: Cancer (Philad.), 1953, 6, 57.

CRoFT, P.B. and WILKINSON, M.: Brain, 1969, 92, 1.

CROME, L.: Proc. R. Soc. Med., 1972, 65, 587.

CROTII, A.: "Diseases of the Thyroid, Parathyroids and Thymus", 1938, Kimpton. London.

CROWDER, R.V., THOMPSON, W.T. and KuPFER, H.G.: Arch. intern. Med., 1959, 103, 445.

CRUIKSHANK, A.H.: J. Clin. Path., 1965, 18, 391.

CuDWORTH, A.G., WooDROW, J.C. and GAMBLE, D.R.: Lancet, 1975, 2, 29.

CuDwORTH, A.G. and ELLIS, A.: Brit. med. J., 1972, 3, 291.

CuENCA, C.R. and BEcKER, K.L.: Arch. intern. Med., 1968, 121, 159.

CUILJERET, J., jANIN, N., GouNoT, R. et al.: Lyon Chir., 1973, 69, 451.

C'uLBF.RTSON, C.G., EASMINGER, P.W. and OVER-TON, W.M.: Amer. J. din. Path., 1972, 57, 375.

CuLBERTSON, e.G., SMITH, J.W., CoHEN, D.V.M. and MINNER, J.R.: Amer. J. Path., 1959, 35, 185.

CuNLIFFE, W.J., IfALL,-R., STEVENSEN, C.J. and WEIGHTMAN, D.: Brit. J. Derm., 1969, 81, 877.

CuRRIE, S. and URICH, H.: J. Neurol. Neurosurg. Psychiat., 1974, 37, 598.

CuRTH, H.O.: Arch. Derm. Syph., 1936, 34, 353.

CuRTH, H.O.: Arch. Derm. Syph., 1948, 57, 158.

CuRTH, H.O., HILBERG, A.W. and MAcHACHEK, G.F.: Cancer, 1962, 15, 364.

CURTIS, A.C., BLAYLOCK, H.C. and HARRELL, E.R.: J. Amer. med. Ass., 1952, 150, 844.

CuRTON, R.J.R., HARLAND, D.H.C., HosFORD, J. and PIKE, C.: Brit. J. Surg., 1956-7, 44, 561.

DACIE, j.V.: "The Haemolytic Anaemias, Congenital and Acquired", 1!162, 2nd. Edit., Part 2. "The Auto-immune Anaemias", Grune and Stratton, New York.

DACIE, J.V., BRAIN, M.C., HARRISON, C.V., LEWIS, C.V. and WoRLLEDGE, S.M.: Brit. J. Haematol., 1969, 17, 317.

DAILEY, M.E., LINDSAY, S. and SKAHEN, R.: Arch. Surg., 1955, 70, 291.

DALGAARD, J.B. and KXss, A.: Acta. path. Microbial. Scand., 1955, 37, 465.

DALLAIRE, L., KINGSMILL-FLYNN, D. and LEBO-EUF, G.: Canad. Med. Ass. J., 1969, 100, 1.

DALY, J.J. and jACKSON, E.: Brit. med. J., 1964, i, 748.

DALY, J.J. and RicKARDs, D.F.: Lancet, 1964, i, 1415.

DAMESHEK, W.: In "Conceptional Advances in Immunology and Oncology", 1963, Hoeber Med. Div., Harper and Row, New York.

DAMESHEK, W. and SAHWARTZ, R.S.: Blood, 1959, 14, 1151.

DAMRON, M.A., CLARK, R.B., CZADO, L. and PowERS, C.W.: Amer. J. Proctol., 1965, 16, 107.

DAVIES, A.G.: Lancet, 1971, ii, 161.

DAVIDSON, F.: Brit. J. Dermatol., 1962, 74, 439.

DAVIDSON, S.L. and SMALL, J.M.: J. Neurol. Psychiat., 1960, 23, 176.

DAVIS, A.E. Jr.: J. Amer. med. Ass., 1960, 173, 153.

DAvrs, H.: Brit. J. Derm., 1922, 34, 12.

DAVIS, J.S. Jr., WEBER, F.C. and BARIFIELD, H.: Ann. int. Med., 1957, 47, 10.

DATTNER, R.: Wien Klin. Wschr., 1937, 2, 87.

DAwBER, R.P.R.; Brit. J. Dermatol., 1968, 80, 275.

DAwsoN, M.A.: Amer. J. Med., 1972, 52, 406.

DAwsoN, P.J. and HARRISON, C.V.: J. din. Path., 1961, 14, 219.

DEATON, J.G. and LEVIN, W.C.: Arch. intern. Med., 1967, 120, 345.

DELANEY, W.E. and BALOGH, K.: Cancer, 1966, 19, 853.

DELLON, A.L., CHRETIEN, P.B., PoTVIN, C. and RocRENT!NE, G.N.: Arch. Surg., 1975, 110, 156.

DELMAS MARSALET, Y., LEDUC, M., LERCHE, E. and GoNDEMAND, M.: Presse Med., 1969, 77, 821.

DENOIX, P.F., ScHWARZ, D. and ANGUERA, G.: Bull. Ass. fran. Cancer, 1958, 45, 1.

DEUTSCH, H.J.: Ann. Otolaryng., 1967, 76, 1074.

DEvlc, E. and ToLoT, G.: Rev. med., 1906, 26, 255.

DrcK, A. and KELLETT, H.S.: Brit. J. Surg., 1951, 39, 257.

DrI'BIAR. K., KocHwA, S., ZucKER-FRANKLIN, D. and WASSERMAN, L.R.: Blood, 1968, 31, 81.

DJAIDANE,A., MAYER,G., LEDERLIN,P. et al.: Tunis Med., 1972, 50, 207.

DJALDETTI, M., PINKHAS, J. and De VRIES, A.: Blood, 1968, 32, 336.

DoBROSSY, L., MoLNAR, L. and RONAY, P.: Magy. Onkol., 1972, 16, 41.

DoE, W.E., EvANs, D.J., HoBBS, J.R. and BooTH, C.C.: Gastroenterology, 1972, 60, 970.

DoE, W.F., HoBBs, J.R., HENRY, K. and DowLING, R.H.: Quart. J. Med., 1970, 39, 619.

DoHAN, F.C.: In "Schizophrenia. Current Concepts and Research". Edit. S. Sankar, New York, P.J.D. Publications, 1969.

DoiG, J.A., WHALEY, K., DICK, W.C., NuKr, G., WILLIAMSON, J. and BucHANAN, W.W.: Brit. med. J., 1921, 4, 460.

DoLL, R. and KINLEN, L.: Brit. med. J., 1970, 4, 420.

DoLMAN, C.L. and CAIRNS, A.R.M.: Neurology, 1961, 11, 349.

DoNIAcH, D., GRANT, D. and NEwNS, G.H.: Proc. R. Soc. Med. 1972, 65, 488.

DoNIACH, D. and RorTT, I.M.: In "Clinical Aspects of Immunology", 1918, Edit. by Gell, P.G.H. and Coombs, R.R.A., 2nd. Edit., Blackwell, Oxford.

DoNIACH, D. and RaiTT, I.M.: In "Textbook of Immunopathology", 1969, Edit. by Miescher, P.A. and Miiller-Eberhard, H., Grune and Stratton, New York.

DoNIACH,D., RmTT, I.M. and HuoSON, R.V.: Lancet, 1958, ii, 265.

DoNIACH, D., ROITT, I.M., WALKER, J.G. and SHERLOCK, R.S.: Clin. exp. Immu nol., 1966, 1, 237.

DoNIACH, D., RaiTT, I.M. and TAYLOR, K.B.: Brit. med. J., 1963, i, 1374.

DoNIACH, I. and SHINER, M.: Brit. J. Radial., 1960, 33, 238.

DosTALOVA, O., ScHON, E., Ku BELKA, V. and HouK, F.: Neoplasma (Bratisl.), 1970, 17, 231.

DouGLAS, A.S. and RIFKIND, B.M.: Scot. med. J., 1966, 9, 469.

DouRov, N., STERNON,J., De CosTER, A. and CHALLY, P.: Ann. Anat. Path., 1968, 13, 201.

DoWNES, J.M., GREENWOOD, B.M. and WRAY, S.H.: Quart. J. Med., 1966, 35, 85.

DoxiAoES, T.: Brit. med. J., 1962, i, 187.

CoxiADES, T.A., Dou KAS, E., YoTsAs, Z. and PoNTIDEs, E.: Gastro(en terology, 1971, 60, 658.

DREYFUS, B., SALMO N, C., ROEHANT, H., GERBAL, A. and SuLTON, C.: Bull. Soc. Med. Hop. Paris. 1966, 117, 675.

DRIESSEN, A.P.P.M. and ScHERPENISS E. L.A.: Ned. T. Geneesk., 1970, 114, 2041.

DRUET, P., DRYLL, A., RYCKEWAERT, A., de SE.zE, S., and KAHN, M.F.: Sem. des Hop. Paris, 1969, 45, 489.

DRYLL, A., RoussELET, F., RYCKEWEART, A. et a!.: Sem. Hop. Paris, 1969, 45, 2135.

DuBE, V.E. and JoYcE, G.T.: Cancer (Philad.), 1971, 27, 434.

DuBLIN, W.B.: "Fundamentals of Neuropathology", 1954, C.C. Thomas, Springfield, Illinois.

DuBois, E.L.: "Lupus Erythematosus", 1966, McGraw-Hill, New York.

Du.sols, E.L., FRION, G.J. and CHA.NDOR, S.: J. Amer. med. Ass., 1972, 220, 515.

Due, M., Due, M.L., FwQUET, J. et a!.: Ann. Med. Nancy, 1973, 12, 1467.

Ducms, P., CoLOMB, L. and AMBLARD, P.: Lyon Med., 1967, 217, 1953.

Ducms, P., AMBIARD, P., LEGER, J. et a!.: Bull. Soc. franc;. Derm. Syph., 1970, 77, 285.

DuKE-ELDER, S.: "Textbook of Ophthalmology", 1954, Kimpton, London.

DuNN, D.C.: Brit. med. J., 1971, 2, 84.

DUNNING, W.F. and CuRTIS, M.R.: Cancer Res., 1946, 6, 668.

DuNNING, W.F. and CuRTIS, M.R.: Cancer Res., 1953, Proc. 1, 13.

DuRANCE, R.D.: Proc. R. Soc. Med., 1971, 64, 61.

DuRANT, J.R., BARRY, W.E. and LEARNER, N.: Lancet, 1966, i, 119.

DuTHIE, J.J.R.: In "Textbook of Rheumatic Diseases". 1969, Edit. by Copeman, W.S.C., 4th. Edit., Livingstone, Edinburgh.

DuTHIE, J.J., BRowN, P.E., TRUELOVE, L.H., BARACAT, F.D. and LAWRIE, A.J.: Ann. R heum. Dis., 1964, 23, 193.

DucA, del, V. and MoRNINGSTAR, W.A.: J. Amer. med. Ass., 1967, 199, 671.

DYER, N.H., KE NDALL, M.J. and HAwKINS, C.F.: Ann. Rheum. Dis., 1971, 30, 626.

DvMocK, I.W.: Brit. J. Cancer, 1966, 20, 236.

EAKINS, D., Fu LTO N, D. and HADDE N, D.R.: Gut, 1964, 5, 315.

EASSON, E.C. and R ussELL,M.H.: Brit. med. J., 1963, 1, 1704.

EASTMA N, R.D. and YoEMA N, W.B.: Acta med. Scand., 1960, 166, 241.

EoER, M.: Schweiz. z. allg. Path. Bact., 1953, 16, 155.

EDWARDS, F.C. and TRUELOVE, S.C.: Gut, 1964, 5, 1.

EnsTROM, G.; Acta med. Sca nd., 1939, 99, 228.

EGGE N, R.R.: Amer. J. din. Path., 1963, 39,3.

EISEMAN N, G. and DAMASHEK, W.: New Eng. J. Med., 1954, 251, 1044.

EisE N, G.: N.Y. Med. Rec., 1900, 58, 6.

ELLERKER, A.G.: Med. Press, 1956, 235,280.

ELus, J.R., MARSHALL, R., NoRMAND, I.C. and PENROSE, L.S.: Nature, 1963, 198; 411.

ELLWOOD, M., IRVINE, W.J. and HARTOG, M.: Proc. R. Soc. Med., 1972, 65, 490.

ELsnoN-DEw, R.: Brit. J. Hasp. Med., 1972, 8, 175.

ELTRINGHAM, J.R. and KAPLAN, H.S.: Nat. Cancer Inst. Monogr., 1973, 36, 107.

ELY, L.W., REED, A.C. and WYcKOFF, H.A.: Calif. State Jour. Med., 1922, 20, 59.

EMANUEL, I., SEVER, L.E., MrLHAM, S. and TauLNIC, H.C.: Lancet, 1972, ii, 361.

EMERSON, C.H. and UnGER, R.D.: New Eng. J. Med., 1972, 287, 328.

ENGEL, A.G. and STICKNEY, J.M.: Arch. int. Med., 1962, 109, 168.

ENGFELDT, B. and ZEITERSTRoM, R.: Acta. med. Scand., 1956, 153, 337.

ENGLAND, J.M., CHANARIN, 1., PERRY, J. and SzuR, L.: Brit. J. Haematol., 1968, 15, 473.

ENGQUIST, A. and PocK-STEEN, O.C.: Lancet, 1971, ii, 438.

ENTWHISTLE, C.C., FENTON, P.H.H. and JA-coBs, A.: Brit. med. J., 1964, ii, 1504.

EREZ, S.E., RicHART, R.M. and SaETTLEs, L.B.: Amer. J. Obstet. Gynec., 1965, 92, 273.

EsTRIDGE, M.N.: Bull. Los Angeles Neural. Soc., 1950, 15, 87.

ETcaEVERRY, R., GusMAN, C., LusADA, M., RE-GONEsr, C. and MaRANDA, M.: Arch. int. Rheum., 1959, 2, 124.

EvANS, H.J.: In "Human Population Cyto-genetics". Edit. by Jacobs, P.A., Price, W.H. and Law, P., 1970., Williams and Wilkins, Baltimore, Maryland.

EvANs, R.W.: "British Encyclopaedia of Medical Practice". 1961. Edit. by Lord Cohen of Birken head, Butterworth, London.

EvANS, R.W.: "Histological Appearances of Tumours". 1966, 2nd. Edit., Livingstone, Edinburgh.

EwiNG, J.: "Neoplastic Diseases", 1940, 4th. Edit., Saunders, Philadelphia.

FABER, M. and BoRUM, K.: Brit. J. Haemat., 1962, 8, 313.

FADEM, R.S.: Cancer, 1952, 5, 128.

FAIRFAX, A.J. and LEATHAM, A.: Brit. med. J., 1975, 4, 322.

FAIRLEY, G.H.: Brit. J. hasp. Med., 1971, 6, 433.

FAIRLEY, G.H. and ScoTT, R.B.: Brit. med. J., 1961, 2, 920.

FArRLEY, G.H. and MAcKm, F.: Brit. med. J., 1937, i, 375.

FAIRMAN, RD.: Proc. R. Soc. Med., 1972, 65, 347.

FALCK, I. and BRUSCHKE, G.: Aertzl. Wschr., 1958, 13, 374.

FARID, N.R. and EvERED, D.C.: Brit. med. J., !1971, 4, 233.

FAsco, F.A., MATTIOLI, F. and BERTOccHI, I.: First Meeting of European Division of Intern. Soc. Haematology, 1971, Abstr., No. 343.

FATOURECHI, V., McCoNAHEY, W.M. and WooL-NER, L.B.: Mayo Clin. Proc., 1971, 46, 682.

FATEH MoGHANDAM, A., BELL, E. and LAMERZ, B.: Dtsch. med. Wschr., 1971, 96, 539.

FAUST, E.C. and RussELL, R.F.: "Clinical Parasitology", 1957, 6th. Edit., Kimpton, London.

FAuVERT, R., BorvrN, P., MALLAME, J. and NrcoLLo, F.: Nouv. Rev. frant;. Hemat., !1961, 1, 459.

FEDERMAN, J., GoLDSTEIN, M.E. and WEINGAR-TEN, B.: Amer. J. Roentgen., 1963, 89, 771.

FELMAN, Y.M., SaAl'IRO, L. and MosER, H.S.: Dermatologica (Basel), 1969, 138, 444.

FENSTER, L.F., BucHANAN, W.W., LAsTER, L. and BuNrM, J.J.: Ann. intern. Med., 1964, 61, 498.

FENYOHAZI, L., WALACHER, L. and MEDGYES, A.: Zeitsch. f. Rheumaforsch., 1970, 29, 153.

FEREMANS, W.: Bull. Cancer (Paris), 1966, 53, 415.

FERGUSON, F.R.: Proc. R. Soc. Med., 1962, 55, 49.

FERNANDEZ-HERLIHY, L. and KoTT, S.: Laryng. Clin. Found. Bull., 1967, 16, 165.

FERRARo, A.: J. nerv. ment. Dis., 1959, 128, 279.

FERRIER, P., FERRIER, S., STALDER, G., BuHLER, E., BAMAITER, F. and KLEIN, D.: Lancet, 1964, i, 80.

FEUTEM, P.H. and JAcoBs, A.: Brit. med. J., 1964, ii, 1540.

FIALKOw, P.J.: Lancet, 1964, i, 474.

FIALKOW, P.J.: Lancet, 1967, i, 1106.

FIALKOW, P.J., THULINE, H.C., HECHT, T. and BRYANT, J.: Amer. J. human Genet., 1971, 23, 67.

FIALKOW, P.J., UcHIDA, I.A., HECHT, F. and MDTULSKY, A.G.: Lancet, 1965, 2, 868.

FIEYTEs, M.A. and CARRI, J.H.: Heta Gastro-enterol Latineam, 1973, 5, 61.

FruPE, M.l. and CooKE, K.B.: J. din. Path., 1974, 27, 315.

FrLrPPOVA, L.A.: Arkh Pat. (Mask.), 1973, 351, 724.

FrNK, C.W., WINDMILLER, J. and SARTAIN, P.: Arth. Rheum., (N.Y.), 1972, 15, 347.

FrsHER, J.C. and KETCHAM, A.S.: W. Va. Med. J., 1966, 62, 137.

FISCHER, T., LAuTENSCHLAEGER, J. and PoETT-GEN, W.: Dtsch. Med. Wschr., 1974, 99,

1867.

"Fiagyl", 5th. Edit., 1967, May and Baker, Dagenham, England.

FLANNERY, G.R., RoLLAND, J. . and NAIRN, R.C.: Lancet, 1975, 1, 751.

FLASTER, R.: R. Soc. Med. Symposium, June 7th., 1972.

FLAVELL MATTS, S.G.: Lancet, 1958, 2, 102.

FJ.EINFELDER, H. and BRACHARZ, H.: Klin. Wschr., 1956, 34, 512.

FoDoR, F. and KRuTsAv, M.: Full. Orr-Gegegy6g., 1964, 10, 138.

FoRSHAW, J.W.B. and MooRHOUSE, E.H.: Brit. med. J., 1964, 2, 94.

FosscREEN, J.: Acta. path. Microbial., Scand., 1962, 56, 143.

FowLER, E.F., MAJARAKIS, J.D. and Cot£, w.H.: Arch. Surg., 1961, 82, 925.

FowLER, P.B.S., SwALE, J. and ANDREWS, I.I.: Lancet, 1970, ii, 488.

Fox, B. and RisDON, R.A.: J. Clin. Path., 1968, 21, 486.

FRAIRE, A.E. and GREENBERG, S.D.: Cancer, 1973, 31, 1078.

FRAISSE, H., MoREL, P. and GIRARD, M.: J. med. Lyon, 1952, 33, 295.

FRANIs, R., GERMAIN, D., RAcLE, P. and MOREAU, P.: Pediatric., 1966, 21, 47.

FRANKLIN, J.: "French's Index of Differential Diagnosis". 8th. Edit., Edit. by Douthwaite, A.H., Wright, Bristol, 1960.

FRANKS, L.M.: Proc. R. Soc. Med., 1972, 65, 672.

FRANZEN, S., JoHANSsoN, B. and KAJGAS, M.: Acta. Med. Scand., 1966, 179 (Suppl. 445), 336.

FRASER, N.G.: Brit. J. Derm., 1970, 83, 609.

FRAUMENI, J.F. and GLAss, J\.G.: J. Amer. med. Ass., 1968, 206, 825.

FRAUMENI, J.F. Jr., VocEL, C.L. and de VrrA, V.T.: Ann. intern. Med., 1969, 71, 279.

FRAVETZ, R.E., Van NooRDEN, S.I. and SPIRO, H.M. : Lancet, 1967, 1, 235.

FRAZER, K.T.: Med. J. Aust., 1969, 56, 298.

FREDERICKSON. D.S.: J. din. Endocrinol., 1957, 11, 766.

FREUND, H.: Munchen med. Wschr., 1919, 66, 84.

FRIED, B.M.: Arch. Surg., Chicago, 1958, 77, 730.

FRIEDBERG, S.A., EDWARDS, R.H. and HAss, G.M.: Ann. Otol. (St. Louis), 1957, 66, 830.

FRIEDMANN. G. and MuLLER, W.: Zbl. Neuro-chir., 1967, 28, 147.

FRIEDMA N. H.B., SILVER, G.M. and BROWN, C.H. : Ann. J. Dig. Dis., 1968, 13, 910.

FRtOU, G.J.: Ann. N.Y. Acad. Sci., 1974, 230, 23.

FRY, L.: Brit. med. J., 1971, 4, 172.

FRY, L. and RussELL, B.F.: Proc. R. Soc. Med., 1968, 61, 240.

FUDENBERG, H.H., GERMAN, J.L. and KUNKEL, H.G.: Arth. Rheum., 1962, 5, 565.

FuKUHARA, A., MoRITA, S., TAKAHASI, S. and WATANABE, S.: J. Jap. Soc. intern. Med., 1963, 51, 57.

Futo, H.: Lancet, 1960, ii, 1029.

FuLTON, J.F.: "Physiology of the Nervous System", 1943, 2nd. Edit., Oxford University Press, London.

FuNc, W.P., TAN, K.K., Yu, S. F. and KHo, K.M.: Gut, 1970, ii, 212.

FuRszYFER, J., KJERLANo, L.T., McCoNAHEY, W.M. and ELVEBACK, L.: Mayo Clin. Proc., 1970, 45, 636.

FuRszvFER, J., KIERLAND, L.T., WooLNER, B., B., ELVEBACK, L. and McCoNAHEY, W.M.: Mayo Clin. Proc., 1970, 45, 586.

FURSZYFER, J., McCoNAHEY, W.M., KIERLAND, L.T. and MALDONADO, J.E.: Mayo Clin. Proc., 1971, 46, 37.

FuTCHER, P.H.: Bull. Johns Hopk. Hosp., 1959, 105, 97.

GABRIELsoN, A.E., CooPER, M.D., PETERsoN, R.D.A. and Goon, R.A.: In "Textbook ot Immunopathology". Vol. II. Edit. by Miescher, P.A. and Miiller-Eberhard, H.J. Grune and Stratton, New York and London, 1969.

GAGEL, O.: 1936, In "Handbuch der Neurolo-gie"., Edit. Bumke, O. and FoP.rster, O. Springer, Berlin, 5, p. 682.

GAL, I. and LISKA, G.: Magy Onkol., 1970, 14, 134.

GAL, P.: J. nerv. ment. Dis., 1957, 125, 574.

GALBRAITH, R.F. et al. : New Eng. J. Med., 1964, 270, 229.

GALEWSKY, E.: In "Handbuch de Haut-und Gcschlechtsk rankheiten", 1933, Band 12, Teil 1. J. Springer, Berlin.

GALLI, T. and CHrri, E.: Ann. rheum. Dis., 1955, 14, 271.

GALL!ARD, H. and MALLARMt, J.: Le Sang, 1955, 26, 526.

GALT, J., HuNTER, R.B. and HuLL, J.M.: Amer. J. med. Sci., 1952, 223, 61.

GAMBILL, E.E.: In Paper read at 51st. Annual Session of the American College of Physicians at Philadelphia, 1970, April 12th-17th.

GARCIN MoRTEO, O., PoRRINI, A. and MALDONADE Cocco, J. : Arch. Argent. Rheuatol., 1971, 34, 27.

GARo. S.: Special Lecture, London University, 1964.

GARDNER, D.L.: "Pathology of the Connective

Tissue Diseases", 1965, Arnold, London.

GARDNEa, D.L.: Honyrnan-Gillespie Lecture, University of Edinburgh Medical School, 1966.

GARD NER, D.L.: In "A Companion to Medical Studies", Vol. II, Edit. Passmore. R. and Robson, J.S., Blackwell, Oxford, 1968.

GAaDNER, D.L.: In "Textbook of the Rheumatic Diseases", 1969, 4th. Edit., Edit. by Copeman, W.S.C., Livingstone, Edimburgh.

GARDNER, D.L.: "The Pathology of Rheumatoid Arthritis", 1972, Edward Arnold, London.

GARDNJ::R, L.W.: Arch. Path., 1955, 59, 372.

GARIJO, J.M., ScRIA, M.F., AMOROS, R.E. and PAscuAL, M.A.: Medicam enta (Madr.), 1973, 61, 39.

GARaon, O. and CLARKE, P.: Proc. R. Soc. Med., 1966.

GASCARD, E., REGIS, M., MouLAaD, J.C. and MuLLER, G.: Marseille Med., 1969, 106, 329.

GASTEAU, C.F., MYERS. .W.R., ARNOLD, J.W and McCoNAHEY, W.M.: Proc. Mayo Clin., 1964, 12, 939.

GEHRMANN, G. and ENGSTFELD, G. : Dtschr. Med. Wschr., 1965, 90, 1328 and 1335.

GELBSHTEIN, M.I. and NABAKOV, S.A.: Arkhpat. (Mosk.), 1968, 30, 24.

GEMMA, G.B.: Minerva Pediat., 1963, 15, 314.

GEMMA, G.B., BERNARDINI, R. and GLEzzr, P.: Minerva Med., 1968, 58, 3587.

GEPTS, W.: Diabetes, 1965, 14, 619.

GERARnv, W.: Z. Rheumaforsch., 1959, 18, 407.

GERBEa, M.A., BRODIN, A. and STEINBERG, D. et al.: New Eng. J. Med., 1972, 286, 14.

GeaEB, T.: Arch. Psychiat., 1953, 191, 134.

GHARIB, H. and GASTINEAu, C.F.: Proc. Mayo Clin., 1969, 44, 217.

GHAZI, A.: Brit. med. J., 1972, i, 144.

GHOSH, L. and MuERLICKE, R.C.: Ann. intern. Med., 1970, 72, 379.

GIAcovAzzo, M., IPPOTIro, A., SPONGE, G. and CARDONE, U.: Rass. Fisiopat. Clin. Ter., 1967' 39, 277.

Gruss, D.D. and PRYOR, J.S.: Proc. R. Soc. Med., 1961, 54, 590.

GrERSTEN, J.: Acta. pa th. Microbiol. Scand., 1956, 38, 439.

GrLBERT, E.F., HARLEY, J.B., ANmo, V., MENGO!.!, H.F. and H UGHES, J.T.: Amer. J. Med., 1968, 44, 820.

Gn.BERT, T.T., EvJY, J.T. and EDELSTEIN, L.: Ca ncer (Philad), 1971, 28, 293.

GILBERTSO N, V.A.: Proc. of VIII International Pigmen t Cell Conference. March 1972, p. 176 (Abstr.), Sydney.

GrLLV, R., CHAMFEVIL, R., CuRCIER, H. et al. : Marseille Med., 1969, 106, 603.

GrTTLER, R.D., ZucKER, G., ErsENGER, R. and SroTTER, N.: New Eng. J. Med., 1958, 258, 932.

GJoNE, E. and NoRooY, A.: Brit. med. J., 1970, 1, 610.

GLAss, H.G., WALDRON, G.W. and BROWN, W.G.: Cancer (Philad.), 1956, 9, 310.

GoDFREY, S.: Brit. med. J., 1964, i, 1159.

GoLDBERG, L.S., SHu sTER, J. and FuDENBERG, H.H.: J. Lab. Clin. Med., 1969, 73, 249.

GoLDENBURG, G.J., PARASKEVAS, F. and IsRAEI.s, L.G.: Arth. Rheum., 1969, 12, 569.

Gor.oFARB, B.L. and COHEN, S.S.: J. Amer. Med. Ass., 1970, 211, 1525.

GoLDING, P.L.: Brit. med. J., 1970, 3, 278.

GoLDING, P.L., BowA, R., MASON, A.M.S. and TAYLOR, E.: Brit. med. J., 1970, 4, 340.

GoLDsMITH, R.E.: Lancet, 1970, ii, 881.

GowsTEIN, J. and HAar, J.T.: Tubercle (London), 1959, 40, 119.

GoLDSTEIN, W.B. and PoKER, N.: Gastroenterology, 1966, 51, 87.

Goon, M.S.: Proc. R. Soc. Med., 1971, 64, 224.

Goon, R.A.: Minn. Med., 1962, 68, 634.

Goon, R.A., GABRIELSON,: Minn. Med., 1966, 57, 725.

Goon, R.A. and RoTSTEIN, J.: Bull. Rheum. Dis., 1960, 10, 203.

GooDMAN, L.S. and GILMAN, A.: "The Pharmacological Basis of Therapeutics", 4th. Edit., 1971. The Macmi llan Co., New York.

GoonwrN, P. and FRY, L.: Proc. R. Soc. Med., 1973, 66, 625.

GoooWIN, P.T.: Cancer (Philad.), 1952, 5, 1089.

GoRDON, H.W. and RvwuN, A.M.: Gastroenterology, 1966, 50, 248.

GoRDON-TAYLOR, G.: Brit. med. J., 1959, i, 455.

GoRnON, R.D.: Aust ralasian Ann. Med., 1963, 12, 202.

GoRDON, R.R. and CooKE, P.: Lancet, 1964, ii, 1212.

GoTHA-!!. G., WAaASTJ ERNA, C. and }EGLENSK Y, B.: Acta med. Scand., 1965, I, 177.

GoTTLIEB, S.K.: J. Amer. med. Ass., 1969; 209, 1963.

Govoi£, R.B., ANDERSON, J.R. and GRAY, K.G.: J. Path. Bact., 1959, 77, 389.

Goi.:nrr::, R.B., BoYLE, I.T., STUART-SMITH, D.D. and FERG usoN, A.: Lancet, 1969, i, 186.

GorniE. R.B. and PINKERTON, P.K.: J. Path. Bact., 1962, 83, 584.

Got:GEROT, H. and D uPERaAT, B.: Ann. Derm. Syph. (Paris), 1942, Be Ser., p. 193.

GouGH, K.R., READ, A.E. and NAISH, J.M.: G ut, 1962, 3. 232.

GRACE, J.R. and DAo, T.L.: Cancer, 1959, 12, h48.

GRADER, J. and MoYNIHAN, J.W.: J. Amer. Med. Ass., 1961, 176, 685.

GRAHAM, A. and McCuLLAGH, E.P.: Arch. Surg., 1931, 22, 548.

GRALNICH, H.R., HARBOR, J. and VoGEL, C.: Blood, 1971, 37, 152.

GRAMPA, G., Bosrsro, M.B., BERGAMINI, F. and ARLOTTA, P.: Path. Europ. (Brux.), 1970, 5, 470.

GRAVANo, L., ScHAJOwrcz, F., MENZANI, A. and VACCARO, A.: Pres. Med. Argent., 1970, 57, 1659.

GREEN, D.: Proc. Int. Cancer Conference. March 1972, p. 52 (Abstr.), Sydney.

GREEN, F.H.Y. and CARTY, J.E.: Lancet, 1976, i, 964.

GREEN, 1., LITWIN, S., ALDERSBERG, R. and RUBIN,!.: Arch. int. Med. 1963, 118,592.

GREEN, I., LITWIN, S., ALDERSBERG, R. and RuBIN, I.: Arch. int. Med., 1966, 118, 592.

GREEN, 1., LITWIN, S., ALDERSBERG, R. and RuBIN, I.: Acta Haematol., 1966, 37, 100.

GREEN, M. and LrM, K.H.: Lancet, 1971, i, 1159.

GREEN, P.A., WoLLAEGER, E.E., SPRAGUE, R.G. and BROWN, A.L.: Diabetes, 1962, 11, 388.

GREENBERGER, N.J., JoNEs, W.A. and IssELBA· CHER, K.J.: Arch. intern. Med. (Chicago}, 1965, 115, 488.

GREENE, R. and OLIVER, L.C.: Brit. med. J., 1968, 4, 412.

GREENFIELD, J.G.: "The Spino-Cerebellar Degenera tions", 1954, Blackwell, Oxford.

GREENWOOD, B.M.: La ncet, 1968, ii, 380.

GREENWOOD, B.M.: Ann. Rheum. Dis., 1969 (a), 28, 488.

GREENWOOD, B.M.: Ann. Rheu m. Dis., 1969 (b) , 28, 617.

GREENWOOD, B.M.: Quart, J. Med., 1969(c), 38, 295.

GRECORIE, H.B., OTHER SEN, H.B. and MooRE, M.P.: Amer. J. Surg., 1962, 104, 577.

GRESHAM, G.A. and AcKERLEY, A.G.: J. Clin. Path., 1958, 11, 244.

GRoB, P.J. and HEROLD, G.E.: Brit. med. J., 1972, 2, 561.

GROPP. A., JussEN, A. and OouN JO, F.; Lancet, 1964, i, 1167.

GROTH,: Virchows Arch., 1864, 29, 602.

GRozrNGER, K.H., DALIENBACH, F. and HEISKI, H. : La ngenbecks Arch. Surg., 1969, 326, 47.

GRUNDY, D.J.: Proc. R. Soc. Med., 1972, 65, 167.

GRYMINSKI, J. and SzYMANSKA, D.: Gruzlika Cha r. Pluc., 1970, 38, 1001.

G u LATA, an d VAISHNAVA,: Pa per read at VII Europea n Congress of Rheuma tology, Brighton, Jun e 7-11th. 1971.

GuMPEL,J.M.: Proc. R. Soc. Med., 1971, 64, 397.

GuM PEL, J.M.: Proc. R. Soc. Med., 1972, 65, 877.

GuNTHER, H.N.C.: Proc. R. Soc. Med., 1965, 58, 579.

GuNz, F.W., FITZGERALD, P.H., CRoSSEN, P.E., MACKENZIE, I.S., PowLEs, C.P. and jENSEN, G.R.: Blood, 1966, 27, 482.

GuPTE, S.P., PERKASH, A., MAHAJAN, C.M. et a!.: Amer. J. Dig. Dis., 1971, 16, 939.

CuRLING, K.J., BARON, D.N. and SMITH, E.J.R.: J. din. Endocrinol., 1959, 19, 717.

GUTMANN, L., CROSBY, T.W., TAKAMORI, M. and MARTIN, J.D.: Amer. J. Med., 1972, 33, 354.

GwrEZDZINSKI, Z. and SzvszYMAR, B.: Przegl Derm., 1972, 59, 37.

HADDAD, R. and MASSARO, D.: Amer. J. Med., 1968, 45, 211.

HAGGAN!, M.T. and HoLTI, G.: Acta. Derm. Venera!. (Stokh.), 1973, 53, 369.

HAJJAR, E.T. and SALTI, I.S.: J. Med. Liban., 1973, 26, 247.

HALBERG, P., BERTRAM, U., S!iSBORC, M. and NERUP, J.: Acta. med. Scand., 1965, 178, 291.

HALDENMANN, R.: Z. Geburtsh. Gynak., 1970, 173, 323.

HALL, G.H.: Lancet, 1971, ii, 935.

HALL, J.F.: Proc. R. Soc. Med., 1968, 61, 871.

HALL, R., SAXENA, K.M. and OwE NS, S.G.: Lancet, 1962, ii, 1291.

HALL, R. and STANBURY, J.B.: Clin. exp. lmmunopa th., 1967, 2, 719.

HALL, R., TuRNER-WARwicK, M. and DoNIACH, D.: Ciin. exp. Immunol., 1966, 1, 285.

HAL LEN, J.: Acta. med. Scand., 1966 (Suppl. No. 462).

HAMBLETON, G.: Proc. R. Soc. Med., 1969, 62, 1095.

HAMILTON, E.B.D. and BYWATERS, E.G.L.: Ann. Rheum. Dis., 1961, 20, 353.

HAMILTON, J.R., LYNCH, M.J. and REILLY, B.J.: Quart. J. M ed., 1969, 38, 135.

HA MSHER, J.B., FARRAR, T. and MooRE, T.D.: J. Urol. Bait., 1958, 80, 299.

HANDLE, W. and CREAMER, B.: Brit. med. J., 1965, ii, 455.

HANISCH, C.M.: Bull. Hasp. Joint Dis, 1950, 11, 43.

HARDEN, R. MeG, CHISHOLM, C.J.S. and CANT, J.S.: Metabolism, 1967, 16, 890.

HARITOPOULos, K.M., DELIKARrs, P.G. and KARAMANAKos, P.P.: Hellin Chir., 1973, 45, 621.

HARNDEN, D.G.: Proc. R. Soc. Med., 1976,

69, 41.

HARRIS, J. and BAGAI, R.C.: Med. Clin. N. Amer., 1972, 56, 501.

HARRIS, P.W.B. and CoLLINS, J.V.: Lancet, 1971, i, 1349.

HARRIS, J., JEssoP, J.D. and de SAINTONGE, D.M.C.: Brit. med. J., 1971, 4, 463.

HARRIS, O.D. and CooKE, W.T.: Brit med. J., 1967, i, 756.

HART, F.D.: Brit. med. J., 1969, 3, 131.

HART, F.D.: Brit. med. J., 1970, 2, 747.

HARVARD, C.W.H.: Brit. med. J., 1972, 1, 360.

HARVEY, A.M.: In Cecil-Loeb "Textbook of Medicine", 1967, 12th. Edit., Edit. by Beeson, P.B. and McDermott, W., Saunders, Philadelphia.

HARVEY, A.M., SauLMAN, L.E., TuMULTY, P.A., CoNLEY, C.L. and ScHOENRICH, E.H.: Medicine (Baltimore), 1954, 33, 291.

HAsLocK, D.I., WRIGHT, V. and HARRIMAN, D.G.F.: Quart. J. Med., 1970, 39, 335.

HAUSMANOVA-PETMSEVlcz, 1., CHoRZELSKI, T. and STRUGALSKA, H.: J. Neural. Sci. (Arnst.), 1969, 9, 273.

HAwKINs, S.E.: In "The Biology of Amoeba", Edit. Jeon, K.W. Cell Biology Monographs, 1973, Academic Press, New York and London.

HAWLEY, P.R., JoHNSTON, A.W. and RANKIN, J.T.: Brit. med. J., 1967, 3, 208.

HAY, D.R.: N.Z. Med. J., 1964, 63, 90.

HEATH, C.W. Jr. and MoLONEY,: New Eng. J. Med., 1965, 272, 882.

HEATHFIELD, K.W.G. and WILLIAMS, J.R.B.: Lancet, 1960, i, 1157.

HEATON, A.M.: Proc. R. Soc. Med., 1962, 55, 479.

HEATON, J.M.: Brit. med. J., 1959, i, 466.

HEATON, J.M.: Amer. J. Ophthalmol., 1963, 55, 983.

HECHT, F., KoLER, R.D. RrGAS, D.A., DAHNKE, G.S., CAsE, M.P., TISDALE, V. and MILLER, R.W.: Lancet, 1966, ii, 1193.

HEDLEY, A.J., Ross, I.P., BEcK, J.S., DoNALD, D., ALBERT-RECHT, F., MICHIE, W. and CROOK, J.: Brit. med. J., 1971, 4, 258.

HEGEWALD, G. and HAGEMANN, H.: Z. ges inn. Med., 1966, 21, 471.

HEIDELBERGER, K.P. and LEGoLVAN, D.P.: Cancer (Philad.), 1974, 331, 280.

HEIMANN, R.: Lancet, 1971, ii, 101.

HEIMER, R., LEVIN, F.M. and Ruoo, E.: Amer. J. Med., 1963, 35, 175.

HEINLE, E.W. Jr., SARSASTI, H.O., GARCIA, D., KENNv, J.J. and WAsTERMAN, M.P.: Arch. intern. Med. (Chicago), 1966, 118, 351.

HELLGREN, L.: Acta rheum. Scand., 1969, 15, 311.

HEMPELMANN, L.H.: In Cecil-Loeb "Textbook of Medicine", 1971, 13th. Edit., Edit. by Beeson, P.B. and McDermott, W., Saunders, Philadelphia.

HENCH, P.S.: Ann. Rheum. Dis., 1949, 8, 90.

HENCH:, P.K., MAYNE, J.G., KIELY, J.M. and DocKERTY, M.B.: Arth. Rheum., 1962, 5, 301.

HENDERSON, A.H. and MAFIA, G.: Thorax, 1960, 24, 124.

HERMANS, P.E. and HUizENGA,: Ann. intern. Med., 1972, 76, 605.

HrFT, W., MosHAL, M.G. and PrLLAY, K.: Lancet, 1973, i, 570.

HIJMANS, W., DoNIAcH, D., RorrT, I.M. and HoLBOROW, E.J.: Brit. med. J., 1961, ii, 909.

HrJMANs, W., VALKENBURG, H.D., MuLLER, A.S. and GRATAMA, S.: Ann. Rheum. Dis., 1964, 23, 45.

HILLS, J.R.: In Cecil-Loeb "Textbook of Medicine", 1967, 12th. Edit., Edit. by Beeson, P.B. and McDermott, W., Saunders, Philadelphia.

HILTON, A.M. and WHITAKER, R.S.: Brit. med. J., 1972, 3, 827.

HrNz, C.F.: Ann. int. Med., 1957, 47, 544.

HrRABAYAsHr, R.N. and LINDSAY, S.: Surg. Gynec. Obstet., 1965, 121, 243.

HIRAKI, K. and KIMURA, I.: Clin. All round, 1962, 11, 807.

HIRAKI, K., KrMURA, 1., 0TA, Z., AsANo, K., KAGEYAMA, H., SaiBUYA, K., KoTANI, H., MATSUURA, R., Tsu cHIDA, J., SEZAKI, T., HoRAOKA, T., HIMEI, H., MoRITANI, Y. and YAMANA, M.: J. Oka yama med. Ass., 1963, 75, 297.

HIRAKI, K. and KIMURA, I.: Acta. med. Okayama, 1964, 18, 87.

HITZENBERGER, G.: Folia haemat. (Frankfurt), 1958, 2, 203.

HoBBs, J.R.: Sci. Basis Med. Ann. Rev., 1966, pp.106.

HoBBs, J.R.: Brit. J. Hasp. Med., 1970, 3, 669.

HoFFBRAND, B.I.: Brit. med. J., 1964, i, 1156.

HoFFBRAND, B.I.: Brit. med. J., 1965, i, 1592.

HoFFBRAND, B.I. and BEcK, E.P.: Brit. med. J., 1965, i, 1273.

HoFFMANN, D.C. and BRooKE, B.N.: Dis. Colon Rec., 1970, 13, 119.

HoFFMANN, D., MAsT, H. and FAUSTMANN, T.: Z. Geburtsh. Gynak., 1969, 171, 39.

HOGAN, J. and SIMONS, C.E.: J. Ural., 1957, 78, 212.

HoLBOROW, E.J.: In "Clinical Aspec ts of Immunology", 1963, Edit. by Gell, P.G.H. and Coomb, R.P.A., Blackwell, Oxford.

HoLDSTOCK, D.J. and 0LEESKY, S.: Brit. med. J., 1970, 4, 369.

HoLDSWORTH:, C.D., HALL, E.W., DAwsoN, A.M.

-460-

and SHERLOCK, S.: Quart. J. Med., 1965, 34, 211.

HoLLANDER, J.L.: "Arthritis and Allied Conditions", 1960, 6th. Edit., Kimpton, London.

HoLLANDER, J.L.: "Arthritis and Allied Conditions", 1971, 7th. Edit., Edit. by Hollander, J.L., Kimpton, London.

BoLLARD, D., MoREL, P. and REVOL, L.: Lyon. med., 1966, 215, 1373.

BOLLARD, D., MuLLER, J.M., LEGER, J. and DER!ES, M.B.: Lyon med., 1965, 213, 967.

HoLLY, H.L., HAMMACK, W.J. and DoUGLAS, C.: Amer. J. Med. Sci., 1961, 242, 331.

HoLMAN, H.R.: Arth. Rheum., 1963, 6 (Suppl.), 513.

HoLMES, F.F., STUBBS, D.W. and LARSEN, W.E.: Arch. intern. Med., (Chicago), 1967, 119, 302.

HoLD, J.M., RoBB-SMITH, A.H.T. and CALLENDER, S.T.: Quart. J. Med., 1970, 39, 629.

HoLZMANN, H. and FtuscH, W.: Aerztl. Forsch., 1970, 24, 129.

HoLZMANN, H. and HtRZ, L.; Aerztl. Forsch., 1969, 23, 335.

Hoo, D.G.: Geneesk. Gids., 1954, 32, 528.

HooD, J. and MASON, A.M.S.: Lancet, 1970, i, 445.

Hoon, C., RoELs, H. and DEvos, E.: Lancet. 1969, ii, 1192.

HooK, F.B. and YUNis, J.J.: Amer. J. Dis. Child, 1965, 110, 551.

HoRN, L. and HoRN, H.L.: Lancet, 1971, ii, 466.

HoRNBAKER, J.H., FosTER, E.A., WILLIAMS, G.S. and DAVIS, J.S. IV.: Arch. intern. Me::!., 1966, 118, 449.

HoRwrrz, C., PoLEsKY, H., STILLMAN, T., WARD, P.C.J., HENLE, G. and HENLE, W.: Brit. med. J., 1973, 1, 591.

HosKINS, E.O.L.: Proc. R. Soc. Med., 1967, 60, 729.

HosKI Ns, L.C., WrN AWER, S.J., BRITMAN, S.A., GoTTLIEB, L.S. and ZAMCHECK, N.: Gastroenterology, 1967, 53, 265.

HosTER, H.A. and DRATMAN, M.B.: Cancer Res., 1948, 8, 1.

HouRA, V. and ALLISON, A.C.: Lancet, 1966, i, 848.

HowARD, F.M. Jr., SILVERSTEIN, M.N. and Mu LDER, D.W.: Amer. J. Med. Sci., 1965, 250, 518.

HowARD, J.M., Moss, N.H. and RHOADS, J.E.: Int. Abst. Surg., 1950, 90, 417.

HowELL, A.: Proc. R. Soc. Med., 1972, 65, 881.

Howrrz, J. and ScHWARTz, M.: Lancet, 1971, i, 1331.

HowQUA, J. and MACKAY, I.R.: Blood, 1963, 22, 191.

HRNCiA, Z., MAzAK, J., MATfJA, F., VANASEK, J. and TicHY, M.: Neoplasma (Bratislava), 1970, 17, 197.

Hsu, L.Y.F., SHAPIRO, L.R., GERTNER, M., LtEBER, E. and HIRsCHHORN, K.: J. Pediat., 1971, 79, 12.

HuANG, C.H. and MASUDA, K.: Amer. J. Surg., 1968, 115, 564.

HuRHEs, L.E. and MAcKAY, W.D.: Brit. med. J., 1965, ii, 1346.

HuoHES, G.R.V. and WHALEY, K.: Brit. med. J., 1972, 4, 533.

H uLsE, E.V.: Brit. J. Haemat., 1959, 5, 278.

HuMBLE, J.G., jAYNE, W.H.W. and PuLVERTAET, R.J.V.: Brit. J. Haematol., 1956, 2, 283.

HuME, A. and ADAMS, J.F.: Scot. Med. J., 1968, 13, 372.

HuME, A. and RoBERTs, G.H.: Brit. med. J., 1967, ii, 548.

HuRD, E.R., SNYDER, W.B. and ZIFF, M.: Amer. J. Med., 1970, 48, 273.

HusKISSON, E.C.: Proc. R. Soc. Med., 1970, 63, 30.

HuTT, M.S.R. and TEMPLETON, A.C.: Proc. R. Soc. Med., 1971, 64, 962.

HYMAN, G.A. and SoMMERS, S.C.: Blood, 1966, 28/3, 416-427.

HYU N-HAHK KJM and WILLIA MS, T.J.: Proc. Mayo Clin., 1972, 47, 39.

IBBRTSON, H.K. and FRASER, R.; Proc. R. Soc. Med., 1956, 49, 831.

IBoH, F. and MARICH, N.: Lancet, 1975, ii, 1119.

ILLINGWORTH, M.D.: Lancet, 1963, ii, 947.

ILLINGWORTH, C.F.W. and DtcK, B.M.: "Surgical Pathology", 1956, 7th. Edit., Churchill, London.

ILYAs, M.: Lancet, 1968, i, 248.

IMAHORr, S. and MooRE, G.E.: N.Y. St. J. Med., 1972, 72, 1625.

IMAIZUMI, M. et al.: Jap. J. Thorac. Surg., 1974, 27, 417.

INGRAM, J.T.: Lancet, 1964, i, 121.

INNIS, M.D.: Nature, 1968, 210, 972.

INNIS, M.D.: Lancet, 1963, ii, 947.

IRVINE, W.J.: Proc. R. Soc. Med., 1968, 61, 271.

IRVINE, W.J., CHAN, M.W.W. and ScARTH, L.: Clin. exp. Immunol., 1969, 4, 489.

IRviNE, W.J., CHAN, M.W.W., SCARTH, L., HARToo, M., BAvuss, R.I.S. and DRURY, M.I.: Lancet, 1968, ii, 883.

IRvi NE, W.J., CLARKE, B.F., ScARTH, L., CuLEN, D.R. and DuNcAN, L.J.P.: Lancet, 1970, n, 163.

IssAcs, R.: J. Amer. Med. Ass., 1954, 156, 1491.

IsoMAIO, H. and KREus, K.E.: Ann. Allergy, 1968, 26, 61.

ITO, T., ONoDERA, T., TvRA, Y., et al.: Jap. J. Cancer Clin., 1968, 14, 585.

ITo, S., TAMURA, T. and NISHIKAWA, M.: Metabolism, 1968, 17, 317.

IvE, F.A.: Proc. R. Soc. Med., 1963, 56, 910.

jABLONSKA, S., STAcHoR, A. and DABROSKA, H.: Ann. Derm. Syph., 1967, 94, 121.

JACCOTTET, M.A. and RAMEL, C.r.: Praxis, 1965, 54, 302.

JACOBS, A. and KILPATRICK, G.S.: Brit. med. J., 1964, ii, 79.

JACOX, R.F. et al.: New Engl. J. Med., 1964, 271, 1091.

jAEGER, M. and LAPP, R.: Helve Med. Acta., 1970, 35, 266.

JAGER, B.V. and STAMM, W.P.: Lancet, 1972, ii, 1343.

JAMIESON, A. and ANDERSON, K.: Lancet, 1974, i, 261,

JANLAN, K.N., MAcLEAN, N., PATH, M.C. et al.: Gastro-enterology, 1969, 56, 583.

JANEWAY, C.A.: In Cecii-Leob, "Textbook of Medicine", 1971 13th. Edit., Edit. by Beeson, P.B. and McDermott, W., Saunders, Philadelphia.

JAR.viNEN, K.A.J.: Ann. med. inst. Fenniae, 1950, 30, 1 (suppl. 5).

jAY, B.: Brit. J. Ophthalm., 1965, 49, 359.

jEFFERSON, M., SMITH, W.T., TAYLOR, A.B. and VASTERis, K.: Thorax, 1954, 9, 291.

jENSEN, K.B., GoLTERMANN, N., JARNUM, S., WEEKE, B. and WESTERGAARE₁ H.: Gut, 1970, 11, 223.

jERNSTROM, P. and MURRAY, C.I.: Cancer, 1966, 19, 60.

jERUSALEM, C.: Tropenmed. Parasite!., 1968, 19, 94.

JoHANssoN, H. and HoLINGVEST, B.: Opusc. med. (Stockh.), 1963, 8, 113.

JoHNE, H.O., DANGLER, H. and PRATJE, A.: Arch. Klin. Exp. Derm., 1955, 201, 36.

JoHNSON, M.L.: Proc. R. Soc. Med., 1965, 58, 425.

JoHNSON, F.D., jACOBs, E.M. and Wooo, D.D.: Calif. Med., 1966, 104, 479.

JoHNSON, G.j., SuMMERSKILL, W.H.J., ANDERsoN, V.E. and KEATING, F.R. Jr.: New Engl. J. Med., 1967, 277, 1379.

JoHNSTON, A.W. and PENROSE, L.S.: J. Med. Genet., 1966, 3, 77.

JosEPH, R.R., ToASTELLOTTE, C.D., BARRY, w.E., SMALLEY, R.V. and DuRANT, J.R.: Ann. intern. Med., 1970, 72, 699.

JosEPH, R.R. and ZARAFONETIS, C.J.D.: J. Amer. Geriat. Soc., 1967, 12, 787.

JosEPH, R.R., ZARAFONETIS, C.J.D. and DuRANT, J.R.: Amer. J. Med. Sci., 1966, 251, 417.

JosEPHY, H.: 1930, In Bumke, O. and Foerster, O., Handbuch der Geisteskrankheiten Spez Teil. p. 763, Springer, Berlin.

JosLIN, E.P., LoMMRD, H.I., BuRRows, R.E. and MANMY, M.D.: New Engl. J. Med., 1959, 260, 486.

JossERAuo, A., DARGENT, M. and MAYER, M.: Press Med., 1948, 56, 674.

KAmN, M.E., DoNALDSON, S.S. and DoRFMAN, R.F.: New Eng. J. Med., 1970, 283, 859.

KALINOWSKI, M.: Pol. Arch. Med. Wewnet., 1965, 35, 393.

KALISH, A.J. and MAcGREGOR, G.A.: Lancet, 1970, ii, 330.

KALTREIDER, H.B. and TALAL, N.: Ann. int. Med., 1969, 70, 757.

KANTOR, G.L., BICKEL, Y.B. and BuRNETT, E.V.: Amer. J. Med., 1969, 47, 433.

KAPLAN, H.S.: Cancer Res., 1954, 14, 535.

KAPLAN, H.S.: Brit. J. Cancer, 1971, 25, 620.

KAPLAN, J.: J. Mt. Sinai Hosp., 1935, 2, 64.

KAPLAN, H.S. and RIGLER, L.G.: Amer. J. med. Sci., 1945, 209, 339.

KAPLAN, L., KATZ, A.D., BEN IssAc, C. and MAsSRY, S.G.: Cancer (Philad.), 1971, 28, 401.

KAPLAN, M.H.: In "Textbook of Immunopathology", 1969, Edit. by Miescher, P.A. and Miiller-Eberhard, H.J., Grune and Stratton, New York.

KAPPELER, R., KREBS, A. and RrvA, G.: Helv. med. Acta., 1968, 25, 54.

KARLisH, A.J.: Proc. R. Soc. Med., 1969, 62, 1942.

KARTEN, I. and HARTFIELD, H.: J. Amer. med. Ass., 1962, 179, 162.

KAsooN, S.C.: Amer. J. Obst. Gynec., 1949, 67, 282.

KAsE, N.: In Cecil-Loeb "Textbook of Medicine", 1971, 13th. Edit.; Edit. by Beeson, P.B. and McDermott, W., Saunders, Philadelphia.

KATARIA, M.S. and RAo, D.B.: Brit. med. J., 1964, i, 1384.

KATZ, A. and DIGBY, J.W.: Canad. med. Ass. J., 1965, 93, 1367.

KAuFMAN, R.L., VIETTL, T.J. and WABNER, C.I.: Birth Defects orig. art. ser., 1974, 10, 191.

KAwAoA, A., TAKADA, Y., NrsHrwAKI, M., MoRJ, S., NovE, S. and TABAIWA, A.: Dermatologica, 1969, 138, 19.

KAY, M.M.B. and KADIN, M.: Lancet, 1975, 1,

750.

KAYE, J., DuRBAcH, D. and NOTMAN, J.: Med. Proc. (Johannesb.), 1971, 17, 284.

KEELEY, J.L., ScHAIRER, A.E. and KEELEY, R.E.: Surgery, 1963, 54, 526.

KEELING, J.H. and OcHsNER, A.: Cancer N.Y., 1959, 12, 596.

KErL, E.: Krebsarzt., 1965, 20, 269.

KEIL, H.: Arch. int. Med., 1940, 66, 169.

KELLETT, H.S. and SuTHERLAND, T.W.: J. Path. Bact., 1949, 61, 235.

KELLNER, R., OTTO, S., PuMP, K. and KovEcs, G.L.: Haematologia. (Budap.), 1968, 2, 371.

KEMP, T.: Lancet, 1961, ii, 488.

KENNEDY, C.B., QuiNN, S.E., HENNINGTON, V.W. and PERRETT, W.J.: South med. J., 1963, 56, 700.

KENNEDY, W.R. and JrMrnEz-PABON, E.: Neurology (Minneap.), 1968, 18, 757.

KENT, T.H.: Arch. Path. Lab. Med., 1964, 78, 97.

KENYON, R. and AcKERMAN;L.V.: Cancer, 1955, 8, 964.

KESSLER, I.I.: J. Nat. Cancer Inst., 1970, 40, 673.

KEssr.ER,I.I.: J. chron. Dis., 1971, 23, 579.

KHORSAND,D.: J. Ural., 1965, 93, 445.

KrBEL, M.A.: Brit. med. J., 1965, i, 1674.

KIERLAND, R.R.: Proc. Mayo Clin., 1964, 39, 53.

KrLBY, P.E.: Cancer, 1965, 18, 947.

KILTON, L. and GoTTLIEB, J.A.: Lancet, 1971, ii, 707.

KIMURA, 1., MoRITANI, Y., TsucHmA, J. and MATSUURA, K.: Jap. J. Allerg., 1962, 11,88.

KINSELLA, T.D., MAcDoNALD, F.R. and joHNSON, L.G.: Canad. med. Ass. J., 1966, 95, 1.

KINTNER, E.P.: J. Indiana med. Ass., 1951, 44, 304.

KrssEL, P., DuREux, J.B., RAUBER, G., BEUREY, J., PETERS, A. and ANTHOINE, D.: Nouv. Rev. d'Hematol., 1961, 1, 625.

KJELDSEN, K., CLANSEN, J. and FROLAND, A.: Acta. med. Scand., 1969, 186, 209.

KLAYMAN, M.I. and BRANDBERG, L.: New Eng. J. Med., 1955, 253, 808.

KLEIN, G.: Brit. med. J., 1970, 4, 418.

KLEIN, M.B. et a!.: Arch. Dermatol., 1974, 110, 602.

KLEIN, J.J., GoTTLIEB, A.J., MaNEs, R.J., APPEL, S.H. and OssERMAN, K.L.: Arch. intern. Med., 1964, 113, 142.

KLIJN, L.C.: Folia med. Neerl., 1961, 4, 65.

KLINGENM, G.H.: Cancer (Philad.), 1965, 18, 157.

KuNcMULLER, G. and VoELAENDER, K.O.: Munch. med. Wschr., 1965, 107, 467.

KLIPPEL, J.H., DECKER, J.L., GRIMLEY, P.M.,

EvANS, A.S. and RoTHFIELD, N.: Lancet, 1973, ii, 1057.

KNIGHT, P.O.: Southern med. J., 1967, 60, 119.

KNoTH, W.: Hautarzt, 1954, 5, 289.

KNox, J.M., LAMB, J.M., SHELMIRE, B. and MoRGAN, R.J.: J. invest. Dermatol., 1954, 22, 11.

KoBAYASHI, N., FuRUKAWA, T. and TAKATSU, T.: Paediat. Univ. Tokyo., 1968, 16, 31.

KocHER, A.: In Kraus und Brugsch's "Spezielle Pathologie und Therapie der inner Krankheiten", Vol. 1, Urban and Schwarzenberg, Berlin and Vienna, 1919-27.

Kororo, C.A., BoYERs, L.M. and SwEZY, O.: Univ. Calif. Pub!. Zoo!., 1924, 26, 165.

KoFOm, C.A. and SwEzY, O.: Univ. Calif. Pub!. Zool., 1922, 20, 301.

Korom, C.A. and SwEzY, O.: Univ. Calif. Pub!. Zoo!., 1922, 20, 309.

KoFOKO, G.W., BAMGANA, N., KNIGHT, E.M. and TIBEMANYA, J.: E. Afric. Med. J. 1969, 46, 414.

KamE, O. and KocuRE, T.: Acta. Path. Jap., 1959, 9 (Suppl.), 1005.

KOLB, L.E., LANGWORTHY, O.R. and CARKTOVA, M.: Amer. J. Hyg., 1942, 35, I.

KoMORN, R.M., FEcHNER, R.E., ALFORD, B.R. et al.: Arch. Otol. laryng., 1973, 97, 420.

KoRNREICH, W., MALOUF, N.N. and HANSON, V.: J. Pediat., 1971, 79, 27.

KoROTNEFF, ; Sporozoen als Krankheiten, 1893, Berlin.

KRArN, L.S.: Brit. J. Dermatol., 1974, 90,397.

KRAtN,L.S. and BIERMAN, S.M.: Cancer, 1974, 33, 1091.

KRAuss, S. and SaKAL, J.E.: Amer. J. Med., 1966, 40, 400.

KRUEGER, F.J. and MEYER, O.O.: J. Lab. din. Med., 1936, 21, 682.

KucERA, J.: J. ment. Defic. Res., 1971, 15, 77.

Kuoo, R.R.: "Protozoology", 1954, 4th. Edit., C.C. Thomas, Springfield.

KuiTUNEN, P., MAENPAA, J., KROHN, K. and VtsAKORPr, J.K.: Scand. J. Gastroent., 1971, 6, 335.

KUMAR, P.J.: Proc. R. Soc. Med., 1973, 66, 428.

KuMAR, P., LANcASTER-SMITH, M., CLARK, M.L. and DAwsoN, A.M.: Case shown at Clinical Meeting of the Royal Society of Medicine, London, March 12th., 1973.

KuMAR, S. and BHARGAVA, M.: Acta. Haematologica. (Basel), 1970, 43, 21.

KuNIN, A.S., MAcKAY, B.R., BURNS, S.L. and HALBERSTAN, M.J.: Amer. J. Med., 1963, 34, 856.

KuTSCHERA, H. and FALDINI, A.: Zbl. Allg. path. Path. Anat., 1965, 107, 288.

KwAsNICKA, A.: Neoplasma, 1965, 12, 1.

KYLE, R.A.: Mayo Ctin. Proc., 1975, 50, 29.

LANCASTER-SMITH, M.J. and STRICKLAND, I.D.: Lancet, 1970, 2, 1091.

LANCASTER-SMITH, M.J. and STRICKLAND, I.D.: Lancet, 1971, i, 1294.

LANDING, B.R., PETTIT, M.D., WIENS, R.L., KNoWLEs, H. and GuEsT, G.M.: J. Clin. Endocrin., 1963, 23, 119.

LANGENBECI(, B.: Dtsch. Klin., 1862, 14, 1.

LANGSTON, J.D., WAGMAN, G.F. and DICKEN-MAN, R.C.: Arch. Path., 1959, 68, 367.

LANSBURY, J.: Ann. Rheum., 1953, 12, 3Bl.

LARRAURI, J., NrsTAL, M., CAPDEVILA, A. and Rios, M.J.: Med. Exp., 1973, 69, 454.

LARRAURI, J., PATRON, M., LoPEZ, R.F. et al.: Patologia, 1974, 7, 55.

LARssoN, O.: Acta. med. Scand., 1962, 172, 195.

LARSSON, O.: Lancet, 1963, ii, 665.

LARSSON, S.O., HAGELQUIST, E. and COOTER, C.: Acta. Haemat., 1961, 26, 50.

LATTES, R.: Cancer, 1962, 15, 1224.

LAUCHLAN, S.C. and WALSH, M.J.: Canad. med. Ass. J., 1963, 88, 891.

LAWRENCE, J.S. and DoNALD, W.G. Jr.: Ann. int. Med., 1958, 49, 43.

LAYANI, F., AscHKANASY, A. and SEBAOUH, J.: Bull. Soc. Mem. H p. Paris, 1952, 6B, 987.

LAZLO, J. and GROVE, H.E.: Cancer, 1967, 20, 545.

LEA, A.J.: Ann. Rheum. Dis., 1964, 23, 480.

LEBLAY, R., LAUNOis, B., GuERIN, D. et a!.: Presse. Med., 1969, 22, 1150.

LE CoMPTE, P.M.: Arch. Path., 1958, 66, 450.

LEE, A.K.Y., RowLEY, M. and MACKAY, I.R.: Brit. J. Cancer, 1970, 24, 454.

LEE, F.I. and BRAJN, A.T.: Lancet, 1962, ii, 693.

LEE, F.I., jENKINS, G.C., HuGHES, D.T.D. and KAZANTZIR, G.: Brit. med. J., 1964, i, 59B.

LEE, R.A. WELcH, J.S. and DocK.ERTY, M.B.: Amer. J. Obstet., 1963, 86, 957.

LEE, S.L.: J. Mt. Sinai Hosp. N.Y., 1955, 22, 74.

LEFKOVITS, A.M. and FARROW, I.J.: J. Ann. Rheum. Dis., 1955, 14, 162.

LEGRE, J., PIToT, G. and SERRATRICE, G.: Rev. Oroneurophthal., 1959, 31, 423.

LEMENAGER, J., TANGREY, A., BENARD, Y. et al.: Rev. Tuberc. (Paris), 1972, 36, 966.

LENo-Ltvv, J., LENG, B., MAoENDIE, P., LACUT, J. and BARGUES, J.F.: Bull. Soc. fran. Derm. Syph., 1967, 74, 105.

LEICHTY, R.D., HoDcEs, R.E. and BuRKETT, J.: J. Amer. med. Ass., 1963, 183, 30.

LENORMAND, Y., STERIN, D., BARGE, J. and BoMN, P.: Scm. Hop. Paris, 1972, 48, 387.

LEoNARDT, T.: Acta. med. Scand., 1964, 176 (Suppl. 412), 1.

LEoPOLD, J.G. and Moco, R.A.: Proc. R. Soc. Med., 1964, 57, 933.

LEPPARD, B.: Proc. R. Soc. Med., 1971, 64, 391.

LERMAN,].: In "Endocrinology of Neoplastic Diseases", 1947, Edit. by Twombley, G.H. and Pack, G.T., .N.Y., Oxford Univ. Press.

LERNER, A.B.: In Cecil-Loeb "Textbook of Medicine", 1967, 12th. Edit., Edit. by Beeson, P.B. and McDermott, W., Saunders, Philadelphia.

LEssoF, M.H. and GLYNN, L.E.: Lancet, 1959, i, 799.

LEVENE, A.: Proc. R. Soc. Med., 1972, 65, 137.

LEVENE, S.A. and LADD, W.S.: Bull. Johns Hosp., 1921, 32, 254.

LEVINE, S. and SHEARN, M.A.: Arch. intern. Med., 1964, 113, 826.

LEvo, Y., Korr, E. and ATSMON, A.: Eur. Neurol. (Basel), 1975, 13, 245.

LEVY, R.L., SHUH-WEN HUANG, BACH, N., BAcH, F.H., HoNG, R., AMMAN, A.J., BeRTIN, M. and KAY, H.E.M.: Lancet, 1971, ii, 898.

LEWIS, E.C. and BRowN, H.E.: Arch. intern. Med., 1957, 100, 296.

LEWIS, S.M. and s uR, L.: Brit. med. J., 1963, i, 472.

LHERMITTE, F., GAUTIER, J.C. and EscouRELLE, R. et al.: Presse Med., 1970, 78, 257.

LIGHTwooo, R. and BRIMBLECOMBE, F.S.W.: "Sick Children", 8th. Edit., 1963, Cassell, London.

LrMPER, M.A.: Kentucky Med. J., 1939, 37, 97.

LrNDER, D.: Proc. Nat. Acad. Slusa., 1969, 63, 699.

LINDSAY, S. and DAILEY, M.E.: J. din. Endocrinol., 1955, 15, 1332.

LINDSTROM, F.D., WILLIAMS, R.D. Jr. and BRUN-NING, R.D.: Arch. int. Med. (Chicago), 1968, 112, 526.

LINKE, A.: Schwartz. med. Wschr., 1965, 95, 1492.

LrNQUETTE, M., DuPONT, A., GAsNAULT, J.P. and MoN'Tms, R.: Lille Med., 1967, 12, 1346.

LIPSMEYER, E.A.: Arch. Rheum., 1972, 15, 183.

LITTLE, T.M.: Lancet, 1972, ii, 400.

LITWIN, S.D., ALLEN, J.C. and KuNKEL, H.D.G.: Arth. Rheum., 1966, 9, 865.

LIVINGSTONE, J.L., LEwis, J.G., REm, L. and }EFFERSON, K.E.: Quart. J. Med., 1964, 33, 71.

LLOYD, O.C.: J. Path. Bact., 1946, 58, 699.

LLOYD, O.C. and URICH, H.: Lancet, 1959, ii, 529.

LoHMANN, D. and GLA.sER, A.: Z. ges. int. Med., 1965, 20, 104.

LOHRMANN, H.P., SCHNEIDER, G., MERTEN, K. and TENBAUM, A.: Blut, 1972, 24, 356.

LoNGCOPE, W.T.: J. Amer. med. Ass., 1928, 90, 1.

LoRBER, J.: Brit. J. Hosp. Med., 1972, 8, 37.

LouGHBRIDGE, L. and LEWIS, M.G. : Lancet, 1971, i, 256.

LouYOT, P., PouREL, J. and BAUMGARTNER, J.C.: Ann. Med. Nancy, 1971, 10, 121.

LowE, C.R.: Brit. med. J., 1972, 3, 515.

LowENTHAL, M.N. and HuTT, M.S.R.: E. African Med. J., 1968, 45, 100.

LowRY, W.S., CLARK, D.A. and HANNEMANN, J.H.: Lancet, 1972, i, 1290.

Lu ccHELU, P.D. and BERETTA, G.M.: Rheumatisma, 1962, 12, 351.

LuccHELLI, P.D. and NATANGELO, R.: Osped. Maggiore, 1964, 59, 731.

LucKEY, E.H.: In Cecil-Loeb "Textbook of Medicine", 1967, 12th. Edit., Edit. by Beeson, P.B. and McDermott, W., Saunders, Philadelphia.

LUMERMAN, H., FREEDMAN, P. and CARACCIOLo, P.: Oral. Surg., 1975, 39, 953.

LuNDMARK, K.M., THILtN, A. and VAHLQUIST, B.: Acta. Paediat. Scand. (Uppsala), 1967, Suppl. 172, 200.

LU POVITCH, A., KALASSE, R.Y., RANDALL, H.P. and BELLAMY, M.D.: J. Amer. med. Ass., 1965, 192, 285.

LuXTON, R.W.: Proc. R. Soc. Med., 1957, 50, 943.

LuxTON, R.W. and CooKE, R.T.: Lancet, 1956, ii, 205.

LYELL, A.: Brit. J. Dermatol., 1969, 87, 228.

LYNCH, H.T.: Med. Clin. N. Amer., 1969, 53, 923.

LYNCH, H.T. et al.: Surg. Gynecol. Obstet., 1974, 138, 717.

LYNCH, H.T. and KRUSH, A.J.: Cancer, 1971, 27, 1505.

LYNCH, H.T., KRuSH, A.J. and LARsEN, A.L.: Amer. J. med. Sci., 1967, 254, 322.

LYNCH, P.G.: Brit. med.]., 1974, iii, 577.

LYNCH, W.J. and JosKE, R.A.: J. din. Path., 1966, 19, 461.

MABERY, J.D. and STONE, O.J.: Arch. Dermato!., 1967, 95, 210.

McALLISTER, R.M., GILDEN, R.V. and GREEN, M.: Lancet, 1972, i, 831.

McCoMAS, A.]., UPTON, A.R.M. and SrccA, R.E.P.: Lancet, 1973, ii, 1477.

McCoMBS, R.P.: J. Amer. med. Ass., 1965, 194, 1059.

McCUDRY, D.K., CoRNWELL, G.C. and De PRATTI, V.J.: Ann. int. Med., 1967, 67, 110.

M cDONALo, G.F. and HILL, R.W.: 1967, Presented 10th. April at the 48th. Annual Session of the American College of Physicians, San Francisco.

McDoNALD, H.G. and MooRE, M.M.: J. Amer. med. Ass., 1965, 193, 199.

McDouGALL, I.R., GREIG, W.R., GRAY, H.W. and SMITH,].F.B.: Brit. med. J. 1971, 4, 275.

McEACHERN, D. and PARNELL, J.L.: J. Clin. Endocrin., 1948, 8, 822.

McFARLAN, H. and NwoKOLO, C.: J. Clin. Path., 1966, 19, 603.

McGAw, B. and McGOVERN, V.J.: Orst. J. Derm., 1956, 3, 115.

McGILL, P.E.: Brit. med. J., 1971, 2, 679.

MAcGREGOR, G.A.: Lancet, 1972, ii, 931.

McHARDY-YouNG, S., DoNIACH, D. and PoLANI, P.E.: Lancet, 1970, ii, 1161.

MACKAY, I.R. and BuRNET, F.M.: "Auto-immune Diseases", 1963, C.C. Thomas, Springfield, Illinois.

MACKAY, I.R., MASEL, M. and BARNET, F.M.: Aust. Ann. Med., 1964, 13, 5.

MACKAY, I.R., TAFT, L.I. and CowLING, D.C.: Lancet, 1956, ii, 1323.

MACKAY, I.R. and RITCHIE, B.: Thorax, 1965, 20, 200.

MACKAY, I.R. and WooD, I.J.: Quart. J. Med., 1962, 31, 485.

MACKENZIE, A.H. and ScHERBEL, A.L.: Geriatrics, 1963, 18, 745.

MACKINTOSH, T.F., GIRDWOOD, T.G., PARKER, D.J. and STRACHAN, I.N. : Brit. J. Ophthal., 1968, 52, 846.

McLARTY, D.G., BRowNLIE, B.E.W., ALEXANOER, W.D., PAPAPETROU, P.D. and HORTON, P.: Brit. med. J., 1973, 2, 332.

MAcLAURIM, B.P.: Lancet, 1971, i, 1670.

M cNrcoL, G.P.: Amer. J. med. Sci., 1961, 241, 336.

M cNuTT, D.R. and FuDENBERG, H.H.: Arch. intern. Med., 1973, 13f, 731.

MACSWEEN, R.N.M., GOUDIE, R.B., ANDERSON, J.R., ARMsTRONG, E., MuRRAY, M.A., MASON, D.K.,] AsANI, M.K., BovLE, J.A. BucHANAN, W.W. and WILLIAMSO N, J.: Ann. Rheum. Dis., 1967, 26, 402.

MAcsWEEN, R.N.M.: Lancet, 1965, i, 460.

MAGANT de DEUCHAISN.ES: Schweiz. med. Wschr., 1960, 90, 889.

MAGGIONI, G. and GrANNONE, R.: Osped. Maggiore, 1969, 64, 902.

MAHAUX, J., PAEPE, J. de. and NAETA, J.P.: Lancet, 1961, ii, 551.

MAILLoux, M. : Presse Med., 1959, 67, 906.

MAINZER, K., ScHMAHI., F.W. and HILL, K.: Med. Welt. (Stultz.), 1968, 19, 1259.

MAJOR, R.H. and LEGER, L.H.: J. Amer. med.

Ass., 1939, 112, 260.

MALDONADO. J.E., BAYRD, E.D. and KIELY, I.M.: Proc. Mayo Clin., 1964, 39, 60.

M...LINS, J.: "Clinical Diabetes Mellitus", 1968, Eyre and Spottiswoode, London.

MALLINSON, W.J.W.: Proc. R. Soc. Med., 1971, 64, 1305.

MANNY, N., RosENMAN, E. and BENBASSET, J.: Brit. med. J. 1972, 2, 291.

MANSSON, T.: Acta Derm. Venerol. (Stockh.), 1971, 51, 397.

MANTOVANI, M. and METRI, G.: Chir. Turac., 1973, 26, 44.

MARANO, R., DAMMACO, F., PASTORE. G. and ScHIRALDI, O.: Digestion (Basel), 1970, 3, 294.

MARCHAL, G. and DuHAMEL, G.: Sem. Hop. Paris, 1965, 41, 129.

MARCHAL, G., MAaouoEA U, D., DuHAMEL, G. and DAUM, S.: Presse Med., 1954, 62, 662.

MARKSON, J.L. and MooRE, J.M.: Brit. med. J., 1962, i, 1352.

MARSDEN, P.D.: In Cecil-Loeb "Textbook of Medicine", 1971, 13th. Edit., Edit. by Beeson, P.B. an:i McDermott, W., Saunders, Philadelphia.

MARSDEN, P.D. and HAMILTON, P.J.S.: Brit. med. J., !969, i, 99.

MARSHALL, A.H.E.: "Cytology and Pathology of the Reticular Tissue". 1956, Oliver and Boyd, Edinburgh.

MARsHALL, A.H.E.: Proc. R. Soc. Med., 1964, 57, 151.

MARSHALL, A.H.E. and WHITE, R.G.: Lancet, 1962, ii, 120.

MARTINAzzr, M., CARNAVALL, L. and BuccHETTA, A.: Arch. de Vecchi Anat. Path., 1968, 51, 279.

MARTIROSYAN, V.V., KoLDYNSKAYA, L.A. and ZAPRUDSKAYA, D.S.: Vop. Neirokhir, 1970, 5, 45.

MAsoN, A.M.S. and GoLDING, P.L.: Lancet, 1970(a), ii, 1104.

MAsoN, A.M.S. and GoLDING, P.L.: Brit. med. J., 1970 (b), 3, 143.

MASON, A.S.: Proc. R. Soc. Med., 1956, 49, 831.

MATHEws, H.M., FisHER, G.V. and KAGAN, I.G.: Amer. J. Trap. Med. Hyg, 1970, 19, 581.

MATHEWS, J.D., WHITTINGHAM, S. and MAcKAY, I.R.: Lancet, 1974, ii, 1423.

MATZNEZ, M.J., TRACHTMAN, B. and MANDELBAUM, R.A.: Amer. J. Gastroent., 1963, 39, 31.

MAWHINNEY, H. and TOMKIN, G.H.: Lancet, 1971, ii, 121.

MAXWELL, J.H.: Trans. Amer. Acad. Ophthal.

Otolaryng., 1960, 60, 225.

MAY and BAKER: Booklet, 1950, Dagenham, England, "Cuprimyl".

MAYcocK, R.L., BERTRAND, P., MoRRISON, C.E. and Scorr, J.H.: Amer. J. med. Sci., 1963, 35, 67.

MAzAR, S.A. and STRAUS, B.: A.M.A. Arch. int. Med., 1951, 88, 819.

MAZZAFERRI, E.L. and PENN, G.M.: Arch. int. Med. (Chicago), 1968, 122, 521.

MEADows, A.T., LICHTENFELD, J.L. and KooP, C.E.: New Engl. J. Med., 1974, 291, 23.

MEIJERS, K.A.E.: Folia med. Neerl., 1969, 12, 194.

Mu.TZER, M. and FRANKLIN, E.C.: Amer. J. Med., 1966, 40, 828 and 837.

MENDELOW, H. and JENKINS, G.: J. Mt. Sinai Hosp., 1954, 21, 48.

MERRICK, D.K., CARR, D.T., PAYNE, W.S. and WooLNER, L.B.: Geriatrics, 1972, 27, 71.

MERRITT, H.H.: "Textbook of Neurology", 1955, Kimpton, London.

METCALF, D.: Brit. J. Cancer, 1965, 15, 769.

METCAI.F, D.: Med. J. Australia, 1971, 2, 739.

METCALFE, W.J. and ScLARE, G.: Brit. J. Surg., 1961, 48, 541.

MEsCON, H. and Cr.ARK, W.H. Jr.: New Eng. J. Med., 1964, 271, 733.

METTERs, J.S.: Proc. R. Soc. Med., 1968, 61, 679.

MEYER, E.C. and LIEBow, A.A.: Cancer, 1965, 18, 322.

MEYER, zum BiiscHE NFEI.DE, BEILREND, H. and BREMER, A.J.: Deutsches Arch. Klin. Med., 1965, 211, 243.

MEYER, J. SMIELOWSKI, B. and WERNER, B.: Genek. Pol., 1970, 41, 917.

MEYERSON, L.B.: Arch. Derm., 1967, 95, 501.

MicHALANY, J.: Int. J. Leprosy, 1966, 34, 274.

MzcHEL, P.J., CRETIN, J. and MoNNET, R.: Bull. Soc. fran,.. Derm. Syph., 1970, 77, 280.

MICHETTE, L. an:i VAUSL!PPE, J.: Acta. Rheum. Scand., 1959, 5, 148.

MICHI.MOYER, G., GUNTHER, R., LEDERER, B. and HuBER, H.: Med. Klin., 1973, 68, 180.

Micoi.ONGHI, T. and MEISSNER, G.F.: Ann. Surg., 1958, 147, 124.

MH:zocH, F.: Ost. arztztg., 1969, 24, 843.

MIECZYNSKA WoJ CK, Z.: Przegl Derm., 1972, 59, 63.

MIGUERES, J., Ducos, J., JovER, A. and TREMOULET, M.: J. Med. Montpelier, 1968, 3, 59.

MIKAL, S.: Surgery, 1964, 55, 233.

MIKHAI.ICHENKO, V.A., BRUK, B.B., RAVENSKAYA, N.M. and TAMARKIN, M.A.: Vopr. Onkol., 1974, 20, 57.

MILLEN, P.J.: Case shown at meeting of the

Royal Society of Medicine (Pediatrics Section), London, 1971, Oct. 22nd.

MILLER, D.G.: Ann. int. Med., 1967, 66, 507.

MILLER. G.A.K., THoMAs, M.L. and MEnD, W.E.: Brit. med. J., 1962, i, 771.

MILLER, H.G., FosTER, J.B., NEwELL, D.J., BARwicK, D.D. and BREWIS, R.A.L.: Brit. med. J., 1963, i, 1436.

MILLER, M. and CHonos, R.B.: Arch. int. Med., 1966, 117, 432.

MILLER, O.J., BERG, W.R., ScHrcKEL, R.D. and TRETTER, W.: Lancet, 1961, ii, 78.

MILLER, P.J.: R. Soc. Med. (Paediatrics Section), October 22nd., 1971.

MrLLER, R.W.: L.A.R.C. Sci. Publ., 1973, 4, 175.

MILLER, R.W., FRAUMENI, J.F. Jr. and MANNING, M.D.: New Eng. J. Med., 1964, 270, 922.

MILLER, T.N.: Proc. R. Soc. Med., 1971, 64, 807.

MILLS, J.A.: J. Chron. Dis., 1963, 16, 797.

MITcHELL, A.B.S.: Brit. J. Hasp. Med., 1973, 9, 605.

MoERTEL, C.G., ANDERSON, H.A. and BAGGEN-STOSS, A.H.: Dis. Chest, 1959, 35, 343.

MoERTEL, e.G., DocKERTY, M.B. and BAGGEN-sross, A.H.: Cancer, 1961, 14, 221.

MOERTEL, e.G. and HAGEDORN, A.B.: Blood, 1957, 12, 788.

MoESMANN, G.: Acta. Rheum. Scand., 1969, 15, 193.

MoLONEY, W.C., GoooMAN, M. and BLocK, K.J.: New Eng. J. Med., 1970, 283, 1332.

MoNOD, J.: "Chance and Necessity". 1972, Collins, London.

MoNTGOMERY, R.D., STIRLING, G.A. and HARMER, N.A.J.: Lancet, 1964, .i, 586.

MoNTI, M.: Schweiz med. Wschr., 1973, 103, 1023.

MooRE, D. and SARKAR, N.: Nature, 1972, 236, 103.

MoRE, J.R.S., DAwsoN, D.W., RALsToN, A.J. and CRAIG, I.: J. din. Path., 1968, 21, 661.

MoRGAN, L.O.: Proc. Ass. Res. Nerv. Ment. Dis., 1940, 20, 753.

MoRGAN, M.Y.: Proc. R. Soc. Med., 1973, 66, 1112.

MoRGAN, W.S. and CAsTLEMAN, B.: Amer. J. Path., 1953, 29, 471.

MoRI, W.: Cancer (Philad.), 1967, 20, 627.

MoRTEO, O.G., FRANKUN, E.S., McEwEN, C., PHYTHYON, J. and TANNER, M.: Arth. Rheum., 1961, 4, 356.

MoRRIS, J.N.: "Uses of Epidemiology", 2nd. Edit.. 1964, Williams, E. and Wilkins, C.O., Baltimore.

MoRRis, P.J.: Gut, 1965, 6, 176.

MoRsE, W.I., CocHRANE, W.A. and LANDRIGAN, P.L.: New Eng. J. Med., 1961, 264, 1021.

MoRsON, B.C.: Proc. R. Soc. Med., 1971, 64, 959.

MosBECH, J.: "Heredity 1953, in "Pernicious Anaemia", Copenhagen, Einar, Munksgaard.

MosBECH, J.: Folia Haemat. (Leipzig), 1959, 76, 487.

MOTALSKY, A.G., WEINBERG, S., SAPHIR, O. and RosENBERG, E.: Arch. int. Med., 1952, 90, 660.

De MowBRAY, R.R.: Proc. R. Soc. Med., 1965, 58, 578.

MoxoN, W.: Guy's Hasp. Rep. 3rd. Series, 1875, 20, 437.

MucciA, F.M. and ULTMANN, J.E.: Lancet, 1971, i, 805.

MULLER, S.A. and WINKELMANN, R.K.: J. Amer. Med. Ass., 1963, 18, 206.

M u NICHOODAPPA, C. and KozAC, G.P.: Diabetes, 1970, 19, 719.

MuRPHv, J.B. et al.: J. Exp. Med., 1921, Vol. 33.

MuRRAY-LYoN, I.M., THoMPSON, R.P.H., ANSELL, I.D. and WILLIAMs, R.: Brit. med. J., 1970, 3, 258.

MusTAKALLIO, K.K., LAssus, A. and WAGER, O.: Int. Arch. Allergy, 1967, 31, 417.

MYERSON, L.B.: Arch. Dermatol., 1967, 95, 501.

MYKING, A.O.: Nord. Med., 1971, 85, 645.

NAGINGTON, J., WATSON, P.G., PLAYFArR, T.S., McGILL, J., JoNEs, B.R. and STEELE, A.D. Mcc.: Lancet, 1974, 2, 1537.

NAKAHARA, W.I. and FuKUOKA, F.: Gann., 1949, 40, 455.

NAKAHARA, W.I. and FUKUOKA, F.: Gann., 1950, 41, 47.

NAPIORSKOWSKA, W.: Pol. Tyg. Lek., 1966, 21, 1780.

NAVARRETE, v.N., ROJAS, C.E., ALGER, C.R. and PANIAGUA, H.E.: Lancet, 1970, ii, 993.

NERUP, J., BENDIKEN, G. and BINDER, C.: Lancet, 1970, ii, 610.

Nuo, R.P.D., STEINBERG, A., KRoN, S.D. and RAcHMAN, R.: Postgrad. Med., 1968, 44, 161.

NIELSON, N. and LANSBURY, J.: Amer. J. Med. Sci., 1961, 241, 700.

NILSEN, L.B., MisSAL, M.E. and CoNnEMI, J.J.: Cancer (Philad.), 1967, 20, i930.

NrxoN, D.W.: South Med. J. (Birmingham, Alabama), 1972, 65, 305.

NoBL,: In "Handbuch de Haut- und Geschlechtskrankheiten", 1933, Band 4, Teil 2, J. Springer, Berlin.

NoRGAARD, O.: Brit. J. Cancer, 1971, 25, 417.

NovAK, F.J., III.: Arch. Otolaryngol., 1947, 45, 477.

NovER, A. and GLEEs, M.: Klin. Wschr., 1966, 44, 462.

Novis, B.H., BANK, S., MARKS, I.N., SELZER, G., KALIN, L. and SEALY, R.: Quart. J. Med., 1971, 40, 521.

NuGENT, F.W., ZUI!ERI, S., BuLAN, M.B. and LEGG, M.A.: Lahey J. Clin, Found. Bull., 1972, 21, 104.

NYMAN, C.P.: Proc. R. Soc. Med., 1972, 65, 688.

OAKLEY, W.G., PIKE, D.A. and TAYLOR, K.W.: "Clinical Diabetes and its Biochemical Basis", 1968, Oxford and Edinburgh Blackwell Scientific, Oxford.

OBERLING and GuERIN,: Quoted by Ewing, J. "Neoplastic Diseases", 1940, 4th. Edit., Saunders, Philadelphia.

OnEJJERG, B.: Acta. Med. Scand., 1965, 177, 129.

OETTLE, A.G.: Int. Path. (Wash.), 1967, 8, 23 and 8, 55.

OGRYZLO, M.A.: Canad. med. Ass. J., 1956, 75, 980.

OKA, M.: Acta. rheum. Scand., 1969, 51, 29.

OLEINICr<, A.: Blood, 1967, 29, 144.

OLEN, E. and KLINCK, G.H.: Arch. Path., 1966, 81, 531.

OLMER, J., GABRIEL, B. and GEVANDAN, M.T.: Marseille Med., 1970, 107, 957.

O'NEILL, P.B.: Amer. J. Dig. Dis., 1961, 6, 1069.

ORCHARD, W.: Lancet, 1961, ii, 312.

ORLOFF, M.J.: Int. Abstr. Surg., 1956, 103, 521.

ORMEROD, W.L.: In Cecil-Loeb "Textbook of Medicine", 1967, 12th. Edit., Edit. by Beeson, P.B. and McDermott, W., Saunders, Philadelphia.

OsSERMAN, E.F.: Parasitology, 1958, 71, 157.

OsSERMAN, E.F.: New Engl. J. Med., 1959, 261, 952.

OsSERMAN, E.F.: In Cecil-Loeb "Textbook of Medicine", 1967, 12th. Edit., Edit by Beeson, P.B. and McDermott, W., Saunders, Philadelphia.

OsSERMAN, E.F.: In Cecil-Leob "Textbook of Medicine", 1971, 13th. Edit., Edit. by Beeson, P.B. and McDermott, W., Saunders, Philadelphia.

OsTERBERG, G. and RAusrNG, A.: Acta. med. scand., 1970, 188, 497.

OwEN, D.S. Jr., WALLER, M. and TooNE, E.: Arth. Rheum., 1967, 10, 302.

OwEN, J.A., PITNEY, W.R. and O'DEA, J.F.: J. clin. Path., 1959, 12, 344.

PAnOVAN, Q.: Riv. Pat. din. Spcr., 1962, 3, 105.

PAGE, F.: Lancet, 1951, ii, 755.

PAGE, F.C.: J. Protozoal., 1967 (a), 14,499.

PAGE, F.C.: J. Protozoal., 1967 (b), 14, 709.

PAGE, A.G., HANSEN, A.E. and Goon, R.A.: Blood, 1963, 21, 197.

PAICE, E.: Clinical Meeting, Royal Society of Medicine, Feb. 14th. 1975.

PALMER, H.M.: Brit. J. Derm., 1974, 91, 476.

PANIZO, A., joRDA, J., FIDALGO, B. and HERMANDEZ, F.: Med. Clin. (Barcelona), 1974, 63, 377.

PAPATESTAS, A.E., OssERMAN, K.E. and KARK, A.E.: Brit. J. Cancer, 1971, 25, 635.

PAPATESTAs, A.E., OssERMAN, K.E. and KARK, A.E.: Lancet, 1972, i, 691.

PAPILION, J., CROIZAT, P., CASSARO, J.L. et al.: Cali. Med. Lyon, 1971, 47, 317.

PAROLARI, P.: Path. Ita!. Otol., 1963, 74, 710.

PARAF, A. and BRAGARD, M.: Sem. Hop. Paris, 1962, 38, 1638.

PARANT, M., CAYRON, R. and HoxsE, G.: Rev. Stomatal. (Paris), 1970, 71, 749.

PARK, D.M., JoHNsoN, R.H., CREAM, G.P. and RoBINSON, J.E.: Brit. med. J., 1972, 3, 510.

PAR :Es, T.G., BussEY, H.J.R. and LocKHART MuMMERY, H.E.: Gut, 1970, 11,323.

PARRISH, R.A., KARsTEN, M.B., McRAE, A.T. and MoRETz, W.H.: Amer. J. Surg., 1968, 115, 371.

PARTRIDGE, R.E.H. and DuTHIE, J.J.R.: Brit. med. J., 1963, i, 89.

PASQUALINI, C. and BAzzocCHI, F.: Riv. Pat. Clin., 1.968, 23, 33.

PALLIS, C.A. and ScoTT, J.T.: Brit. med. J., 1965, i, 1141.

PAUDERs, J.T. and LEEII:sMA, H.W.: Ned. T. Geneesk., 1963, 107, 811.

PAULINE-NETTO, A., DREILING, D.A. and BARONOFSKY, I.D.: Ann. Surg., 1960, 151, 530.

De Ia PAvA, S., KNuTSON, G.H., MuKHTAR, F. and PrcKREN, C.W.: Cancer (Philad.), 1965, 18, 790.

PAvERo, A. and DELIA PIETRA, S.: Arch. E. Maragliano Pat. Clin., 1966, 22, 541.

PEARSON, R.S.B.: Gut, 1961, 2, 210.

PEASE, P.E.: "L. Forms, Episomes and Auto-immune Disease", 1965, Livingstone, Edinburgh.

PENA, P., ENRIQUEz, L., SANTos, L.M. and GuRciA, E.: Rev. Clin. Esp., 1970, 118, 447.

PENN, I.: Cancer (Philad.), 1974, 34, 858.

PENROSE, L.S. and DELHANTY, J.D.A.: Lancet, 1961, i, 1261.

PERCY-ROBB, I.W. and CoLLE£, J.G.: Brit. med.

J., 1972, 3, 813.

PERLMAN, M., LEVIN, M. and WITTELS, B.: Cancer (Philad.), 1975, 30, 1212.

PERLMANN, P. and GROBERGER, O.: In "Textbook of Immunopathology", 1968 Edit. by Gell, P.G.H. and Coombs, R.R.A.. 2nd . Edit., Blackwell, Oxford.

PERLMUTTER, I. and STRAIN, R.E.: Neurology (Minneapolis), 1954, 4, 398.

PERLMUTTER, M., ELLISON, P.R., NoRSA, L. and KANROWITZ, A.R.: Amer. J. Med., 1956, 21, 634.

PERRETT, A.D., HIGGINS, G., jOHNSTON, H.H., MASSARELIA, R.G., TRUELOVE, S.C. and WRIGHT, R.: Quart. J. Med. N.S., 1971, 40, 211.

PETERKIN, G.A.G. and McMILLAN, J.B.: Arch. Dermat., 1959, 80, 564.

PETERSON, M.L.: In Cecil-Loeb "Textbook of Medicine", 1967, 5th. Edit., Edit. by Beeson, P.B. and McDermott, W., Saunders, Philadelphia.

PETERSON, R.D.A., CooPER, M.D. and Goon, R.A.: Amer. J. Med., 1965, 38, 579.

PETERSON, R.D.A., KELLY, W.O. and Goon, R.A.: Lancet, 1964, i, 1189.

PETRO. A.B. and HARDY, J.D.: Ann. Surg., 1975, 181, 118.

PETTIT, M.D., LANDING, B.R. and GuEST, G.M.: J. Clin. Endocrin., 1961, 21, 209.

PETITJEAN, R., BURCHARD, G., STRAMPLER, G. and FIEVEZ, M.: J. franc;. Med. Chir. Thor., 1968, 22, 43.

PETERSSON, T., WEGEuus, O. and SKRIFVARs, B.: Acta med. Scand., 1970, 188, 139.

PHIUJPS, P.E.: J. exp. Med., 1971, 134, 313.

PicK, G.J. and DAvis, J.: Surgery, 1961, 49, 347.

PrERCE, J.C., MADGE, G.E., LEE, H.M. and HuME. D.M.: A. Amer. med. Ass., 1972, 219, 1593.

PrERCE, L.E., HossErNIAN, A.H. and CoNsTANTINE, A.B.: Blood, 1967, 29, 540.

PrROFSKY. B.: Ann. intern. Med., 1968, 68, 109.

PIROTTE, J.H.: Amer. J. Gastroent., 1974, 62, 230.

PnK E!*THLY, D.A. and CoOMES, E.N.: Ann. rheum. Dis., 1966, 25, 127.

PnoT. H.C.: J. Nat. Cancer Inst., 1974, 53, 905.

PJTT:11AN, F.E. and HoLUB, D.A.: Gastroenterology, 1965, 48, 869.

PrrTM..N,J.A.: New Eng. J. Med., 1972, 287, 356.

PLAt:T, J.A.: Ann. Surg., 1942, 116, 43.

PLuM, F.: In Cccii·Loeb "Texabook of Medicine", 1971, 13th. Edit, Edit. by Beeson, P.ll. and McDemott, W., Saunders, Philadelphia.

PLUNKETT, E.R., LANGECROFT, G. and HAEGY, F.C.: J. Ment. Defic. Res., 1964, 8, 21.

PoE, R.H., CABLE, G.E. and JARRoLD, T.: Arch. intern. Med., 1966, 118, 199.

PoMPE, K.: Cs Derm., 1972, 47, 172.

PoNo, C.W.: Ann. Otol. Rhin. Larynx, 1940, 49, 500.

PooLE-WILSON, P.A.: Proc. R. Soc. Med., 1972, 65, 561.

PoPERT, A.J., MEIJ ERS, K.A.E., SHARP, J. and BIER, F.: Ann. rheum. Dis., 1961, 20, 18.

PoPov, E.A. and K uRILOVICH, V.K.: Arkh. Pat. (Mosk.), 1973, 35, 70.

PoPHRISTOV, P. and CESMEDZIEV, Z.: Savr. med., 1959, 10, 96.

PoRCELLINI, M., MATTIOLI, P.L. and CACCAVALE, P.: Diagn. Lab. Clin., 1971, 21, 356.

PoRTO, A. and SALDANHA, M.H.: J. Med. (Porto), 1969, 68, 725.

PosNER, J.E.: In Cecil-Loeb "Textbook of Medicine", 1971, 13th. Edit., Edit. by Beeson, P.B. and McDermott, W., Saunders, Philadelphia.

PoTALSKY, A.L., HEATH, C.W. Jr., BucKLEY, C.E. and RoWLANDS, D.T. Jr.: Amer. J. Med., 1971, 50, 42.

PoTTER, E.L.: "Pathology of the Foetus and the New Born", 1952, The Year Book Publishers, Chicago.

PowELL, D.E.B. and THOMAS, F.W.: Brit. J. Geriat. Pract., 1968, 5, 235.

PowELL, L.W. Jr., GADDY, C.G. and McGovERN, F.H.: Nebrasks Med.]., 1964, 49, 303.

PowLEs, R.L. and MALPAs, J.S.: Brit. med. J., 1967, 3, 286.

PRJ£, W.H., MacLEAN, N. and LITTLEWOOD, A.P.: Lancet, 1976, i, 807.

PRINGLE, J.S.: Brit. J. Dermato!., 1900, 12, 1.

PRIOR, J.T. and FAIRCHILD, R.D.: Amer. J. Surg., 1963, 106, 57.

PRITCHARD, P.B. and NETSKY, M.G.: Neurology (Minneap.), 1973, 23, 215.

PR UZANSiu, \V., UNDERDOWN, B., SILVER, E.H. and KATZ, A.: Amer. J. Med., 1974, 57, 259.

RABE N, A.C., BoGENOVITCH, N.K. and GoLOCHEVSKAYA, V.S.: Prob. Hematol., 1962, 6, 763.

RAcz, S.: Acta. U. int. Caner., 1960, 16, 910.

RAoJ., J., MAsOPUST, J., VoRTEL, V. and TouSEK. M.: Z. ges. inn. Med., 1965, 20, 107.

RADKE, R.A.: South med. J. (Birmingham, Alabama), 1952, 45, 1027.

RA AGE, }.H. and KrNNEAR, W.F.: Brit. J. Ophthalrnol., 1956, 40, 416.

RAMOT, B., SHAKIM, N. and BABis, J.J.: Israel J. Med., 1965, 1, 221.

RANKIN, J.G., SKYRING, A.P. and CouLsToN, S.J.M.: Gut, 1964, 5, 1.

RANSTROM, S.: Acta. chir. Scand., 1957, 113, 185.

RAPPAPORT, E.M., RossiEN, A.X. and RosEN-BLUM, L.A.: Ann. int. Med., 1951, 34, 1224.

RAusiNo, A. and TRELL, E.: Acta. med. Scand., 1971, 189, 1310.

RAwLs, W.E., IwAMOTO, K., AnAM, E., MELNICK, j.L. and GREEN, G.H.: Lancet, 1970, ii, 1142.

RAZJs, D.V., DIAMOND, H.D. and CRAVER, L.F.: Ann. int. Med., 1959 (a), 51, 933.

RAzls, D.V., DIAMOND, H.D. and CRAVER, L F.: Amer. J. Med. Sci., 1959 (b), 238, 327.

READ, A.E.: Brit. med. J., 1970, 3, 278

READ, A.E., SHERLOCK, S. and HARRISON, W.: Gut, 1963, 4, 378.

READETT, M.D.: Brit. J. Derm., 1964, 76, 126.

RECANT, L. and LACEY, P.: Amer. J. Med., 1964, 37, 578.

REICFI, C. and BRODSKY, A.E.: J. Bone Joint Dis., 1948, 30, 642.

REINERT DILTFIEY, I.: Zhaut-Geschl., -Kr., 1970, 45, 241.

REINLEIN,].M.A. and NAVARRO, V.: Europa Medica, 1967, I, 7.

REISNER, D.J. and ELLSWORTH, R.M.: Ann. int. Med., 1955, 43, 1116.

REPERT, R.W.: J. Mich. mel. Soc., 1952, 51, 1315.

RETHORNE, M.O., PRIEUR LECUYER, A.M., GRISCEILLI, C. et al.: Ann. Genet., 1971, 14, 193.

REWCASTLE, N.B. and ToM, I.: J. Neural. Neurosurg. Psychia t., 1962, 25, 51.

REYNOLDS, T.B., DENISON, E.K., FRANKEL, H.D., LIEBERMAN, F.L. and PETERs, R.L.: Amer. J. Med., 1971, 50, 302.

RicH, A.R.: Med. Hyg. Geneva, 1951, 205, 400.

RicH, M.L. and ScHIFF, L.: Ann. int. Med., 1936, 10, 252.

RicHARDS, A.J.: Brit. J. Clin. Pract., 1971, 25, 34.

RicHMOND, J., GARDNER, D.L., RoY, L.M.H. and DuTHIE, J.J.R.: Ann. Rheum. Dis., 1956, 15, 217.

RicHARDSON, E.P. Jr.: New Engl. J. Md., 1961, 365, 815.

RicFEs, E.T.: Diseases of the Body of the Testis or Epididymis. In French's Index of Differential Diagnosis. Edit. by Douthwaits, A.H., 8th. Edit., 1960, Wrigh t, Bristol.

RmDOCH, G.: In "The Hypothalamus", 1938, Oliver and Boyd, Edinburgh.

RIGBY, P.G., RosENLOF, R.C., PRATT, P.T. and LEMON, H.M.: J. Amer. Med. Ass., 1966, 197, 25.

RINEHART, R.E.: Northwest Med. (Seattle), 1952, 51, 225.

RINGEL, s.P., BENDER, A.N., ENGEL, w.K. and SMITH, H.J.: Lancet, 1975, 2, 1388.

Rio, DEL, A., NovA, M., ALVAREZ-PRECHONs, A. and de OYA, j.C.: Lancet, 1971, ii, 104.

RIVF.R, G.L. and ScHORR, W.T.: Arch. Derm. (Chicago), 1966, 93, 432.

RoBBINS, R.: Amer. J. med. Sci., 1967, 254, 848.

RoBINsoN, S.S. and TAsKER, S.: Arch. Derm. Syph., 1947, 55, 749.

ROBINSON, T.J.: Brit. med. J., 1976, 1, 745.

RoBINSON, W.D.: In Cecil-Loeb "Textbook of Medicine". 1971, 13th. Edit., Edit by Beeson, P.B. and McDermott, W., Saunders, Philadelphia.

RoBINSON, W.D.: In Cecil-Loeb "Textbook of Medicine", 1967, 11th. Edit., Edit. by Beeson, P.B. and McDermott, W., Saunders, Philadelphia.

RomouEz, E., De BoNAPATE, P. and MoRGEN-FRLD, M.C. et al.: Int. J. Leprosy, 1968, 36, 203.

RoMEY, R. and MosKOWITZ, M.: Chest, 1973, 64, 371.

RHODE, R.A.: Lancet, 1964, ii, 149.

RoiTT, I.M. and DoNIAcH, D.: In "Textbook of Immunopathology", 1969, Edit. by Miescher, P.A. and Muller-Eberha rd, Grune and Stra tton, New York.

Ros.E, A.L. and WALTON, J.N.: Brain, 1966, 89, 747.

RosE N, R.B. and TEPLITZ, R.L.: Blood, 1965, 26, 148.

RosE NBERG, S.A., DIA MOND, H.D., JAsLOWITZ, B. and CRAVER, L.F.: M edicine, 1961, 40, 31.

RosENKRANTz, J.A. and GLUCKMAN, E.C.: Amer. J. Roentgen., 1957, 78, 30.

RosENKRA NTZ, J.A., WOLF, J. and KAICKER, J.J.: Arch. int. Med., 1952, 90, 610.

RosEN MANN, E.: Israel J. Med. Sci., 1966. 2, 269.

RosENTHAL, F.D., BEELEY, J.M., GELsTHORPE, K. and DouGHTY, R.W.: Quart. J. Med., 1974, 43, 187.

RosE NTHAL, M.C., PISCIOTTA, A.V., KoMMINOS, Z.D., GoLDENBERG, H. and DA MESHEK, W.: Blood, 1955, 10, 197.

RossBERG, J.: Dtsch. Gesundh., 1963, 18, 36.

RoTSTEIN, J. and GooD, R.A.: Ann. Rheum. Dis., 1962, 21, 202.

RoTHMAN, S.: Arch. Derm. Syph., 1925, 149, 99.

ROTHMAN, S.: J. Amer. Med. Ass., 1954, 156, 242.

RoTHMAN, S., BLocK, M. and HAUSER, F.V.:

Arch. Derm. Syph (Chicago), 1951, 63, 642.

RoTMAN, M., DoRFMANN, H., De SEzE, S. and KAHN, M.T.: Nouv. Presse Med., 1972, 1, 853.

Rou zAND, M., LEROUX, M.E., LAMISSE, F. et al.: Sem. Hop. Paris, 1969, 45, 2931.

RowLAND, E.P.: In Cecil-Loeb "Textbook of Medicine", 1971, 13th. Edit., Edit. by Beeson, P.B. and McDermott, W., Saunders, Philadelphia.

RowLAND, L.P. and GREER, M.: Neurology (Minneap.), 1961, 11, 367.

RoWLAND, L.P., OssERMANN, E.F., ScHARFMAN, W.B. et al.: Amer. J. Med., 1969, 46, 599.

Rowi NSKA, ZAKREWSKA, E., LAZAR, P. and BuRTIN, F.: Ann. inst. Pasteur, 1970, 119, 621.

RowLEY, D. and JENKINs, C.R.: Nature (Lond.), 1962, 193, 151.

RuBIN, C.E., EIDELMAN, S. and WERNSTEIN, W.M.: Gastro-enterology, 1970, 58, 1009.

RuDNEw, : Virchows Arch., 1866, 35, 600.

RuEBNER, B. and BRAMHALL, J.L.: Arch. Path., 1960, 60, 110.

RuNDLF, L.G. and SPARKs, F.P.: Arch. Path., 1963, 75, 276.

RuNDLE, L.G. and SPARKS, F.P.: Arch. Path. (Chicago), 1963, 75, 276.

RusciAN, L. and AMERIO, P.L.: Gazz. int. Med. Chir., 1971, 76, 252.

RussELL, D.S. and RUBINSTEIN, L.J.: "The Pathology of the Nervous System", 1959, Arnold, London.

Ru ssELL, J.M. and CocHRAN, N.J.: Lancet, 1973, ii, 1215.

RYAN, G.P., JAMES, R.A. and Mr LAzzo, S.C.: Australia-N.Z. J. Med., 1974, 4, 287.

SAATI, V. and PnNAR, T.: Turk. J. Pediat., 1970, 12, 24.

SAcHSE, H.H. and PosER, H.: Z. Alternsforsch., 1961, 15, 191.

SACK, W.: In "Handbuch der Haut-und Geschlechtskrankheiten", 1933, Band 4, Teil 2, J. Springer, Berlin.

SACREZ, R., FROHLING, L., HEUMANN, G. and CAHN, R.: Arch. franc. Pediat., 1954, 11, 141.

SADIEwrcz, A., PoREBSKI, Z. and J ARZEMOWSKI, J.: Wiad. Lek., 1970, 23, 1597.

SAGE, R.E. and FoRBEs, I.J.: Blood, 1968, 31, 536.

SAGEBEL, R.W., McFARLAND, R.B. and TAFT, E.B.: Amer. J. Cjir. Path., 1963, 40, 516.

SAGO£, A-S.: Brit. med. J., 1970, 3, 378.

SAITA, G., BARONI, M. and TENTORIO, A.: Haematologica, 1969, 54, 179.

SAHA, T.K.: J. Indian Med. Ass., 1964, 42, 478.

SALEM, S.N. and TRUELOVE, S.C.: Brit. med. J., 1965, i, 827.

SALEM, S.N., TRUE LOVE, S.C. and RICHARDS, W.C.D.: Brit. med. J., 1964, i, 394.

SALMON, M.A. and AsHwoRTH, M.: Lancet, 1970, ii, 1085.

SALO, O.P. and RASANEN, J.A.: Ann. Clin. Res., 1972, 4, 173.

SALTSTEIN, S.L. and AcKERMAN, L.V.: Cancer, N.Y., 1959, 12, 164.

SALZBURGER, M.B. and WoLF, J.: "Dermatologic Therapy in General Practice", 1940, Chicago Year Book Publishers, Inc. SAKULA, A.: Brit. J. Cancer, 1963, 17, 206. SAMS, w.M.Jr.: Proc. Mayo Clin., 1967, 42, 300.

SAMs, W.M. Jr., HARVILLE, D.D. and WINKELMANN, R.K.: Brit. J. Dermat., 1968, 80, 555.

SANDBANK, M., GRUNEBAUM, M. and KATZENBOGEN, I.: Arch. Dermatol., 1966, 94, 432.

SANKALE, M., Sow, A.M., AcBETRA, M. and TEYSSIER, P.: Bull. Soc. Path. Exot., 1973, 66, 646.

SANNICAUDRo, F.: Med. Wschr., 1963, 148, 629.

SANTY, P., BERNARD, M., GALY, P. and CouRAJNE, R.G.: J. franc. Med. Chir. Thorac., 1954, 8, 119.

SAUVEzrr: B., MrssiOux, D., Le Rov, V. et al.: Rev. Rheum., 1974, 41, 449.

SAvrc, D., SPALAJKOVIC, M. and LAZAREVIC, D.: J. franc. Oto-rhino-larynx., 1966, 15, 117.

SAXENA, K.M. and CRAWFORD, J.D.: Pediatrics, 1962, 30, 917.

ScAODINc, J.G.: Proc. R. Soc. Med., 1967, 60, 737.

ScADDING, J.G.: Proc. R. Soc. Med., 1969, 62, 227.

ScADUING, J.G.: Brit. med. J., 1970, 60, 737.

ScARABICCHI, S., MAsSIMO, L. and ToRTOROLo G.: Minerva Pediat. (Torino), 1960, 12, 1368.

ScHAisoN, G., NAJEAN, Y., SELIMANN, M. et al.: Nouv. Rev. franc. Hemat., 1969, 9, 419.

ScHALLER, J., BEcKWITH, B. and WEDGwooo, R.J.: J. Pediat., 1970, 77, 203.

Sc HALLER, J.: J. Pediat., 1971, 79, 139.

Sc HALLER, J.: J. Pediat., 1972, 81, 793.

Sc.HAPIRA, H.E. and OPPENHEIMER, G.D.: J. Mt. Sinai Hosp., 1963, 30, 228.

ScHAPIRO, P.F.: Arch. Neurol. Psychiat. Chicago, 1930, 24, 509.

ScHAUB, F.: Schweiz. med. Wschr., 1953, 83, 1256.

ScHEFF, W., SYMONS, J., VAN CAM P, K., DANIELS, R. and DE LEEUW-DELVIGAE, C.: Brit. med. J., 1974, i, 78.

Sc HEINBERG, L.C.: In Cecil-Loeb "Textbook of Medicine", 1971, 13th. Edit., Edit. by

Beeson, P.B. and McDermott, W., Saunders. Philadelphia.

ScHENER-KARPIN, R.: Brit. med. J., 1972, 3, 116.

ScHEN ER-KARPIN, R.: Proc. 7th. Cong. Europea n Soc. Haematol., London, Part II, Karger, 1959, Basle.

ScHE NER-KARPIN, R. and D'IliuRE usE-GER- HARDT, R.: Israel J. Med. Science, 1965, 1, 819.

ScHERBEL, A.L., McCoR M AcK, L.J., MAcKEN- ZIE, A.H. and ATDJEAN, M.: Postgrad. Med., 1964, 35, 619.

ScHERER, H.E.: J. Beige. Neuro!. Psychia t., 1938, 38, 1.

ScHIEWE, R.: Monatschr. Unf allheilk., 1966, 69, 394.

ScHIEWE, R. and KocH, W.: Arch. Geschwulst- forsch., 1967, 29, 85.

ScHrMPFF, S.C., ScHIMPFF, C.R., BRAGER, D.M. and WrERNIK, P.H.: Lancet, 1975, i, 124.

ScHLECL, B. and ANDERS, G.: Arztl. Wschr., 1959, 14, 670.

ScHLESINGER. M.H., ALMY, T.P. and BAER, D.P.: Amer. J. Mecf., 1953, 15, 666.

ScHLICK£, C.P., HILL, J.E. and ScHULTZ, G.F.: Surg. Gynec. Obstet., 1960, 111, 552.

ScHMAMAN, A. and IssAACSON, C.: S. Afr. med. J., 1960, 34, 761.

ScHMIDT, W. and GEBHARDT, R.: Med. Welt. (Stuttg.), 1969, 69, 567.

ScHNACK, H. and STEFENELLI, N.: Wien. med. Ws.,hr., !954, 66, 862.

ScHNEIDERBAUER, A.: Wien. med. Wschr., 1954, 104, 472.

ScHOTTENFELD, D. and BERG, J.: J. Nat. Can- cer Inst., 1971, 46, 161.

ScHREINER, B.F. and MULTICK, W.L.: J. Cane. Res., 1924, 8, 504.

ScHUERMANS, Y.: Lancet, 1975, i, I11.

ScHULTHEss, G. Von.: Pract. oto-rhino-laryng., 1968, 30, 314.

ScHWARTZ, R.S. and BELDOTTI, L.: Science. N.Y., 1965, 149, 1511.

ScLARE, G. and NICOL, A.: J. Clin. Path., 1964, 17, 438.

ScoTT, B.B. and Losow:SKY, M.S.: Lancet, 1975, ii, 956.

ScoTTO, J., STRALIN, H. and CARou, J.: Gut, 1970, 11, 782.

Scu RR, J.A.: Proc. R. Soc. Med., 1972, 65. 725.

SEARS, W.G.: Guy's Hosp. Rep., 1932, 82, 40.

SEODON, J.A.: Brit. med. J., 1960, i, 1185.

SEGURA, R. and ZrECLER, D.K.: Dis. Nerv. System. 1973, 34, 284.

SEIGNON, B., CAULET, T., HoPFER, C. and Gou- GEON, J.: Sem. Hop. Pa ris, 1972, 48, 903.

SEIFERT, G. and GEILER, G.: Dtsch. med. Wschr., 1967, 82, 1415.

SELYE, H.: "Textbook of Endocrinology", 1947, Acta Endocrinologica, Montreal.

SENTI, P.A., CANEDO, A.R., PuLIDo, L.R. et a!.: Rev. Cuba Med., 1964, 3, 560.

SEIl.RE,H. and SJMON, L.: Rev. Rheum., 1959, 26, 347.

SHAMMY, H.K.: Proc. R. Soc. Med., 1963, 56, 904.

SHANBROM, E.: Amer. J. din. Path., 1963, 40, 67.

SHANDS, W.C.: Ann. Su rg., 1960, 151, 675.

SHAPER, A.G., KAPLAN, M.H., MoDY, N.J. and MciNTYRE, P.A.: Lancet, 1968, i, 1342.

SHARLANo, D.E.: Proc. R. Soc. Med., 1971, 64, 397.

SHARP, G.C., IRVIN, W.S., TA N, E.M., GouLD, R.G. and HoLMAN, H.R.: Amer. J. Med., 1972, 62, 148.

SHARVILL, D.: Proc. R. Soc. Med., 1958, 51, 934.

S HAW, R.C. and SMITH, F.B.: Brit. J. Surg., 1925, 13, 93.

SHEARN, M.A.: "Sjogren's Syndrome", 1971, Saunders, London.

SHEEHAN, H.L. and Su MMERS, V.K.: Quart. J. Med., 1949, 18. 319.

SHEINWELL, R.E.: J. La. Med. Soc., 1971, 12, 409.

SHELooN, T.K.: Proc. R. Soc. Med., 1939, 32, 255.

SHELLY, W.B. and HuRLEY, H.J.: Arch. Der- ma to!., 1960, 81, 889.

SHEMWELL, R.E.: J. LA., me<k Soc., 1971, 123, 409.

SHERLOCK, S.P.V.: "Diseases of the Liver and Biliary System", 1968, 4th. Edit. Oxford and Edinburgh, Blackell Scientific.

SHERMA1;',J.D., BANAS, J.S. Jr., EowARDS, T.L. et al.: Gastro-enterology, 1966, 51, 681.

SHERMAN, R.L., SARTIA NO, G.P., VINCIGNERRA, V.P. and BECKER, E.L.: Ann. intern. Med., 1970, 72, 805.

SHERMAN, W.R.: In Cecil-Loeb "Textbook of Medicine", 1967, 12th. Edit., Edit. by Beeson, P.B. and McDermott, W., Saunders, Phila- delphia.

SHERRY, M.G.: Amer. J. din. Path., 1968, 50, 398.

SHIOJI, R., FuRUYAMA, T., ONODERA, S., SArro, H., Iro. H. and SASAKI, Y.: Amer. J. Med., 1970, 48, 456.

SHOOKHOFF, H.B.: In Cecil-Loeb "Textbook of Medicine", 1963, 11th. Edit., Edit. by Beeson, P.B. and McDermott, W., Saunders, Philadelphia.

SHORT, G.L., BAUER, W. and REYNOLDS, W.E.:

1957, Harvard University Press, Cambridge, Mass.

SHUCKSMITH, H.S. and DossETT, J.A.: Brit. med. J., 1965, i, 1495.

SHUCKSMITH, H.S. and DossETT, J.A.: Lancet, 1966, ii, 909.

SIBLEY, W.K.: Brit. J. Dermatol., 1915, 27, 52.

Smr, E. and REINBERG, A.: Lancet, 1960, ii, 842.

SrEGEL, M., LEE, S.L., WmELOCK, D., GrvoN, N.V. and KRAVITZ, H.: New Eng. J. Med., 1965, 273, 893.

SILBERMAN, H.R., McGINN, T.G. and KREMER, W.B.: J. Amer. med. Ass., 1965, 194, 597.

SILBERSTEIN, E.: Brit. med. J., 1970, 3, 445.

SILTBACH, L.E.: In Cecil-Loeb "Textbook of Medicine", 1971, 13th. Edit., Edit. by Beeson, P.B. and McDermott, W., Saunders, Philadelphia.

DaSILVA HoRTA, J. and MoRAis, D.A.: Gaz. med. post., 1958, 11, 175.

SILVER, H.M., NACHNANI, G. and BRESLow, A.: Amer. Rev. Resp. Dis., 1967, 96, 290.

SILVERMAN, B.B., O'NEILL, R.T. and MIKUTA, J.J.: Surg. Gynec. Obst., 1972, 134, 244.

SIMONELLI, C.: Clinotorinolaring., 1971, 23, 365.

SIMPSON, J.A.: J. Neurol., 1964, 27, 485.

SIMPSON, J.A.: Ann. N.Y. Acad. Sci., 1966, 135, 506.

SIMPSON, J.R.: Proc. R. Soc. M ed, 1953, 46, 288.

SmcLAm, R.J.G. and CRUIKS HANK, B.: Quart. J. Med., 1956, 25, 331.

SINGER, W. and SAHAY, B.W.: Brit. med. J., 1966, i, 904.

SINGH, R.N.: Aust. Ann. Med., 1969, 18, 55.

SINGH, B.N. and DAs, S.R.: Phil. Trans. Roy. Soc. B., 1970, 259, 435.

SrRRIOGE, MS.: Ann. int. Med., 1960, 53, 380.

SIURALA, M. and IKKALA, E.: Ann. Med. intern. Fenn., 1965, 54, 43.

SIUR ALA, M., LEHTOLA, J. and I HAMAKI, T.: Cs. Gastroent. Vy2, 1974, 28, 106.

SwRALA, M. and SEPPALA, K.: Acta med. Sca nd., 1960, ! 66, 455.

SruRALA, M., TULKUNEN, H., ToiVONEN, S., PELKOMEN, R., SAXEN, E. and PrTKANEN, E.: Acta med. Sca nd., 1965, 178, 13.

SIURALA, M., VuoRINEN, Y. and SEPPALA, K.: Acta med. Scand., 1961, 170, 151.

SJoGREN, H.: Acta Opjtjal. (K bh.), 1951, 29, 33.

SKLARZ, E.: Z. Haut. v Gescglkr., 1955, 19, 321.

SLATER, E. and RoTH, M.: In Mayer-Gross' "Clinical Psychiatry", 1969, 3rd. Edit., Baillicre, Tinda ll and Cassell, London.

SLAUGHTER, D.P. and CRAVER, L.F.: Amer. J. Roentgenol., 1942, 47, 596.

SLEISENGER, M.H.: In Cecil-Lobe "Textbook of Medicine", 1967, 12th. Edit., Edit. by Beeson, P.B. and McDermott, W., Saunders, Philadelphia.

SLOMSKA, J.: Nowotwory, 1967, 171, 59.

SMART, G.A. and OwERs, S.G.: J. Chron. Dis., 1961, 14, 537.

SMITH, C.K., CAssiDY, J.T. and BoLE, G.C.: Amer. J. Med., 1970, 48, 113.

SMITH, J.P. and GATES, P.O.: J. Path. Bact., 1955, 70, 111.

SMITH, M.J.L., BENSON, M.K. and STRICKLAND, I.D.: Lancet, 1971, i, 473.

SMITHERS, D.W.: Brit. med. J., 1967, ii, 263.

SNEDDON, LB.: Brit. med. J., 1963, ii, 405.

SoDERSTROM, N.: Lancet, 1960, ii, 947.

SoFTie, N.: Nouv. Rev. fran\<· d'Hematol., 1964, 4, 458.

SoKOLOFF, L.: Amer. Heart J., 1953, 45, 635.

SoKOLOFF, L.: In "The Peripheral Blood Vessels", 1963, Edit. by Orbison, J.H. and Smith, D.E., Baltimore.

SoKOLOFF, L.: In "Arthritis and Allied Conditions", 1966, 7th. Edit. by Hollander, J.L., Kimpton, London.

SouGNAC, H., CAsTANY, J., BARTHELEMY, Y. et a!.: Nouv. Presse Med., 1972, 1, 729.

SoLOMON, D.H. and CHOPRA, I.J.: Proc. Mayo Clin., 1972, 47, 803.

SéLTOFT, J. and LIND, K.: Acta path. Microbial. Sca nd., 1968, 93, 13.

SoM MERs, S.C.: Lab. invest. (Philad.), 1955, 4, 160.

SoNADJEAN, J.V., SILVERSTEIN, M.N. and TITus, J.L.: Cancer (Philad.), 1968, 22, 1221.

So KEN, P.H.: Brit. J. Hosp. Med., 1972, 7, 151.

SoRRELL, T., FoREEs, I.J., BuRNESS, F.R. and Ru-:cH RIETH, R.H.C.: La ncet, 1971, ii, 1233.

SoUTHAr, C.M.: Ca ncer Res., 1968, 28, 1433.

SPAIN, D.M.: Ann. Rev. Tuberc., 1957, 76, 559.

SPARAGANA, M.: Post grad. med., 1970, 47, 209.

SPARKEs, R.S. and MoTU LSKY, A.G.: Lancet, 1963, i, 947.

SPENCER, H.: "Pathology of the Lung", 2nd. Edi t., 1968, Pergamon Press, Oxford.

SPERUNG, I.L.: Minerva Med., 1961, 2, 590.

SPERRYN, P.N.: Proc. R. Soc. Med., 1971, 64, 58.

SPICKARD, A.: Bull. Johns Hop. H osp., 1960, 107, 234.

SPĿSRERG, I. and MEYER, G.J.: Art hr. Rheu m. (I'.'.Y.), 1972, 15, 630.

SPrNIVASA, R.K. and SHARMA, : Indian J. Path. Bact., 1968, 11, 8.

SPRACKLEN, F.: Proc. R. Soc. Med., 1963, 56, 167.

SPRINKLE, P.M. and YARINGTON, C.T. Jr.: Sth. Med. J. {Birmingham, Ala.), 1968, 61, 971.

SsoBELow, (Quoted by Plaut, J.A., 1942).

SrAJANO, C.: Sisterma Vegetativo y neurosis tropica. Montevideo, 1933.

STALDER, A.: Schweiz. rued. Wschr., 1972, 102, 192.

SrALEWSKI, R., SrR, J. and FIWEK, J.: Nowoto-wory, 1965, 15, 203.

STAMM, W.P.: Trans. R. Soc. trop. Med. Hyg., 1972, 66, 210.

STAVRAKY, K.M., WATSON, T.A., WHITE, D.E. and MILES, E.M.: Cancer (Philad.), 1970, 26, 410.

STEEL, S.J.: Amer. Rev. resp. Dis., 1964, 89, 736.

STEGLEDER, G.K.: Hautaizt., 1955, 6, 89.

STEINBRJNCK, W.: Z. Klin. Med., 1941, 139, 67.

STEINER, I.E.: Amer. J. Path., 1937, 13, 109.

STEINER, J.W. and GELBLOOM, A.J.: Arth. Rheum., 1959, 2, 537.

STEINBERG, A.D. and TALAL, N.: Ann. int. Med., 1971, 74, 55.

STEPHENS, M.E.M. and SKINER, M.: Lancet, 1971, ii, 431.

STERNE, E.H. Jr., ScHIRO, H. and MoLLo, W.: Amer. J. Med. Sci., 1941, 202, 167.

STEVANIVJC, D.V.: Arch. Derm. Syph., 1968, 82, 96.

STEWART, A.L., KEAY, A.J., JAcoBs, P.A. and MELVILLE, M.M.: J. Pediat., 1969, 74, 449.

STEWART, G.G.: Arch. int. Med., 1929, 44, 772.

STEWART, I.A. and SruART, A.E.: J. Laryng., 1971, 85, 1069.

STICHER, R.M., HERST, A.N., SOLOMON, W.M. and WoLPAW, R.: Amer. J. Hum. Genet., 1953, 5, 118.

STICKLER, G.B., PEYLA, T.L., DowER, J.C. and LoGAN, G.B.: Clin. Pediat., 1965, 4, 276. STITT, R.B. and COLAPINTO, V.: J. Urol., 1966, 96, 733.

STOBBE, H.: Acta Haema t., 1962, 27, 180.

STOKER, T.A.M.: Proc. R. Soc. Med., 1971, 64, 661.

SroHR and RrsAK (Quoted by Plaut, J.A., 1942).

SroLTZE, C.A., HANLOW, D.G., PEASE, G.L. et al. : Arch. int. Med., 1960, 106, 513.

STREET, E.W.: Lancet, 1972, ii, 381.

STRANDBERG, B.: Scand. J. Rheumatol., 1974, 3 Sup. 5, 14p.

STRANDBERG, B. and }ARLøv, N.V.: Arch. Phys. Med., 1961, 42, 273.

STRANG, L.B.: Brit. med. J., 1960, i, 167.

STRAuss, A.J.L.: Brit. med J., 1965, i, 1245.

STRONG, R.P.: International Clinics, 1931, 4, 68.

STUART, A.E. and ALLAN, W.S.A.: Lancet, 1958, ii, 47.

STuRROCK, R.D., CowDEN, E.M., HowrE, E., GRENNAN, D.M. and WATSON-BucHANAN, W.: Brit. med. J., 1975, 4, 92.

SuMMERLEY, R.: Brit. J. Derma tol., 1964, 76, 370.

SuMMERS, G.W. and SrssoN, G.A.: Trans. Amcr. Acad. Ophthal. Otola ryng., 1972, 76, 1387.

SuMMEY, T.J. and PRESSLEY, C.L.: Ann. Surg., 1946, 123, 135.

SuRY, B. and VESTERDAL, E.: Acta rheum. Scand., 1969, 14, 309.

Su zuKr, Y., IwAI, H., TAKASAKI, A., MoNYE, T. and KARAI, H.: Oto-rhino-laryng., (Tokyo), 1960, 32, 121.

SwANK, R.L.: Neurology {Minneap.), 1958, 8, 497.

SwENSON, S.A. and OMEL, J.L.: Henry Ford Hosp. Med. J., 1974, 22, 153.

SwiFT, M.: Nature (Lond.), 1971, 230, 370.

SnrAN, W.E., RoHN, R.J. and BoND, W.H.·: Amer. J. Med., 1957, 234, 160.

SvMMERS, D.: Arch. int. Med., 1944, 74, 163.

SzEGEDl, G., NAGY, E. and DAR6czi, P.: Z. Ha ut. Geschl-krkh., 1968, 43, 363.

SzLEZAK, L. and PRzYBORA, L.: Otolar. Polska, 1957, 11, 303.

TABAKOvA, T.V.: Klin. Med. (Mosk.), 1966, 7, 122.

TAFT, A.E.: Rev. Neurol. Psychiat., 1916, 14, 57.

TAKENCHI. S. and PICKREN. J.W.: Cancer (Philad.), 1967, 20, 1000.

TALAL, N. and BuNIM, J.J.: Amer. J. Med., 1964, 36, 529.

TALAL. N., SoKOLOFF, L. and BARTH, W.F.: Amcr. J. Med., 1967, 43, 50.

TALAL, N., ZisMAN, E. and ScHUR, P.H.: Arth. Rheum., 1968, 11, 774:.

TALLENT, M.B., SIMMONS, R.L. and NAJARIAN. J.S.: Amec J. Obstet. Gynec., 1971, 109, 663.

TALLEY, R.W., DoHERTY, J.E. and SHuKERs, C.F.: South rned. J., 1952, 45, 559.

TAN. R.S-H.: Proc. R. Soc. Mcd., 1974 (a), 67, 195.

TA;, R-S-H.: Proc. R. Soc. Med., 1974 (b), 67, 196.

TAN, E.M. and CHARPLIN, H.Jr.: Jox. san-guine, 1968, 15, 161.

TAN, R.S.H., BuTTERWORTH, C.D., McLAUGHIN,

H. et a!.: Brit. J. Derm., 1974, 91, 607.

TANAKA, J. et al.: J. Neurosurg., 1975, 43, 80.

TANNEBERGER, S. and BAciGALUPO, G.: Arch. Gescgwulstforsch., 1967, 29, 266.

TAYLOR, C.R.: Lancet, 1974, ii, 802.

TAYLOR, R.T.: Brit. J. Hosp. Med., 1970, 4, 653.

TAYKJ, H. and KEELE, D.: Amer. J. Roentgen., 1962, 88, 432.

TEEs, J.G.: Brit. med. J., 1961, ii, 383.

TEITELMAN, S.L. and BRILL, N.R.: Amer. J. Surg, 1960, 99, 247.

THIEDE, H.A.: Modern Medicine, 1967, 11, 929.

TRIERs, H. et a!.: Bull. Soc. fran. Derm. Syph., 1969, 76, 578.

TrWMA, G.W.: Amer.]. med. Sci., 1964, 247, 427.

TrroMPSON, D.M.: Proc. R. Soc. Med., 1974, 67, 26.

TrroMPSON, D.M.: Proc. R. Soc. Med., 1974, 67, 1010.

THRUSH, D.C.: Brit. med. J., 1970, 4, 474.

TIC.FIY, J., PROCHAZKA, J. and BAYER, A.: Cas. Lek. Ces., 1962, 101, 999.

TmKus, G.S. and DEKKER, A.: Cancer, 1970, 25, 121.

ToMASI, T.B., FuNDENBERG, H.H. and FINBY, N.: Amer. J. Med., 1962, 33, 293.

ToMKIN, G.H.: Brit. J. Derm., 1969, 81, 213.

ToMKIN, G.H., MAwFIINNEY, H. and NEVIN, N.C.: Lancet, 1917, ii, 124.

T ROK, L.: In "Handbuch der Haut-und Geschlechtskrankh eiten", 1933, Band 6, Teil 2, J. Springer, Berlin.

ToRREY, E.F. and PETERSON, M.R.: Lancet, 1973. ii, 22.

TouRNIAIRE, J., ORciAzzi, J., DAzoRo, A. et a!.: Ann. Endocrin. (Paris), 1972, 33, 97.

TowNsEND, S.R.: Canad. Med. Ass. J., 1949, 61, 417.

TRABUcco, A. and MARQUEZ, F.: Rev. Argent. Urol., 1947, 16, 500.

TRIPP, C.D.: N.Y. St. .f. Med., 1967, 67, 1907.

TRUELOVE. S.C. and WRIGFIT, R.: In "Clinical Aspects of Immunology". Edit. by Cell, P.G.H. and Coombs, R.R.P. 2nd. Edit. 1968, Blackwell, Oxford.

Tsuzi, l. et al.: Stomach Intest. (Tokyo), 1970, 5, 1679.

Tu, W.H., SrrEARN, M.A., LEE, J.C. and HooPER,]. Jr.: Ann. int. Med., 1968, 69, 1163.

TuFFANELLI, D.L. and WINKELMANN, R.K.: Amer. J. med. Sci., 1962, 243, 133.

TuRNER, J. and NIGRISOLI, P.; Zbl. allg. Path. Path. Anat., 1957, 96, 161.

TuRNER-WARWICK, M.: Quart. J. Med. N.S.,
1968, 37, 133.

TuRNER-WARWICK, M. and DoNIACFI, D.: Brit. med. J., 1965, i, 886.

TuRNER-WARWICK, M. and PARKEs, W.R.: Brit. med. J., 1970, 3, 492.

TwAST, M. and SruRALA, M.: Acta Med. Scand., 1956, 154, 211.

TwoMEY, J.J., JoRDAN, P.H., LAUGHTER, A.H., MEUWISSEN, H.J. and Goon, R.A.: Ann. int. Med., 1970, 72, 499.

TwoMEY, J.J., LAUGHTER, A.H. and VILLANUEVA, N.D. eta!.: Arch. intern. Med., 1971, 128, 846.

TwoRT, C.C.: J. Path. Bact., 1930, 33, 539.

TYLER, A.: In "Analysis of Development" by Willier, B.H., Weiss, P.A. and Hamburger, V. (1955), Saunders, Philadelphia.

ULRICH, H. and WrLLKINSON, M.: J. Neurol. Neurosurgpsychiat., 1970, 33, 398.

ULRIGFI, J. and WuTHRICH, R.: Eur. neurol. (Basel), 1974, 12, 65.

ULTMANN,].E., FISH, W., OsSERMAN, E. and GELLHORN, A.: Ann. int. Med., 1959, 51, 501.

UtTMANN,].E., HYMAN, G.A. and CALDER, B.: Blood, 1963, 21, 282.

UNGAR, B., STOCKS, A.E., MARTIN, F.I.R., WHITTINGHAM, S. and MACAY, I.R.: Lancet, 1968, 2, 415.

UNITED KINGDOM REPORT,·. Lancet, 1969, i, 163.

URBACH, E.: Arch. Derm., 1942, 45, 697.

URBACH, E. and GoTTLIEB, P.M.: "Allergy", 1944, Heinemann, London.

URBAIN, G. and CARROLL,].: Rev. med. Chir. mal. foie., 1959. 6, 299.

VALLANCE-OWEN, J.: Diabetologica, 1966, 2, 248.

VALLOLLEN, M.B. and FoRBES, D.P.: Lancet, 1967, i, 648.

VAN der SAR, A., BosscHIETER, E., RuGENHOLTZ, M.J. and VAN. der HoEVEN, L.: Documenta de Med. Georg. Trop., 1956, 8, 85.

VAN ScoTT, E.J. and REINERTSON, R.P.: J. invest. Derm., 1961, 36, 109.

VAN ToNGEREN, J.H.M.: Ned. Tijdschr. Genecsk., 1962, 106, 1017.

VAN ToNGEREN, J.H.M.: Lancet, 1966, i, 1266.

VAN de WAL, A.M., HuRziNGER, E., ORIE, N.G.M., SHUTER, H.J. and de VRIES, K.: Scand. J. Resp. Dis., 1960, 47, 161.

VARJ A, L., SzABO, M. and LAIZLO, A.: Orv. Hetil., 1962, 105, 1076.

VAUGFIAN, B.F.: Brit. J. Radio!., N.S., 1958, 31 (361), 45.

VAUGHAN, J.H.: In "Arthritis and Allied Conditions". 1960, 6th. Edit., Edit. by Hollander, J.L., Kimpton, London.

VAuzANT, F.R., ALVAREZ, W.C., EusTERMAN, G.B., DuNN, G.B. and BERKSON,}.: Arch. int. Med., 1932, 49, 345.

VAZQUEZ,J.J.: Quoted by Bloch, K.H., Wohl, M.J., Schipp, I.J., Oglesby, R.B. and Bunim, J.J. Arch. Rheum., 1960, 3, 287.

VEHAvE,J.H.: Ned. T. Genesk., 1926, 70, 1082.

VErGA FERNANDES, F. and CELESTINO DA CosTA, J.: J. Med. (Porto), 1969, 69, 313.

VELVE, K., HuBER, J. and SLrKKE, L.V. Van der.: Ann. intern. Med., 1966, 65, 554.

VELEz GARCIA, E., SANTIAGO, J.V. and MALONADO, N.: Ann. intern. Med., 1969, 70, 1219.

VENABLES, C.W.: Proc. R. Soc. Med., 1966, 59, 426.

VEssEv,M.P. and DoLL,R.: Brit. J. Cancer, 1972, 26, 53.

VETTORI, G. and ERLE, G.: Arch. E. Maragliano Pat. Clin., 1967, 23, 391.

VIALLET, A., BENHAMON, J.P., BERTHELEB, P., HARTMANN, L. and FAUVERT, R.: Gastroenterology, 1962, 43, 88.

VIANNA,N.J. and EssMAN,L.J.: Cancer (Philad.), 1971, 27, 1337.

VIANNA, N.J., GREENWALD, P. and DAVIES, J.N.P.: Lancet, 1971, I, 73"3.

VIANNA, N.J., GREENWALD, P. and DAVIES, J.N.P.: Lancet, 1971, I, 1209.

VIDAL, C.E.: Bull. Roswell Park Memorial Inst., Buffalo, N.Y., 1956, I, 105.

VIDEBACK, A.: "Heredity in Human Leukaemia and its Relation to Cancer". Ejnar. Munksgaad, Copenhagen, 1947.

VrcNON, G., CHAPUY, P. and BrEo, J.C.: Rev. Prat. (Paris}, 1969, 19, 945.

VrLAN, J., RHYNER, K. and GANZONI, A.: Lancet, 1971, ii, 51.

VrRSHUP, A.M. and SLrwiNSKT, A.J.: Arth. Rheum. (N.Y.), 1973, 16, 388.

VISAKORPI, J.K.:Lancet, 1969, ii, 1192.

VmcHOW, R.: Virchow's Arch., 1864, 29, 608.

du VMER, A. and MuNRO, D.D.: Brit. med. J., 1975, 1, 191.

VLADUTIU, A.O. and SIELSKI, L.: Lancet, 1973, 1, 1122.

VoRLAENDER, K.O.: Med. Welt., 1960, 45, 2376.

WAGER, O. and RAsiiNEN, J.A.: Proc. Int. Symposium on Immune Complex Diseases, 1970, p. 140.

WAGNER, K. and NEUN, H.: Krebsarzt., 1955, 10, 34.

WALACH, N. and HoRN, Y.: J. Amer. Med. Ass., 1973, 226, 201.

WALDER, B.K., RoBERTSON, M.R. and jEREMY, D.: Lancet, 1971, ii, 1282.

\VALDRAM, R, KoPELMAN, H., TsANTOuLAS, D. and WILLIAMS, R.: Lancet, 1975, 1, 550.

WALFORD, R.L.: "Etiology and Pathogenesis of Aging", 1969, Williams and Wilkins, Baltimore.

WALKER, F.C. and WEAVER, J.P.A.: Brit. J. Surg., 1964, 51, 475.

WALKER-SMtrH,].A. and GRICOR, W.: Lancet, 1969, i, 1021.

WALL, R.L. Jr.: Amer. J. Obstet. Gynec., 1958, 76, 803.

WALLACE, A.F.: Brit. J. Surg., 1957, 45, 165.

WALLACE, D.C.: Lancet, 1969, ii, 1138.

WALLER, J.V., ScHAPIRO, M. and PALTAN; F.R.: Amer. Heart J, 1957, 53, 479.

WALSH, E.G.: "Physiology of the Nervous System", I 957, Longmans, Green and Co., Ltd., London.

Wi\LSHE, F.: Lancet, 1961, ii, 993.

WALT, A.J., WOOLNER, L.B. and BLACK, B.M.: J. din. Endocrin., 1957, 17, 45.

WALTER, L.H., SzuR, L. and LEwis, S.M.: Brit. med. J., 1958, ii, 859.

WALZER, S., BREAU, G. and GERALD, P.S.: J Paediat., 1969, 74, 438.

WANEBO, H.J. and CLARE.SON, B.D.: Ann. int. Med., 1965, 62, 1025.

WANEBo, H.J, BENUA,R.S. and RAwsoN,R.W.: Cancer (Philad.), 1966, 19, 1523.

WARD, H.N. and REINHARD, E.H.: Ann. int. Med., 1971, 75, 193.

WARD, H.W.C.: Lancet, 1976, 1, 294.

WARTN, A.P.: Proc. R. Soc. Med., 1973, 66, 621.

WARNER, A.H.: N.Y. St. J. Med., 1962, 62, 18.

WARREN, K.W.: Surg. clin N. Amer., 1959, 39, 725.

WARREN, S. and GATEs, O.: Amer. J. Cancer. 1932, 16, 1358.

WARREN, S., LECOMPTE, P. and LEGG, M.A.: "The Pathology of Diabetes Mellitus", 1966, 4th. Edit., Lea and Fibiger, Philadelphia.

WARWICK, M.J.: Brit. J. Hosp. Med., 1973, 9, 19.

WATERHOusE, J.P. and DoNIACH, I.: J. Path. Bact., I 966, 91, 53.

WATKINS, S.M.: Proc. R. Soc. Med., 1970, 63, 622.

WATI<INS, S.: Lancet, 1973, i, 1254. WATSON, A.A.: J. clin. Path., 1972, 25, 240. WEAVER, A.L., DIVORTIE, M.B. and Trrus, JL.: Proc. Mayo C!in., 1967, 42, 754.

WEBSTER, A.D.B.: Proc. R. Soc. Med., 1973, 66, I126.

WEBSTER. A.D.B.: Clinical Meeting, Royal Society of Medicine, Feb. 14th. 1975.

WEGELJUS, O., FYHRQUIST, F. and ADNER, P.L.: Acta. rheum. Scand., 1970, 16, 184.

WEGELius, O., SKRIFVARS, B. and ANDERSSON, L.: Acta. med. Scand., 1970, 187, 133.

WEGLENKA, L.C., WuEPPER, K.D., KoMARMY, L.E. and FoRSHAN, P.R.: Lancet, 1966, i, 741.

WEIGL, L.S.: Zeitsch. f. d. ges inn. Med., 1970, 25, 621.

WEITZEL, R.A.: Cancer, N.Y., 1958, 11, 546.

WELCH, J.W., CHESKY, V.C. and HELLWEG, C.A.: Surg. Gynec. Obst., 1958, 106, 70.

WELcH, J.L. and EPSTEIN, E.: J. Amer. Med. Ass., 1952, 148, 1221.

WELCH, C.E. and HEDBERG, S.E.: J. Amer. Med. Ass., 1965, 191, 815.

WELLs, H.G.: Arch. Path., 1940, 30, 593.

WENYON, L.M.: "Protozoology", 1926, Bail-Here, Tindall and Cox, London.

WERNER, S.C.: Proc. Mayo Clin., 1972, 47, 696.

WERNER, S.C. and STEWART, W.B.: J. din. Endocr., 1958, 18, 266.

WERTilAMER, S., }ABUSH, M. and ScHULMAN, J.: J. Amer. Med. Ass., 1961, 175, 558.

WEWALKA, F.: Lancet, 1966, i, 1150.

WHALEY, K., CHISHOLM, D.M., DAVIE, W.W., DicK, W.C. and WILLIAMSON, J.: Arch. rheum. Scand., 1968, 14, 298.

WHALEY, K., WILLIAMSON, J., CHISHOLM, D.M., WEBB, J., MAsoN, D.K. and BucHANAN, W.W.: Quart, J. Med., 1973 (a), 42, 279.

WHALEY, K., WEBB, J., McAvoR, BA., HuGHEs. G.R.V., LEE, P., MAcSwEEN, R.N.M. and BucHANAN, W.W.: Quart. J. Med., 1973 (b), 42, 513.

WHALEY, K., GoUDIE, R.B., WILLIAMSON, J. NuKr, G., DicK, W.C. and BucHANAN, W.W.: Lancet, 1970, 1, 861.

WHEELER, C.E.: In Cecil-Loeb "Textbook of Medicine", 1967, 12th. Edit., Edit. by Beeson, P.B. and McDermott, W., Saunders, Philadelphia.

WHELTON, M.J.: Brit. J. Hosp. Med., 1970, 3, 243.

WHISNANT, J.P., EsPINOSA, R.E., KIERLAND, R.R. and LAMBERT, E.H.: Proc. Mayo Clin., 1963, 38, 50l.

WHITBY, L.E.H. and BRITTON, C.J.C.: "Disorders of the Blood", 1969, lOth. Edit., Churchill, London.

WHITE, R.G., BAss, E.H. and WILLIAMS, W.: Lancet, 1961, i, 368.

WHITEHOUSE, J.M.A. and HoLBOROW, E.J.: Brit. med. J., 1971, 4, 511.

WHITELAW, D.M.: Canad. Med. Ass. J., 1968, 99, 291.

WHITTINGHAM, S., MATHEWS, J.D., MACKAY,

I.R., STOCKS, A.E., UNGAR, B. and MARTIN. F.I.R.: Lancet, 1971, i, 763.

WIEDMANN, H.R., ToLKENDORF, M. and HANSET, H.G.: Lancet, 1964, i, 1166.

WIENER, K.: "Skin Manifestations of Internal Disorders", 1947, Kimpton, London.

WINKELMANN, R.K., MuLDER, D.W., LAMBERT, E.H., HowARD, F.M. Jr. and DIESSNER, G.R.: Proc. Mayo Clin., 1968, 43, 545.

WINKELMANN, R.K., SGHEEN, S.R. and UNDERDAHL, L.O.: J. Amer. Med. Ass., 1960, 174, 1145.

WILKINSON, J.F.: Brit. med. J., 1945, ii, 664.

WILKINSON, J.f.; Brit. med. J., 1950, ii, 576.

WILLIAMS, D.I.: Proc. R. Soc. Med., 1965, 58, 423.

WILLIAMs, E.D. and DoNIACH, L: J. Path. Bact., 1962, 83, 255.

Wn.LIAMS, E. and Woon, C.: Arch. Dis. Child, 1959, 34, 302.

WILLIAMS, E.D.: J. din. Path., 1965, 18, 288.

WILLIAMS, E.R.: Brit. J. Clin. Pract., 1968, 22, 461.

WILLIAMs, M.H., BROSTOFF, J. and RorTT, I.M.: Lancet, 1970, ii, 303.

WILLIAMS, M.H., BROSTOFF, J. and RoiTT, I.M.: Lancet, 1970, ii, 277.

WILLIAMS, R.C.: Ann. intern. Med., 1959, 50, 1174.

WILLIAMS, R.W.: "Textbook of Endocrinology", 1962, Saunders, Philadelphia.

WILLIER, B.H., WErss, P.A. and HAMBURGER, V.: "Analysis and Development", 1955, S: unders, Philadelphia.

WILLIS, R.A.: "The Spread of Tumours in the Human Body", 1952, 2nd. Edit., Butterworth, London.

WILLIS, R.A.: "The Borderland of Embryology and Pathology", 1958, Butterworth, London.

WILLis, R.A.: "The Pathology of Tumours", 1967, 4th. Edit. Butterworth, London.

WILMOT, A.J.: "Clinical Amoebiasis", 1962, Blackwell Scientific Publications, Oxford.

WILNER, D. and SIIERMAN, R.S.: Medical Radiography and Photography, 1966, 42, 35.

WlsLOCKI, G.B. and KING, L.S.: Arner. J. Anat., 1936, 58, 421.

WILSON, R.: Bull. Vancouver med. Ass., 1948, 24, 273.

WILSON, S.A.K.: "Neurology", 1940, Arnold, London.

WrLsoN, E., FINLEY, A.G. and KrLLINGBACK, M.: Brit. med. J., 1965, 2, 80.

WrLSON, F.C. and ORTt:N, L.S.: J. Bone Jt. Surg., 1965, 47, 1609.

WILTSHAW, E.: Brit. med. J., 1971, 2, 327.

WINTROBE, M.M.: "Clinical Hematology", 1967, 6th. Edit., Kimpton, London.

WJsEMAN, C. and LIAo, K.J.: Cancer (Philad.), 1972, 29, 1705.

WISHJEWSKI, M. and ToKER, C.: Mt. Sinai J. Med., 1973, 40, 681.

WISKETICH, S.T. and SIEGMUND, G.: Wien. klin. Wschr., 1961, 73, 473.

WoLFE, A.M. and BLACK, W.C.: Rocky Mountains med. J., 1941, 37, 581.

WOLF, J.K.: New Eng. J. Med., 1962, 266, 473.

WoLF, S.M.: Brit. med. J., 1972, I, 380.

WooD, C.B.S.: Proc. R. Soc. Med. Lit., 1963, 34, 1103.

WooLLEY, P.B.: Lancet, 1944, i, 85.

WooLNER, L.B., McCoNAHEY, W.M. and BEAHRS, O.H.: J. din. Endocrinol., 1959, 19, 53.

WoorNER, L.B., McCONAHEY, W.M., BEAHRS, O.H. and BLACK, B.M.: Amer. J. Surg., 1966, III, 502:

WoRLLEDGE, S.M., BRAIN, M.C., CooPER, A.C., HoBBS. JR. and DACIE, J.V.: Proc. R. Soc. Med., 1968, 61, 1312.

WRIGHT, D.J.M., DoNIACH, D., LESSOF, M.H., TuRK, J.L., GRIMBLE, A.S. and CATTERALL, R.D.: Lancet, 1970, i, 740.

WRIGHT, J.J. and RICHARDsON, P.C.: Brit. med. J., 1967, i, 530.

WRIGHT, R. and TRUELOVE, S.C.: Amer. J. Dig. Dis., 1966, 11, 831.

WRIGHT, R. and TRUELOVE, S.C.: Gut, 1966, 7, 32.

WRIGHT, V. and WATKINSON, G.: Amer. J. Proctol., 1966, 17, 107.

WRUBLE, L.D. and KAISER, M.H.: Amer. J. Med., 1964, 37, 118.

WvnuRN·MASON, R.: "Trophic Nerves", 1949, Kimpton, London.

WveuRN-MASON, R.: Brit. med. J., 1955, ii, 1106.

WvnURN·MASON, R.: Brit. med. J., 1957, ii, 615.

WvnuRN-MAsoN, R.: "The Reticulo-endothelial System in Growth and Tumour Formation", 1958, Kimpton, London.

WvnuRN-MAsON, R.: "A New Protozoon. Its Relation to Malignant and Other Diseases". 1964, Kimpton, London.

WvnuRN-MAsoN, R.: Lancet, 1966, i, 1266.

WvnuRN-MASON, R.: Proc. IXth. Int. Congress Chemotherapy, 1976, Vol. 6, Plenum, New York.

WvnURN-MAsON, R.: Lancet, 1976, i, 489.

WvNDER, E.L., LEMON, F.R. and BRoss, I.J.: Cancer (Philad.), 1959, 12, 1016.

WvsE, E.P., HILL, C., BRANEZ, M.L. and CLARK, R.L: Cancer (Philad.), 1969, 24, 701.

YAMAMOTO, T., CHANDOR, S., YoKOYAMA, M. et al.: Hawaii med. J., 1970, 29, 288.

YAKOLEVA, V.L.: Arkh. Patol., 1958, 20, 67.

YosHIKAWA, T. et al.: Acta Med. Bioi., Japan, 1960, 8, 1.

YosHIRO YAst:: Lancet, 1972, 2, 292.

YouNc. L.E.: In Cecil-Loeb "Textbook of Medicine", 1971, 13th. Edit., Edit. by Beeson, P.B. and McDermott, W., Saunders, Philadelphia.

ZACHAU-CHRISTIANSEN, B. and CHRISTIANSEN, H.E.: Acta. Path. Microbiol., Scand., 1966, 68, 343.

ZADEK, I.: Ergebn. ges Med., 1927, 10, 355.

ZAIDI, Z.H. and de BELLEFEUILLE, P.: Dis. Chest, 1960, 38, 343.

ZALIN, A.M., WEEPLE, J. and GuMPEL, M.: Brit. med. J., 1970, 4, 804.

ZARAFONETrS, C.J.D. et al.: Blood, 1957, 12, 1011.

ZAWADSKI, Z.A. and BENEDEK, T.G.: Arth. Rheum., 1969, 12, 555.

ZAWADSIU, Z.A., BENEDEK, T.G., EIN, D. and EASTON, J.M.: Ann. intern. Med., 1969, 70, 335.

ZAWADSKI, Z.A. and EDwARDS, G.A.: Amer. J. Med., 1970, 48, 196.

ZEROMSKI, J.O., GoRNY, M.K. and jARCZEWSKA, K.: Lancet, 1972, ii, 1035.

ZETZEL, L.: In Cecil-Loeb "Textbook of Medicine", 1971, 13th. Edit., Saunders, Philadelphia, 1971.

ZIEGLER, J.L., CoHEN, M.H. and Hurr, M.S.R.: Brit. med. J., 1969, 3, 15.

ZIEGLER, J.L. and STAIVER, R.C.: Brit. med. J., 1972, 3, 79.

ZocRAPHOV, D.G.: Acta. haematol. (Basel), 1962, 27, 60.

ZsAKO, S. and KAPLAN, A.R.: Amer. J. ment. Defic., 1968, 72, 809.

ZuFFA, M., KABANCOK, J., HoRVATH, A. et al.: Neoplasma (Bratisl.), 1972, 19, 141.

Additional References

AcKERMAN, N.B. and ARRJBAs, R.F.: Amer. J. Surg., 1976, 132, 660.

Aaus, B., KRisTT, D., GuMPORT, S.L. and SuN-sHINE, A.: N.Y. St. J. Med., 1975, 75, 1538.

BEHAN, P.O., DuRWARD, W.F. and DICK, W.: Lancet, 1976, ii, 803.

BERGERET, G., ALBOUY, R., BENE, P. et al.: Sem. Hop., Paris, 1975, 51, 1525.

BROOKS, A.P. and HARRINGTON, C.I.: Brit. med. J., 1977, ii, 739.

CHECKLEY, S.A. and BIRLEY, J.L.T.: Lancet, 1977, ii, 1258.

CuowoRTH, A.G. and WooDRow, J.C.: Brit. med. J., 1976, ii, 846.

DENT, C.E., JoNES, P.E. and MuLLAN, D.P.: Lancet, 1975, i, 1161.

EDGESK.JOLD, E-M., GRAUDAL, H., SoRENSEN, H.T. and PERMIN, H.: Lancet, 1977, ii, 456.

ETTINGER, D.S., HuMPHREY, R.L. and SKINNER, M.D.: Johns Hopkins Med. J., 1975, 137, 88.

EvERs, J.A.: Proc. R. Soc. Med., 1976, 69, 943.

FAIRFAX, A.J.: Proc. R. Soc. Med., 1977, 70, 327.

FODOR, J. and BonROGI, I.: Neoplasma (Bratisl.), 1975, 22, 445.

FowLER, J.M. and THOMAS, D.J.B.: Brit. med. J., 1976, 2, 737.

FRAUMENI, J.F. Jr., WECTELECKI, W., BLATTNER, W.A. et al.: Amer. J. Med., 1975, 59, 145.

GrRANDON, B., YvER, L., SunRE, Y. et al.: Nouv. Presse Med., 1976, 5, 137.

GoDEAU, P., HERREMAN, G., LANOE, R. et al.: Sem. Hop., Paris. 1975, 31, 2415.

GoaBAR, J.P.: Lancet, 1977, i, 1010.

GRADIENT, S.E. and KALFAYAN, B.: Oral. Surg., 1975, 40, 391.

GREGOR, R.T.: S. Afr. Med. J., 1976, 50, 1447.

GuM PEL, J.M. and CRow, J.: Case presented at the Royal Society of Medicine. London, on October 8th. 1976.

HALL-SMITH, P.: Proc. R. Soc. Med., 1976, 69, 380.

HECKMAYR. M., SEIFERT, G. and DoNATH, K.: Laryng. Rhinal. Otol. Grenzgeb., 1976, 55, 593.

HENRIKSSON, K.G., HALLERT, C. and WALAN, A.: Lancet, 1976, ii, 317.

HER NANDEZ PEREZ, E.: Med. Cutanea Ibero. Lat. Am., 1975, 3, 47.

HoRTON, W.A.: Birth defects orig. Art. Sci., 1976, 12, 91.

KoEPPEN, A.H., BisHOP, M.B. and Kou DOURis, S.: J. Neurol. Sci. (Arnst.), 1976, 27, 123.

LAPRESSLE, J., RADADOT, J. and SAID, G.: J. Neural. Sci. (Arnst.), 1976, 28, 249.

LENDER, M., LAWRENCE, A.M. and PALOVAN, E.: Lancet, 1977, i, 1110.

LowE, W.C.: N.J. St. J. Med., 1976, 76, 926.

LuNo-OLESEN, K.: Curr. Ther. Res., 1977, 21, 704.

LuTWYCHE, V.U.: Chest, 1976, 70, 292.

LYNH, H.T., LYNCH, J. and LYNCH. P.: Arch. Surg., 1975, 110, 1227.

MACAK, J.: Acta Univ. Palacki Olomuc. Fac.

Med., 1975, 73, 229.

MciNNES, G.T.: Brit. med. J., 1977, i, 685.

MACKENZIE, A.H.: Arth. Rheum., 1970, 13, 280.

NARASIMHAM, P., JAGATHAMBAL, K., ELIZALDE, A.M. and RosNER, F.: Arch. int. Med., 1975, 135, 729.

NILsEN, K.H.: N.Z. Med. J., 1976, 83, 320.

NrME, F.F.A., COOPER, H.S. and EccLESTON, J.C.: Cancer (Philad.), 1976, 37, 906.

OTTERNEss, I. and NIBLACK, J.: Lancet, 1976, 1, 148.

PACHMAN, L.M., JoANASSON, O., CANNON, R.A. and FRIEDMAN, J.M.: Lancet, 1977, 2, 1238.

PHILLIPS, R.N., RETSAS, S. and NEwTON, K.A.: Brit. med. J., 1977, i, 1447.

PINcHING, A.J., PETERS, D.R. and DAvrs, J.M.: Lancet, 1976. ii, 1373.

RAr, G.S., HAMLYN, A.N., DAHL, M.G.C., MoRLEY, D.R. and Wn.KINSON, R.: Brit. med. J., 1977, i, 817.

RATNAKAR, K.S., LAKSHMINARAYAN, C.A., RAMACHANDRAIAH, U. and RAcHu, C.R.: Indian J. Surg., 1976, 38, 254.

RooNEY, P.J., BALLANTYNE, D. and BucHANAN, W.W.: 1975, in Clinics in Rheumatic Disseases. Edit. E.G. Bywaters, Saunders, London.

SANDSTROM, C.: Acta Path. Microbial. Scand. Sect. A., 1976, 84, 317.

SANY, J., MoRLOCK, G., CLOT, J. et al.: Rev. Rheum., 1976, 43, 1.

ScoTT, J.S.: Lancet, 1976, 1, 78.

SEGAr., A.W., LEvi, A.J. and LoEwr, G.: Brit. med. J., 1977, ii, 555.

SuMNER, P. and DwEK, J.H.: N.Y. St. J. Med., 1976, 76, 94.

TAGAMI, H., IMAMURA, S., NozucHI, S. and NISHITANI, H.: Dermatologica (Basel), 1976, 152, 181.

TsuDA, H., FuKUSHIMA, S., TAKAHASHI, M. et al.: Cancer (Philad.), 1976, 37, 1831.

TwERSKY, J., TwERSKY, N. and LEHR, S.: Clin. Radiol, 1976, 22, 203.

TwoMEY, J.J., RossEN, R.D., LEwrs, V.M. et al.: Proc. Nat. Acad. Sci. U.S.A., 1976, 73, 2106.

VIETA, J.O. and DELGADO, G.E.: Dis. Colon Rect., 1976, 19, 56.

WALKER, W.R. and KEATs, D.M.: Agents and Actions, 1976, 6, 454.

WELLINGS, F.M., LEwrs, A.L. and AMuso, P.T.: Lancet, 1977, i, 199.

WrLLAERT, E. and STEVENs, A.R.: Lancet, 1976, ii, 741.

WYBURN-MAsON, R.: Lancet, 1976, 1, 489.

ZEROMSKI, J., ZrELESKIEwrcz, M. and KRYZSKO, R.: Ann. Immunol. (Poznan), 1975, 7, 137.

-479-

These are Roger Wyburn-Mason's after-thoughts once his book was published!

Page 11: Kirby J, and Munro D.D. Proc. R. Soc.Med., 1977, 70, 748. report a case with overlap of several collagen diseases. Ramos-Niembro F., Alancon-Segovia D. and Hernandez-Ortiz J. Arth. Rheum. 1979, 22, 43.discussed 28 cases of mixed connective tissue disease with arthropathy, SLE, Scleroderma or polymyositis with positive rheumatoid factor in the serum. MCTD is also discussed in Mixed Connective tissue disease—a decade of growing pains, Alarcon-Segovia D. J. Rheumatol. 1981, 8 535-540.

Page 15: Crisp, A.J., Hoffbrand, B.I. , J. Roy.Soc. Med. 1980, 73, 60-61, report a case of Sjogren's syndrome which developed ulcerative colitis with negative RA, ANF and autoantibodies in the blood. The patient was treated with prednisolone and sulphasaalzine and afterwards developed rheumatoid arthritis, tender subcutaneous patches and nodules on the face, scalp and limbs with surrounding hair loss. The serum ANF was now positive. Skin biopsy showed vasculitis. She then developed pyrexia, chest pain and an enlarged cardaic shadow and bilateral basal pleural effusions. The serum, ANF and RF were now positvie. The sulphasalazine was stopped and antibiotics and steroids given with speedy recovery and the patient remained well for 4 years.

Addendum: Brooks, A.P. and Paulley, J.W. Brit.Med.J., 1980, 280, 480, describe the case of a male patient with antibody positive hypothyroidsim and hypertension who was given hydrallazine and afterwards developed polyarthraglia, fever, malaise, chest pains, haemoptosis, vasculitis, anaemia, raised ESR and ANF in the serum. Symptoms regressed with withdrawal of hydrallazine.

Page 16: Montiero, E., Ceboleiro. C. and Galvas-Teles, D. Lancet, 1979, 2. 797 report that in 90 cases of adult rheumatoid arthritis, 13 of juvenile rheumatoid arthritis and 27 of ankylosing spondylits 18%, 27% and 17% respectively of ant-microsomalthyroid antibodies were demonstrated by immunofluorescence.

Page 17: Reid, J.M. and Murdoch, R., Brit. Heart. Journ. 1979, 41, 628-629 report a case of complete heart block occurring 4 years after the onset of polymyositis.

Addendum: Dermatomyositis associated with fibrosing alveolitis was described by Plowman, P.N. and Stableforth, D.E. (Proc. R. Soc. Med., 1977, 70, 738). Another case of dermatomyositis without apparent myositis, but com- plicated by fibrosing alveolitis was reported by Fernandes, L. and Goodwill, C.T., J. Roy. Soc. Med ., 1979, 72, 777.

480

Page 21: Rheumatoid nodules formatoin within the choroid plexus. Report of a second case. Kim RC, Collins, GH, Paris, JE. Arch PatholLab Med 1982, 106, 83 - 84

Page 22: Benign rheumatoid nodules may occur in children. Roggins DL, Moore, TL, Naguwa SM Clin. Rheumatol. 1982, 1/ 2104-111 In the absence of obvious rheumatoid disease.

Addendum: Rheumatoid nodules also occur in systemic sclerosis (Bywaters, E.G.L., Journ. Rheumatol 1979, 6, 243-246)

Page 26: Rheumatoid lymphoedema. Kyle VM, de Silva M, Hurst G. Clinical Rheumatology 1982, 1 /2 126·7. This occurs in upper limbs due to abnormalities of the lymphatics resulting from lymphangitis secondary to the inflammatory process of the disease. The demonstration of lymphatic channels on wrist arthrography in rheumatoid disease with particular reference to associated lymphoedema. Wu g, Whitehouse GH, Littler TR, Lwasowe Hosp. LiverpoolUK. Rheumatol. Rehabil1982, 21, 65-71.

Page 30: Hamilton, D.V. (J.R. Soc.Med., 1978, 71, 147) describes a woman of 68 with S.L.E. with rheumatic symptoms, myxoedema due to Hashimoto's thyroiditis and atrophic gastritis and pernicious anaemia. Her mother was crippled with rheumatoid arthritis and the patient's twin brothers have Hashimoto's thyroiditis and one diabetes.

Page 31: Blizzard, R.M., Clee, D., ft Davis, W., Clin. Exp. lmmunol. 1966, 1, 119, reported idiopathic hypoparathyroidism, Addison 's disease, diabetes mellitus and ovarian failure together. E monds,.0.E· Sa u.ers,, A., Sturrock, R.D., j. Roy. Soc. Med., 1979, 72, 856·8, described a case of rheumatoid arthntis wlth SJogrens syndrome and hypoparathyroidism.

Page 32: Botazzo, G.F. and Doniach, D., J. Roy. Soc. M.D., 1978, 7, 43, and Gleson e. t., Arch.- ah. Lab. Med., 1978, 102, 46, also describe cases of lymphocytic hypophyslits either associated With thyroiditis, gastritis or adrenalitis or with unexplained arthralgias.

Page 33: Dr. M.C.J. Rudolf at the Annual American Diabetes Association, 1980, reported from the Yale Regional Center of the Connecticut Program for Children with Diabetes (InternationalMedicalNews Service, 1980) a group of diabetic children developing the adult form of rheumatoid arthritis with positive RF or significant titers of anti-nuclear antibodies or mitochondrialantibodies in 6 or 7 children. These clinical and serological features were often associated with auto-immune disorders related to SLE, Type I diabetes pellitus is often associated with auto-immune thyrogastric disorders as they were in the above cases, six of the 7 patients had organ-specific antibodies to either thyroid microsomes, tyroglobulin, parietalor adrenalcells. Six children had the HLA alleles DRw3 or DRw4 which have been associated with HSKS for type I diabetes mellitus and RA.

Page 37: Mycarditis may occur in scleroderma patiels with inflammatory infiltrates with muscle fibre destruction in skeletal and heart muscle.

Congenital heart block often with endomycardial fibrosis occurs in neonatal SLE often born of mothers with active connective tissue disease (Esscher, E. and Scott, J.S. (Brit. med. J., 1979, 1, 1235, Hardy, J. et al., Arch. Dis. Childlt., 1979, 54, 7)

Immunogenetics and Essential Hypertension. Leading Article, Lancet, 1978, ii, 409. People with essential hypertension are more likely than normotensive controls to have RF, thyroid and other auto-antibodies a nd raised IgG and IgA in their serum , raising the possibility that essential hypertension a nd some of the immuno- logical changes share genetic and environmental causes and that some immunological changes are contributory causes of essential hypertension. Hypertensive patients with raised IgG concentrations or wit h serum auto·antibodies more commonly give a family history of h ypertension than patients

without immunological changes. H LA lin ked genes are also probably important in the aetiology of essential hypertension.

Page 39: Epstein, O., Thomas, H.C. and Sherlock, S., Primary Biliary Cirrhosis is a dry gland syndrome with features of Chronic Graft-Versus-Host disease. Lancet, 1980, 1, 1166-1168. Primary biliary cirrhosis is part of a disease complex characterized by dry eyes, dry mouth and both biliary and pancreatic hyposecretions: it is a "dry gland" syndrome resulting from damage to ductular epithelium. Additional extraglandular features include scherodermatous skin changes, skin pigmentation, Raynaud's phenomena and associated with other auto-immune diseases, especially rheumatoid arthritis and Hashimoto's thyroidis, and evidence of Sjchallenge. Large concentrations of circulating immune responses IgM, IgG, and anti-antibodies may be found. The whole picture resembles either a chronic graft-versus-host disease or a chronic antigenic stimulation. The disease in fact forms part of the rheumatoid disease complex.

Page 41: Descam ps, Ch., Gillain , P., Van Heuverzwyn , P. et al. Acta gastro-ent. belg., 1977, 40, 55, descnbe a case of ulcerative colitis with cholecystitis and progressive sclerosing cholangitis. They point out that ulcerative colitis is often associated with coeliac disease, chronic active hepatitis, biliary cirrhosis (all auto-immune dieseases), sclerosing cholangitis and chola ngiocarcinoma.

Page 44: Venous ulcers. Thurtle OA, Cawley MID. Lancet 1982, ii 722.Patients with RA twice as liable to leg uclers as OA controls and in a prospective study of 15 patients with RA and leg ulceration six had ulcers that were venous in appearance. Of these only one had severe VVS but the other 5 had marked RA of ipsilateral ankle joint, which by contrast was only slightly involved in patient with severe VVs. Severe ankle joint dysfunction might seriously impair calf muscle venous pump and might this have a haemodynamic effect on the dermal capillary bed similar to that resulting from incompetent perforating veins, predsiposing these patients to a "venous" type of leg ucleration.

Page 48: Acne link with arthritis. Davis DE et al. J. Rheumatol1981 8 2 317-320. Acne may be linked with rheumatoid arthritis.

Page 62: Giardiasis *and severe jejunal abnormality*. Blenkinsopp, W.K., Gibson, J.A. and Haffenden, G.P., Lancet, 1978, i , 994, describe the case of a 65 year old woman, who developed watery diarrhoea 3 weeks after returning to England from a tour of the Far East. She lost weight, developed pitting oedema of the ankles, low serum albumin and high faecal fat excretion. Six stoolspecimens were negative for parasites. Jejunal biopsy revealed severe partial villous atrophy and a dense plasma-cell infiltration of the lamina propria. There was a heavy infiltration with *Giardia Iamblia*. A course of metronidazole rapidly cured the patient, the jejunal mucosa returned to normal and the Giardia disappeared.

Page 65: Boss JM Peachey RDG, Easty DL, Thomsitt J. Peripheral corneal melting syndrome with psoriasis. A report of two cases. Brit. med. J ., 1981, 282, 609-10. The syndrome consists of marginal corneal thinning, sometimes to the extent of perforation . It is often seen in rheumatoid arthritis, Sjogren's syndrome, polyarteritis nodosa or psoriasis.

Addendum: Retinal vasculitis may occr in RD and SLE or in the absence of these diseases with RF in the serum. It is possibly due to raised concentration of circulating immune complexes. Retinal vasculitis in RA. Martin MFR, Scott DGI , Gilbert C, Dieppe PA, Easty DL. Brit med J 1981 282 1745-6.

Page 67: Relapsing polychondritis. This condition appears to be "auto-immune" in nature (Clayton, R.N. and Hoffenberg, R., Brit. med. J., 1978, 2, 999). It may affect aural, nasal, trachael and articular cartilage producing deafness and arthropathy. It may be associated with Hashimoto's thyroiditis with myxoedema, goitre, expohthalmos and ophthalmoplegia, diabetes mellitus, vitiligo and arthropathy. Auto-antibodies to human cartilage, thryoglobulin, intrinsic factor and gastric parietal cells may be present in the serum.

Page 70: Pure red cell aplasia may be associated with SLE, thymoma, autoimmune hypothyroidism or multiple endocrine insufficiency.

Page 71: Waugh, D, Ibels, L. Malginant scleroderma associated with autoimmune neutropenia. Brit. med. J., 1980, 280, 1577-8 reported a case of scleroderma developing autoimmune neutropenia and mentioned that autoimmune haemolytic anaemia, thrombocytopenia and pancytopenia may occur in patients with scleroderma.

Page 77: Acquired haemophilia. Leading Article, Lancet 1981, i, 255. This condition may occur especially in elderly females. There is a well recognized association with autoimmune or allergic diseases, including rheumatoid arthritis a nd other collagen-vascular diseases, cancer, pemphigus, ulcerative colitis and asthma or as a side effect of drug therapy. The blood contains a circulating anticoag ulant with special activity against Factor VIII in the blood. It is an antibody usually of the IgG class and evidently arises in response to the organism producing rheumatoid and autoimmune diseases. Acquired haemophilia. Duran-Sua rez JR, Pigra u-Serra llach C, Bosch-Gil JA, Triginer-Boixeda J, Lancet 1981, i, 723. report that 46 of 6,000 patients had circulating anticoagulants, (against Factor VIII in 27) 8 of these 27 patients had acquired haemophilia and the rest had other diseases, including active chronic hepatitis, SLE and cancer.

Page 79: Galli, M., Landi, G., Rastelli, D.L. and Scarlato, G. Myasthenia gravis with a monclonal gammopathy. Report of a case, J. Neurol. Sci., 1980, 45 /1, 103-108. The authors report the fourth case of an elderly man with myasthenia and monclonal gammopathy.

Page 83: Rheumatoid periostitis of calcaneus responds to drilling treatment. Cheu Boaxing and Li Zumou. Chinese Med. J. 1981, 94. 5. 288·290 Rheumatoid periostitis is well recognized.

Addendum: Adult onset hypogammaglobulinaemia may be associated with various autoimmune diseases, namely primary hypothyroidism and hyperthyroidism; atrophic gastritis with pernicious anaemia; vitiligo; alopecia areata; diabetes; Coombs·positive haemolytic anaemia; autoimmune neutropenia; idiopathic thrombocytopenia and coeliac disease. Relatives more commonly than normal subjects show organ-specific autoantibodies in their blood. Development of insulin-dependent diabetes in adult onset hypogammaglobulinaemia. Young. RJ, Duncan LJ, Paton L. Yap PL. Brit. med. J., 1981, 2.82, 1668.

Page 90: Guyer, P.B. and Chamberlain A.T. Paget'a dis ease of bone into American cities. Brit. med. J., 1980, 280, 985. Paget's disease of bone is rare among African Blacks. The authors investigated its incidence in two American cities, New York and Atlanta, Georgia, in both Blacks and Whites and also at different latitudes in both sexes. The incidence proved the same in both cities, sexes, and cool countries. This provides evidence of the influence of environment in the aetioolgy of the disease and is in favour of the organsimal nature of the disease rather than a metabolic one.

Addendum: Guyer PB. Radiology in Paget's disease. Clinical and aetiological significance. Hospital Update, 1980, 6, 1079-1091. The author points out that the disease varies in frequency in different parts of the world and different parts of the country.. There is no evidence for its cause by an environmental factor.

Addendum: Solomon I.R. (Brit. med. J., 1979, i, 931) points out that Paget's disease often occurs at sites of pressure, recalling r a similar phenomenon in the case of rheumatoid nodules, psoriasis (often assocaited witth rheumatoid dsi ease), syphyilis and the localization of pathogens to such sites mentioned by Pasteur, Koch and also by Burrows (1932), suggesting the organismal nature of Paget's disease.

Addendum: Lievre, J.A. (La Presse Medicate, 1936, 3, 45 and J. Beige de Rhumatol et Med. Physique Acta, Med. Be ge., 1974, 29, 322), Solomon, I.R. (Brit. med. J., 1979, i, 931) and Gasper T.M. (Ibid, 1217) point out that Paget's disease (often occurs at sites of pressure, recalling a similar phenomenon in the case of rheumatoid disease), syphilis and the localization of pathogens to such sites mentioned by Pasteur, Koch and also by Burrows (1932), suggesting the organismal nature of Paget's disease.

Page 107: Crisp, A.J., Hoffbrand, B.I., J. Roy.Soc. Med. 1980, 73, 60-61, report a case of Sjogren's syndrome which developed ulceratvie colitis with negative RA, ANF and autoantibodies in the blood. The patient was treated with prednisolone and sulphasalaznie and afterwards developed rheumatoid arthritis, tender subcutaneous patches and nodules on the face, scalp and limbs with surrounding hair loss. The serum ANF was now positive. Skin biopsy showed vasculitis. She then developed pyrexia, chest pain and an enlarged cardiac shadow: and.bilateral scalp effusions. The serum ANF and RF were now positive. The sulphasalazine was

485

stopped and antibiotics given with speedy recovery and the patient remained well for 4 years.

Addendum: Brooks, A.P. and Paulley, J.W. Brit. Med. J., 1980, 280, 480, describe the case of a male patient with antibody positive hypothyroidsim and hypertension who was given hydrallazine and afterwards developed polyarthralgia, ever malaise, chest pains, haemoptosis, vasculitis, anaemia, raised ESR and ANF in the serum. Symptoms regressed with withdrawalof hydrallazine.

Page 110: :Schweiger F. (International Medical News, October 1st. 1980) stated at a meeting of the RoyalCollege of Physicians and Surgeons of Canada that the aetiology of RA is unlikely to be associated with the genetic marker HLA—DRw3 or 4 or with virus infection.

Page 116: Arthritis and arthralgia associated with toxocaral infestation. Williams D, Roy S. Brit. med. J., 1981 283, 192, The authors report cases of toxocaral infection with transient arthropathy and also arthritis and arthralgia with various filarial infestations cured by diethyl-carbamazine.

Page 118: Species of free-living amoebae may be non-pathogenic or pathogenic to different animals including man.
Addendum: Elsdon-Dew, R. (Lancet, 1979, i, 1038) points out that pathogenic Entamoeba histolytica produce cytotoxins, toxins and specific iso-enzymes and that the body produces serum antibodies to the pathogenic type. The same may be true of some species of free-living amoebae.

Page 125: A leading Article, Brit. med. J., 1978, ii, 379, emphasizes false-positive identification of entamoeba histolytica in mistake for leucocytes in sections or vice versa failure to diagnose amoebiasis by clinicians of lab- oratories to regard amoebae as leucocytes. Identification requires skill and diligence. Amoebae are easily missed in routine histological sections and requires immunofluorescent techniques by an expert.

Page 137: Bruusgaard, A. and Andersen, R.B., Lancet, 1976, 1, 700, reported that the administration of chenodeoxycholic acid chemically closely related to deoxycholic acid, 750-1000 mgm. daily for 3-11 weeks to 16 patients with rheumatoid arthritis caused initial exaggeration of the joint and general condition, some- times rather severe, and accompanied by fever. This was followed by obvious remission in the disease and fall in the ESR.

Page 179: The beneficial effect of jaundice and bile salts and their derivatives in rheumatodi patients has been confirmed by Sulilvan SN. The effect of jaundice on rheumatoid arthritis J Rheuymatoid 1980., 7. 417-418 and Famaey J-P J.

486

Rheumatol 1981 8 181.

Page 197: Relief first time for many years and after this single [dose] daily normal motions. The abdominal aching gradually decreased and disappeared over the next week and at the end of which time the evidence of arthropathy in the fingers had largely disappeared the joints being cool and no longer reddened or swollen. She was followed up and able to return to a normal diet and ceased taking Salasopyrin. The symptoms and signs in the knees disappeared. She has remained well without bowel or joint symptoms over a year when a repeat barium enema was normal and her anxiety depressive symptoms had disappeared.

Addendum: That ulcerative colitis and its not uncommonly associated arthropathy are the result of free-living amoebic infection is shown by the results of treatment of patients suffering from this disease with 5-nitroimidazoles as exemplified by the following case. Female, aged 67 years. No family history of rheumatoid disease. At the age of 51 years hysterectomy for fibroids resulting in Menorrhagia and anaemia. At the age of 24 she began to suffer from intermittent bouts of diarrhoea with the passage of large amounts of slime and occasionally of blood. On investigation at the age of 65 years she showed the presence of the typical radiological changes of ulcerative colitis confirmed by rectal biopsy. Throughout the course of this disease she had been affected by depression and anxiety symptoms requiring anti-depressant drugs. After the diagnosis of ulcerative colitis she was treated with a low residue diet and Salasopyrin, which controlled the abdominal symptoms reasonably well. Three years before being seen she developed pain, redness, swelling and restriction of movement of the peripheral interphalangeal joints of all her fingers, but not the thumb, pain and hotness of both knees with some restricted flexion and some pains in the neck. She was treated with Tinidazole 2 grams on two successive evenings. This resulted in influenzal-like symptoms after the first dose with mild pyrexia and sweating, a constant ache across the abdomen and increased pain and swelling of the affected finger joints with involvement of the. midinterphalangeal joints of the fingers with pain redness and swelling. On the day after the first dose of Tinidazole she had three normal motions for the first time for many years and after this single [dose] daily normal motions. The abdominal aching gradually decreased and disappeared over the next week and at the end of which time the evidence of arthropathy in the fingers had largely disappeared the joints being cool and no longer reddened or swollen. She was followed up and able to return to a normal

487

diet and ceased taking Salasopyrin. The symptoms and signs in the knees disappeared. She has remained well without bowel or joint symptoms over a year when a repeat barium enema was normal and her anxiety depressive symptoms had disappeared.

Page 203: *Chenodeoxycholic acid in the prevention of migraine.* Levy, V.G., Nusinovici, V., Roner, D. and Darnis, F. New Eng. J.Med., 1978, 298, 630. Chenodeoxycholic acid is closely related chemically to bile acids and has similar properties. The above authors report markedly favourably on the effects of this substance on cases of migraine in doses of 200 mgms. three times daily. In a personal case a doctor, now aged 67 years old, who had suffered from migraine with speech difficulties all his life, took copper sulphate 25 mgms. three times daily for three weeks with immediate cessation of migraine over the next year. The author, therefore, tried the effect of this form of treatment over four weeks as compared with a placebo on 25 cases each of typical migraine not helped by other treatment. In all but two of the cases treated with copper sulphate there was an immediate cessation of migraine attacks lasting *over* 9-12 months. In other words two cases the frequency and severity of attacks was markedly lessened.

Page 205: Addendum: The effects of tinidazole on various manifestations of rheumatoid disease is the following: <u>Female, aged 67 years.</u> Born with a pigmented mole on the dorsum of the right hand. At puberty the left breast became notably larger than the right. From early life she had frequent cracks on the skin of the finger pulps. At her only pregnancy at the age of 21 years the left breast became even larger than the right, tender and swollen, but yielded no milk through the nipple, even with a pump. From that time it always remained larger than the right with periods when it became painful and tender and required extra support. There was never any abnormality with the right breast. From time to time painful areas could be detected in the left breast. The difference in size persisted even after the menopause. From the time of the pregnancy she noticed that the left upper eyelid would droop prinicipally round the time of the menses, but also when tired. At the age of 47 years a lipoma as big as a walnut appeared at the lower aspect of the right shoulder blade. She also developed attacks of acute cholecystitis with pain and tenderness in the right hypochondrium, pyrexia, sweating, severe pain in the region of the left shoulder blade and later became mildly jaundiced. The pain was of such severity as to require morphine injections. At operation an enormously dilated gall bladder was found adherent to the transverse colon, duodenum and liver, but

488

no gall stones. The common bile duct was, however, found to be thickened. A diagnosis of cholecystitis with sclerosing cholangitis was made. from that time she suffered from irregular attacks of severe pain in the region of the left shoulder blade appearing for no apparent reason and requiring morphine or they were relieved by nitroglycerine tablets. The attacks lasted up to 24 hours. These appeared to be resulting from the sclerosing cholangeitis. About the same time she developed marked thickening if the skin of the soles of the feet which became very tender and developed severe painful cracks with extreme dryness of the skin. She also developed pads of fat on the anterior aspect of both legs just below the knees. From the time of the menopause at the age of 56 years she was subject to occasional attacks of right-sided sciatica lasting 2-3 weeks eased by aspirin compounds. X-rays of the lumbar spine were normal. Blood count and ESR were normal and RF negative. She was given a single dose of 2G tinidazole and in about 4 hours she felt shivery, but otherwise there were no symptoms. One week later she suddenly awoke in the night with sweating, generalized headache and pain in the back of the peck with nausea and severe pain in the region of the left shoulder blade. This lasted about 4 hours and after which time the patient was symptomless except for a generalized sensaton of gooseflesh and a shivery feeling, but no temperature or sweating. Ten days after taking tinidazole the left breast became extremely painful, tender and hot, especially in the inferior segment where there appeared a red discolouration beneath the skin over an area of tenderness suggesting an inflammatory change. The pain extended into the axilla and down the upper arm. The symptoms lasted for several days before gradually disappearing. From this time the thickened, cracked skin of the soles of the feet disappeared as did the drooping of the left eyelid, sciatica and the fatty lumps below the knees became tender but smaller. Nineteen days after taking tinidazole she developed marked generalized itching of the skin which persisted. There was notable diuresis and the feet becane smaller requiring two sizes smaller in shoes. The inflammatory mastitis had now almost disappeared. She also experienced during the first 3 weeks fleeting pains and crepitus in the finger joints. After 5 weeks she was symptomless and the attacks of sciatica, pain in the region of the left shoulder blade and the drooping of the left eyelid disappeared completely. The lipoma was no longer palpable. In addition the congenital pigmented mole on the back of the dorsum of the right hand and numerous acquired senile keratoses and pigmented sopte on the

489

dorsum of both hands and sides of the neck became depigmented and the keratoses disappeared. She now felt and looked extremely well. This case indicates the beneficial effects of tinidazole on sclerosing cholangeitis, chronic cystic mastitis, myasthenic like symptoms of the eyelid, thickening and cracking of the skin of the feet and fingers, sciatica in the absence of bony changes in the lumbar spine, congenital and acquired pigmented lesions of the skin and keratoses and a lipomata. Follow up over the course of a year showed no recurrence.

Addendum: In 1922 (a) and (b) the eminent Californian protozoologists Kofoid and Swezy reported on the finding of an amoeba in the bone marrow in cases of rheumatoid arthritis and in the affected lymph nodes in cases of Hodgkin's disease. The amoeba was distinguished from other normal human cells by its mitotic processes and by the fact that it appeared to contain only 6 chromosomes. They suggested a causal relationship of the organism to the two diseases. At first they considered the amoeba to be an aberrant form of *Entamoeba histolytica*, but later that it was a free-living amoeba. Kofoid CA, Swezy 0. Mitosis in *Endamoeba dysenteriae* in the bone marrow in arthritis deformans. Univ. Calif. Publ. Zool. 1922 (a) 20, 301-7. Kofoid CA, Boyers LM, Swezy 0. Endamoeba dysenteriae in the lymph glands of man in Hodgkin's disease. Univ. Calif. Publ. Zool. 1922 (b), 20, 309-12.

Addendum: Several patients who had suffered from chronic cholecystitis accompanied by sclerosing cholangitis were treated by chole-cystectomy, but the sclerosing process in the bile ducts led to recurrent obstructive jaundice treated surgically on several occasions. They were then given tinidazole 2G. at two weekly intervals. This led to immediate influenzal-like symptoms and 6-10 days later to symptoms identical with those of cholangitis with nausea, vomiting, pain between the shoulder blades and fever, but without jaundice. These lasted six days on the first occasion and then gradually became less severe and shorter with successive doses, finally disappearing, the patient becoming completely symptomless and remaining so while being observed over 18 months, suggesting healing of the sclerosing process in the bile ducts.

Addendum: The effect of metronidazole or tinidazole on migraine. Not infrequently in the author's experience typical unrelated headache, constituting migraine or other forms of headache, were found to occur in cases of rheumatoid disease and treatment of the latter with either tinidazole or metronidazole relieved both the rheumatoid disease and caused disappearance of the headache during observation over one to two years.

The effect of metronidazole or tinidazole on endogenous asthma. As already indicated endogenous asthma not infrequently occurs in patients with rheumatoid disease. The asthma usually persists in spite of all known treatment. In such cases it was found that treatment of the rheumatoid disease resulted in the complete disappearance of the asthmatic attacks while under observation. This began with the first dose of the drug. The author, therefore, treated 20 cases of endogenous asthma in the absence of evidence of rheumatoid disease and compared, in a double blind trial, the effect of metronidazole with a placebo. While the latter had no effect on the incidence of the asthmatic attacks, in the patients treated with metronidazole asthma ceased immediately and during the period of observation of 1-2 years did not return.

Addendum: Cervical spondylitis, lumbago and sciatica. It has been seen that rheumatoid infection may involve any or all parts of the spine, including the cervical and lumbar regions. In cases of rheumatoid disease this may show itself as backache or stiffness, occipital headache, lumbago and sciatica forming part of the general disease. In such cases there are at first no radiological changes. Successful treatment of the disease causes the above symptoms to disappear. When nitroimidazole drugs are administered to cases of rheumatoid disease not exhibiting these symptoms the Herxheimer response may include temporary neckache and stiffness, lumbago and sciatica, which disappear in a few days. In 20 subjects of lumbago and sciatica not exhibiting radiological changes or evidence of rheumatoid disease in which all other treatment had failed, it was found that in all cases administration of a single 2G dose of metronidazole or tinidazole either caused a temporary increase in symptoms for a few days and then their rapid disappearance or their complete disappearance within a few days without return wnile under observation. This was often accompanied by short-lived peripheral arthropathy or tenosynovitis, headache and sweating, typical of rheumatoid infection. identical reaction occurred in all of 32 cases of cervical spondylitis with symptoms. Thus, this condition and lumbago and sciatica in the absence of radiological changes thus usually a manifestation of rheumatoid disease of the lumbar spine.

Addendum: Williams, B.D., Lockwood, C.M., Pussell, B.A., Brit. med. J., 1979, 2, 235-238, reported typical Herxheimer reactions 18 hours after injections of gold salts into cases of rheumatoid arthritis and pointed out that gold not only reduces symptoms, but may slow or even halt the disease. The author found that, like copper, gold salts had a markedly inhibitory reaction on Naegleria in vitro.

Addendum: The effect of 5-nitro-

491

imidazoles on cases of psoriasis. As indicated in Part I of this monograph cases of true rheumatoid arthritis are not uncommonly associated with psoriasis quite apart from the separate condition of psoriatic arthropathy. In all the cases of rheuma- toid arthritis combined with psoriasis treated by 5-nitroimidazoles (22 in number) with the rapid lessening of activity of the rheumatoid disease the skin lesions disappeared completely and did not recur again even after completion of treatment. This suggested the possibility that psoriasis in the absence of arthropathy might perhaps respond to therapy with 5-nitro-imidazole drugs. Ten such cases, all of long standing, and all of which had received various forms of therapy without benefit, were treated with weekly doses of 2G. of tinidazole or metronidazole. in most cases the first one or two doses produced an Herxheimer reaction in the form of influenzal-like symptoms and in two cases transient swelling of one or more joints. After three weeks treatment the psoriasis showed considerable improvement and in three of the ten cases after two months the skin lesions had practically disappeared but it was found necessary to continue the treatment, otherwise the skin lesions would tend to recur in various degrees. In all the other cases it was necessary to give daily ultra violet ray treatment to the body in order to obtain partial or almost complete disappearance of the skin lesions which,

however, reappeared when the ultra violet treatment was stopped. One case failed to respond to either the single or combined form of treatment.

Addendum: The effect of 5-nitro-imidazoles on cases of coeliac disease. When 5-nitro-imidazoles, such as tinidazole, in doses of 2G. once weekly, are administered to cases of coeliac disease which are symptomless as a result of taking a gluten-free diet, within a few hours they induce a constant central abdominal aching lasting for several days. This recurs with repeated doses until it eventually disappears. This procedure was carried out in five cases of coeliac disease, who had first been diagnosed before the ages of one year and up to six years and who had been on a gluten-free diet and symptomless for as long as 20 years. Prior to beginning weekly treatment with 2G. of 5-nitro- imidazoles subtotal villous atrophy of the jejunal mucosa was present in spite of the dietary restriction. After weekly treatment with 5-nitro-imidazoles for about 2 months challenged with a normal diet did not cause symptoms of coeliac disease and a repeat of the jejunal biopsy showed completely normal appearances. The cases have been followed through for two years with a monthly dose of the drug, on a normal diet, without recurrence of symptoms. In several patients following early treatments there occurred short-lived pain and swelling of various joints

492

and the skin became markedly smooth. If the treatment is stopped, however, after three months the jejunal abnormalities reappear.

Addendum: Effect of 5-nitro-imidazoles on Paget's disease of bone. In an 83 year old male with Paget's disease of the upper end of both femora and of both sides of the pelvis and an ESR of 55mm. per hour with some degree of aching in the affected region, the administration of weekly doses of tinidazole alternating with metronidazole produced an Herxheimer reaction in the affected region with increase in pain the day after the weekly dose. This was followed by lessening of the Herxheimer reaction and of the naturally occurring pain followed by a fall in the ESR to normal.

Addendum: Other features of rheumatoid disease which were encountered and which were not present in the patient prior to treatment with 5-nitroimidazoles were as follows: a). painful rheumatoid nodules appearing round the elbows, around the sacrum and elbows in a very thin long-standing case. These disappeared three months after treatment. b). an area of cystic mastitis in a patient recurring at the same site as a cystic mastitis mass had been previously removed and which gradually disappeared within a month of commencing treatment and has remained absent. c). in an advanced case of rheumatoid disease which reoccurred swelling of the left parotid gland had

occurred over 10 years, treatment resulted in a severe reaction with the reappearance of left sided slightly tender salivary gland enlargement and lacrimation from both eyes. In addition bilateral olecranon bursitis and Baker's cysts of both knees developed. All these symptoms died down in a period of 4-6 weeks. d). The case described by Descamps et al (1977) on page 41 suffering from ulcerative colitis and progressive sclerosing cholangitis and cholecystitis in whom cholestectomy had been carried out under the writer's care because of recurrent sclerosingcholangitis. He was treated with two courses of tinidazole at monthly intervals of 2G. on 2 successive days after the evening meal taken with milk. This resulted in the first occasion in an activation of the cholangitis with pain and temporary jaundice, nausea and vomiting and symptoms lasting for 5 days. On the second occasion the symptoms were minimal. For the last three years he has had no recurrence of symptoms of cholangitis and the symptoms of coeliac disease have cleared.

Addendum: Interesting observations were made in other cases of rheumatoid disease treated by metronidazole 2G on two successive evenings. One was in a female patient aged 60 years with severe long-standing rheumatoid disease, chair-bound and completely unable to use her hands and arms. she had suffered from atlanto-axial

493

subluxation of the cervical spine and wore a collar permanently. For the last 5 years she had suffered from severe cough and sputum with shadowing in the left lung radiologically. Extensive investigations both at the Massachuaetts Cameral Hospital and in this country failed to reveal the nature of the condition. The metronidazole produced a severe Herxheimer reaction but was followed by a marked generalized improvement in all joint movements, including those of the neck, which returned to normal. After six weeks the chest symptoms ceased and the radiological shadows disappeared. She, however, developed numerous rheumatoid nodules over the sacrum and elbows, hard and painful at firsts but later disappearing and also transient dryness of the eyes, conjunctivitis and punctate keratitis, which later cleared. All joint pain disappeared and the sedimentation rate returned to normal.

Addendum: Another significant case was the following. Female, aged 84 years with a 12 year history of creaking of the neck with pain and restricted movements, pain, swelling and restricted movements of the wrists, fingers and elbows, pains and swelling of the knees, ankles and feet. Four years previously she began to suffer from late-onset diabetes which was controlled by a low carbohydrate diet on which the urine showed intermittent passage of sugar sufficient to give a yellow colouration with the strip test.

She was treated with 2G. metronidazole on 2 successive evenings which caused some degree of increased pain, hotness and swelling of the affected joints with sweating. Over the next week every specimen of urine gave a yellow reaction with the strip test although she remained on the same diet. The sugar content of the urine gradually diminished until after four weeks it ceased and has not returned. The pain, swelling and restricted movements of the joints disappeared completely after six weeks enabling her to walk normally, use her wrists and fingers and regain full movements of the head. She has remained in this condition for the last 6 months. This shows that late onset diabetes like RA responds to antiprotozoal drugs. A further significant case is the following. Male, aged 74 years. Twenty years history of seropositive RA affecting especially the wrists, elbows, shoulders, neck. knees and ankles with present signs of active disease. In addition over the last 8 years there had been recurrent attacks of painless swelling of the left parotid gland each lasting several months. He was treated with tinidazole 2G. on 2 successive evenings which caused a violent exacerbation of activity in the affected joints and increase in the swelling already swollen of the left parotid gland which became somewhat tender. He ran a pyrexia of 100 degrees F. After 7 days the joint pains, hotness and swelling rapidly

494

subsided and by 14 days the swelling, and pain in the parotid gland had ceased. During the next three months there was a dramatic disappearance of all the joint pains and swelling and the parotid swelling did not recur. This shows that Sjögren's syndrome responds like the other manifestations of RD to antiprotozoal drugs.

Page 206: In practice after trials of different dosages of 5-nitro-imidazoles in active rheumatoid disease the author found that since the drugs remain in the blood in sufficient concentration to kill amoebae for 3-4 weeks or more the best mode of treatment is to administer 2G of the drug on two successive evenings with a meal and to prevent the exacerbation of symptoms by administering indometha- cin at the same time. After waiting for all the manifestations of the Herxheimer reaction t o di e down in 6-8 weeks the process i s repeated until the drugs produce no Herxheimer reaction. Afterwards 5-nitro-imidazoles should be used to prevent the emergence of resistant mutant amoebae.

Addendum: Review article. Intestinal biopsies operations for obesity. MacLean, Canadian J. Surg. 1976: 19; 387-399. Poly arthritis in obese patients with intestinal bypass. Shagrin JW, Frame B, Duncan H, Ann Int Med., 1971: 75; 377-380 Polyarthropathy may occur in about 23 per cent of patients undergoing small bowel shunt for obesity and all affected patients had a jejunal colostomy rather than a jejuno-iliostomy. Usually the arthropathy is transient lasting only about two months. (This leaves a blind loop without bile salts entering). May be severe and last two or more years. The affected joints are the wrists, fingers, knees and ankles and tenosynovitis of the fingers and hands. RF, AMP, LE cells are absent. The symptoms may respond to salicylates and rest or to steroids but sometimes it is necessary to revise the intestinal shunt before the arthropathy appears. Antibiotics have no effect The second authors recall that arthropathy which may complicate Whipple's disease, ulcerative colitis and Crohn's disease and that which may complicate certain intestinal infections with bacterial such as salmonella, shigella, etc. In two cases of administration of tinidazole rapidly cured the condition.

Addendum: Other antiprotozoal drugs and rheumatoid disease. Allopurinol has antiprotozoal properties. It has been shown to be effective against species of Leishmania and trypanosome cruzi as well as *Crithidia fasciculata*. It has proved effective in the treatment of Leishmaniasis and trypanosomiasis cruzi in man. (Allopurinol treatment for protozoon infections?. J A M A 1978 240 Medical News 1941-42. Allopurinol the ribonucloeside as an anti-Leishmanial agent. Nelson D J et al. J. Biol. Chemistry

1979, 254, 11544-49). The writer tried the effects of this drug in doses of 300 mgms. t.d.s. for 10 days in cases of active rheumatoid disease and found it produced the same effect as 5-nitro-imidazoles with a marked Herxheimer reaction and often violent sweating and very high temperature. The symptoms began after 3-4 days and lasted for about a week with genrral malaise and severe arthritic pain. The effect of the treatment seems more certain than 5-nitroimidazoles. Furazolidone is an antiprotozoal drug active against *E histolytica*, *Giardia lamblia* and other protozoa. It is poorly absorbed from the gut and only about 5% of the dose administered by mouth enters the body tissue. It is in general use as an antiamoebic drug in USA and elsewhere in the world. It was found that administration of the drug in doses of 100 mgm. 4 times daily for a week produced a typical Herxheimer reaction in cases of active rheumatoid disease with beneficial effects possibly superior to that of 5-nitro-imidazoles.Refampicin is an amoebistatic drug in vitro (Cursons RTM, Donald JJ, Keys EA, Brown TJ. Acanthamoeba Conference, Colombus Ohio June 14-16 1978). Administration of refampicin in doses of 600 mgms. daily to cases of active rheumatoid disease was found to induce a typical Herxheimer reaction after 3-4 days lasting up to two weeks. It was followed by gradual disappearance of disease activity comparable to that of 5-nitro-imidazoles, allopurinol and furazolidone.

Addendum: Goudie, R.B., Spence, J.C., MacKie, R., Lancet 1979, ii, 393-395, point out that vitiligo may be distributed in certain anatomical regions corresponding to the internal structures affected in some of the auto-immune and rheumatic diseases, such as a) the skin of the eyelids and lower front of the neck, reminiscent of the anatomical distribution of thyroid lesions with exophthalmos, b) the skin over the vertebral column, shoulder girdle and tibial tuberosities recalling ankylosing spondylitis, c) butterfly distirbution of the cheeks, brow and chin, suggestive of SLE, d) total vitiligo, recalling multiple endocrine failure with pernicious anaemia, hepatitis, arthritis. keratitis, alopecia and moniliasis, e) patches over the anterior surfaces of ankles, knees, lateral surface of hips, posterior surfaces of shoulders, elbows, metacarpophalangeal and interphalangeal joints and in the perioral and submental regions resembling rheumatoid arthritis, f) the skin of the hair line, extensor surfaces of the skin of arms and distal phalanges of the fingers. In vitiligo the skin exhibits loss of pigment cells and since it has been shown that the auto-immune and rheumatoid lesions appear to be due to infection with free-living amoebae in the neighbouring structures it seems possible that secretions of the amoebae extend to

496

affect the dermal melanocytes, just as they do neuro-transmitters.

Page: 207: Two recent reports, one from the Cedars-Sinai hospital, Los Angeles, concerned 12 severe cases of rheumatoid arthritis for whom medications, including gold and penicillamine, provided no relief, who were treated with plasmaphoresis or lymphoplasmaphoresis (removing lymphocytes and plasma cells from the blood) in 20 sessions over 11 weeks and the others from the National Institute of Health, Bethesda, Maryland, where four patients were treated with lymphophoresis three times a week for 5-6 weeks. Two of the Los Angeles cases showed no improvement, but all the others obtained marked benefit in relief of stiffness and pain over periods averaging several months and some patients also obtained help from drugs previously ineffective. Tenenbaum, J. et Annals. Rheum. Dis. 1979, 38, 40-44 reported on 2 similarly treated cases with some temporary improvement and variable or no alterations in serologic tests. These observations indicate that the humoral and lymphocytic response to the presence of Naegleria plays some part in the production of symptoms of rheumatoid disease.

Addendum: RA and food. A case study. A L Farke, GRU Hughes. Brit. med. J., 1981, 282, 2027-29. The authors through a case of a 38 year old female with 11 yr. history of progressive, errosive seronegative RA unresponsive to any treatment with a history of multiple drug allergies and rashes related to elastoplast and detergents but no asthma. She had never noticed exacerbation of her arthritis accompaning these allergies. Her mother also suffered from RA and was also reactive to elastoplast, detergents, penicillin, aspirin and nickle. Her sister and niece both had asthma. Avoidance of milk, cheese and butter in the diet produced remarkable resolutions in the RA symptoms beginning three weeks after commencing the diet. Symptoms reappeared on resuming a normal diet within 24 hours with the development of leucocytosis and change in the concentration of circulating immune complexes. The IgE antibodies to milk and cheese protein negative before the challenge became positive. (In the absence of evidence of allergy to milk and its products these findings could be explained on the presence in milk and its products of FL amoebae and their secretion, the latter being absorbed through the wall of the gastro-intestinal tract. An arthritis almost indistinguishable from RA is well known to complicate some cases of amoebic colitis and disappears with cure of the latter.

Addendum: Apart from the enormous amount of evidence adduced above showing

497

the amoebic nature of rheumatoid disease further complete proof of this has been found. Metronidazole has recently been produced for parenteral injection in bottles of 500 mgms per 100 mls. In 5 patients suffering from active rheumatoid disease involving both knee joints with effusions, 500 mgms. was injected into one joint to replace some of the intra-articular fluid and the same volume of saline into the other and one week later the knees were compared. It was found that the knee injected with the drug became slightly hotter and more painful for two days after injection, but within 8-10 days the swelling and signs of inflammation disappeared completely with return of joint mobility to normal. The knee injected with saline remained unchanged. This showed the antiprotozoal drug, which has no anti-inflammatory properties effectively killed the organism in the joint causing the inflammation. Since there is no evidence that an anaerobic bacterium causes rheumatoid disease, this proves the protozoal (amoebic) nature of the inflammation in the knee joint in rheumatoid disease.

Page 209: Aortic atheroma, abdominal aneurysm and auto-immune and rheumatoid disease. In syphilitic aortitis there occur collections of lymphocytes around the vasa vasorum of the adventitia and media of the aorta and an eventual weakening of the wall of the vessel and stretching to form an aneurysmal dilatation. Hurst, J.W., Cecil-Loeb,Textbook of Medicine, 13th. Edit., 1971, Saunders, London, points out that rheumatoid aortitis may occur in a small percentage of patients with rheumatoid arthritis producing aortic regurgitation. It is to be differentiated from syphilitis aortic valve disease. The lesions in the aorta usually do not extend beyond the ascending portion and consist of plaque-like lesions. Similar aortitis may occur in association with scleroderma and Hodgkin's disease. Mitchell, J.R.A., Lancet, 1978, 2, 583, points out that large vessel atheroma correlates in severity and extent with the systemic arterial pressures recorded in life and there is a close correlation between the severity and nature of athermatous plaques and focal collections of lymphocytes in the adjacent adventitia. These collections of cells when found in other organs, such as the thyroid gland, are thought to indicate the operation of an auto-immune process. Again there are significant increases of serum IgG and IgM levels in patients with proven atherosclerotic vascular disease. In the abdominal aorta extensive atheromatous areas are associated with weakness of the vessel wall and the tendency to aneurysm formation, which is increased when a persistently high blood pressure exists. Niarchos, A.P. and Finn, R., Brit. Med. J., 1973,

498

4, 110, pointed out that auto-immunity could well be implicated in some cases of abdominal aneurysm and reveals the high frequency of the latter in cases of myxoedema. The old name for atheroma was "endarteritis chronica deformans" but the inflammatory element has been increasingly forgotten. The link between atheroma and auto-immunity or rheumatoid disease may thus be highly significant. The changes of atherome of the aorta and large vessels with its associated lymphocytic infiltration and vascular dilatation or aneurysm formation would appear to be produced by amoebic infection of the vessel wall increasing in severity with age and resembling syphilitis aortitis. That this is so appears to be shown by the effect of metronidazole or tinidazole 2G on successive evenings on patients with abdominal aneurysm resulting in abdominal pain. This gives rise after 3 successive doses at weekly intervals to disappearance of the abdominal pain and lessening of the pulsation.

Addendum: Immunogenetics, atherosclerosis and essential hypertension. Reference has been made to the possible relationship of essential hypertension to genetic and environmental causes and that immmmunological changes presumably from amoebic infection are contributory. Gualde, N., Michel, J.P. and Safar, M.E., Lancet, 1978, ii, 890, found and refer to other workers findings that HLA B8 and B15 antigens are significantly more common in hypertensives. This suggests the possibility of connections between essential hypertension, diabetes and auto-immune disease. The humoral theory of the causation of essential hypertension postulates the presence in the blood of a vasoconstrictor substance, the nature of which is unknown. However, Talpos. G. et al., Lancet, 1978, i, 416, describe five patients with severe Raynaud's disease, a manifestation of collagen disease, which were unresponsive to other treatments, but in which plasmapheresis induced a striking improvement in their condition with opening up of the digital vessels, indicating the presence in the blood of a vasoconstrictor substance, presumably derived from amoebae. The author found that successful treatment of rheumatoid disease by 5-nitroimidazoles in patients also exhibiting essential hypertension may result in reduction of the blood pressure to normal or to a considerably lower level than previously. On the other hand, in treating normotensive patients it was found that in a proportion of cases there was a sudden transient rise in the blood pressure from the normal to a level of 200-220/100-110 mms. lasting for several days. These observations could be explained by the liberation of a vasoconstrictor substance into the blood from dying amoebae, probably identical with that found in Raynaud's syndrome and the blood pressure lowering effect of antiprotozoals is in accord with the humoral theory of essential hypertension and suggest the origin of the humor from living amoebae. Lambrecht, A.J. et al., Lancet, 1978, i, 1206, and Maurois, P., et al., Lancet, 1978, ii, 629, reported that in cases of plasmodium vivax infection in man there occurred a transient rise in the plasma chylomicrons, low density lipoproteins (L.D.L.) and very low density lipoproteins (V.L.D.L). This was correlated with parasitaemia. These changes were also found during therapy with chloroquine in *P. vivax, P. ovale and P. falciparium* infections. A patient of the author's, a male aged 36 years, had suffered from congenital ichthyosis, especially marked on the shins. He complained of vague intermittent sharp left chest pain and coolness of the left hand, in which he often noticed tingling of the fingers and more recently aching in the left upper arm, unrelated to exertion, and pain in the back of the neck. Examination showed no abnormality apart from the ichthyosis, coldness of the left hand, restricted movements of the neck, and an absent left supinator jerk. E.C.G. was normal. X-ray of the heart was normal, but one of the cervical spines showed loss of lordosis and some anterior osteophytes, more marked on the left side. The serum RF was positive. Serum cholesterol was 310 mgms. per cent (normal 150-280 mgms.). Low density lipoproteins were 610 mgms. per cent (normal 450-650 mgms.); triglycerides 80 mgms/100 mls (normal 0-170 mgms). He was treated with metronidazole 2G. in one dose, which produced a severe Herxheimer response with pyrexia, drenching night sweats and general aching, headache and neck stiffness lasting for 24 hours, following which his symptoms disappeared completely. Seven days later a repeat fasting serum examination showed cholesterol 330 mgms. per cent, low density lipoproteins 880 mgms. per cent, triglycerides still within normal limits, representing the changes of type IIa hyperlipoproteinaemia. These changes gradually reverted to normal during the next six months. The ichthyosis disappeared within one month. Similar observations were made in other cases of rheumatoid disease treated in this way, which taken with those on infection with the protozoon, plasmodium, mentioned above are in line with the protozoal aetiology of rheumatoid disease. An interesting observation was made on a number of cases of rheumatoid disease who also suffered from primary hyperlipoproteinaemia, type IIa. This condition is well known to be associated with an excessive tendency to vascular thromboses in the coronary, cerebral, iliac, axillary and other vessels and by an excessive liability of such vessels to atheromatous change. This condition is familial in nature and characterized by increased concentration of

500

low density lipoproteins in the plasma, by the deposition of xanthomas in various tissues and by an early onset of corneal arcus. The level of the serum cholesterol may also be raised. There is little or no increase in triglycerides. A case of type IIa hyperlipoproteinaemia, a male aged 40 years, gave a family history of recurrent coronary thromboses in his father and his father's sister, who also had recurrent cerebral thromboses. His brother suffered from coronary thrombosis at the age of 34 years. The patient himself had sustained coronary thromboses at the ages of 34. and 38 years. All these patients exhibited in their fasting serum a raised level of cholesterol and low density lipoproteins. While taking atromid S, 2G. three times daily, the fasting serum cholesterol in the patient was 300 mgms. per cent (normal 150-260 mgms.). Low density lipoproteins were 600 mgms. per cent (normal up to 650 mgms. per cent), triglycerides 19 mgms. per cent. He then developed a "frozen" shoulder with considerable pain. The serum RF was positive. Xanthomata were present round the eyes. He was treated with 2G. tinidazole, which produced a most intense reaction with drenching night sweats, pyrexia of 105 F, headache, generalized aching and stiffness and enlarged right cervical lymph nodes accompanied by right-sided trigeminal neuralgia. These symptoms persisted with diminishing severity for 10 days, at the end of which time, however, the shoulder had become completely mobile and painless. Repetition of the tests in the fasting serum two weeks after beginning treatment now showed cholesterol 340 mgms. per cent; low density lipoproteins 990 mgms. per cent. Six months later the readings were cholesterol 260 mgms. per cent, low density lipoproteins 600 mgms. per cent. He was able to give up taking atromid S. Similar findings were obtained in two other cases of type II hyperlipoproteinaemia. This suggests the possibility that bothh the serum abnormalities and the tendency to atheroma in this condition are due to toxic products of infection with free-living amoebae, to which these patients exhibit an inherited sensitivity. Since amoebic infection also appears to predispose to hypertension and this is a well known factor in inducing atheroma, it must be concluded that atheroma may also be caused primarily by infection with free-living amoebae, the effects of which appear increasingly with increasing age as do other manifestations of amoebic infection.

Page 211: Reference has been made earlier to the fact that infectious organisms introduced into the body tend to localize in areas of trauma or chronic inflammation. This obviously applies to amoebic infection, since not infrequently rheumatoid disease starts in an injured joint.

Page 215: Muggeo M. R JG, Ham LC and w England J. Med. 1979, 300, 477-480- Treatment by.

Page 217: Proof of the suggested nature of motor neurone disease is forthcoming in the following case. A male, aged 50 years, Norwegian. Nothing of significance in the family or past history. Six months previously he began to notice involuntary twitching in the thighs and arms followed by weakness of the legs, especially the right, and walking became difficult. No speech, swallowing or urinary difficulties, sphincter disturbance or weight loss were found. Examination showed no abnormalities in the cranial nerves or in the upper limbs except for fibrillation in the upper arms and forearms. The tendon reflexes in the upper limbs were normal. Tendon reflexes in the lower limbs were very brisk, plantar reflexes were flexor. There was generalized fibrillation in the buttocks and through-out the lower limbs, especially on the right side with generalized weakness and inability to walk on his heels. He was unable to stand on his right foot. The right buttock was wasted. EMG findings were consistent with motor neurone disease. A diagnosis of motor neurone disease was made. A blood count and ESR were completely normal, RF and LE cells were negative. The pati ent wished to have a second opinion and went to Mount Sinai Hospital, New York, where the diagnosis was confirmed but no treatment was offered. He was treated with metronidazole 2G in one dose weekly. The effect of this was to halt the progress of the disease and the fibrillation ceased. There was no further wasting, though the weakness of the muscles of the lower limbs persisted. He was now able to drive his car again: The improvement in the power of the lower limbs and the cessation of the fibrillation suggested that the progress of the disease had been halted by the anti-amoebic treatment.

Addendum: <u>Trigeminal neuralgia and free-living amoebic infection</u>.

As indicated many anti-amoebic drugs when administered to cases of rheumatoid infection may induce an Herxheimer reaction. It was found that in one case the administration of bile acids induced an attack of intense left-sided trigeminal neuralgia in a woman of 57 years, which lasted for a considerable time after omission of the bile acids and was eventually controlled with specific drugs. At a later date she was given metronidazole 2G. and this again precipitated a less severe attack of neuralgia than previously, which died down as the effects of the metronidazole wore off. In five further cases of rheumatoid disease the administration of either metronidazole or tinidazole was found to induce short-lived attacks of typical trigeminal neuralgia dying down with the Herxheimer reaction produced by the imidazole drugs. On the other hand in 4 patients with trigeminal neuralgia uncontrolled by drugs administration of metronidazole or tinidazole caused cessation of the pain within 48-72 hours, In spite of extensive research the causation of trigeminal neuralgia has been a mystery, but the above observations suggest that in some way it is the result of infection with free-living amoebae and this indicat e s a new method of treatment with anti-amoebic drugs.

Page 222: Heath, R.G., Krupp, I.M., Schizophrenia as an immunologic disorder. Arch. Gen. Psychiat., 1967; 16: 1-9 put forward the auto-immune hypothesis of schizophrenia. They found a protein (globulin) fraction in the sera of schizophrenics, which was called taraxein, which leads to EEG and psychotic disturbances like schizophrenia when introduced intravenously into macacque rhesus monkeys. It causes fluorescence in certain parts of the brain of schizophrenics with antigammaglobulin serum, but not in normal brains. Normal sera do not do so, but sera from cases of SLE and rheumatoid arthritis also cause similar fluorescence in the brains of schizophrenics or normal brains with antigammaglobulin sera. The findings suggest the presence of abnormal substance in the serum of schizophrenics similar to that in SLE and rheumatoid arthritis and this acts on certain brain cells.

Addendum: Two other cases treated by the author are significant. The first was a woman of 45 years, who two years previously had developed aching in the back of the neck and head spreading to the shoulders and down the dorsal and lumbar spine. This was particularly marked on waking, but varied in severity and was accompanied by gross depression which varied with the severity of the pain. Examination showed marked tenderness on pressure over the cervical nerve roots and the muscles in the back of the neck, the trapezii and over the dorsal and lumbar spine. An x-ray of the cervical spine showed complete loss of lordosis and the RF in the blood was positive. The blood pressure was 110/70 mms. A diagnosis of rheumatoid spondylitis was made. She was treated with a single dose of tinidazole 2G. with the complete disappearance of her symptoms, both physical and mental next day. They did not return during observation over the next 6 months. The second patient was also a woman, aged 60 years, who had spent the last ten years in a mental hospital suffering from severe endogenous depression with withdrawal, guilt feelings, delusions and periods of mutism. These failed to respond to any treatment. Three months, prior to

503

coming under observation she developed severe obstructive jaundice due to gall stones and during this period her mental symptoms suddenly disappeared completely. At operation a gall stone was removed from the ampulla of Vater and the jaundice disappeared, but the mental symptoms then returned as before. She was then treated with dehydrocholine (bile acids) 1G. three times daily with rapid disappearance of her mental symptoms after a few days. This treatment was continued for 3 months and then stopped. She remained well while being observed over the next six months. The effect of the obstructive jaundice with its rise in circulating bile salts and acids on the mental state and the later effect of bile acids point to the fact that the endogenous depression in this case was probably due to the effect of circulating secretions of amoebae as causing the mental symptoms.

Addendum: Mathe, A.A., Sedvall, G., Wiesel, F.A. and Nybäck, H. Lancet, 1980, i, 16-18, described an increased content of immunoreactive prostaglandin E in the cerebro-spinal fluid of patients with schizophrenia as compared with normals. This is compatable with the presence of an inflammatory process somewhere in the body, which, of course, occurs in infections with free-living amoebae and is consistent with a causative relationship of the latter with schizophrenia.

Page 226: Pinching, A.J. (Brit. J. Hosp. Med., 1978, 20, 552) reviewing plasma exchange, showed that it is beneficial in myasthenia gravis, idiopathic thrombocytopenic purpura (auto-immune), thrombotic thrombocytopenic purpura, hypogammaglobulinaemia, SLE, cutaneous vasculitis, Raynaud's disease with or without scleroderma and in homozygonus familial hypercholesterolaemia lowers the blood cholesterol and lipoproteins. This indicates the presence in the blood in these conditions of a substance presumably derived from free-living amoebae which produces the above manifestations.

Addendum: Many mammals, including dogs and horses, suffer from polyarthritis and/or tendinitis. The latter is especially common in racehorses for which so-called "firing" of the tendon is carried out by veterinarians. The infection causes a "race horse to "break-down" and to become useless for racing. It is treated by cortisone or butazolidine. The author found that metronidazole or tinidazole in appropriate weight for weight doses at 2 weekly intervals would cure polyarthritis and tendonitis in both these animals readily and could be used as a prophylactic.

Addendum: Dandona, P. et al., (Brit. med. J., 1979, i, 374) describe a rapidly

504

successful treatment of exophthalmos and pretibial myxoedema in a patient with Graves' disease by plasmapheresis? due to removal of abnormal immunoglobulins.

Addendum: Maternal autoimmune thrombocytopenia and the newborn. Van Leewen, E.F., Helmerhorst F.M., Engel C.P., von dem Borne A.E.G. Brit. med. J., 1981, 283, 104. The authors recall that maternal autoimmune thrombocytopenia may be transmitted to the new born producing transient manifestations of the same condition which pass into the foetal circulation where IgG but not IgM autoantibodies pass through the placenta.

Addendum: Levy, R.L., Newkirk, R., 0choa, J., Lancet, 1979, ii, 259-260 treated a case of chronic relapsing Guillain-Barre' syndrome by plasma exchange with dramatic and permanent improvement of symptoms, suggesting the syndrome may depend on humoral and cellular components in response to an infection. The author treated a similar such case with copper salts and obtained a similar result.

Addendum: Psoriasis is a feature of some cases of rheumatoid arthritis, ankylosing spondylitis and as psoriatic arthropathy. Webster et al., Brit. med. J., 1978, i, 478, report the remission of psoriasis during haemodialysis in a number of cases. This indicates that the skin lesions are due to circulation in the blood of some substance affecting the skin and presumably derived from amoebae.

Addendum: Taipos et al., Lancet, 1978, i, 416, describe five patients with severe Raynaud's disease, unresponsive to other treatments in which plasmapheresis produced a striking improvement in their condition with opening up of the digital vessels. This indicates the presence in the blood of a vasoconstrictor substance, presumably derived from amoebae.

Addendum: Intrinsic asthma may accompany rheumatoid disease. Gartmann, J., Grob, P. and Krey, M., Lancet, 1978, ii, 40. report the case of a 50 year old female severely asthmatic with atopic asthma beginning at the age of 6 months and now invalided over the last 20 years. After repeated plasmophoresis the asthma improved dramatically with striking fall in serum IgE and marked improvement in lung function tests. She was able to give up treatment with prednisolone and other drugs. This suggests the presence in the plasma of some substance inducing bronchospasm. As asthma may be associated with rheumatoid arthritis this could be derived from amoebae.

Page 234: Lobo, E. de H., Kahn, M. and Tew, J. Community Study of Hypothyroidism in Down's Syndrome, Brit. med. J., 1980, 280, 1253. Down's syndrome is associated with auto-immune dsi eases affecting the thyroid, pancreas, gastric mucosa and adrenal glands and patients have an increased tendency to produce antibodies. They may also develop hyperthyroidism or diabetes.

Page 241: Cossman, J., Sdhnitzer, B., and Deegan, M.J., Amer. J. Clin. Pathol., 1978, 70, 409-415, report the case of a man of 45 years, who suffered from two distinct lymphomas in separate sites. One was a nodular poorly differentiated lymphocyitc lymphoma and the other a diffuse histiocytic lymphoma. This is in accord with a common causation for all forms of lymphoma.

Page 243: Rubins J., Sischy B, Lee T C K. Am. J. Clin. Pathol. 1980, 74/5 696·700. Non-Hodgkin's lymphoma following treatment for Hodgkin's Disease. Case report and review of the literature. Authors report non-Hodgkin's lymphoma appearing following treatment for HD.

Addendum : Leinkram C, Chou S T. Lser J, SaliA. Med. J. Aust 1980, 1/7, 309·11 Multiple primary cancers arising from different organs and tissues. Report a case of lymphoma and adenocarcinoma of the stomach in the same patient and a metastatic squamous carcinoma in the axillary nodes from an unknown primary.

Page 245: Prat. J. and Scully, R.E., Cancer (Philadelphia) 1979, 44, 132, 1331. Sarcomas in ovarian mucinous tumours. A report of two cases. The authors report two cases of ovarian cysts. One a cyst adenocarcinoma in which the walls contained solitary nodules of sarcoma. It shows a common aetiology of sarcoma, adenoma and adenocarcinoma.

Addendum: Peyhonen, L, Heikkinen, J and Vehkalaht, S. Two different primary tumours of the brain in a patient wtih breast cancer. Eur. J. Nucl. Med., 1979 4/ 6 483-484. The authors report a case who had primary breast cancer and later meningioma and a glioblastoma multiforme were found at autopsy.

Page 246: Milano, CT, Deppe G, Delidisch I and Cohen C.T. Multiple primary neoplasms of the upper female genital tract. Gynecol. Oncol. 1980 9/ 1 120-124. The authors report that synchronous multifocal primary malignant neoplasms of the upper female reproductive system are more commonplace. They report an unusual combination of ovarian carcinoid, ovarian cystadenoid carcinoma and uterine adenosquamous carcinoma suggesting an area response of embryologically related organs in the genesis of the tumours, that is a field response.

Page 247: Multiple primary malignant neoplasia in three members of a family. Kenyon G S.J. Roy Soc Med 1981 74 601-4. Three of 5 sibs in adult life presented with a succession of malignancies. There were no known premalignant conditions present and no immune incompetence was found. The cases were 1) of 52 year old female with a caecal carcinoma followed by uterine carcinoma, carcinoma of the renal pelvis and distal ureter and anal cancer. 2) a male aged 26 years with carcinoma of the caecum then melanoma of the choroid, carcinoma of the duodenojejunal flexion, carcinoma of the transverse colon and finally a separate carcinoma of the pancreatic head. 3) 50 year old female with papilliferous adenocarcinoma of the ovaries followed by carcinoma of the rectum. Their mother died of uterine carcinoma and an uncle of carcinoma of the bronchus.

Addendum: Lynch, H., and Albano, W., of the Creighton School of Medicine, writing in the Journal of the Amer. Med. Ass., 1979, regard about 20 per cent of all breast cancers as familial and dependent on a genetic abnormality in the females of the family.

Addendum: Li, F.P., Marchetto, D.J. and Vawter, G.F. Acute leukaemia and preleukaemia in eight males in a family. A X-linked disorder?. Amer. J. Hematol., 1979, 6, 61-69 described acute leukaemia and preleukaemia in eight males in a family.

Addendum: Vaccari, E. Testicular seminoma in father and son. Andrologia, 1979, 11, 250-254, described a father and son suffering from seminomas, the father on the right and the son bilaterally. This is the fifth report of testicular malignancies in father and son. There are 26 reports of testicular malignancies occurring in closely related family members.

Addendum: Philipp, E.G. Familial carcinoma of the ovary. Brit. J. Obstet. Gynaecol., 1979, 86, 152-153 reports five relatives dying of ovarian cancer.

Addendum: Walker, J.P., Weiter, J.S., Albert, D.M. et. al. Uveal malignant melanoma in three generations of the same family. Am. J. Ophthalmol., 1979, 88/4, 723-726. The authors report three patients in three seccessive generations of the same family who had choroidal malignant melanoma. The third generation had multiple primary malignancies.

Addendum: Li, F.P., Marchette, D.J. and Vawter, C.F. Acute leukaemia and prelaukaemia in eight males in a family. An X-linked disorder? Am. J. Hematol. 1979, 6/1 61-69 The authors describe 8 males in a family who died of acute leukaemia or a potentially preleukaemic blood disease. Three patients were descendents of the man through his first wife and the others through his second wife suggesting X-linked inheritance through the two wives. No detectable enviromental leukaemogens were observed.

Addendum: Riaberg B, wife Nickels J, Wagermark J, Familial clustering of malignant mesothelioma. Cancer 1980,

45(9) 2422-2427. The authors report malignant mesothelioma in a father, 3 sons and a daughter suggesting heredity is an important predisposing factor in the genesis of this tumour.

Addendum: Genetics, etiology and human cancer. Lynch HT Prev Med 1980 9/2 231-243. The authors suggest that hereditary factors account for 5-10% of all human cancers, but myriad exogenous and endogenous factors influence the induction and promotion of both single gene and polygenically determined varieties of cancer

Addendum: Landthaler, M. and Braun-Falco, 0., Familial hereditary malignant melanoma. Med. Klin. (Munich) 74, 353-357 report the existence of familial-hereditary malignant melanoma inherited as an autosomal-dominant character. Such patients have numerous inherited, clinical and histological atypical naevi with a high incidence of malignant melanoma beginning early in life with a high incidence of multiple lesions and other malignant tumours in the family.

Addendum: Wilm's tumour in 5 cousins. Cordaro J F Li F P Holmes L B Gerald P S. Wilm's tumour has been reported in 5 cousins. Pediatrics 1980 66/5 716-9

Page 248: Identical cancers in sibs or twins sometimes uniovular or nonidentical cancers and congenital anomalies in sibs have been recorded. Pelgram et al. (Neurology, 1977, 27, 1058), described astrocytome of identical structures in three sisters; Napoli, V.M. and Campbell, W.G.J. (Cancer, Philad.), 1977, 39, 2647) hepatoblastoma in infant brother and sister; Joishy, S.K. et al. (Ann. intern. Med., 1977, 87, 447) alveolar cell carcinoma in identical twins with identical time of onset, biochemistry and site of metastases; familial Waldenstrom's macroglobulinaemia in father and offspring by Gelaz, E.P. and Staples;. W.G. (S. Afr. Med. J., 1977, 51, 891) (Literature); and double primary cancers in 2 sibs (glioblastoma and non-Hodgkin's lymphoma in one at 11 years and brain tumour and acute leukaemia at 6 years in another) with myelogenous leukaemia at 3 years in a third and cyanotic congenital heart disease with dextrocardia in a fourth sib at eleven weeks. Each child had at least one hamartomatous skin lesion. Such observations show the interaction of hereditary factors in causing both malignant change and congenital anomalies.

Addendum: Culliton, B.J. and Waterfall, W.K., Symposium on Genetics, Brit. Med.., 1979, 2, 1059-1060 recall that a miniscule deletion on the short arm of chromosome 11 is associated with the so-called AGR triad (aniridia, genitourinary abnormalities and mental retardation) and in about half the cases with Wilm's tumour. This linkage indicates that Wilm's tumour has a locus close to that or aniridia. Possession of chromosome 11p poses only a 50 per cent chance of developing the tumour and is step 1. An unknown step 2 is necessary to produce the tumour. As will be seen later this could well be infection with free-living amoebae.

Addendum: Van Der Riet-Fox, M.F., Relief, A.E. and Van Niebeck, W.A. (Cancer, Philadelphia), 1979, 44, 2108-2119. Chromosome changes in neoplasms studied with banding. These authors found chromosome abnormalities in all of the 17 malignancies studied and notably in chromosome I. Their findings suggest widespread involvement of this chromosome in this malignancy.

Addendum: Russ, J.E. and Scanlon E.F. (Surg. Gynaecol. Obstet. 1980, 150, 664-6) state that identical cancers have been found in 11 married couples, in all but 3 of the spouses developed cancer within 5 years of their partners. The cancer included breast, kidney, nasopharnyx, mouth, colon and rectum, melanoma and fibrosarcoma.

Addendum: Foster, J.H., Donohue, J.A., Berman, N.M., New Eng. J. Med., 1978, 299, 239-241 described a family with at least four members with liver cell adenomas, all being diabetic. Two also had sclerocystic ovaries and two ancestors who died with hepatocellular carcinoma.

Page 249: Geographic patterns of multiple myeloma; Racial and industrial correlation. AGU VU, Christensen BL, Baffler PA. J. Nat Cancer Inst. 1981, 65/4 735-738. The authors data supports previous findings by another investigator of a strong association between farming occupations and death from multiple myeloma. Farmers are close to animal faeces and the surface layer of the earth where amoebae are found.

Addendum: Drinking water and liver cell cancer. An epidemiologic approach to the etiology of this disease in China. Delong S. Chin. med, J. (Peking) 1979, 92, 748-756 The author found high frequency areas of liver cell cancer restricted to the coastal zones in Jiangsu Province of China. The frequency of the liver cancer varies with the origin of the drinking water being high where its origin is highly polluted ditch water and low when the origin is from wells.

Addendum: Burmeister LF Cancer Mortality in Iowa farmers. 1971-8. J N C I 66 461-464. Burmeister found that in Iowa state farmers were more likely to die from leukaemic, myelomatosis, lymphomas prostatic cancer than non-farmers. Although the overall cancer death rate for farmers was lower then people in other occupations this was because farmers do not contract fatal smoking related cancers as often since they rarely smoke due to the danger of fires. Similer figures were found in Washington and Oregon states. Burmeister suggested that they originate from the dust from hay and soilage from chemicals or animal viruses. Workers in other countries have found similar link between myloma and poultry formers. Such findings could be explained if lymphomas, leukaemias and mylomas were due to close contact with surface soil end its free-flying amoebae which occurs in farmers.

Addendum: Farming and mortality from non-Hodgkin's lymphoma: a case control study, Cantor KP. Int. Cancer 1982, 29, 239-247. Found farming a more common occupation in non-Hodgkin's lymphoma. Epidemiological risk factor in Hodgkin's disease. Szele Cyeck J, Kolosza Z. Nowtoory 1981, 31, 169-174. Hodgkin's disease commoner in rural areas. Allergic and rheumatic diseases were nearly twice as frequent in the parents of patients with FD than in controls.

Page 251: Sauer, O. and Spelger, G. (Monatschr Kinderheilkd., 1977, 125, 885) describe Duo: ᵓ itz's syndrome in 2 sisters, one had hypogammaglobulinaemia and neurobal stome, the other complete IgA deflclency and malignant lymphoma.

Page 253: *Protozoal infection and cancer.* Infection with protozoa may predispose to malignant change. Thus heavy malarial infection is an important factor in the development of African lymphoma, both in Africa and New Guinea, while cancer of the oesophagus, uterine cervix and urinary system appears to be more common in sufferers from Chaga's disease than in non-Chaga's subjects. Association of Chaga's disease and cancer. De Lustig ES, Puricedi L, BalE and LanzettiJC. Medicina (B. Aires) 1980, 40, 43-96. Furthermore trichomonas vaginails infect on of the vagina may cause atypicalcell alterations of the cervix. Trichomonas vaginalis and cytologicalfindings. Hotho H. Arch, Geschwulstforsch. 1977, 471, 455-461.

Page 271: Addendum: The treatment of carcinoma with oral copper sulphate. The following case is of considerable interest as regards the effects of antiamoebic drugs in cases of cancer. Male, aged 65 years, Italian, inhabitant of Brooklyn, New York, USA. He presented at Coney Island Hospital with a history of tiredness, anorexia, cough, sputum, haemoptysis, shortness of breath and the loss of 20 lbs. in weight over 6 weeks. On x-ray of the chest showed a right supra-hilar mass measuring 2 cms. in diameter without significant calcification. Bronchial biopsy yielded a histological diagnosis of poorly differentiated small cell carcinoma of the right main bronchus composed of nests of small ovoid cells with hyperchromatic nuclei, some of which were elongated while others irregular. Tumour cells invaded the subcutaneous stroma and there was inflammatory reaction of plasma cells and lymphocytes around. A diagnosis of oat cell carcinoma was made. No evidence of metastases was found. The ESR was 60 mms. per hour with some degree of hypochromic anaemia. He was given a course of radiation treatment to the mass and one dose of cyclophosphamide, methotrexate, adriomycin and CCNU and sheduled for further treatment. The patient however, became so ill that he was nauseated, continually vomited, had complete anorexia and continued to lose weight totalling 40 lbs. in all. On his return to hospital he was told of the diagnosis and prognosis and sent home to die. A repeated chest x-ray under the writer's care showed increase in the size of the suprahilar shadow had occurred. There was no other evidence of metastases. Some 6 weeks after his last hospital treatment he began treatment with copper sulphate tablets 50 mgms. daily with the most dramatic improvement in his condition. Within a few days the nausea ceased and after 2 weeks his appetite began to return. Gradually his condition returned to normal with a gain in weight of 20 lbs over the next 4 months, at the end of which time he was symptomless. At 6 months chest-x-ray and sedimentation

rate had returned to normal. His treatment lasted for six months and at the end of this time he was leading a perfectly normal existence. He retired from his work and went to live in Florida where he remains well four years later.

Page 352: Multiple myeloma in primary biliary cirrhosis. Blade J. Moserrat E, Brugnera Metal. Scand J. Haematol 1981; 26/1; 14;18. The authors point out that both conditions are the result of chronic stimulation of reticuloendothelial system.

Addendum: Fine, J.M., Lambin, P., Derycke, C. et al., Rev. Fr. Transfus. Immuno-Haematol., 1978, 21, 973-979, record that in the serum of 36,015 blood donors an incidence of monoclonal gammopathies of 0.14 per cent, 86 per cent of which were asymptomatic and 14 per cent were malginant melanoma or Waldenstrom 's macroglobulinaemia.

Page 353: Mandel E.M. et at. (Acta Haematol., 1977, 58, 120) describe multiple myeloma associated with Kaposi's sarcoma. Law, I.P. and Blom, J. (Oncology [base 1]), 1977, 34, 20) report 7 patients with myeloma, four of whom developed acute leukaemia, one renal cancer and 2 with combined adenocarcinoma of another organ and a carcinoma of the bronchus. Smith, A.G. and Cumming, R.L.S. (J. ctni , Path., 1977, 30, 1053) describe myelomatosis with oat-cell carcinoma of the bronchus and stress the linking of multiple myeloma with a higher incidence of other cancers than in the normal population.

Addendum: Parathyroid adenoma and tight chain myeloma. Chisholm RC, Weaver YJ, Chung EB and Townsend JL. J. Natl. Med. Assoc.1981 73 875·880.

Page 356: Robin, A., Adenis, L.P., Loubet, R. et. al Bull. Med. Soc. Fr. Ophthalm., 1977, 89, 300-306 described a man of 61 years suffering from Sjögren's syndrome and relapsing lymphocytic pleuritis, culminating in a diffuse lymphosarcomatosis and diffuse amyloidosis.

Addendum: Hochberg, M.C., Shulman, L.E., Johns Hopkins Med.J., 1978, 142, 211-214, report acute leukaemia following Sjögren's syndrome.

Addendum: Sjögren's syndrome. J.M. Gumpel. Leading Article BMJ 1982, 25, 1598. Sjögren's syndrome may occur in RA and AI disease, lymphoma or leukaemia. It may be called an exocrinopathy when other glands are involved and may be accompanied by lung lesions, renal tubular acidosis, hyperglobulinaemia and purpura and vaginal dryness.

Page 357: Familial Warthin's tumour. NovekAM, Prilzker KPH, Greyson ND et al J. Otolaryngeol., 1980, 90-96

The authors suggest that Wartin's tumour is suggested as a hypersensitivity disease.

Addendum: Squamous cell carcinoma arising in benign adenolymphoma (Warthin's tumour) of the parotid gland. Baker M, Yuzon D and Baker BH. J. Surg. Oncol. 1980, 15/1, 1-10.

Page 360: Yamashitta, N., Maruchi, N. and Mori, W. Hashimoto's thyroiditis: a possible risk factor for lung cancer among Japanese women. Cancer Lett. 1979, 7, 9·13. report an increased incidence of lung cancer among Japanese women with Hashimoto's thyroiditis, though the relationship with breast cancer was not significant.

Page 361: Rose, D.P. and Davis, T.E. Plasma triiodothyronine concentration in breast cancer. Cancer (Philadelphia) 1979; 43, 1434-1438, found a proportion of breast cancer cases who were mildly hypothyroid.

Page 364: Vogel J.M. et al. (N.Y. State J. Med. 1977, 72, 2255) report the occurrence of 5 cases of concomitant chronic lymphocytic leukaemia among 1300 myasthenics, coinciding with previous reports of a high overall incidence of extrathymic neoplasms in non-thymectomized patients with myasthenia gravis.

Addendum: Hassan,M.M. (Childs Brain, 1977, 3, 65) reports the case of a child aged 3 with myasthenia and ganglia· neuroblastoma of the mediastinum and mentions one similar report in

512

the literature.

Page 365: Histologically, the orbital changes consist of oedema and fatty deposition and in particular collections of lymphocytes and plasma cells with the formation of germinal follicles, that is changes identical with those of rheumatoid disease. In addition, as previously pointed out, these changes may be reversed by the administration of the antiamoebic drugs, chloroquine or metronidazole, which is further evidence for the rheumatoid nature of the malignant exophthalmos. Knowles and Jakobiec (1980) studied 60 cases of malignant exophthalmos which histologically they divided into 1) inflammatory pseudotumour, 2) reactive lymphoid hyperplasia, 3) atypical lymphoid hyperplasia and 4) malignant lymphocytic lymphoma. There was no clinical difference between them. Twenty-eight of those of any group developed systemic lymphoma. This shows the relationship of rheumatoid and autoimmune disease to lymphoma. Knowles DM, Jakobiec FA, Cancer (Philadelphia) 1980, 45, 576-580. Orbital lymphoid neoplasms. A clinico- pathologic study of 60 patients.

Addendum: Malignancy associated with dermatolyositis with fibrosing alveolitis. Holmes R, Black M M, Farebrother MJB and van Gratten M. Clin. Exp. Dermatol. 1980 5/4 415-20. A case of dermatolyositis associated with carcinoma of the bronchus developed fibrosing alveolitis.

Page 371: Addendum: Musculoskeletal syndromes associated with malignancy. Caldwell DS. Semin. Arthritis Rheum. 1982 10/3, 198-223. The author refers to primary connective 44 tissue diseases associated with malignancies.

Addendum: Banks, P.M., Witrak, G.A. and Conn, D.L. Lymphoid neoplasia following connective tissue disease. Mayo Clin. Proc., 1979, 54, 104-108 report 29 cases of connective tissue disease followed by malignant lymphoma, myeloma or chronic lymphatic leukaemia.

Addendum: Chromosomal aonormalities. Findings in a patient with lymphoma and rheumatoid arthritis treated with intra-articular gold. Goli K., Jacox R.F. and Anderson F.W. Arch. Pathol. Lab. Med., 1980, 104/9, 473-75.

Addendum: Remission in systemic lupus erythematosus after combination chemotherapy for Hodgkin's disease. Goodwin J.S. J. Am. Med. Ass. 1980, 244/17, 1962.

Page 373: Cohen, S.R., Landing, B.H., Isaacs, H., et al. Ann. Otol. Rhinol. Laryngol., 1978, 87, H. Supple. 52. 11. report the case of a soiltary plasmocytoma of the larynx and upper

513

trachea developing in a patient with systemic lupus erythematosus of nine years standing.

Addendum: Wallach, H.W., Arch. Intern. Med., 1977,137, 532-535 reported 2 patients with locally advanced cancer of the breast treated with radio-therapy which was followed in a year by the lupus syndrome.

Page 377: Carassone, Y., Bonvenot, G., Gastant, J.A. and Sebahour, G. The association of myeloma and Paget 's disease. Ann.Med. Interne., 1979; 130, 177·184, remark on the frequent association of Paget's disease and myeloma in recent reports and emphasize that the former may also be associated with macroglobulinaemias or other monoclonal gammapathies.

Page 380: Cairns et al., (Brit. med. J., 1978, ii, 474) report 2 cases of Henoch‑Schtinlein purpura with polyarthritis who later developed squamous carcinoma of the bronchus. Maurice, T.R. and also Hoffbrand (Ibid p. 831) report similar cases clearing after tumour resection.

Page 384: Another case of vitiligenous achromia developing malignant melanoma was reported by Perrot, H., Ortonna, J.P. and Schmitt, D. (Arch. Dermatol. Res., 1977, 357·273).

Addendum: Albert D.M., Sober, A.J., Fitzpatrick, T.b. Arch. Ophthalmol (Chicago), 1978, 96, 2081·4 described two patients with vitiligo, malignant melanoma and uveitis.

Page 385: Maddin W.S. and Wood W.S. Multiple Keratoacanthomas and squamous cell carcinomas occurring at psoriatic treatment sites. J. Cutaneous Pathol. 1979, 6, 96-100.

Page 390: Borochowitz D., Dutz W., Kohont E. and Vessal, K. lst. J. Med. Sci., 1979, 15, 397-404 Gastro-intestinal mucosa and primary gastro-intestinal lymphoma. The authors report that in Shiraz (Iran) gastro-intestinal lymphoma affects the upper duodeno-jejunal area and is associated with atrophy of the surrounding non-lymphomatous area and formation of lymph follicles. This is frequently linked to repeated gastro-enteritis leading to mucosal atrophy, mutation of plasma cell precursors a nd secretion of alpha-heavy chain proteins. In USA gastro-intestinal lymphoma affects the stomach and is accompanied by superficial perifovealar plasma cell gastritis of the surroundi ng mucosa or in preformed lymphoid tissue of the ileo-colon surrounded usually by normal mucosa. In both areas the lesions are suggestive of a parasitic infection.

Page 391: Coeliac Dsieases and malignancy. C Swinson, G Slavin, E C Coles, C Booth. Lancet 1983, i, 111-115. Patients with coeliac disease

514

seem more prone to develop malignancy especially lymphoma, than a general population —— 235 patients. developed 259 malignancies of which 133 were lymphomas particualrly histiocytos s of the small intestine but also a greatly increased risk for the development of small intestinaladenocarcinomas. Amomg 116 nonylmphomatous malignancies there were 19 small intestine adenocarcinomas compared with the expected 0.25 and more oesophagealand pharyngeal squamous carcinomas. Malignant lymphoma may also develop in extra-intestinal sites.

Addendum: Dermatitsi herpetiformis and lymphoma. Gawkrodger DJ and Barnetson R St. C. Lancet 1982 2 987. A record of patients with dermatitis herpetiformis and villus atrophy of the small intestine in which ymphoma of the intestine or generalized lymphoma develops.

Addendum: Parker, A.C. and Bennett, M. (Eng. Scand. J . Haemat, 1976, 17, 395) report 2 cases of pernicious anaemia with lymphoproliferative disease.

Page 393:: Hsi tiocytic lymphoma in chronic ulceratvi e colitis. BashitiHO and Kraus FT. Cancer (Philadelphia) 1980 46/7 1695·1700 colonic lymphoma and adenocarcinoma occurred in a man with long-standing ulcerative colitis.

Addendum: Atkinson A.R., Buchanan, K.D.,Carson, D.S., et al. Brit.Med. J. 1978, 2, 1397·1398, also report an insulinoma developing in a diabetic. Page 42.

Addendum: Reference was made earlier to the fact that infectious organisms introduced into the body tend to localize in areas of trauma or chronic inflammation. This applies to free-living amoebae and readily explains the fact that malignant disease may begin at the site of trauma or chronic inflammation, an observation to which reference has been made previously. Obviously this only occurs in subjects with a labile genetic state.

Addendum: Feingold , N., Bull, Cancer (Paris), 1978, 65, 79-82 in considering the relationship of the HLA system to malignant diseases found a significant geographical association between some cancers and specific HLA antigens and considered this evidence for a genetic background of susceptibility or resistance to cancer.

Page 405: Mueller, 5. et at., (J. Pediat, 1978, 127, 219) describe a case of hemihypertrophy and hamartomas with Wilma's tumour and adrenocorticalcarcinoma.

Page 407: Knudson, A.G,Jr., Mutation and Human Cancer, Avd Cancer Res., 1973, 17, 317-352, and Genetics and the Aetiology of Childhood Cancer, Pediatr. Res., 1976, 10, 513-517, has put forward the two mutation model of carcinogenesis, according to which the non-hereditary form of cancer can develop through two somatic mutations in a single cell. The hereditary form of the

515

same cancer develops through one germinal prezygotic mutation present in all somatic cells and one additional, somatic mutation. This applies to retinoblastoma, neuroblastoma, tumour, phaeochromocytoma, and several other neoplasms. This second somatic mutation may well be induced by amoebic infection. Boczkowski, K. and Piatkowski, J., Familial occurrence of gonadal tumours in women with 46 XY karyotype. Endokrynol. Pol. 1978, 527-535 described three sisters in a family showing a male 46 XY karyotype, in two of which dysgerminomia of the dysgenetic gonads was found.

Addendum: Geraedts, J.P.M., Mol, A., Briët. E, Hadtgrink-Groeneveld, C.A, Van Ottolander, C.T., Lancet, 1980; 1; 774 point out the increased incidence of acute leukaemia in Klinefelter's and Down's syndromes.

Page 413: Multiple myeloma after phenytoin therapy. Aymard JP, Lederlin P. Witz Fet al. Scand.J. Haematol. 1981, 26 330-332 Authors report a case of multiple myeloma in a 4 year old woman treated with phenytoin 55 months. Association may be fortuitous but depressive effect of drug on immune responses would account for blood changes.

Addendum: Mougeot-Martin,M., Krulik, M., Haronsseau, J.L., et al., Ann.Med, Interne., 1978, 129, 175-80, collected more than thirty

examples of acute leukaemia following immunosuppressive therapy for multiple sclerosis and for Behcet's syndrome. The leukaemia was often preceded by a preleukaemic phase.

Addendum: Matzner Y and Polliack A. Monoclonal gammopathy and subsequent multiple myeloma in a patient on chronic diphenylhydantoin therapy. lsr. J. Med. Sci. 1978, 14, 1265 -1267 Page 414:

Addendum: Cancer following successful cadavaric donor renaltransplantation. Sheil A G, Mahoney J F, Hovath J S, Johnson J R, Tiller D J. Transplant Proc. 1981 13 733-5 Of 459 patients who survived with functional renal grafts for at least six months following cadacaric donor renal transplantation 87 (24%) developed cancer, especially of the skin when it is often multiple, recurrent and aggressive or generalized. Cancers other than of the skin included reticulum cell sarcoma and other lymphomas and cancer of the genitourinary or gastrointestinal tracts respiratory and haemopoietic systems. These increased in number with the duration of the transplant. Cancer is a major cause of mortality following transplants.

Addendum: Immunosuppression and skin cancer. Penn I. Clin. Plast. Surg; 7, 361-368, 1980. 906 organ transplant recipients developed 959 malignancies over an 11.5 year period. 399 were skin tumours (squamous, or basal cell carcinoma mixed, non-Kaposi's sarcoma,

516

Kaposi's sarcoma and multiple primary tumours in 53 recipients (lymphomas, carcinoma of colon, lungs, parotid or thyroid). The use of immuno-suppressive therapy for disorders with an autoimmune basis should be avoided.

Addendum: Kinlen, N.J., Shiel, A.G.R., Peto, J., Doll, R., Brit. Med, J. 1979, 2, 1461-1466, report there is no clear evidence that immuno-suppressive drugs produce the increased risk of most of the common cancers that might be expected from the simplest interpretation of impaired "immunosurveilance".

Addendum: Cancer following successful cadaveric donar renaltransplantation. Sheil AGR,Mahony JF, Horvath JS. et al. Transplant Proc. 1981, 13 / 1 733-735. Cancer is a major cause of morbidity or mortality after renal transplant. Its exact infection remains to be determined. Addendum: Borzy,M.S., Hong, R., Horowitz, S.D. et al., New Eng. J. Med., 1979, 301. 565-8, found fatal lymphoma developed in 5 of 30 cases after transplantation of cultures of thymus cells in children with combined immunodeficiency disease.

Addendum: Leading Article, Brit. med. J., 1979, i, 509, points out that lymphoma may occur after cardiac transplantation (6 of 143 patients).

Page 422: Cutaneous granulomas in malignant lymphnoma. Randle HW, Banks PM, Winkelmann RK. Arch. Dermatol1980, 116/ 4, 441-443 Two patients with massive localized dermaland subcutaneous epithlioid granulomatous masses were finally diagnosed after a years investigation as Hodgkin's disease by lymph node biopsy.

Page 423: Complete, partial or minor spontaneous regression may be found in cases of non-Hodgkin's lymphoma. It occurred in 18 out of 140 cases of nodular lymphoma and in 2 of 68 with diffuse lymphoma. It may last a few weeks up to many years. Spontaneous remission in non-Hodgkin's lymphoma. Gattiker HH, Wiltshaw E and Galton DG. Cancer (Philadelphia) 1980, 45, 2627-32.

Addendum: Simultaneous Hodgkin's disease in 3 siblings with identical HLA genotype. Torres A, Martinez F, Gomez P. et. al. Cancer (Philadelphia) 1980 46/4 838-845 Three siblings in a family of 7 children had Hodgkin's disease contemporaneously and one of these had an idiopathic thrombocytopenia. Both genetic and environmental factors were concerned in the pathogenesis.

Addendum: Rosenbaum D.J., MacCarty C.S. and Buettner H. Uveitis and cerebral reticulum cell sarcoma {large cell lymphoma) J. Neurosurg, 1979, 50, 660-664 describe a case of long-standing uveitis (a manifestation of amoebic infection) which developed cere- bral reticulum cell sarcoma.

517

Page 426: The association between chronic eosinophilia, phenumonia and histiocytic lymphoma. Brenner BE, Thorgeri sson G. Amer. J. Med. Sci 1979 279 83-88. An eosinophil eukaemia with pneumonic changes was treated by cortico-steroids for 10 months when diffuse histiocytic lymphoma was diagnosed.

Addendum: Gravelau, P., Perot, R., Mornet, P. and Morin, M. Neuv. Presse Med., 1978, 7, 3909 report the case of a patient with small intestinal tumours and mesenteric lymph nodes exhibiting the changes of an eosniophilic granuloma over four years and eventually the lesions became those of Hodgkni 's disease.

Page 438: Risberg B. Nickels J, Wagermark, J. Familialclustering of malignant mesothelioma. Cancer 1980, 45(9) 2422-2427. The authors report malignant mesothelioma in a father, 3 sons and a daughter suggesting herdity is an important predisposing factor in the genesis of this tumour.

Page 441: Palma, L., DiLorenzo, N. and Guidetti, B., J. Neurosurg., 1978, 49, 854-861, emphasize the frequency of lymphocytic infiltrates in primary glioblastomas and ricid vous gliomas.

Addendum: Horten , B.C., Urich, H . and Stefoski, D. Meningiomas with conspicious plasma cell lymphocytic components. Report of 5 cases. Cancer (Philadelphia), 1979; 43, 258-264 describe 5 cases grossly resembling meningioma, but histologically containing meningothelial cells together with abundant plasma cells and lymphocytes.

Page 443: Both rheumatoid and auto-immune diseases appear to be due to infections. Recent reviews on the nature of multiple sclerosis also regard. the disease as due to an immunological disturbance. Brain, W.R. and Wilkinson, Y., Brain, 1957, 80, 456 studied 17 patients with both cervical spondylitis and multiple sclerosis. In some cases the symptoms were solely due to multiple sclerosis with signs confined to evidence to damage to the spinal cord. In others symptoms of both diseases are present. The author observed a case of a female, aged 58 years. who 4 years previously began to get aching and stiffness of the neck and shoulders. X-rays revealed spondylosis. Later she developed lumbar pain and further x-rays showed lumbar spondylosis. Soon after the appearance of the neck symptoms there was an onset of progressive spinal multiple sclerosis without evidence of neurological disease above the cervical cord. Since it appears that spondylosis is a manifestation of rheumatoid disease the result of free-living amoebic infection such cases point to the auto-immune nature of the lesions of multiple sclerosis in the cervical cord region.

Addendum: A patient with multiple

sclerosis and polymyositis with mild rheumatoid arthritis, in whom the multiple sclerosis had been stable for 20 years, was treated with the 5-nitroimidazole Nimorazole, in a single 2G. dose for the polymyositis. The next day there was a rapid exacerbation of the multiple sclerosis symptoms with confusion, slurred speech, incontinence of urine and faeces, marked increase in weakness of the lower limbs and pyrexia of 100 degrees F. All these symptoms were short lived and disappeared within two days. They indicate an Herxheimer reaction in a case of multiple sclerosis with increase in neurological symptoms when treated with an anti-Naeglerial drug and point to the possible Naegierial cause of the neurological disease.

Addendum: A patient with multiple sclerosis and polymyositis with mild rheumatoid arthritis, in whom the multiple sclerosis had been stable for 20 years, was treated with the 5-nitroimidazole Nimorazole, in a single 2G. dose for the polymyositis. The next day there was a rapid exacerbation of the multiple sclerosis symptoms with confusion, slurred speech, incontinence of urine and faeces, marked increase in weakness of the lower limbs and pyrexia of 100 degrees F. All these symptoms were short lived and disappeared within two days. They indicate an Herxheimer reaction in a case of multiple sclerosis with increase

in neurological symptoms when treated with an anti-Naeglerial drug and point to the possible Naelgerial cause of the neurological disease.

Addendum: Association of ulcerative colitis with MS. Rang EH, Brooke BN, Taylor JH. Lancet 1982 ii 555. MS noted as P.S. The neurological complications of A spondylitis Mathews WB, J. Neurol. Sc. 1968, 6, 561-73. Nervous system involvement in S. spondylitis Brit. med. J., 1974, i, 148-50. Thomas DJ, Kendall MJ, Whitfield AGW. AS and MS a possible association. Khan MA, Kushner I Arthritis Rheumatol 1978, 22, 784-6.

Addendum: Three further cases of multiple sclerosis associated with glioma was reported by Spaar, F.W. and Wikstroem, J. (J. Neurol., 1978, 218, 23). Zimmerman, H.M. and Netsky, M. in Multiple Sclerosis and the Demyelinating Diseases (Williams and Wilkins Co., Baltimore, 1950, Page 271) report on the autopsy of 40 cases of multiple sclerosis and found that no less than 10 had associated malignancies, of which one was a glioblastoma multiforme of the cerebrum and another a cerebellar haemangioblastoma. The remainder had carcinoma of the stomach, breast (2 cases), kidney (2 cases), liver, pancreas and bladder. An incidence of malignancy of 25 per cent in cases of multiple sclerosis is far higher than the expected number and the particular association of CNS malignancies related to demyelination in CNS is noteworthy.

Addendum: Gliomatous transformation and demyelinating diseases. Anderson M, Hughes B , Jefferson M et al. Brain 1980 103/3, 603-622 Three patients with M.S. with neoplastic glial transformation in areas of demyelination.

Addendum: Combination of multiple sclerosis and cerebral glioblastoma. Lahl R. Eur. Neural., 1980: 1973 192-197. The tumour margins appeared in the neighbourhood of multiple sclerosis plaques.

Addendum: Kalimo H. ,Frey H., Raine C.S. et al. Late-onset malignant astrocytoma in a case of sclerosis. multiple sclerosis. Acta Neuropathol. 1979. 46, 231-234 report a further case of cerebral glioma developing in a case of multiple sclerosis.

Addendum: Sibley, W.A., Bamford, C.A. and Laguna, J.F. (Neurology, 1978, 28, 125) found a significant relationship between familial multiple sclerosis and neoplasia.

Addendum: Recent reviews on the nature of multiple sclerosis regard the disease as due to an immunological disturbance.

Page 443: Both rheumatoid and auto-immune diseases appear to be due to infections. Recent reviews on the nature of

multiple sclerosis also regard. the disease as due to an immunological disturbance. Brain, W.R. and Wilkinson, Y., Brain, 1957, 80, 456 studied 17 patients with both cervical spondylitis and multiple sclerosis. In some cases the symptoms were solely due to multiple sclerosis with signs confined to evidence to damage to the spinal cord. In others symptoms of both diseases are present. The author observed a case of a femele, aged 58 years. who 4 years previously began to get aching and stiffness of the neck and shoulders. X-rays revealed spondylosis. Later she developed lumbar pain and further x-rays showed lumbar spondylosis. Soon after the appearance of the neck symptoms there was an onset of progressive spinal multiple sclerosis without evidence of neurological disease above the cervical cord. Since it appears that spondylosis is a manifestation of rheumatoid disease the result of free-living amoebic infection such cases point to the auto-immune nature of the lesions of multiple sclerosis in the cervical cord region.

Addendum: A patient with multiple sclerosis and polymyositis with mild rheumatoid arthritis, in whom the multiple sclerosis had been stable for 20 years, was treated with the 5-nitroimidazole Nimorazole, in a single 2G. dose for the polymyositis. The next day there was a rapid exacerbation of the multiple sclerosis

520

symptoms with confusion, slurred speech, incontinence of urine and faeces, marked increase in weakness of the lower limbs and pyrexia of 100degrees F. All these symptoms were short lived and disappeared within two days. They indicate an Herxheimer reaction in a case of multiple sclerosis with increase in neurological symptoms when treated with an anti-Naeglerial drug and point to the possible Naegierial cause of the neurological disease.

Addendum: A patient with multiple sclerosis and polymyositis with mild rheumatoid arthritis, in whom the multiple sclerosis had been stable for 20 years, was treated with the 5-nitroimidazole Nimorazole, in a single 2G. dose for the polymyositis. The next day there was a rapid exacerbation of the multiple sclerosis symptoms with confusion, slurred speech, incontinence of urine and faeces, marked increase in weakness of the lower limbs and pyrexia of 100degrees F. All these symptoms were short lived and disappeared within two days. They indicate an Herxheimer reaction in a case of multiple sclerosis with increase in neurological symptoms when treated with an anti-Naeglerial drug and point to the possible Naelgerial cause of the neurological disease.

Addendum: Association of ulcerative colitis with MS. Rang EH, Brooke BN, Taylor JH. Lancet 1982 ii 555. MS noted as P.S.

The neurological complications of A spondylitis Mathews WB, J. Neurol. Sc. 1968, 6, 561-73. Nervous system involvement in S. spondylitis Brit. med. J., 1974, i, 148-50. Thomas DJ, Kendall MJ, Whitfield AGW. AS and MS a possible association. Khan MA, Kushner I Arthritis Rheumatol 1978, 22, 784-6.

Addendum: Three further cases of multiple sclerosis associated with glioma was reported by Spaar, F.W. and Wikstroem, J. (J. Neurol., 1978, 218, 23). Zimmerman, H.M. and Netsky, M. in Multiple Sclerosis and the Demyelinating Diseases (Williams and Wilkins Co., Baltimore, 1950, Page 271) report on the autopsy of 40 cases of multiple sclerosis and found that no less than 10 had associated malignancies, of which one was a glioblastoma multiforme of the cerebrum and another a cerebellar haemangioblastoma. The remainder had carcinoma of the stomach, breast (2 cases), kidney (2 cases), liver, pancreas and bladder. An incidence of malignancy of 25 per cent in cases of multiple sclerosis is far higher than the expected number and the particular association of CNS malignancies related to demyelination in CNS is noteworthy.

Addendum: Gliomatous transformation and demyelinating diseases. Anderson M, Hughes B, Jefferson M et al. Brain 1980 103/3, 603-622 Three patients with M.S.

with neoplastic glial transformation in areas of demyelination.

Addendum: Combination of multiple sclerosis and cerebral glioblastoma. Lahl R. Eur. Neural., 1980: 1973 192-197. The tumour margins appeared in the neighbourhood of multiple sclerosis plaques.

Addendum: Kalimo H. ,Frey H., Raine C.S. et al. Late-onset malignant astrocytoma in a case of sclerosis. multiple sclerosis. Acta Neuropathol. 1979. 46, 231-234 report a further case of cerebral glioma developing in a case of multiple sclerosis.

Addendum: Sibley, W.A., Bamford, C.A. and Laguna, J.F. (Neurology, 1978, 28, 125) found a significant relationship between familial multiple sclerosis and neoplasia.

Addendum: Recent reviews on the nature of multiple sclerosis regard the disease as due to an immuninsertological disturbance.

Addendum: Fulford, K.W.M., Catterall, R.D., Delhanty, J,J., Doniach, D. and Kremer, M., Brain, 1972, 95, 373, described the condition of "lupoid sclerosis" in 6 young female patients showing clinical evidence of multiple sclerosis. In one the neurological disease was associated with fever, arthropathy and pleural effusions, in another with vitiligo, arthropathy and food allergies, in another with arthropathy and urticaria, in another with photosensitivity of the skin and in yet another with iridocyclitis; one was psychotic. The ESR was usually raised. In most LE cells and ANF were present in the blood. The Lange curve was usually paretic or tabetic in type and false WR's occurred in the blood. The IgM content of the serum was usually markedly raised. Three cases showed a moderate titre of thyroid auto-antibodies and two gastric parietal cell auto-antibodies. The CSF protein was sometimes increased, but RF was absent in the serum in all cases. The authors suggest a possible relationship between SLE and multiple sclerosis in most cases. Holmes, F.F., Stubbs, D.W. and Larsen, W.R., Arch. int. Med., (Chicago), 1967, 119, 302, reported monozygotic twins of which one developed MS at 15 years and the other SLE at 19 years. Fantelli, F.J., Mitsumoto, H. and Sebak, B.A., Lancet, 1978, 1, 1039, report a case of a 50 year old female with malabsorption, severe diffuse villous atrophy and small intestinal inflammation with MS and quote Lange, L.S. and Shiner, M., Lancet, 1976, ii, 1319, who report 12 cases of MS with small intestinal changes at biopsy. Two had partial or subtotal villous atrophy and five mucosal chronic inflammatory infiltrates. Thompson, R.A. and Jones, M., Neurology (Minneap.), 1969, 19, 885, describe remitting demyelinating disease associated with a myeloproliferative syndrome and histiocytosis of the spleen. All these observations point to a possible amoebic cause of MS. As indicated above the cause of trigeminal neuralgia may lie in amoebic infection. It is well known that the one disease which may be complicated by trigeminal neuralgia is MS again suggesting the possibility of a free-living amoebic cause of the demyelinating disease. Shepherd, D.I. and Downie, A.E., Brit. med. J. 1978, 2, 314, point out the remarkably similar geographical distribution of MS and HLA antigens A3 and B7 in N.E.. Scotland, where there is a remarkably high incidence of the disease, suggesting that the appearance of MS in the patient is related to the existence of specific HLA antigens together with an essential additional environmental factor.

t

How to Get Well from Rheumatoid Disease

Many doctors worked with Roger Wyburn-Mason's breakthrough treatment for rheumatoid disease and found that there can be numerous factors that cause the condition. They certainly accepted his protocol, but they added more areas for the rheumatoid affected to explore. Of course not all people are going to be affected by all possible stresses that bring about the disease. Some will find only one or perhaps two conditions that have affected them. A few will need to explore numerous avenues, and we list here for the benefit of the health professional and the rheumatoid victim. So here it is, the major factors that should be explored.

How Do I Cure My Rheumatoid Arthritis?

1. How Do I Cure My Rheumatoid Disease?

You start the cure by learning what Rheumatoid Disease is, where it's located in the body, and what causes it. The very first thing to learn is that it is a disease of the whole body, not of your joints. This is true no matter how much your joints ache or how insistent is your friendly neighborhood rheumatologist.

2. Where is Rheumatoid Disease Located in my body?

Rheumatoid Disease is a "systemic" disease. This means that whatever ails you is actually a problem of your whole body — cells, organs, systems — the whole works. If you suffer from Rheumatoid Arthritis, for example, this systemic disease is manifesting itself in your joints. If you suffer from a differently named Rheumatoid Disease, then the target area of your body is given a new name, one different from Rheumatoid Arthritis. In fact, there are about 100 differently named diseases that have essentially the same causes but are known under totally different names as shown at the "Articles" tab, "Arthritis Classifications" at our website http://www.arthritistrust.org.

Professor Roger Wyburn-Mason, M.D., Ph.D., explained this astounding fact by describing the medical profession's past technique for naming tuberculosis before discovery of the tuberculin germ. There were about 100 unique names for apparently different diseases depending upon the part of the

523

body affected. Once the tuberculin bacillus was discovered, all of those names collapsed into TB of the bone, TB of the lung, TB of the skin, and so on.

We think Rheumatoid Disease is a cluster of symptoms named differently — 100 unique names — that can now be understood from the viewpoint of a single, systemic disease. (See "Arthritis Classifications" tab at http://www.arthritistrust.org.)

3. But what about my immune system? My doctor says that Rheumatoid Arthritis (or Rheumatoid Disease) is caused by a defective immune system?

There may be some folks who have a defective immune system, but these are probably rare. We believe that your immune system is doing exactly what it was constructed to do. By analogy, consider the camel with too many straws on its back. If you remove those straws one or two at a time eventually the camel will be able to stand again. Our recommended treatment protocol does exactly that — removes the stressors from your immune system until your body (and immune system) functions properly again.

Professor Roger Wyburn-Mason again constructed a useful analogy citing past medical history. Prior to the discovery of the syphilis spirochete, the disease of syphilis was often considered a "defective immune system" disease. It displayed all of the characteristics of an immune system gone awry. Once the spirochete was found it was clear to all that this was an infectious disease problem.

Current internal medicine books will often provide two hypotheses for the cause of Rheumatoid Disease: (a) Something is wrong with the immune system, the body is attacking itself; (b) There is one or more microorganisms inside the body producing a reaction on the rheumatoid disease victim's tissues, thus causing the manifestation of the disease.

Billions of dollars worth of research following up the "something is wrong with the immune system" has never produced a cure. Whereas tens of thousands — stemming from the 1960s — have gotten well following up on the second, that is that the body is responding to one or more microorganisms.

4. What microorganism causes this terrible disease? Is there only one that affects everyone the same?

When we started the Arthritis Trust of America (The Rheumatoid Disease Foundation) in 1982 we believed that there was but one nasty microorganism, an amoeba. This was according to the presumed findings of Professor Roger Wyburn-Mason and a world-class amoebologist, Dr. Stamm. Dr. Wyburn-Mason was convinced because his treatment designed on the basis of their alleged amoebic findings worked in the large majority of cases. We conducted numerous studies coming at last to the realization that Dr. Wyburn-Mason's treatment protocol was indeed working, but that his belief in an amoebic origin was not necessarily the best answer.

Meanwhile, independently, Thomas

524

McPherson Brown, M.D. had concluded that a mycoplasm was the culprit in the creation of Rheumatoid Disease. (See "Thomas McPherson Brown, M.D. Treatment of Rheumatoid Disease," at "Articles Important" tab of http://www.arthritistrust.org.)

There are treatments predicated on both of these hypothesis, except that we've added additional, necessary wellness-serving treatment protocols. These are the necessity of correcting nutritional intake, Candidiasis, food allergies, root canal infections, mercury toxification, herbicide and pesticide accumulations, hormone balancing, and so on.

We now believe that Rheumatoid Disease is caused by many factors (multi-factored) and that there can be one or more out of tens of thousands of invasive microorganisms to which a genetically sensitive person's tissues will respond — either to the microorganisms' protein products or to their waste products. This is known as a "genetic susceptibility" to the toxins or protein products of the microorganism.

5. Should I have tests for these microorganisms, these pathogens?

Unless a health professional has some reason to search for a particular pathogen we feel it is a waste of money and time looking for any specific invader by the taking of blood tests or other traditional tests designed to find pathogens that might be the causative agents for rheumatoid disease. However, Computerized Electrodermal Screening or applied kinesiology are two low-cost, often accurate means for making such a determination, if you wish to make the effort.

Experience has shown, however, that broad-spectrum anti-microorganism treatment, coupled with investigation of all the other known causes and assisting treatments, is usually successful, at least 80% of the time.

Here's an example of a patient where our recommended anti-microorganism drugs did not work, but, by following our principles, the patient recovered from Ankylosing Spondilitis, one of the 100 or so named Rheumatoid Diseases. Reason: he was exposed to a whole different type of invading microorganism than normally found in the United States, *Schistosomiasis bilharzia*, a parasite obtained by swimming in Zimbabwe waters at an altitude where the waters are known to harbor this organism. He was able to get well by using the proper pharmaceutical created for this specific microorganism together with proper application of our other treatment recommendations — that is, unloading the immune system. (See http://www.arthritistrust.org, "Newsletters" "Spring 2005.")

We know patients who achieved wellness using only our recommended anti-microorganism treatments.

We also know of patients who only needed our other recommendations — not the anti-microorganism protocol — and got well.

Some patients require many or all of our

recommendations to achieve wellness.

But, concentrate on the principles we describe and not on a literal-minded authoritarian approach.

6. How will I know exactly what to do? Take the anti-microorganism treatment or the other treatments?

Your best bet — if you truly want to get well — is to work with one or more knowledgeable health professional, and to remove every single suppressor, every straw on the camel's back! You must learn more than your friendly neighborhood rheumatologist. This will be easy to do, because this group of professionals know absolutely nothing about how to get you well (according to their own statements), and you'll know something!

One drawback is this: There's no one health professional or dentist in the United States who offers all the treatment recommendations you will need to explore. Several clinics come close, but the majority of those are rather limited in what they chose to offer you. So, if you truly want to get well, you should consider several options right at the start.

a. First off, learn everything you can on this website. Especially read the book *Arthritis* by Prosch and di Fabio at Amazon.com. Read it end to end. I'll list other books by our foundation at the end of this article.

If you don't understand some of the words, use "Google" or a dictionary or some other search engine to define them. Don't let words stand between you and a good understanding of the principles for achieving wellness. You won't have to learn your friendly neighborhood rheumatologist's complex medical language, thank goodness, but you'll need to clear up some basic concepts to avoid confusion.

b. After you've learned as much as you feel you can absorb, then start searching for a health professional who will work with you. This could be your family doctor. We'll help her/him to learn, if s/he is open-minded and willing to learn.

Otherwise, you can search for a doctor in your geographical region who is dedicated to or inclined to practice alternative/complementary medicine.

Plan on traveling to another location where exists a health professional who will help — and then plan on traveling to another location to visit another health professional. You will understand this option better when you go over the causes of arthritis, and removal of the straws in the instructions that follow.

By now you're thinking, "Good gosh! This is getting complicated. I only want a pill to make me feel better and to get me well."

That's the kind of thinking encouraged by your present treatment plan, and the very reason that you're not getting well. It's an "authoritarian" approach. Face it! There's no pill that will remove all the straws from the camel's back.

There may be easier ways for achieving wellness, and if you find them, please let us know so we can tell others. Meanwhile, here's our recommended treatment protocol!

7. Proper Nutrition is important! So what is proper nutrition for the Arthritic?

There are numerous animal and plant substances considered to be "food" around the world. No one country has a monopoly on what is right, or even what is right for you.

Regardless of your genetic background, native country, religious bent, or family tradition, you must find a way to change your diet so that your tissues are primarily alkaline rather than acidic. What you eat determines this situation!

To be sure that you're capable of utilizing the nutrients that you take in through the mouth, some physicians will want to test the acidity of your stomach. They'll want to know, "Are you actually absorbing your food?" If not, they'll place you on a proper regimen to handle this common problem. (The stomach is one place that you want acidity. Read Dr. Wright's "Myth of Acid Indigestion — Heartburn & GERD" at http:www.arthritistrust.org under the "Articles Important" tab.)

The health professional may also want to know if your metabolism is capable of operating at the correct rate. Without a proper overall metabolic temperature, essential enzymes will not chemically unfold to manipulate your digested and absorbed nutrients. If low, you'll probably need thyroid supplements — but only the right kind, not the generally administered type given out by traditional medical practitioners. Read "Thyroid Hormone Therapy: Cutting the Gordian Knot" at http:www.arthritistrust.org under the ""Articles Important" tab.

Assuming all the other hormones are functioning properly, then the general dietary principle is simple, but requires a definition of "food," which we now provide.

There are two types of things routinely placed in folks' mouths. One is called "food" and the other is called "non-food." So that you'll better understand "food" we'll first define "non-food."

"Non-food" is everything you place in your mouth that has been packaged, processed, treated, frozen, or otherwise stabilized for long grocery store shelf life.

"Food" is what you get out of the garden, or from the animals that have provided meat that is fresh, untainted, and untreated.

The closer you can eat from the garden (or killed animal) the healthier. Similarly, the further away from the garden (or killed animal) you eat, the unhealthier — especially when your intake derives from substances packaged, processed, treated, frozen, or otherwise stabilized for long grocery store shelf life.

Some call this the "cave-man" diet. But you don't have to be a cave-man as the principles are really not that difficult to follow.

One exception to the "food" vs. "non-food" designation and restriction on "non-foods" is your liberal use of proper supplements. Your friendly neighborhood rheumatologist may tell you that these are simply "expensive urine." Don't disturb her/his authoritarian fantasies! There are very good reasons

527

why properly prepared and packaged vitamins, minerals and essential fatty acids are absolutely essential for your wellness trek, and in any case, the lack of some of these may be weighty straws holding down the camel's back.

For excellent descriptions of appropriate Rheumatoid Disease diets, read the following articles on our website at http://www.arthritistrust.org, under the "Articles Important" tab: "Natural Treatment for Arthritis," Proper Nutrition for Rheumatoid Arthritis," and "The Perfect Health Plan."

8. It's important that I check out Candidiasis Infection. So what is it?

You must determine if you've got systemic Candidiasis and, if so, you must get rid of the infection.

Many excellent books have been written on this subject. We'll not repeat the great deal known about this modern plague, but we'll cover some important essentials.

Candida albicans — among other invasive organisms-of-opportunity — is a yeast/fungus with at least six known "switching mechanisms." A "switching mechanism" is simply a microorganism's method of survival. When the environment is changed surrounding it — say from acid to alkaline, for example — the microorganism switches to a different form and function, one that permits it to survive in the new environment.

Candida albicans (among other invasive organisms) has one very nasty switching mechanism that spreads throughout the intestinal tract, also pushing or growing a "rootlet" right thru your protective intestinal mucosa. This opening permits undigested molecular-sized proteins to go directly into your blood stream where your ever-watchful immune system spots it, recognizes that protein molecule as an invader (antigen), and proceeds to construct an antibody to protect you from it. This "antigen/antibody" relationship results in an increasing number of food allergies.

Food allergies not only produce their own unique health problems, but can also mimic most of the degenerative diseases, including Rheumatoid Diseases.

Candidiasis also results in a yeast production of either alcohol or acetylhyde, the metabolite of alcohol. Acetylhyde is believed to be the part that gives you a hang-over after drinking too much alcohol the night before.

Constant, persistent production of these products, even at a low level, not only create their own special health problems, but can also mimic many of the degenerative diseases.

Some physicians estimate that about 50% of their Rheumatoid Disease patients suffer from Candidiasis. Other physicians estimate a higher rate. We've known one friendly neighborhood rheumatologist to pronounce a patient who suffered only from Candidiasis as having Rheumatoid Arthritis, and proceeded thereafter to prescribe the standard, non-effective and damaging methotrexate. Of course, the patient did not get well for two reasons: (1) She didn't have Rheumatoid Arthritis

528

in the first place; and, (2) Methotrexate at best covers up arthritic symptoms while permitting the disease to rage onward.

The main reason for this pathetic mistake is that traditional medical practitioners do not accept systemic candidiasis as a commonly acquired disease!

So where do folks acquire Candidiasis?

There are several main direct routes to its being acquired: (a) Use of antibiotics administered by medical practitioners for an infection kill off the "good-guys'" intestinal microflora and permits organisms-of-opportunity to flourish; (b) Long stretches of stress brings on their intestinal overburdening; (c) The use of the immune suppressing drugs against Rheumatoid Disease (or other disease states) brings on the overgrowth. Birth control pills are one common example.

So — you must understand — that the very drugs that you've been given by your friendly neighborhood rheumatologist, or your family general practitioner, may have created the unwanted overgrowth. At the very least, it helps this nasty growth to survive.

There are numerous solutions to Candidiasis, some better than others. Read "Candidiasis: Scourge of Arthritics," at http://www.arthritistrust.org under the "Articles Important" tab. Here you'll find that a blood test sent to the proper laboratory can determine infestation, but that normally the health professional will rely on your answers to a specially designed questionaire, as well as other signs and symptoms. The referenced article contains such a questionaire used by Gus J. Prosch, Jr., M.D. before his death for his patients.

You must rid yourself of Candidiasis for many reasons, least of which is that it could be the actual source of your Rheumatoid Disease symptoms. If not the source, then certainly it will be a contributing factor — one of the camel's straws!

By the way, for females, a vaginal infection is generally symptomatic of a systemic infection. Treating only the vagina, as recommended by standard medical advice, is not the general, systemic solution!

9. It's vital that I spot and handle my food allergies. So, how do I do this?

Food allergies may be one of the most common reasons for the manifestation of many kinds of degenerative disease, including Rheumatoid Disease. You've already read how Candidiasis can promote food allergies, but food allergies can also occur in other ways.

One of the most surprising — and distasteful — facts about food allergies is that allergies' biological rules are virtually the same as those of drug addiction! A person called an "alcoholic" has a "food" allergy. S/he's allergic to alcohol!

We "like" and always eat certain foods because we're addicted to them!

We develop food allergies from (a) "foods" most easily digested and assimilated, and (b) those "foods" eaten most often; i.e., the "foods" we really

529

like.

"Foods" that are most easily digested and assimilated are, in their order of ease (a) alcohol, (b) sugar, (c) simple carbohydrates like white flour and products made with white flour.

Complex carbohydrates, such as whole vegetables, and various proteins from meats are not so easily digested and assimilated, but can also be a source of food allergies, especially if eaten regularly, i.e., daily or near daily. If systemic Candidiasis is present most any food can be allergenic.

Warren Levin, M.D. explains the food allergy (drug addiction) phenomena very nicely at http://www.arthritistrust.org at the "Articles Important" tab in his "Allergies and Biodetoxification for the Arthritic." He also provides a 5-day abstinence fasting program together with the keeping of a food intake and symptom log that assists in determining exactly what foods create a problem for you. (Some foods cause reactions immediately while others require three days to kick in, thus, the need for a written calendar "food" intake log.)

William H. Philpott, M.D. also provides a solution to the food allergy problem through the use of benign heavy-duty magnets and a 5-day or 7-day food rotation diet. Go to http://www.arthritistrust.org, "Research" thence to "Research and Letters," and then look for his name at the alphabetized list to the left. You'll find many complete articles of Dr. Philpott's describing the beneficial use of heavy-duty magnets and rotation diets for food allergies.

Some "foods," rather than allergenic, are chemically disturbing to people with a genetic susceptibility to those products. Ed Wendlocher and other scientists have determined the source of arthritic pain for many folks as stemming from hot chili peppers, especially those found in various "food" products as flavor enhancers, but not listed on the labels. Go to http://www.arthritistrust.org to the "Articles Important" tab and read his "Chemicals in 'hot' Chili Peppers Confirmed to be a Cause of Arthritis."

Appropriate blood tests from a properly equipped laboratory can also help determine your food allergies; and, it goes without further explanation that those well trained and experienced in the application of electrodermal screening or applied kinesiology can also help make this determination.

It's very important that you find your food allergies and that you handle them, especially if the allergies are a component of causation — another straw — for your Rheumatoid Disease!

10. Yes, that's all very well, but what about the anti-microorganism treatment? I want to start with that treatment because I've heard so much about it!

Certainly many more Rheumatoid Arthritis victims have gotten well from anti-microorganism treatment than any other treatment used by the accepted medical establishment. Although some few rheumatologists will try Thomas McPherson Brown's anti-mycoplasm treatment and some few

530

will try the Roger Wyburn-Mason anti-microorganism treatment, the mistake both make is in still subscribing to the archaic nineteenth century philosophy that for each disease there is one microorganism. Kill that organism and wellness ensues. This is true for many infectious diseases, but generally not true for the so-called "degenerative" diseases, which are usually multi-factored — caused by many factors.

Generally, though, your friendly neighborhood rheumatologist will not wander from the path laid down by his peers, his hospital, or insurance providers, none of which achieve wellness, but rather, provide you with damaging drugs that permit you to function without pain a little longer while the crippling disease rages onward.

Please consider this: While some of us have gotten free of Rheumatoid Arthritis simply by taking a drug, failures usually occur because the physician or the patient has ignored the rest of the camel's straws. We know, as fact, that Dr. Gus J. Prosch's consistent arthritic cure rate of 80% occurred because he and the patient also tackled other causations at the same time.

So, when you reach this aspect of your treatment program you've got two choices: (a) the Thomas McPherson Brown anti-mycoplasm approach, or (b) the Roger Wyburn-Mason (the Arthritis Trust of America) broad spectrum anti-microorganism approach.

Frankly, we're not selling either one. We're only interested in your wellness!

And, we've had folks call or write to tell us they've been on one or the other approach, and they're still not well.

Frankly, too, practitioners who subscribe to one approach and not to the other both claim about 80% cure rate, sometimes both sides pooh-poohing the other side.

We do, however, recommend that you start with the Arthritis Trust of America (Wyburn-Mason) approach for several rational reasons:

(a) You'll know in about six to twelve weeks whether or not it will work whereas, for the anti-mycoplasm approach you'll know in about a year. If the arthritis broad spectrum anti-microorganism treatment doesn't work, you can still try the anti-mycoplasm approach. The Arthritis Trust of America recommended anti-microorganism approach taking only six to twelve weeks will then require only about 2 or 3 visits to your assisting health professional. Whereas the anti-mycoplasm approach takes periodic visits for a year.

(b) The Arthritis Trust of America anti-microorganism approach is cheaper.

If you're a gambler, and like to play for the jackpot with your paycheck, then try either of these without removing the other straws. Either might work without removing the additional straws — but really, now, don't bet too heavily on it!

11. What is the Arthritis Trust of America anti-microorganism approach?

With some modification by a committee of our referral physicians, it's the same as the Professor

531

Roger Wyburn-Mason, M.D., Ph.D. development begun in the 1960s. He was curing patients worldwide. We'll list the main ingredients here. At the end of this article we'll also list books that you can order through Amazon.com.

Recommended broad spectrum prescription drugs are the following:

(a) Metronidazole - Get from any pharmacy.

(b) Clotrimazole - Get through a compounding pharmacist.

(c) Tinidazole - Get through a compounding pharmacist, except in the American Southwest get from most pharmacies.

(e) Nimorazole - Cannot get in the United States.

(f) Ornidazole - Cannot get in the United States.

Above (a) thru (f) are called the 5-nitroimidazoles.

(g) Allopurinol - Get from any pharmacy.

(h) Furazolidone - Get from any pharmacy.

Here's how they are used to make up a broad-spectrum anti-microorganism treatment:

First, your health professional must be assured that your liver and kidneys can tolerate these drugs in the dosage prescribed. The dosage recommended is by body weight. Do not permit your doctor to lower the dosage below the recommended body weight simply because he thinks you cannot tolerate the drugs. If you can't tolerate the drugs, don't take any of them!

Baseline is 200 pounds. If you weigh 200 pounds, then you should take two grams (2000 mgs) of one of the drugs "a" thru "f" each day for two days in a row, like, for example, Saturday and Sunday. Then you skip taking any drugs for five days, a drug washout period. Then you take 2 grams (2000 mgs) per day for two successive days the next Saturday and Sunday. In all, you repeat this process for six weeks.

During the first seven days you also take 300 mg of allopurinol (item "g") 3 times a day, each day. Then stop! No more allopurinol for this cycle of treatment!

If for some odd reason you're allergic to allopurinol, or your health professional thinks s/he would prefer to have you do so, then take furazolidone (item "h") for the first 10 successive days, 100 mg 3 times per day. Then stop. No more furazolidone for this cycle of treatment!

Important: For each 25 pounds over or under the 200 pound baseline that you weigh, you either add or substract 250 mg (1/4 gram), respectively, to the 5-nitroimidazole prescription.

Some doctors since 1982 have varied this standardized protocol with success. For example, Gus J. Prosch, Jr., M.D. often tried a second cycle of treatments using a different one of the 5-nitroimidazoles. John Parks Trowbridge, M.D. developed a slightly different protocol with success, and he added in the use of DHEA/pregnenolone IV (intravenous natural hormone replacement) plus EDTA chelation IV, whence usually 80-90% are helped. He also monitors blood tests. (Press the tab

532

"Articles Important," and go to the article "Chelation Therapy," on our website http://www.arthritistrust.org for the nature of EDTA chelation IV; and also for "Hormone Balancing: Natural Treatment & Cure for Arthritis.")

It bears repetition! The principles of treatment are important, not the literal-minded interpretation of rules!! If your health professional and you get good results, then both of you know what you're doing!!!

12. My doctor says that metronidazole might cause cancer. Is this correct?

Metronidazole is not carcinogenic. This is one of the most popular discreditations, unrelated to fact. According to a Senator Ted Kennedy joint hearing before the subcommittee on labor and public welfare and the subcommittee on administrative practice and procedure of the committee on the *Judiciary United States Senate Ninety Fourth Congress, July 10, 11, 1975,* Searle (pharmaceutical company) representatives testified that some lab data had been misplaced regarding control group rats, and that carcinogenic symptoms had been observed *in the control group* (the rat group that was not on metronidazole). The FDA, they said, had required them to throw the carcinogenic count into the non control group. [See "First Session On Examination of the Process of Drug Testing and FDA's Role in the Regulation and Conditions Under Which Such Testing is Carried Out," *Preclinical and clinical testing by the Pharmaceutical Industry, 1975,* Published by the U.S. Government Printing Office, Washington, D.C. 1975]

Thus, the *Physicians Desk Reference* now contains the statement that metronidazole may cause cancers in rats. This error has never been corrected on a drug package insert, and probably never will be.

In an address by Wayne Martin [deceased] of Fairhope, Alabama, before the Seattle Chapter of the International Association of Cancer Victims and Friends, he summarized the results of a study of Flagyl (metronidazole) in the treatment of cancer:

In the Seattle area, the Group Health Cooperative of Puget Sound has treated 12,280 patients with Flagyl (metronidazole) mostly for the parasitic disease trichomonoasis, which causes urogenital distress. Of this group, only five patients developed cancer over a 2-1/2 year period, whereas among the 123,620 non Flagyl users, 311 patients developed cancer over the same period of time. On a percentage basis, 0.04% of the Flagyl patients developed cancer, compared with 2.5% of the non Flagyl users - a score of better than 60 to 1 in favor of Flagyl users. When a correction for age was factored in, the score was still 3 to 1 in favor of Flagyl users *(Journal of the American Medical Association,* May 14, 1982, pp. 2498 2499.)

The *Physicians Desk Reference* also states that since 1967 there has never been a reported case of human carcinogenicity or mutagenicity through the use of metronidazole.

According to *The First Metronidazole Conference,* metronidazole is world widely used,

533

often in dosages much higher than our recommendations, and often in hospital settings where it is frequently used intravenously in very high dosages for bacterial infections.

13. My doctor uses intravenous metronidazole in hospitals to kill bacteria. He says he's willing to give me the same treatment since he knows it's safe. Should I use it?

Intravenous dosages of metronidazole will do nothing to halt the progress of Rheumatoid Disease, although it might ease the free radical damage for a short time. Reason: Your "good-guys" microflora must "metabolize" the drug. It's the metabolites of metronidazole that kill the microorganisms, not the drug itself. Your "good-guys" microflora should be supplemented with a good quality grade of supplemental *Lactobaccilus acidophilus & Bifido bacterium*. Such supplementation is important for the proper activation of the metronidazole and other 5-nitroimidazoles.

14. What signs and symptoms should my doctor and I look for?

You should both look for the Herxheimer effect!

In 1902 two research physicians, Doctors Adolph Jarisch and Karl Herxheimer, studied the treatment of syphilis, using various kinds of relatively dangerous drugs. They learned that whenever they killed the syphilis spirochete the patient displayed a series of symptoms similar to "flu." They later concluded that whenever an organism more complex than a simple bacteria was killed within the human body, one had these same symptoms. Subsequently this phenomenon became named the "Jarisch-Herxheimer" or "Herxheimer" effect.

When treating tuberculosis, the Herxheimer occurs, as it also does in treating Leishmaniasis. When treating Leprosy, the same phenomenon occurs, but it's called "Lucio's" phenomenon." Some other rare, tropical diseases also exhibit the Herxheimer when treated by killing the causative organism. Some call it the "die off effect" — for example in treating Candidiasis — as it occurs whenever the invading organism is dying off.

According to the Jarisch-Herxheimer theory, when an invading organism (more complex than a simple bacteria) acts as an antigen (allergy agent) the body prepares antibodies that tend to fight the antigen. This creates products which are the cause of the swelling, heat, and joint damage. One's tissues and immune system responds to the killing of the organism inside the body by producing a serious allergic response inside the body. The products of that allergic response create secondary problems that lead to the additional damage.

If there is a causative organism that creates RD, and if the organism is killed by this medicine, and if you've been sensitized to the protein products of that organism, then more of the protein products resulting from dead organisms will increase the internal allergic response. It follows, therefore, that, just by killing off one of the causative agents of

534

Rheumatoid Disease, the body will have an intensification of the very symptoms that we label as "Rheumatoid Disease." Rheumatoid Disease symptoms <u>are</u> a systemic manifestation of the internal allergy!

The Herxheimer effect consists of these signs and symptoms:

(a.) General and usual: Sweating and especially night sweats, diarrhea, nausea, vomiting, headache, fever, general malaise, flushing of skin, anorexia, aching bones and "flu" symptoms resembling a serum reaction.

(b.) The inflamed and affected tissues become more inflamed and tissues previously unknown to be involved become inflamed.

(c.) If the heart, pericardium or cardiac tissues are infected, patients may develop some paroxysmal auricular tachycardia, premature ventricular contractions or ectopic beats.

(d.) If the urinary bladder tissues are infected the patient may develop signs of full-blown cystitis.

(e.) If the brain or meninges are infected the patient may develop severe (temporary) depression, lethargy, generalized weakness, temporary memory loss, irritability along with headaches.

(f.) If the mouth tissues are infected, a bitter and/or metallic taste may be noted along with mild shedding or peeling of the mucosal tissues. This has also been noted in the rectal tissues. However, <u>it should be noted that Metronidazole and Tinidazole also produce a metallic taste without the Herxheimer effect being present</u>.

(g.) When the periosteal tissues and skeletal muscle tissues are involved, fairly severe bone pain usually accompanied by severe muscle pains and spasms may be observed, usually at night.

(h.) When the lungs and bronchial tissues are infected the patients may develop bronchitis symptoms and occasionally pneumonitis (resembling viral) has been observed.

You and your physician must learn to distinguish between the possible effects of drug toxicity, an allergic reaction to one or more drugs, or the Herxheimer effect. (See http://www.arthritistrust.org, "Articles Important" tab, "The Herxheimer Effect.")

15. What if the Herxheimer effect becomes so strong that I can't tolerate it?

The Herxheimer is a good sign, because then both you and your doctor know that the drug is killing organisms. Something good is really happening! When your body cleans up the antigen/antibody complexes, you'll probably be free of Rheumatoid Disease — assuming the other straws do not need to be removed.

To tolerate the Herxheimer, when we first designed our treatment protocol in 1982 we made certain recommendations related to the taking of small amounts of prednisone or, perhaps, non-steroidal anti-inflammatory drugs. We don't like what prednisone does to the body, but, if no other recourse is available to you, one of those options

535

may be necessary.

But, what we truly know will work favorably is the judicious application of Dr. Pybus' Intraneural Injections!

What we know about the use of intraneural injections simultaneous with your visit to your doctor fills another booklet, which you'll find mentioned at the end of this article.

Indeed, Dr. Prosch's consistent success rate depended upon use of all of the above, including same day use of intraneural injections. The Arthritis Trust of America feels that the booklet, *Intraneural Injections for Rheumatoid Arthritis and Osteoarthritis & The Control of Pain in Arthritis of the Knee,* by Dr. Paul K. Pybus, is a must for all forms of Rheumatoid Disease and arthritis-like pain, and that the use where appropriate of designated intraneural injections decreases the time to wellness, regardless of what other modalities are used on the patient. One important advantage being the ability to get the patient off of damaging pain-relieving drugs while the body is adapting to healing treatments and wellness routines. These easy-to-administer injections address the source of your joint pain, nerve ganglia that lead to the affected joint. (You'll also find a description of Intraneural Injections at http://www.arthritistrust.org, "Newsletters," Spring, Summer, Fall, . . . 2006.)

Englishman Roger Wyburn-Mason, M.D., Ph.D., nerve specialist, was the first to describe the source (not causation) principle of joint damage from tender nerve locations, sometimes called "trigger points," in arthritis and arthritis-like pain.

South African Dr. Paul K. Pybus, his former house physician, learned to implement in clinical practice Wyburn-Mason's theories of intraneural injections, successfully using his discoveries for more than 20 years.

Keith McElroy, M.D. (The New York Orthopaedic Hospital) independently discovered the same principles, and applied them to his patients, also for many years. He called them "Injection Therapy."

Dr. Paul K. Pybus and Gus J. Prosch, Jr., M.D. explored additional key "trigger points," until it became clear to them that a virtual one-to-one correspondence existed between painful neuroma and acupuncture points — but not always so.

Dr. I.H.J. Bourne, a friend of both Dr. Roger Wyburn-Mason and Dr. Paul Pybus, also developed the use of intraneural injections which he published as "Musculoskeletal Disorders: Local Injection Therapy."

Dr. Curt Maxwell of Los Algodones, Mexico uses all injection modalities. While the book does not address itself to inflamed neuroma, he also recommends the W.B. Saunders book, *Atlas of Pain Management Injection Techniques* by Steven D. Waldman, M.D., J.D. as an excellent supplementary book. (It is very convenient for doctors who are into reimbursement via insurance, as it gives the insurance code that is acceptable for each of the injections. The artwork is excellent, and there can be no doubt as to how to do the recommended

536

injections in the various parts of the body. The text is quite appropriate, giving not only the how, but also contra-indications, et. al.)

Of additional major importance, for more than 50 years American Harry H. Philbert, M.D. independently developed the use of what he chose to call "Specific Injection Therapy," covering many of the same aspects as the several intraneural publications reported above. *The Anatomy of Pain: Specific Injection Therapy*, is a well-done report by Dr. Philbert.

To clarify further, your doctor should know how to use any one of several types of injections: (a) Intraneural Injections, (b) Neural Therapy according to Huenke, and (c) Sclerotherapy [Prolo or Proliferative Therapy or Reconstructive Therapy].

Neural Therapy (Injections), developed by Ferdinand and Walter Huenke, also about 90 years ago, addresses the problem of patterns of stored "pain" reflexes which trigger off permanent relief upon injection. These injections are particularly important when addressing scar tissue and the ability of such permanent scars to distort structure.

Sclerotherapy (or Prolo Therapy) is very important for tightening up tendons or ligaments that have become stretched or torn. This eventually applies to all arthritics, but is not germane at this point, except that in any form of arthritis many joint pains do, in fact, stem from stretched or torn ligaments and tendons. This is the only treatment that can permanently solve that problem. (You can read more about it at http://www.arthritistrust.org,

"Articles Important" tab, in "Sclero Therapy — Prolo Therapy," and, if you're a health professional, *Structural Diagnostic Photography*, by James A. Carlson, D.O. as referenced at the end of this article.

When using the intraneural injection protocol, your doctor will probably want you to return in about three weeks. That's about the length of time that the effects of the intraneural injections will last, permitting you and your doctor during the interim to work on removing as many of the camel's straws as possible. At that time, you can receive another set of injections which will safely — and almost miraculously — remove your joint pain for another three weeks.

Once you've rid yourself of the Rheumatoid Disease, you may still need some injections, but each time you receive them there'll be less pain points and the injections will last longer. (This aspect is covered in more detail in the aforementioned Dr. Pybus' book on intraneural injections at our website.)

16. What about the Thomas McPherson Brown, M.D. anti-mycoplasm treatment?

This treatment is predicated on the assumption that the mycoplasm is the cause of Rheumatoid Disease and a form of antibiotic is used to kill this microorganism. Treatment is usually spaced out over numerous visits throughout the year. At each visit a small amount of a specific antibiotic is given. This is called "pulsing." For further information go to our website at http://www.arthritistrust.org, "Articles Important" tab, "Thomas McPherson Brown, M.D. Treatment of

537

Rheumatoid Disease."

17. My doctor has done all of the above, and I'm still not well! What do I do next?

Eighty percent of those treated by Dr. Prosch, and other doctors, have gotten well, many for the first time in years of suffering. You must be one among the remaining 20%. Too bad! But don't give up. It simply means that you've got more straws to remove, and it's important that you know what they are, and how to remove them.

In fact, the successful 80% also should be routinely removing these additional straws to continue strengthening their immune system!!

Some remaining important straws are: (a) root canal cleansing, (b) mercury removal, (c) intestinal cleansing, and (d) detoxification.

18. I've taken very good care of my teeth — spent lots of money. I've got a very good dentist and he says that I don't need any further work on my gums or removal of mercury. He says you folks are crazy!

Well, then, I guess you've got a choice! Stay away from crazy people, or get yourself well!

We've learned over the years that it's more difficult to wean Rheumatoid Disease victims away from their very friendly neighborhood dentist than it is from their friendly neighborhood rheumatologist. We can understand the reasons. You've just gone through a stressful series of dental sessions, and you've put out big bucks, and now you might have to do it all over again? Crazy, indeed!

Here's the problem: Whenever root canal work has been completed, or a tooth has been extracted, the dentist is not taught to remove the tough integument that held the tooth in place. This tough tissue keeps antibiotics from getting into the cavitation formed there. Your friendly neighborhood dentist has not been taught this fact, although it was his trade union's predecessors who funded affirming definitive studies on this subject many years ago. Bacteria that lives in your mouth and that has gotten locked into these cavities mutates from an oxygen-loving form (aerobic) to one that does not love oxygen (anaerobic), and sets up shop behind this tough tissue. It begans manufacturing some of the most deadly toxins in the world, ten times more deadly than botulism. Radioactive substances have traced these poisonous toxins to specific organs in the body with resulting disease states.

Only ten percent of folks are aware of having any microbial growth there, so silently do these organisms work — and, through their stealthy action, they also become the source for persistent gum shrinkage as folks age.

Removing this important straw requires a "biological dentist," one who is trained in identifying this kind of problem, and who can safely cleanse the infected cavitation. No matter how kind and friendly your family dentist, s/he will not have been trained in this area, and will most likely pooh pooh the idea!

Again you can rely on non-invasive electro-dermal screening, or applied kinesiology to make a determination of need for this straw's removal. But

538

in addition, the Biology Department at the University of Kentucky developed a method for the dentist to swab the base of the gums at each tooth and determine whether or not there's an infection in the tooth's root canal.

The Price Pottenger Nutrition Foundation, address and the end of this article, will provide you with names and addresses of biological dentists near you. Caution, however, their list does not show which biological dentists are trained for safe mercury removal and which trained for both cavitation cleansing and safe mercury removal. You'll have to call the various biological dentists on their list and ask.

George E. Meinig, D.D.S., F.A.C.D., one of the nineteen founding members that organized the American Association of Endodontists and a former Twentieth Century Fox Studio dentist, discusses this serious health problem in his book *Root Canal Coverup*.

You should order this book and read it!

19. My dentist says that once mercury has been combined with other metals and placed in my teeth, it's safe and doesn't create any problems. So, why should I redo all that beautiful, expensive workmanship?

Your dentist is demonstrably wrong!

Regardless of which doctor, dentist or organization tells you that mercury is safe once it's placed in your mouth, and saying "it's safe" doesn't make it safe! They're flat out wrong! They haven't done their homework! They're simply repeating a long-standing falsehood!

Let's consider some provable facts:

a. The EPA as well as the American Medical Association states that there is no lower safe limit to the amount of mercury a person can intake.

b. Dentists and their employees are required to handle mercury in special ways that the Environmental Protection Agency considers safe because of mercury's extreme health hazard. This protection is for the benefit of the dentist and her/his employees and their office, not the patient.

c. The two different metals (the amalgam) immersed in an acid or alkaline environment (the mouth) produces an electromotive force which is easily measurable at each filled tooth.

d. This electric current plus the mouth's acidity or alkalinity causes a small amount of the amalgam to vaporize in your mouth. The vapor combines with organic materials to form a very toxic mercury molecule that accumulates in your body.

e. The stored organic mercury compound added to other mercury from the intake of food and from pesticides and herbicides can eventually cause any one of many forms of degenerative disease, including those of Rheumatoid Disease.

f. After many years of resistance, just like the American Dental Association (a protective trade union), the Swedish Dental Association studied the problem, apologized to their citizens, and phased out mercury. Most of the European community has also done so. Only the stubborn, intransigent American Dental Association — probably fearful of expensive accumulating law suits like the tobacco industry — resists.

Three doctors working together in Tijuana, Mexico felt so strongly about the importance of mercury stress on the body that they refused to accept an American Rheumatoid Arthritis patient until he'd cleared his mouth of mercury amalgams through an American biological dentist. Once properly cleared, the American no longer had a need to visit these Mexican doctors as the patient's Rheumatoid Arthritis had magically disappeared!

While perhaps statistically improbable, this true anecdote nicely illustrates the point of safely removing mercury and other metals from your mouth. We say "safely" because, if you should decide it's more convenient and cheaper to have your friendly neighborhood dentist do the job (if he's willing), you could easily end up sicker than when you started. Why? Because the order in which the amalgams are removed is important, and the manner in which you're protected from mercury fumes while removing the amalgams is paramount.

A "biological" dentist has the tools and know how and is important for your health!

We recommend dentist Hal Huggins' *Uninformed Consent* You should order this book from the Price Pottenger Nutrition Foundation and read it end to end! Also don't forget Meinig's *Root Canal Coverup*!

20. After I've safely removed all the metal in my mouth will that take care of all of my mercury?

Probably not. Your body has taken your lifetime to store up mercury from various sources: teeth, food, vaccination shots (preservatives), pesticides and herbicides that surround us everywhere, to name a few major sources.

There's several means for ridding your body of mercury, each requiring help from a knowledgeable health professional, some taking longer than others.

a. Chelate the mercury from your body using proper chelating agents. Periodic urine and hair samples may assist in determining effectiveness. Repeated visits for some time may be necessary.

b. Use chlorella with your other nutritional supplements. This may take a long time.

c. Use applied kinesiology and/or electrodermal screening to determine location of mercury accumulation, and then drive the organic mercury out thru use of either (1) magnetic polarity, or (2) injections of novacaine in the mercury deposits. The novacaine converts to a B vitamin that drives the mercury out of nerve ganglia where stored, according to Lee Cowden, M.D.

21. Is colon cleansing really necessary? If so, what do I do?

Detoxification of the body is one of the most neglected wellness projects, although most health professionals realize that a sick body is a toxic one. Some health professionals feel that the colon is one of the most important organs in the body. Here you'll find the source of many diseases, and you'll also find the lack of desirable microorganisms and many

540

unwanted microorganisms: bacterial, viral, amoebic, mycoplasmic, worms, and yeast/fungus infections. Any one of these can create the tissue sensitivity that brings about your arthritic condition. There are numerous methods for ridding your body of these undesirables, or (replacing the desirables) advocated by various health professionals. If your doctor is unversed in colon cleansing, then seek out an alternative/complementary health professional. More than likely one with an N.D. degree will be knowledgeable in colon cleansing.

Toxic acids are normal products of cell catabolism, and we also take in many toxic products when breathing, eating, and drinking. When toxic products accumulate or come into the body faster than we expel them, we build up serious health problems.

Various parts of the colon as well as "cleansing" for liver, gall bladder, kidney and so on can be seriously explored. There's ozone water enemas, coffee enemas, and so on — a number of recommended, reliable treatments too numerous to mention here, most requiring professional help, but also many that can be learned from professionals and thereafter safely administered to self.

Many of Sherry Rogers' (M.D.) books will include excellent advice in this area.

Tissue Cleansing Through Bowel Management, by Bernard Jenson, D.C., Ph.D. and Sylvia Bell is also an excellent guide.

Various books on alternative medicine or natural medicine also contain recommendations. Seek them out and work with a health professional on appropriate treatment regimens. You can find the above books, and others, via internet search.

22. What about getting rid of herbicides and pesticides? How do I do it?

One of the fastest and surest means is through the use of a sauna.

The basic purpose of a sauna is to cleanse the body through perspiration. This means opening the pores of the skin and flushing out the impurities in the body through the process of sweating. The sauna of Finland is a tradition which some researchers date back over two thousand years. The Finns attribute their endurance and longevity to the tradition of sauna.

What happens to the body during a sauna is quite simple — your metabolism and pulse rate increases, your blood vessels become much more flexible, and your extremities benefit from increased circulation. Physical fitness fans will recognize that some of these changes can also be achieved through strenuous exercise. Not to say that a sauna would put you in excellent physical condition without moving a muscle, but that it brings about the same metabolic results as physical exercise.

The effects of the sauna are numerous and varied. Proponents of dry heat bath mention a feeling of psychological peace and contentment as well as physical rejuvenation. Many people claim that the sauna relieves the symptoms of minor illnesses such as colds, revives the muscles after tough physical exertion, and clears the complexion. The sauna

541

experience will often leave you feeling very much alive. Your senses will be sharpened, and your tactile sensitivity heightened.

All of the above is accurate and true, and normally refers to short periods of sauna exposure, such as one experiences socially for an hour or two.

Zane R. Gard, M.D. was one of the first medical doctors to install a Hubbardian sweat sauna for his medical practice after he, his wife, and daughter were vastly helped from exposure to agent orange. (Go to http://www.arthritistrust.org, "Research" tab, "Research and Letters" tab, and find Zane R. Gard, M.D. in alphabetical list at left of page; Also see "Chemical Exposure" at "Articles Important" tab.)

Numerous scientific studies established the great value of the sauna technique, and both firemen as well as policemen have benefited through its use from accidental exposure to toxic materials.

Several medical doctors have made a sauna program available for their patients.

Regardless of where you receive this type of sauna, a medical exam is required to assure that your heart can sustain the stress. The program requires consecutive daily attendance for 3-1/2 to 4-1/2 weeks under a temperature of 140 degrees to 180 degrees Fahrenheit. You can leave the sauna to cool down for lunch, or a quick shower, if desired, but the idea — as with any sauna — is to sweat copiously over a long period of time.

When sweating, the metabolites and xenobiotics (pesticides and herbicides) that have been stored in the fatty parts of your cells (lipids) mobilize and will start exiting through your sweat pores. These tiny chemical portions are triggering agents for vast responses inside your body that have led to apparent degenerative disease states that have baffled the medical world for generations. For example, you've probably heard of "flashback" caused by the past use of certain illegal drugs, such as LSD. The former LSD user suddenly experiences phenomena as if taking the substances again, when s/he's not actually doing so.

While sweating out these xenobiotic products in the sauna your body/mind/emotions will trigger flashbacks reminding you of operations, sunburn under the beach, drug usage (including prescribed drugs), and so on. These are "triggered" reactions to the activation and expelling of substances previously accumulated in the fatty parts of your cells when your body didn't know what else to do with them.

These xenobiotics (metabolites of pesticides and herbicides), though minimal in size and well stored in the lipids (fatty cells), are also the source of many poorly understood disease states.

A key element for successful use of the Hubbardian sauna (called the "Purif," or Purification Rundown) is that when the vitamins, minerals and essential fatty acids are sweated out, they're replaced daily by an amount determined by the amount of niacin it requires to produce a flush for that day.

Major differences between Hubbard's sauna and that of medical doctors are that (1) The

542

Hubbard's places a partner in the sauna with you who has already been through the experience, and assures that you are experiencing everything OK; and, also the Church has a supervisor review your log of daily events; (2) Unlike the Church, Medical doctors usually take laboratory samples that report on specific xenobiotics and these will be compared against progress in the decrease of your chronic symptoms.

This sauna treatment requires strong will for continued exposure and endurance, but, once you've gone through the initial "want-to-quit" stage, you'll find it easy to endure, and quite beneficial, even restful.

23. After doing all of the above will I be well?

No one knows the answer to such a question!

Keep in mind that you're the camel, and your back is being weighted downward. The key principle to wellness is to began removing the straws that hold you down. How many straws there are, and whether or not you actually remove them is between you and your health professionals. No one — other than you — knows if you've given each straw an honest tug.

Then, too, there may be other straws that we've not mentioned, or we've not known about. One such, for example, might be problems specific to you such as Diabetes (type II normally can be traced to serious food allergy problems); cancer (a serious systemic and metabolic disease; the tumor is not the cancer!), long-standing metallic poisoning from sources we've not mentioned, and so on. (A former welder got well after decontaminating welding rod metals in his body.)

Of course if you're one of those who've been given a patented drug to alleviate a symptom, and then another to alleviate the side-effects of the first drug, and then another to suppress the side-effects of the second drug — ad infinitum — you've been long-conned into the patented drug game which fattens the portfolio of pharmaceutical companies, bottom-line "health" insurance agents and unthinking doctors! In your drugged state of apathy and slow thought you probably don't have much opportunity to become the lead pack dog to govern your own health.

What to do?

Get away from those *disease* practitioners and find a *health* practitioner!

With some critical exceptions, traditional medical practitioners have an accurate ability to diagnose a medical problem and a lousy ability to cure it. Use their keen ability to diagnose, but seriously question their "solution."

For initial and confirming support of undiagnosed problems you can also take advantage of skilled practitioners of applied kinesiology and electro-dermal screening. Once accurate diagnosis is assured, you must become the lead pack dog, not the doctor!

Remember, always avoid the authoritarian "Doctor knows best!" approach.

Be honest enough with yourself and the system you use to see palliative treatment for what

543

it is — treatment of a symptom and not a solution for the disease.

Diagnosis and healing remedies should go hand in hand!

And good luck to your straw removal!

Like the happy, standing camel, we pray that you, too, will be full-standing soon!

By the way. If you find a simpler, faster, cheaper way of getting well, please let us know!

24. OK, so I want to get help in the manner you've outlined. Where do I go? How do I find the right kind of health professional?

You've just asked the toughest question!

We'll try to answer the best we can at this time.

a. You know your family doctor. Is s/he open-minded? Willing to learn? If yes, then go talk to that person first. We'll be glad to give them free information or references. If not, stay away and search further.

b. Look for doctors who advertise as alternative or complementary or even alternative and general practice. Holistic practitioners may be applicable. Preventive medicine practitioners can be confusing. Many hospitals have jumped on the popular bandwagon for providing "preventive" or "complementary" treatment, but, in fact, have little understanding of the difference between treating causes and treating symptoms. Question the practitioner. Is s/he simply treating your symptoms with herbs instead of drugs? Are they providing some form of "emotional" or "visualization" support, rather than hard, solid curative protocols? (Herbs

and other supportive techniques are OK in their place, but, generally, are not solutions to the causes.) After you've absorbed the principles on this website you'll find it easier to distinguish between those who strike for the roots of the disease and those who piddle around its edges.

c. Unfortunately, no one health professional provides all of the medical and dental treatments that may be required for you. Some come close, but regardless of where you live there will most likely be a need to search further for helpful practitioners — several treatments here, several there, and perhaps another far away.

Here are some reputable organizations that can help you find proper physicians or dentists:

To find a biological dentist write or call **The Price-Pottenger Nutrition Foundation**, PO Box 2614, La Mesa, CA 91943-2614; (619) 462-7600.

Or, for a dentist, **American Academy of Biological Dentists**; http// www.biologicaldentistry.org

To find a physician for allergies/chemical sensitivities/addictions **American Academy of Environmental Medicine** call (215) 862-4544)

To find a physician for heart/circulatory problems (chelation therapy) and many other problems write (self-addressed, stamped envelope) **American College for Advancement of Medicine** 23121 Verdugo Dr, Laguna Hills, CA 92653.

The following is a list of books by The Arthritis Trust of America available on Amazon.com.

Arthritis: Osteoarthritis & Rheumatoid Disease, Including Rheumatoid Arthritis
Soft Tissue Arthritis
Arthritis: Little Known Treatments
Rheumatoid Disease Cured. at Last!
The Magic of Magnetic Healing
Absolutely Phenomenal Medical Treatments
A New Diagnostic Tool for Prolo Therapy
Intraneural Injections
Arthritis Treatments That Work!
The Causation of Rheumatoid Disease and Many Human Cancers -- A Précis